Stenson

INTRODUCTION TO CLINICAL ALLERGY

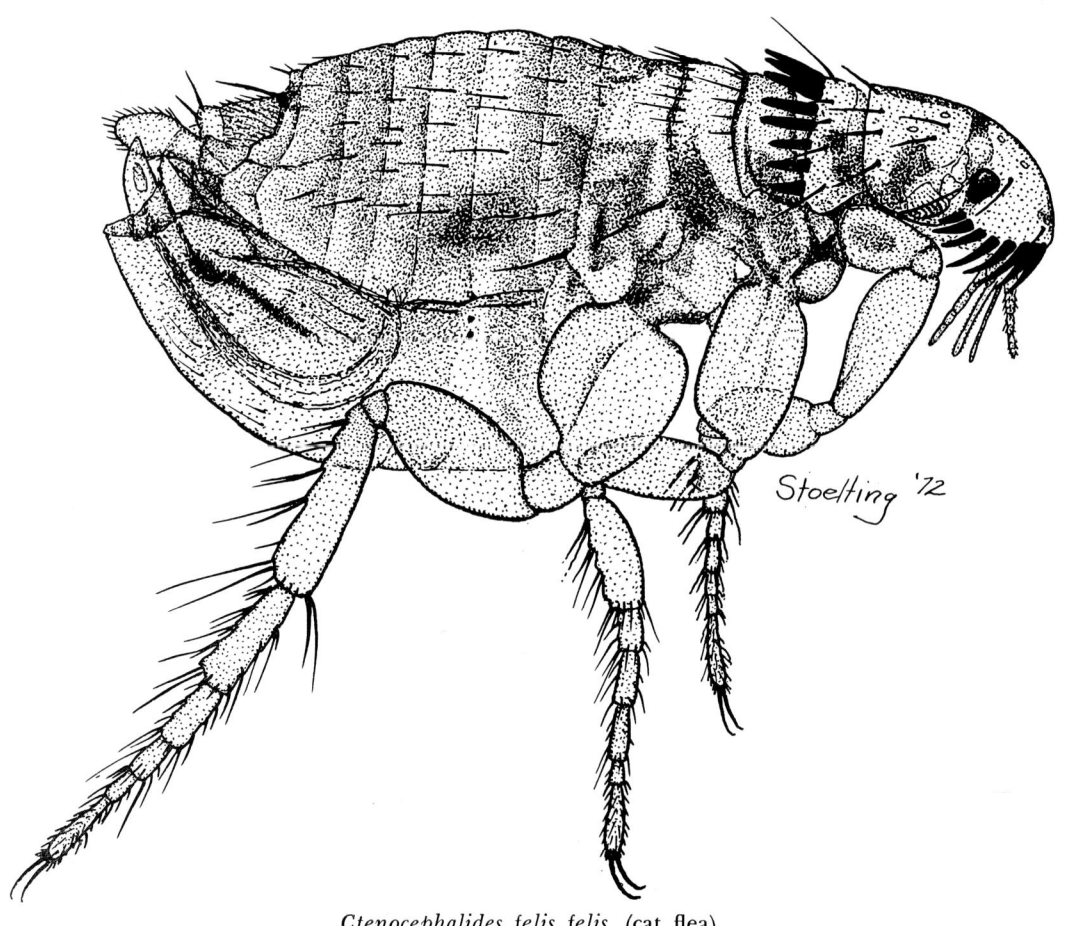

Ctenocephalides felis felis (cat flea)

A hapten derived from cat flea saliva served as a model for studying allergic reactions to insect bites at the Laboratory of Medical Entomology of the Kaiser Foundation Research Institute.

INTRODUCTION TO CLINICAL ALLERGY

By

BEN F. FEINGOLD, M.D.

Chief Emeritus, Allergy Department
Former Director Laboratory Medical Entomology
Former Chairman Central Research Committee
Kaiser Foundation Hospital and Permanente Medical Group
San Francisco, California
Diplomate of American Board of Allergy and Immunology

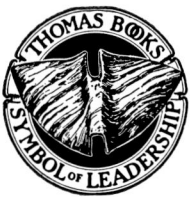

CHARLES C THOMAS • PUBLISHER
Springfield • Illinois • U.S.A.

Published and Distributed Throughout the World by
CHARLES C THOMAS • PUBLISHER
Bannerstone House
301-327 East Lawrence Avenue, Springfield, Illinois, U.S.A.

This book is protected by copyright. No part of it
may be reproduced in any manner without written
permission from the publisher

© *1973, by* CHARLES C THOMAS • PUBLISHER
ISBN 0-398-02797-8
Library of Congress Catalog Card Number: 72-93211

With THOMAS BOOKS careful attention is given to all details of manufacturing and design. It is the Publisher's desire to present books that are satisfactory as to their physical qualities and artistic possibilities and appropriate for their particular use. THOMAS BOOKS will be true to those laws of quality that assure a good name and good will.

Printed in the United States of America
CC-11

*To my wife, Helene,
whose patience, understanding
and encouragement made this
book possible.*

INTRODUCTION

MEDICINE* IS DEFINED as the science and art concerned with the care, alleviation and prevention of disease, and with the restoration and preservation of health.

Like all other branches of medicine allergy is both a science and an art.

Contributions from immunochemistry, immunology, physics, zoology, physiology and genetics have made possible the classification of immune reactions and the tissue responses induced by them. Variations in the immune reactions with their ensuing tissue changes and the resulting symptomatology constitute allergic disease. The tissue reactions in allergic disease are not limited to a select immune mechanism, such as the immediate type of reactivity induced by reaginic allergy, but may involve one or more of the immune responses if they deviate from their norm. Recognizing this, the scope of clinical allergy has broadened and has become more inclusive. Eventually, the specialty of allergy may encompass a variety of immunologic diseases, such as the auto-allergic diseases and perhaps even malignancy and the processes of aging.

The great advances in science have already established allergy as a specialty with formal recognition by the creation of an independent Board of Allergy for certification.

The trend of the future seems to be away from the restricted application of the term "allergy" to a broader, more inclusive concept. The American Academy of Allergy recognized this tendency when the name of the official publication was changed from *Journal of Allergy* to the *Journal of Allergy and Clinical Immunology*. Medical schools are also sensitive to the changing status and are toying with programs to permit broader instruction in the field of clinical immunology. Allergy as practiced presently will no doubt continue, but only as a division of the more comprehensive specialty, clinical immunology. The inclusion of a chapter on auto-allergic diseases recognizes this trend and indicates to the clinician the scope of the practice of allergy in the immediate future.

* *Shorter Oxford Dictionary*, Oxford, Clarendon Press, 1944.

On the other hand, the *Art of Medicine* has suffered from these advances in science which have divided medicine into numerous specialties. The individual personal relationship between the doctor and the patient has been replaced by brief visits with various specialists who often are only attentive to their limited fields with complete disregard of the overall needs of the patient. Prior to the era of specialization, the art of medicine was an important part of the general practitioner's stock in trade. There was no formal training, but the art was administered either through intuition, by precept or by experience. Today, with the great emphasis upon the inadequacies of the delivery of medical care, there is an awareness of the need for emphasis on the *Art of Medicine*. The trend is already being felt by renewed interest in general practice and increased reports of studies on doctor-patient interaction and doctor-patient communication.

It is difficult to define the *Art of Medicine* since criteria have not yet been established. Many variables operate for both the patient and the physician. To be considered for the patient are the nature and the seriousness of the illness, the personality profile and emotional pattern, the socio-economic and cultural status. The personality pattern of the physician as well as his emotional state are also important, while other contributing factors to consider include the reputation of the physician or the institution in which he practices, the physical environment in which he functions, and the paramedical personnel that serves as an intermediary between the patient and the physician.

In spite of the numerous inconstant factors, several studies are attempting to analyze doctor-patient interaction in order to establish greater objectivity and specific guidelines for quantifying the *Art of Medicine*. The success of these investigations may not be realized for a number of years; however, in the meantime the reports of these studies serve to create an awareness of the need for greater emphasis upon the *Art of Medicine* which will lead to its increased application in daily practice.

Management in clinical allergy depends upon the fullest cooperation of the patient to a greater degree than in most other branches of medicine. On the part of the physician, in no division of medicine other than in clinical allergy is a strict uncompromising position so essential for successful patient management. When seeking relief from allergic ailments, the patient is very frequently subjected to difficult and trying experiences which can tax the fullest cooperation between patient and physician. It may be necessary for the patient to resort to long detailed and accurate diaries essential for diagnosis and management; or he may be subjected to long testing procedures, and very often he is required to exercise restrictions on pets to which there are emotional ties and the elimination of foods that can create great inconveniences. Gaining the cooperation of the patient for the careful conduct of these programs may require the full exercise of the *Art of Medicine*. For the physician to compromise may mean failure in the control of the disease, yet rigidity can alienate the patient. In most cases firmness tempered with understanding on the part of both the patient and the physician, coupled with sympathy and compassion can gain the patient's cooperation. There are, as yet, no specific instructions for the physician for the conduct of this patient relationship; however, an awareness of the importance of the *Art of Medicine* in addition to scientific comprehension will contribute much toward solving difficult problems in clinical allergy.

This book is an *Introduction to Clinical Allergy* directed to the physician who does not limit his practice to problems of allergy. A number of the cardinal points in diagnosis and management are stressed and for the purpose of emphasis are frequently repeated.

1. Allergic disease may be induced by any one of the four types of immune response as illustrated by the immediate or reaginic form of tissue response in allergic rhinitis, hay fever, and bronchial allergy; the intermediate or Arthus mechanism which operates in some drug reactions, carditis, vasculitis, arthritis and nephritis; the delayed type of reaction that causes contact dermatitis; and the cytotoxic or cytolytic form of response observed in a number of blood dyscrasias.

2. More than one type of immune response may operate concurrently to produce syndromes as observed in serum sickness and in extrinsic allergic bronchopneumonia.

3. All that looks like allergy clinically may not be allergy. In other words, nonallergic mechanisms may induce clinical patterns which simulate allergic disease as observed with the immune deficiency states, many drug reactions and possibly with food intolerance. Recognizing these possibilities, a chapter on the immune deficiency states has been included, while the respective chapters on foods and drugs have been captioned "Adverse Reactions" to permit the inclusion of nonimmunologic reactions which can resemble allergic responses.

The nature of migraine has been emphasized to point out its importance in the differential diagnosis and management of headache.

A separate chapter devoted to drugs used in allergy and one on immunotherapy offer a holistic approach to therapy. By combining the discussions on the preparation of extracts, the technique of skin testing and the procedure for injection therapy, all facets of definitive therapy are coordinated.

The chapter on the botany of allergy serves as a guide for the physician in the very complex problem of evaluating the offending pollens in the various regions of the country.

The chapter on allergy in infancy is intended to point out the differences in the allergic response in the early months of life which can be attributed to anatomical and immunological immaturity.

The chapters on insect allergy and psychological factors in allergic disease have drawn heavily upon studies supported by U.S.P.H.–N.I.H. grants.

REFERENCES

1. Balint, Michael: *The Doctor, His Patient and the Illness.* New York, Univ Pr, 1957.
2. Bloom, Samuel W.: *The Doctor and His Patient—A Sociological Interpretation.* New York, Russell Sage, 1963.
3. Blum, Richard H.: *The Management of the Doctor-Patient Relationship.* New York, McGraw-Hill, 1960.
4. Francis, Vida, Korsch, Barbara M. and Morris, Marie J.: Gaps in doctor-patient communication: Patients' response to medical advice. *N Engl J Med, 280:* 535, 1969.
5. Freemon, Barbara, Negrete, Vida F., Davis, Milton and Korsch, Barbara M.: Gaps in doctor-patient communication: Doctor-patient interaction analysis. *Pediatr Res, 5:* 298, 1971.
6. Korsch, Barbara M., Gozzi, Ethel K. and Francis, Vida: Gaps in doctor-patient communication, I: Doctor-patient interaction and patient satisfaction. *Pediatrics, 42:* 855, 1968.
7. Swineford, O. Jr.: Allergy, the bastard of medical education. *J Med Educ, 39:* 946, 1964.

ACKNOWLEDGMENTS

THIS BOOK WAS suggested by several of my associates and colleagues but was not given serious consideration until I received the encouragement and support of Doctor Clifford H. Keene, President and Chief Executive Officer of the Kaiser Foundation Health Plan and the Kaiser Foundation Hospitals; Doctor Cecil C. Cutting, Executive Director of the Permanente Medical Group (Northern California) and his assistant, Doctor John G. Smillie.

I am fortunate to have the collaboration of several noteworthy contributors. I am grateful to Doctor Donald F. German for the chapter on the allergic infant; to Doctor Alice D. Friedman for her discussion of elimination diets; to Doctors Alan S. Levin, Lynn E. Spitler and H. Hugh Fudenberg for the chapter on immune deficiency states; and to Messrs. Morris E. Webb, Robert W. Townsend and Ray Nelson for their presentation on the botany of allergy.

I wish to express my appreciation to Mr. Robert Jack and Mrs. Ivanelle Childers of the administrative staff of the Kaiser Research Institute for their assistance with many procedural problems. I owe a debt of special gratitude to Mary Ann Warr Giacona who has carried out many typings of the manuscript and has assisted in all aspects of its preparation. I wish to thank Mr. Eric Stoelting who found time in a very busy schedule to produce the various figures, charts and drawings.

I also wish to make acknowledgment to the numerous authors and publishers who have granted permission for the reproduction of many figures and tables.

Finally, I express my thanks to Messrs. Payne Thomas and Robert Schinneer of Charles C Thomas, Publisher for their interest and cooperation in the publication of this volume.

BEN F. FEINGOLD

CONTENTS

Chapter	Page
Introduction	vii
Acknowledgments	xi
1. THE IMMUNOLOGY OF ALLERGY	3

    Immunology of Allergy
       Definition of Immunity
       Definition of Allergy
       Classification of Immune Responses
           Humoral Response; Cellular Response; Tolerance
       Classification of Allergic Responses
           Immediate Type (Reaginic, Atopic and Anaphylactic Allergy); Intermediate (Arthus Reaction) Type; Delayed (Cellular or Tuberculin) Type; Cytolytic and Cytotoxic; Gell and Coombs Classification
    Elements of Immunity
       Immunogen
       Antigen
           Complete; Incomplete (Hapten)
       Antibodies (Gammaglobulins) (Ig)
           IgA; IgG; IgD; IgM; IgE (Reaginic)
       Antigen-Antibody Complexes
       Cellular Elements
           Lymphocytes; T-cell; B-cell; Mast Cells; Monocytes; Eosinophils
       Mediators
       Complement
       Serum Disease

2. ALLERGIC DISEASES OF THE UPPER RESPIRATORY TRACT	53

    Nose
       Histology
       Pathology
           Allergic Rhinitis; Hay Fever; Polyps
       Throat
           Lymphoid Structures (Waldeyer's Ring); Palate and Fauces
       Sinuses
       Eustachian Tube
       Middle Ear
           Tympanic Cavity; Tympanic Membrane; Serous Otitis
       Allergic Laryngitis
       Diagnosis of Upper Respiratory Allergic Disease
           Laboratory Tests
       Treatment of Upper Respiratory Allergic Disease

3. ALLERGIC DISEASES OF THE EYE	62

    Conjunctivitis
       Reaginic-Atopic
           Acute; Chronic; Treatment

| Chapter | Page |

      Follicular
      Vernal
      Phlyctenular
   Eyelids
      Reaginic-Atopic
      Blepharitis
      Contact Dermatitis
   Cornea
      Superficial Keratitis
      Punctate Keratitis
      Isolated Ulcers
      Ring Ulcer
      Interstitial or Parenchymatous Keratitis
      Kerato-conjunctivitis (Wessely Phenomenon)
   Uvea
      Iritis
      Cyclitis
      Iridocyclitis
      Choroiditis
      Uveitis

4. ALLERGIC DISEASES OF THE LOWER RESPIRATORY TRACT............... 71

   Anatomical Features and Pathophysiology
      Cartilaginous Segment
         Trachea; Bronchi
      Transitional Fibro-muscular Segment
         Bronchioles; Terminal Bronchioles
      Acini—Gas Exchange Segment
   Allergic Diseases of the Bronchial Tree
      Mild Involvement
         Asthmatic Bronchitis
      Moderate Involvement
         Allergic Bronchitis; Asthmatic Bronchitis
      Extreme Involvement
         Bronchial Asthma; Status Asthmaticus
      Asthma in Infancy
   Etiology of Bronchial Allergy and Bronchial Asthma
      Infection
         Bacterial; Viral
      Extrinsic Asthma
      Intrinsic Asthma
      Non-Infectious Agents
         Cold Air; Air Pollutants; Irritating Gases and Vapors; Smoke (including tobacco); Physical Exertion—running, jumping, exercising; Emotional Disturbances—laughing, crying
   Beta-adrenergic Blockade Hypothesis
   Complications of Bronchial Allergic Disease
      Status Asthmaticus
         Bronchitis; Atelectasis; Emphysema
   Treatment of Bronchial Allergy
      Mild and Moderate Involvement
      Severe Involvement—Bronchial Asthma
      Extreme Involvement—Status Asthmaticus
   Pulmonary Function
      Mechanics of Respiration
         Inspiration; Expiration; Elastic Recoil
   Surface Tension and Pulmonary Surfactants

Chapter   Page

    Airway Resistance
    Terms Used in Respiratory Physiology
    Ventilatory Portion of Lung and Gas Exchange
        Partial Pressure of Oxygen (pO_2); Partial Pressure of Carbon Dioxide (pCO_2)
    Blood Oxygen Tension (pO_2)
    Blood Carbon Dioxide (pCO_2) and Acid-Base Balance (pH)
    Hendersen-Hasselbach Equation
    Pulmonary Function in Allergic Bronchial Disease
        Asymptomatic Patient
        Bronchial Asthma
        Hypoxemia
        Respiratory Acidosis and Alkalosis
        Cyanosis
    Allergic Bronchopulmonary Disease (Allergic Alveolitis)
    (Extrinsic Allergic Bronchopneumonia)
        Farmer's Lung
            Etiology; Histopathology; Immunology; Diagnosis; Treatment
        Pulmonary Aspergillosis
            Etiology; Pattern in Atopic Individuals: With Uncomplicated Asthma; Asthma with Pulmonary Eosinophilia (APE); Saccular Bronchiectasis; Fibrosis; Blood Eosinophilia; Sputum; Skin Tests; Precipitins. Pattern in Non-Atopic Individuals: Invasive Form; Treatment; Course of the Disease
        Aspergilloma
        Bird Fanciers Disease

5. GASTROINTESTINAL ALLERGY 116

    Immunological Considerations
    Clinical Considerations
        Incidence
        Etiologic Agents: Pollens; Environmental Factors; Molds; Foods; Drugs and Chemicals

6. ALLERGIC DISEASES OF THE SKIN 120

    Anatomy
        Epidermis
        Corium
    Dermatitis
        Definition
    Eczema
        Definition
    Allergic Dermatitis
        Specific Factors
            Immediate or Reaginic Type of Reaction; Intermediate or Arthus Type of Reaction; Delayed Type of Reaction
        Non-Specific Factors
            Histological Variations; Irritant Factors; Pruritus
        Atopic Dermatitis
            In Infancy; Beyond Infancy; Etiology of Atopic Dermatitis
    Complications of Infantile Eczema and Atopic Dermatitis
        Adenopathy
        Infection
            Bacterial; Viral
        Diagnosis
            Infantile Eczema Differentiated From:
                Contact Dermatitis; Seborrheic Dermatitis; Letterer-Siwe Syndrome (Histiocytosis X); Wiskott-Aldrich Syndrome; Acrodermatitis

| Chapter | Page |

    Atopic Dermatitis or Atopic Eczema Differentiated From:
        Contact Dermatitis; Seborrheic Dermatitis; Neurodermatitis (Lichen Simplex Chronicus); Nummular Eczema
    Treatment of Dermatitis: Topical; Infection; Pruritus
  Contact Dermatitis
    Non-Allergic
      Diagnosis and Treatment
    Allergic
      Etiology; Treatment; "Id" Reaction; Diagnosis and Treatment: In Infants; In Childhood, Adolescence and Adulthood
  Patch Testing
  Poison Oak (*Rhus toxicodendron diversilobia*)
  Poison Ivy (*Rhus toxicodendron radicans*)
    Urushiol—The Active Principle
    Clinical Pattern
    Diagnosis
    Treatment
      Topical and Systemic; Prophylaxis
  Urticaria
    Pathology
    Etiology
    Cholinergic Urticaria
    Chronic Urticaria
    Treatment of Urticaria
  Dermographism
  Angio-Edema
  Hereditary Angio-Edema (Quincke's Disease)

7. **HEADACHES** 139

  Allergic Headaches
  Migraine
    The Migraine Headache
      Distribution; Duration; Intensity; Nausea; Facial Appearance; Ocular Symptoms; Nasal Symptoms; Abdominal Symptoms
    Fluid Retention
    Etiology of Migraine
      Allergy; Vascular Theory; Chemical Theory: Histamine; Acetylcholine; Serotonin; Electrical Theory
    Treatment of Migraine

8. **ADVERSE REACTIONS TO FOODS AND FOOD CHEMICALS** 147

  Adverse Reactions to Foods
    Non-Immunologic Mechanisms
      Enzymatic Deficiencies; Chemical Irritation; Toxic Reactions; Contamination
    Symptomatology
      Immediate; Delayed
    Identification of Foods Involved in Reactions
      Skin Tests: The Positive Skin Test for Food; False Positive Skin Test Reaction; Negative Skin Test Reaction
    Antibodies to Foods
      Milk; Eggs; Meats; Chocolate; Corn
  Food Chemicals
    Non-Intentional Food Additives
    Intentional Food Additives
      Preservatives; Stabilizers and Thickeners; Synthetic Food Colors and Flavors

Diagnosis
  The Aspirin Sensitive Patient
Non-Nutritive Sweeteners
  Saccharin; Sorbitol and Mannitol

9. MANAGEMENT WITH THE ELIMINATION DIET—*Alice D. Friedman* 162

Procedure for Diet Elimination
Role of Inhalant Factors in Dietary Management
The Diet Diary
The Salicylate-free Diet
The Milk-free Diet
The Egg-free Diet
The Milk and Egg-free Diet
The Mold-free Diet
The Corn-free Diet
The Wheat-free Diet
The Wheat-Egg-Milk-free Diet
The Rowe Diet

10. ADVERSE REACTIONS TO DRUGS 171

Classification of Unwanted Drug Reactions
Mechanism of Allergic Drug Reactions
Clinical Manifestations
  Skin
    Urticaria and Angio-Edema; Maculo-papular Eruption; Fixed Drug Reactions; Generalized Involvement; Purpuric Lesions; Contact Dermatitis; Photosensitivity: Non-Allergic; Allergic
Hematological Manifestations
  Bone Marrow Involvement
  Peripheral Involvement
  Thrombocytopenia
  Hemolytic Anemia
Anaphylaxis
Serum Sickness Syndrome
Vasculitis
Exfoliative Dermatitis
Aspirin Sensitivity
  Mechanism Involved
  Diagnosis and Management
Allergic Reaction to Antibiotics
  Penicillin
    Immunological Considerations in Penicillin Reactions; Clinical Patterns of Penicillin Reactions; Tests for Penicillin Sensitivity; Desensitization Procedure for Penicillin; Depot Penicillin; Ampicillin
  Cephalosporins
  Tetracyclines
  Streptomycin
  Sulfonamides
Diagnosis of Drug Sensitivity
Treatments of Drug Reactions
  Prophylactic
  Symptomatic

Chapter	Page
11. PSYCHOLOGICAL FACTORS IN ALLERGIC DISEASE	189

    Introduction
    Hypotheses Concerning the Relationship of Psychological Behavior and Allergic Disease
        I. Psychoanalytic View of Alexander and French
       II. Allergy as Response to Stress
      III. Asthma and Psychoses
      IV. Psychosomatic Specificity
       V. Emotional Precipitation of Allergy Symptoms
      VI. Allergic Persons as Psychologically Heterogeneous Population
        Skin Test Positive Individuals; Skin Test Negative Individuals; Behavioral Disturbances Induced by Food Chemicals
      VII. Relevance of Animal Conditioning Studies to Asthma
    Psychological Treatment of Allergic Individuals

12. INSECT ALLERGY	198

    Allergic Reaction to Biting Insects
      Flea Bites
        Stages of Reactivity; Papular Urticaria; Cross Reactivity; Treatment: Prophylactic; Palliative; Infection; Hyposensitization
      Mosquitoes
      Bed Bugs
      Body Lice
      Sand Flies
      Triatomata (Cone-nosed Beetle)
        The Bite Reaction; Diagnosis; Treatment
    Hymenoptera Stings
      Honey Bees, Yellow Jackets, Wasps, Hornets
        Venoms: Immunology; Cross Reactivity. Clinical Patterns: Local; Constitutional; Delayed. Diagnosis and Identification; Treatment: Emergency Treatment; Hyposensitization
      Urticating (Stinging) Hairs and Spines
      Imported Fire Ants
      (Solenopsis Saevissima Richteri)
        Sting Reaction; Signs and Symptoms; Treatment
    Arthropods as Inhalants
      Species Which Serve as a Source of Antigen.; Silk; Mites

13. THE ALLERGIC PATIENT	220

    Heredity in Allergic Disease
    Patterns of Clinical Allergy
      Tension Fatigue Syndrome
      Infancy
      Childhood
      Adulthood
    Physical Examination

14. ALLERGY IN INFANCY—Donald F. German	227

    The Immune Response
      Fetus
      Neonate
      Infant
    Sensitization

Clinical Manifestation of Allergic Disease in Infancy
   Gastrointestinal
      Incidence; Symptoms; Differential Diagnosis: Coeliac Disease; Cystic Fibrosis; Immune Deficiency Disorders. Treatment; Prognosis
   Respiratory
      Allergic Rhinitis; Pharynx
   The Allergic Ear in Infancy
   Bronchial Allergy
      Pathology; Signs and Symptoms; Laboratory Findings; Diagnosis and Differential Diagnosis: Foreign Body; Vascular Ring; Cystic Fibrosis; Tracheo-esophageal Fistula; Bronchitis; Bronchiolitis; Immunological Disorders; Heiner Syndrome. Treatment of the Acute Condition; Definitive Treatment; Dietary Management; Prophylaxis of Allergy in Infancy

15. DRUGS USED IN TREATMENT OF ALLERGIC DISEASE 240
   Antihistamines
     Absorption, Fate and Excretion
     Adverse Reactions
       Sedation; Gastrointestinal Side Effects; Blood Dyscrasias; Allergic Reactions
     In the Common Cold
   Sympathomimetic Drugs
     Alpha (α) and Beta (β) Receptors
     Catecholamines
       Epinephrine; Isoproterenol (Isuprel®); Levarterenol; Salbutanol
     Non-Catecholamines
       Amphetamine; Ephedrine; Methoxyphenamine (Orthoxine®)
     Aerosol Sprays
   Methylxanthines
     Theophylline
       Aminophylline; Elixophyllin; Oxtriphylline (Choledyl®)
     Theophylline Mixtures
       Tedral®; Marax®
   Expectorants
     Water as an Expectorant
       Steam Inhalation
     Aerosol Inhalation Preparations
     Potassium Iodide (KI)
     Sodium Iodide (NaI)
     Syrup Hydriodic Acid (Syr. H.I.)
     Ammonium Chloride
     Glycerol Guaiacolate (Robitussin®)
     Syrup of Ipecac
     Expectorant Mixtures
   Corticotropin (ACTH)
     Action and Uses in Allergy
   Corticosteroids
     Mineralocorticoids
     Glucocorticoids
       Action of Glucocorticoids
   Indication for Steroid Therapy
     Allergic Rhinitis
     Nasal Polyps
     Hay Fever
     Bronchial Allergy
     Bronchial Asthma
     Urticaria and Angio-Edema
     Drug Allergy
     Allergic Dermatitis

Chapter	Page

    Choice of Preparations
      High Level Dosage
      Maintenance Dose
      Injectable Steroids
      Topical Steroids
          Dermatological; Ophthalmic; Otic
      Rectal Suppositories
    Sedatives
      Upper Respiratory Allergic Disease
      Lower Respiratory Allergic Disease
      Barbiturates
      Non-Barbiturate Sedatives
          Chloral Hydrate; Paraldehyde
      Bromides
    Antianxiety Agents (Minor Tranquilizers)
    Cromolyn Sodium (Disodium Cromoglycate) (DSCG)

16. BOTANY OF ALLERGY—*Morris E. Webb, Robert W. Townsend, Ray Nelson* 267

    Taxonomy
      Definition
      Classification
    Ecology
      Factors Governing Growth
    Pollen
      Production
      Floral Anatomy
      Thommen's Postulates
          Related to the Plant; Related to the Pollen
      Collecting Pollen
    Geographical Distribution and Survey
      Plant Surveys
          Indigenous Plants; Cultivated Plants and Trees
      Changes in Surveys
    Primary Offenders
    Secondary Offenders
    Geographical Regions of the United States
      I through XVII

17. IMMUNOTHERAPY (DESENSITIZATION—HYPOSENSITIZATION) 290

    Definition
      I. Preparation of Extracts
      Pollen Extracts
          Control of Contamination of Pollen Supply; Storage of Pollens
      Extracting Procedure for Pollens
      Standardization of Pollen Extracts
          Noon Units; Protein Nitrogen Units (PNU); Weight by Volume (W/V); IgE Standardization
      Quality Control of Pollen Extracts
      Environmental Factors
          Feathers; Hairs; Vegetable Fibers: Coconut Fiber; Kapok; Jute; Cotton.
      Dust Extracts
      Mites
      Gums
      Silk

Acetone Precipitation Technique
II. Skin Testing
Techniques
    Scratch; Prick; Intradermal (Intracutaneous); Patch
Choice of Allergen for Testing
Choice of Technique for Testing
Concentration of the Test Antigen
Control Test
Skin Test Reaction Rating
Testing Procedure
Mucosal Test
Nasal Test
Ophthalmic Test
III. Injection Therapy
Principles of Immunotherapy
    Blocking IgG Antibody; Reduction of Serum Reagin; Decreased Histamine Release
Efficacy of Immunotherapy
The Clinical Program
    Environmental Control
Injection Procedure
    Formulation of the Treatment Extract; Technique for Administering Antigens; Dosage Schedule for Treatment Extracts; Interval Between Injections; Indications for Perennial, Pre-seasonal and Co-seasonal Treatment; Duration of the Treatment Program; Reactions; Local and Constitutional; Immediate and Delayed
Adjuvant Therapy
    Emulsion Repository Technique; Alum Precipitated Extracts; Pyridine-Alum Precipitated Extracts (Allpyral)
Mold Allergy
    Incidence of Mold Sensitivity
    Immunology of Molds
    Mold Antigens and Antibodies
    Skin Test Reactions to Mold Extracts
    Treatment with Mold Antigens
    Management of Mold Allergy

18. AUTO-ALLERGIC DISEASE 337

Definition
Hypotheses
    (1) Sequestered Protein
    (2) Cross Reactivity of AD for Bacteria and Tissue
    (3) Environmental Factors
        Infection; Drugs and Chemicals; Trauma
    (4) Genetic and Somatic Factors
        Burnett's Theory of the "Forbidden Clone"; Fudenberg's Concept of Immunologic Deficiency
    (5) Breakdown of the Mechanism of Tolerance
Types of Auto Antibodies
    Antinuclear Antibodies
    Anticytoplasmic Antibodies
    Antigammaglobulin Antibodies
        Gm and Inv Specific Antibodies; Rheumatoid Factor (RF); Non-Rheumatoid Type (Milgram Factor); Antibodies to Buried Determinants

| Chapter | Page |

   Anticollagen Antibodies
   Anti-elastin Antibodies
   Disease Associated with Auto-Antibodies

19. IMMUNE DEFICIENCY STATES—*Alan S. Levin, Lynn E. Spitler, H. Hugh Fudenberg* 346
   Introduction
      I. Congenital Immune Deficiency States
      Defective Cellular (T-Cell) System with Intact Humoral (B-Cell) System
         Thymic and Parathyroid Agenesis: DiGeorge Syndrome; Autosomal Recessive Thymic Aplasia with Lymphopenia: "Nezeloff"
      Defective Antibody Mediated (B-Cell) System with Intact Cellular (T-Cell) System
         Infantile X-linked Agammaglobulinemia (Bruton); Selective Immunoglobulin Disorders: Selective IgA Deficiency; Selective IgG Deficiency; Selective IgM Deficiency; Selective Immune Paralysis with Normal Immunoglobulin Levels. Transient Hypogammaglobulinemia of Infancy. Non-Sex Linked Primary Immunoglobulin Aberrations: Adult "Acquired" Hypogammaglobulinemia
      Mixed Deficiencies
         Ataxia Telangiectasia; X-Linked Dual System Deficiency: "Thymic Alymphoplasia"; Autosomal Recessive Dual System Deficiency: "Swiss Type"; Variable Deficiencies: Mucocutaneous Candidiasis: Wiskott-Aldrick Syndrome
      Granulocyte Defects
         Chronic Granulomatous Disease; Job's Syndrome; Chediak-Higashi Syndrome
      II. "Acquired" Immune Deficiency States
      Infectious "Acquired" Immune Deficiency States
         Sarcoidosis; Tuberculosis; Coccidioidomycosis; Leprosy
      Malignant "Acquired" Immune Deficiency States:
         Carcinoma; Sarcoma
   Iatrogenic Immunosuppresive Therapy
      Evaluation of Immunologic Competence
         Humoral Immunity
         Cellular Immunity
      Evaluation of the Procedures Used in the Treatment of Cellular Immune Defects

Index 361

INTRODUCTION TO CLINICAL ALLERGY

Chapter 1

THE IMMUNOLOGY OF ALLERGY

DEFINITION: Allergy cannot be defined without a consideration of the nature of immunity. Immunity involves all the mechanisms concerned with the protection of the individual against the assault of foreign substances. A foreign substance is any material which the body does not recognize as *self*, i.e. a part of itself. If the foreign substances originate outside the body, they are called extrinsic, but if they originate within the body, they are known as intrinsic. Extrinsic materials include bacteria, viruses, fungi, parasites, foreign sera, chemicals, drugs, environmental factors, pollens and even foods. Intrinsic materials are derived from intracellular bacteria or viruses and from tissue components which have been altered in structure by various factors, such as infection, radiation or mutation, and accordingly, the body does not recognize them as *self*.

Immunity includes not only the active protective mechanisms against foreign agents (antigens-allergens) but also the suppression of these mechanisms (tolerance).

There are levels for the degree of response of the immune system which are generally recognized as normal. Any deviation from the norm constitutes the "altered reactivity" which in 1906 was labelled "allergy" by Pirquet. Pirquet termed the baseline for the immune response "ergy" (force). Any deviation above the baseline, which may be either an increased or an accelerated response of the immune mechanism, was termed "hyperergy" or increased force which currently is referred to as hypersensitivity. Reactions below the baseline were called "hypoergy" or decreased force which currently is called "partial tolerance," while complete failure of the immune mechanism to respond was called "anergy" which in current literature is termed "tolerance" (see discussion of tolerance below).

Initially, the interest of Pirquet and Schick in altered reactivity was related to serum disease. At the turn of the century the morbidity for tuberculosis among the Viennese was about 90 percent. Because of this high incidence, the attention of Pirquet and Schick gravitated very naturally toward the altered reactivity as observed in infection, and particularly in tuberculosis. In their early observations reference is made to hyperergy or increased reactivity (hypersensitivity) as observed in tuberculous infection, and anergy or lack of immune response as observed in overwhelming tuberculous infection.

The definition of the term "allergy," as originally stated by Pirquet, avoids restricting the term to the commonly recognized hypersensitivity diseases, such as allergic rhinitis, hay fever, bronchial allergy, bronchial asthma and allergic dermatitis, but permits a broader application which includes various hematological diseases based upon an alteration of the immune response, drug allergy, and auto-allergic disease.

Since allergy is a variation of the basic immune mechanism, a discussion of allergy is actually a consideration of the mechanism of immunity.

Immunological responses are classified as:

(1) The *cell mediated* reaction in which all the activity is induced by cells. It is postulated that antibody is either attached to the wall of the immune cell or is a part of the cell wall. This concept requires further

confirmation. *No humoral antibody* is demonstrable in this class of reactions.

(2) *Humoral response* in which antibodies demonstrable in the blood serum are involved in the tissue reactions.

The two classes of immune response, the cellular and the humoral, participate in allergic disease through four types of allergic reactions.

    I. The *Immediate* type, also called
        (a) Reaginic allergy
        (b) Atopic allergy
        (c) Anaphylactic allergy
   II. The *Intermediate* type, also called the Arthus reaction
  III. The *Delayed* type, also called cellular or tuberculin type
  IV. Cytolytic and cytotoxic

Note: Gell and Coombs propose the following classification of the allergic reactions:

Type I—Anaphylactic
Type II—Cytolytic or cytotoxic
Type III—Inflammatory reaction or response (Arthus reaction or toxic-complex syndrome)
Type IV—Cellular reaction or response (delayed or tuberculin-type sensitivity).

The classification presented in this book does not differ fundamentally from that proposed by Gell and Coombs. Instead of numerical designations, each type of reaction is labelled with a descriptive name, which together with the temporal sequence of classification permits simpler identification. This arrangement necessitates moving the cytolytic or cytotoxic reactions to the fourth position.

Before discussing the four types of allergic response, it is important to consider the elements or building blocks that participate in the various reactions:

    I. Immunogens
   II. Antigens (Ag)
        (a) complete antigens
        (b) incomplete antigens—haptens
  III. Antibodies (Ab)
  IV. Antigen-Antibody complexes (Ag-Ab)
   V. Cellular Elements
        (a) Lymphocytes and plasma cells
        (b) Mast cells and basophils
        (c) Monocytes
        (d) Eosinophils
  VI. Chemical Mediators, including Complement

IMMUNOGEN

Definition: An immunogen is any substance capable of initiating *de novo* an immune response, e.g. (a) committing a lymphocyte to produce specific antibodies when it subsequently encounters its specific antigen, and (b) committing a lymphocyte to respond with the cellular reaction of delayed hypersensitivity when it subsequently encounters an identical antigen.

Requirements for immunogenicity:

(1) The first prerequisite for immunogenicity is the ability of the body to recognize the substance as *foreign* (not self).

(2) Chemical Requirements: Immunogens are usually proteins.

Occasionally carbohydrates such as those found in the capsule of the pneumococcus can act as immunogens, but for practical clinical purposes immunogens can usually be considered to be proteins.

Size and molecular weight are important factors in immunogenicity. It is usually stated that proteins must have a molecular weight of 10,000 or more to be immunogenic, i.e. able to induce an immune response. There are examples of small proteins, such as insulin (6,000 mol. wt.) which are immunogenic. Proteins of low molecular weight are referred to as weak immunogens since they induce an immune response of a low degree. The larger the protein, and the greater the molecular weight, the more active and more immunogenic is the molecule (strong antigen). For example, serum proteins which are of large molecular weight are usually good antigens. In addition to size and molecular weight the steric structure, charges and degree of foreignness of the molecule are conditions that determine immunogenicity.

ANTIGEN*

Antigens are of two types: (1) complete, and (2) incomplete.

(1) Complete Antigens

Complete antigens are:

(a) immunogenic
(b) able to evoke antibody production
(c) able to combine specifically with the antibodies it evokes.

This selective behavior of the antigen in combining with the antibody it evokes is termed *specificity*.

Specificity is governed by both the configuration or shape of the protein molecule and the antigenic determinant.

The antigenic determinant is a restricted or localized portion of the protein molecule which at times may consist of a cluster of as few as four or five amino acids. At times the determinant may only involve a side chain of the amino acid or a radical attached to a side chain.

A protein molecule serving as an antigen may have one or many antigenic determinants on its body. The chemical structure of these determinants may be identical or they may vary. Since each determinant evokes its specific antibody, depending upon its structure, it is possible for a single molecule, i.e. a single antigen, to induce the production of identical antibodies(1) (homogeneity) or a variety of antibodies (heterogeneity).

---

* Allergen is the term applied to antigens involved in reaginic or atopic allergy. The common allergens include foods, pollens, environmental factors (feathers, animal danders, and dusts), and molds.

(2) Incomplete Antigens (Haptens)

Incomplete antigens are not immunogenic, cannot evoke antibody production, but are able to combine with a specific antibody.

It has been indicated that immunogenicity, the ability to induce an immune response, is usually limited to proteins of 10,000 molecular weight or above. However, it is generally recognized that many simple chemicals of low molecular weight, less than 1,000 or even as low as 200, are involved in the induction of immune reactions. For a simple chemical to have the capacity to be immunogenic, it must combine or conjugate with a protein to give it sufficient bulk to induce an immune response. Recent studies have demonstrated that it is possible for low molecular weight compounds to achieve increased size through aggregation and as a result become immunogenic. The protein to which the simple chemical is joined is called a carrier, while the simple chemical is termed a "hapten" (Greek: *haptein*—to touch, to seize upon, or to hold fast). The conjugation of the protein carrier with the hapten forms a *complete antigen*, which may induce an immune response (immunogenic), evoke the production of antibodies, and combine specifically with antibodies it evokes (antigenic).

When the conjugated antigen stimulates antibody production, the antibodies may be of three classes:

(1) specific for the hapten
(2) specific for the carrier
(3) specific for the conjugated antigen

Both the protein carrier and the conjugated antigen have the ability to interact with its specific antibody to form Ag-Ab complexes with the capacity to induce tissue responses.

The isolated simple chemical (hapten) also has the capacity to combine with its specific antibody (antigenicity), but such a union does not initiate a tissue reaction. Actually, when the hapten occupies the com-

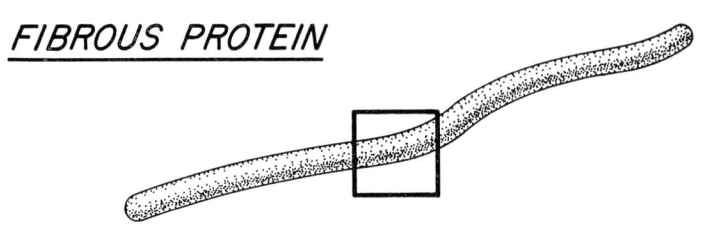

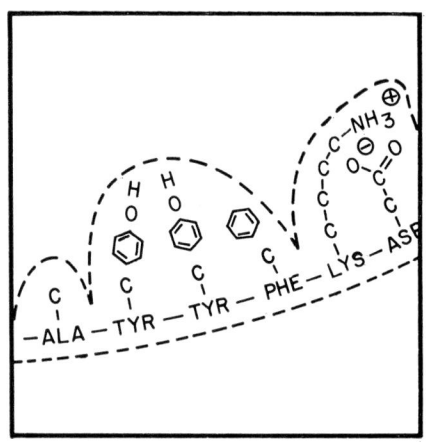

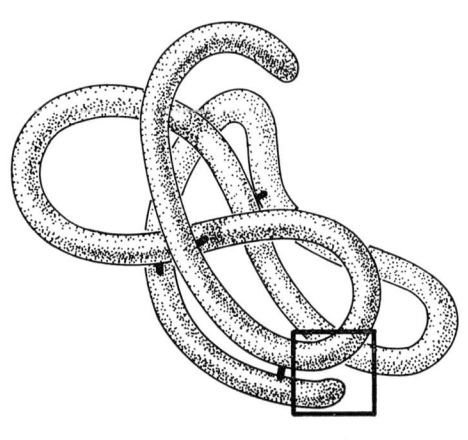

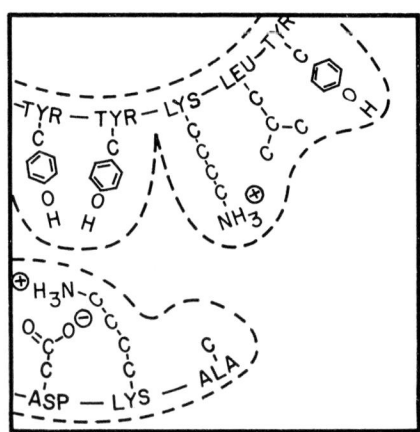

Figure 1-1. Fibrous proteins are linear structures composed of sequences of peptides (a group of amino acid residues). The cut-out (□) on the fibrous protein illustrates the configuration of the molecule governed by the side chains. The position of the side chain is determined by its charge, relative to neighboring side chains. Globular proteins are twisted upon themselves. Their configuration is also determined by the sequence of amino acids and the relationship to neighboring side chains. The loops of the globular protein are held together by disulfide bonds (–). Rupture of a bond permits an alteration in configuration which can influence immunogenicity, antigenicity and specificity. The cut-out (□) illustrates how the apposition of chemical groups provides a cluster which can serve as an antigenic determinant. An antigenic determinant can involve more than one loop of the molecule. Rupture of the disulfide bond permits an alteration which changes the relationship of apposed side chains and in this way can alter specificity.

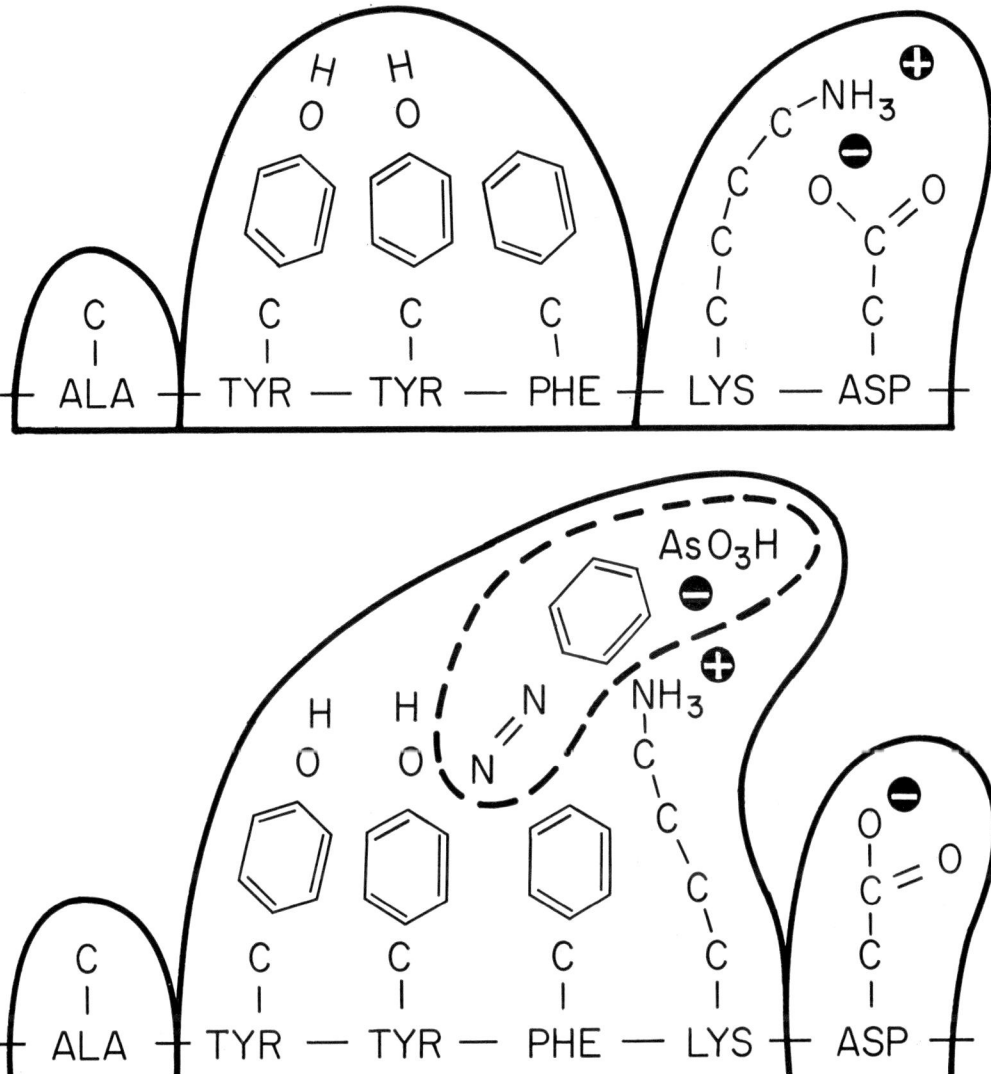

Figure 1-2. The diagrams in Figures 1-2 and 1-3 illustrate a hypothetical polypeptide made up of a sequence of amino acids (residues). The sequence is shown in two dimensions, but the molecule has a steric structure (three dimensions) which must be visualized. The side chains of the amino acids and their relationship to neighboring side chains determine the configuration of the molecule.

The upper diagram illustrates a polypeptide chain consisting of alanyl-tyrosyl-tyrosyl-phenylallanyl-lysyl-aspartic acid. The amino acid side chains are shown with no haptenic attachments. The amino acids in the cluster tyrosyl-tyrosyl-phenylallanyl are attracted towards each other since the components are hydrophobic and of like solubilities. This cluster could serve as a natural antigenic determinant since aromatic centers are usually good antigenic determinants. The positively charged lysine is attracted toward the negatively charged aspartic acid and in so doing uncovers the aromatic center of the phenylalanine, making it more readily available as a determinant site for antibody synthesis.

The lower diagram of Figure 1-2 repeats the same sequence of residues, but by diazotization the hapten, para-aminophenyl arsenilic acid, is conjugated to the radical tyrosyl. As a result the negatively charged arsenilic acid and the neighboring positively charged lysine are attracted towards each other and in so doing the lysine is pulled away from the aspartic acid. As a result, two important changes in the structure occur:

(1) the configuration of the cluster is changed, and (2) the natural antigenic site of the phenylalanine is masked so that it is no longer available as an antigenic determinant.

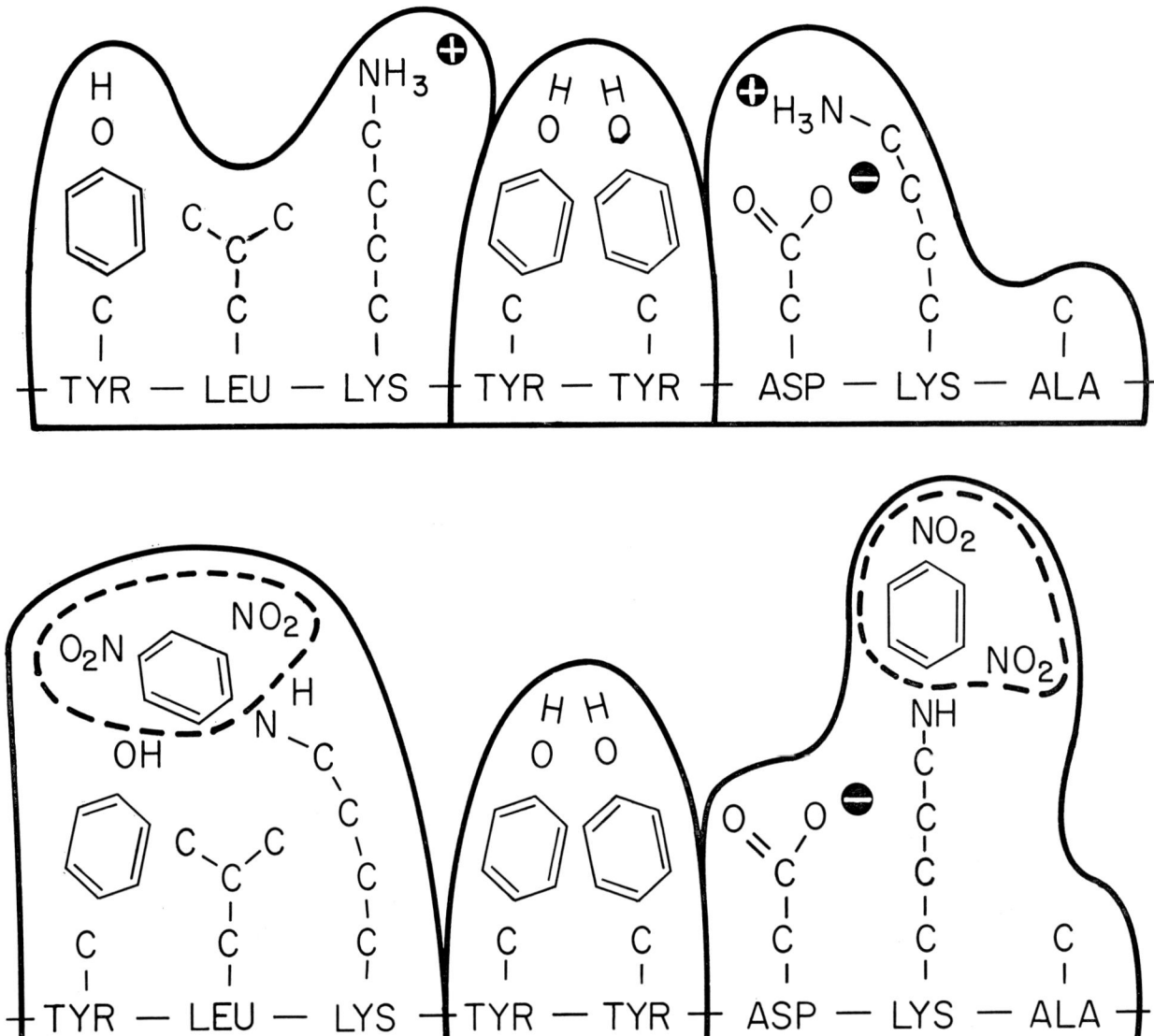

Figure 1-3. This figure illustrates how the amino acid side chains contribute to the configuration of the molecule. (The steric structure or 3-D dimension must be visualized.) The polypeptide is constituted of the amino acids tyrosyl-leucine-lysine-tyrosyl-tyrosyl-aspartic acid-lysine-alanine.

The attachment of an identical haptenic group to diverse positions on the protein molecule changes the configuration of the peptide depending upon the variations in the neighboring amino acids.

In the left grouping of the lower diagram, the hapten, dinitrobenzene, is attached to the lysine side chain. As a result the lysine has lost its charge and is attracted toward the hydrophobic tyrosyl and leucine. The configuration of this cluster of the peptide molecule is altered which changes its specificity from that of the original structure illustrated in the upper diagram.

The grouping on the right in the upper diagram has the identical haptenic group, dinitrobenzene, attached to the lysine side chain (see lower diagram). The lysine again loses its positive charge. However, in this situation the neighbor on the left is the negatively charged aspartic acid, while on the right there is the small alanine radical. As a result the lysine with the conjugated hapten dinitrobenzene sticks straight out from the backbone of the protein molecule which produces a change in the configuration of the cluster.

The identical hapten, dinitrobenzene, has been attached to both the left and right clusters, but their resulting specificity is different because the configuration of the clusters is different. The lysine on the left, pulling away from the tyrosyl radical and the cluster on the right pulling away from the adjacent tyrosol with its aromatic center makes this grouping (tyrosyl-tyrosyl) more readily available as an antigenic determinant.

Summary of Figures 1-2 and 1-3:

(1) A cluster of side chains of the amino acids in a protein may determine an antigenic area.

(2) The sequence of the residues may determine: (a) the shape of the protein, and (b) the antigenic determinant area of the protein through the interaction of neighboring amino acids.

(3) The identical haptenic grouping attached to a side chain of the protein can produce various shapes in the protein depending upon the position of the attachment. This can result in: (a) the masking or covering of a pre-existing natural antigenic determinant site, and (b) the exposure of a natural antigenic determinant group.

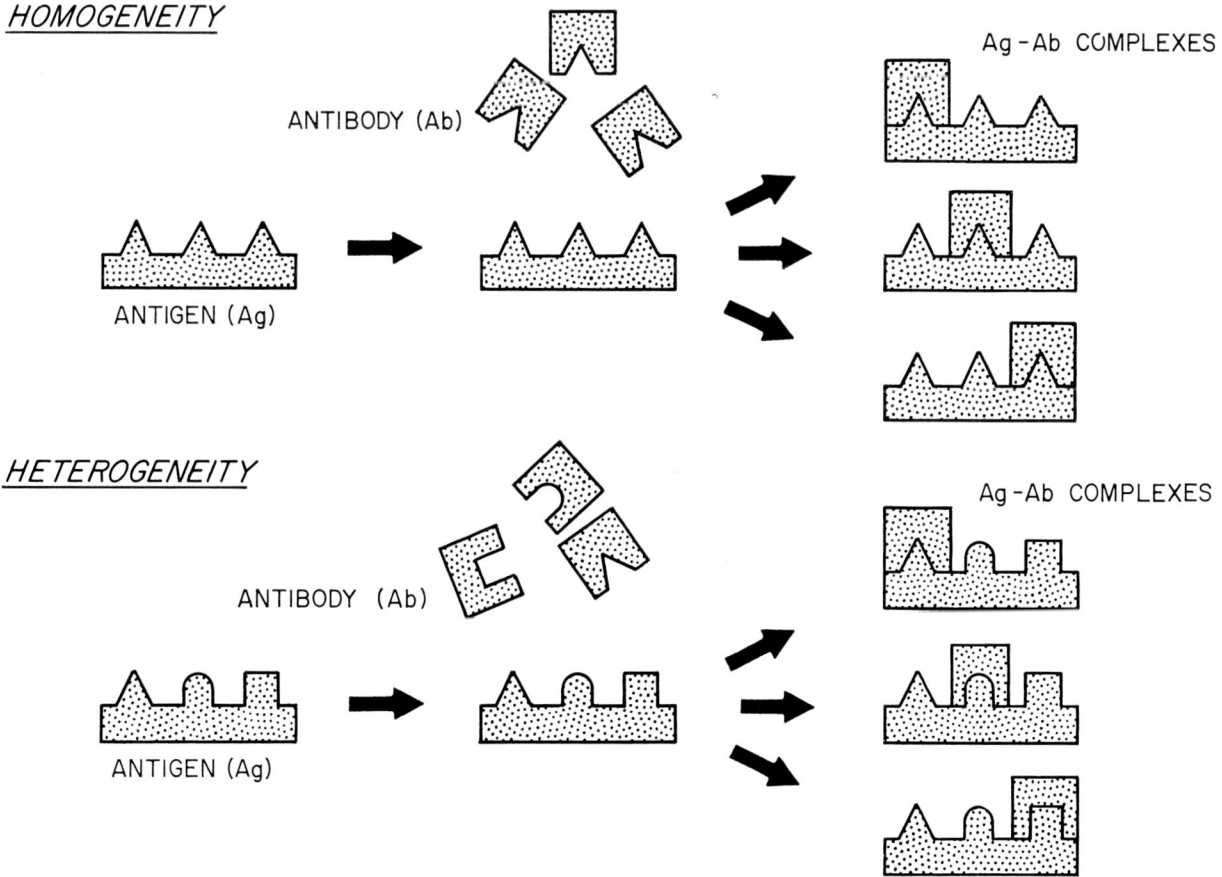

Figure 1-4. An antigen may have identical determinants (repeating sub-units) which evoke identical antibodies—homogeneity.

An antigen may have different determinants which evoke different antibodies—heterogeneity.

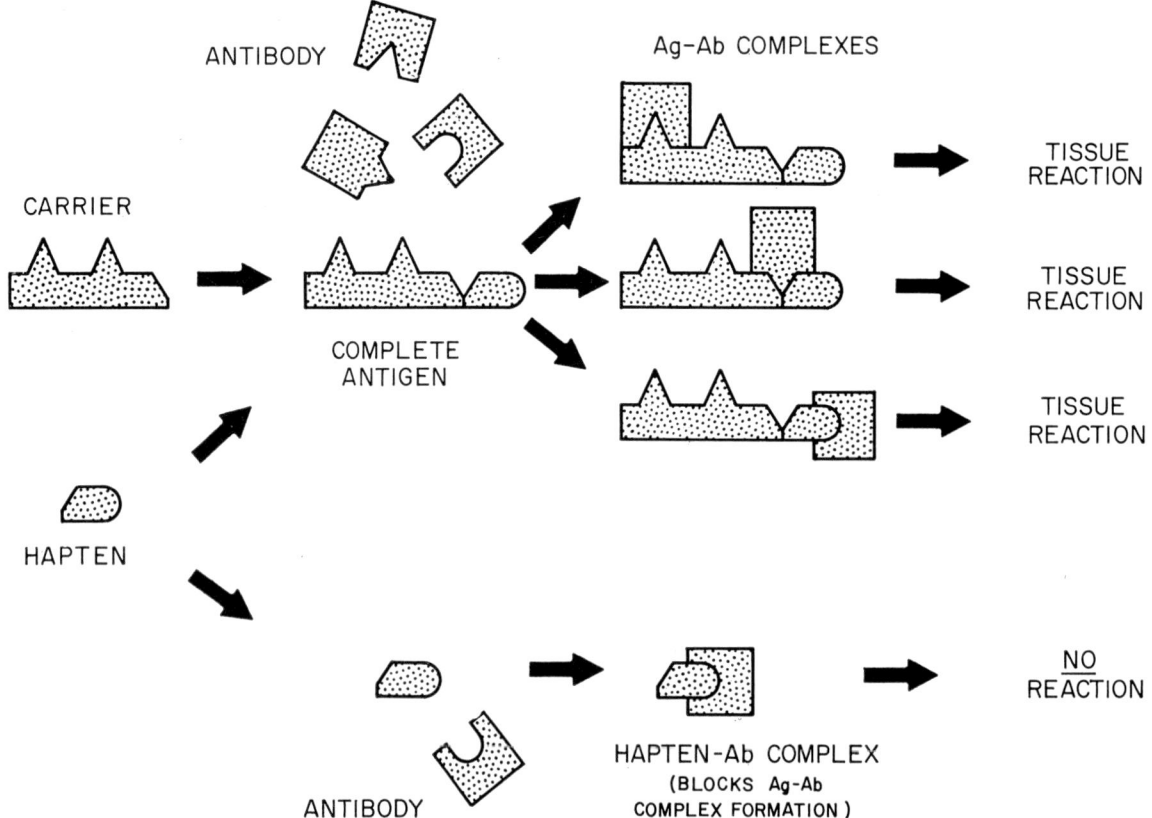

Figure 1–5. A hapten (low molecular substance less than 10,000) combines with its carrier to become immunogenic. Three types of antibodies are produced: (1) antibodies against the carrier, (2) antibodies against the hapten, and (3) antibodies against the conjugate. Antibodies plus the complete conjugate—tissue reaction. Antibodies plus hapten—no tissue reaction. (Actually blocks the formation of Ag-Ab complex).

bining site of the antibody, it makes it impossible for the complete antigen to unite with the specific antibody to form Ag-Ab complexes which have the capacity to induce tissue reactions. Therefore, the union of the hapten with its specific antibody prevents allergic tissue reactions.

Note: In current immunological literature the term "ligand" is appearing. Ligand refers to a molecule with antigenicity, i.e. the ability to combine with antibody. Accordingly, either a complete antigen or a hapten may be referred to as a ligand.

ANTIBODIES

Antibodies are proteins which are produced by small lymphocytes and plasma cells in response to their stimulation by a complete antigen. An antibody can only react with the specific antigen responsible for its production. Conversely, an antigen can only react with the specific antibody which it evokes. This characteristic is referred to as specificity of antigens and antibodies.

The portion of the antibody molecule which combines with the *antigenic determinant* is the combining site. The exact structure of the combining site is not known. However, like the antigenic determinant, the antibody combining site is also a restricted portion of the antibody molecule (a small group of amino acids) which is complementary or specific for the anigenic determinant.

Classification of Antibodies: On the basis of their mobility in an electric field (electrophoresis) and physio-chemical char-

Table 1-I

Ig Class	Mol Wt	Carbo-hydrate	Sed. value	Serum Conc. (mg%)	Compl. Fix.	Cross Placenta	Biol. ½ life	Where formed in highest concentration
IgA	170,000* 400,000†	7.5%	7S–11S	100 – 400	—	—	4-8 days	sero-mucus secretions
IgD	200,000	14.8%	7S	0.3– 4.0	—		2-8 days	interstitial connective tissue
IgE	130,000 to 200,000	10.7%	8.2S	0.1– 0.7‡ μgm/ml	—		2 days	skin and epithelium
IgG	150,000	2.9%	7S–11S	700 –1500	+	+	23 days	serum
IgM	900,000	11.8%	19S	50 – 200	+		5 days	serum

* serum IgA
† secretory IgA
‡ figure is given for normals—considerably elevated in atopic individuals

acteristics, plasma proteins are separated into four main groups:

albumen
alpha (α)
beta (β) } globulins
gamma (γ)

In man, antibodies occur in only the gamma fraction of the globulins. The gamma globulins are produced by lymphocytes and plasma cells which are found in the antibody-producing centers of the reticulo-endothelial system. These include the lymph nodes, the spleen, the intestinal submucosa and Peyer's patches, the tonsils and adenoids, and the lymphoid cells of the respiratory submucosa.

Although the gamma globulins show physio-chemical differences, they have structural characteristics in common which justify their classification in a common group which by international agreement has been labelled with the generic term "immunoglobulin" and designated by the symbol *Ig*.

In man, five main classes of immunoglobulins (Ig) are recognized:

IgA
IgG
IgD
IgM
IgE

IgA

IgA has a molecular weight of about 170,000, a sedimentation coefficient of about 7S, and approximately 7.5 per cent carbohydrate. It constitutes between 10 per cent and 15 per cent of the total Ig in human serum.

IgA does not cross the placenta and does not fix complement.

About 40 per cent of the IgA in the body is found intravascularly, while the remainder which occurs as exocrine IgA is found in the epithelial surfaces of the eyes, the respiratory and gastrointestinal tracts.

Table 1-II: LEVELS OF IMMUNE GLOBULINS IN SERA OF NORMAL SUBJECTS, BY AGE*

	IgG		IgM		IgA		Total Immunoglobulin	
	mg/100 ml	% of Adult Level	mg/100 ml	% of Adult Level	mg/100 ml	% of Adult Level	mg/100 ml	% of Adult Level
Newborn	1,031 ± 200	89 ± 17	11 ± 5	11 ± 5	2 ± 3	1 ± 2	1,044 ± 201	67 ± 13
1- 3 mo.	430 ± 119	37 ± 10	30 ± 11	30 ± 11	21 ± 13	11 ± 7	481 ± 127	31 ± 9
4- 6 mo.	427 ± 186	37 ± 16	43 ± 17	43 ± 17	28 ± 18	14 ± 9	498 ± 204	32 ± 13
7-12 mo.	661 ± 219	58 ± 19	54 ± 23	55 ± 23	37 ± 18	19 ± 9	752 ± 242	48 ± 15
13-24 mo.	762 ± 209	66 ± 18	58 ± 23	59 ± 23	50 ± 24	25 ± 12	870 ± 258	56 ± 16
25-36 mo.	892 ± 183	77 ± 16	61 ± 19	62 ± 19	71 ± 37	36 ± 19	1,024 ± 205	65 ± 14
3- 5 yr.	929 ± 228	80 ± 20	56 ± 18	57 ± 18	93 ± 27	47 ± 14	1,078 ± 245	69 ± 17
6- 8 yr.	923 ± 256	80 ± 22	65 ± 25	66 ± 25	124 ± 45	62 ± 23	1,112 ± 293	71 ± 20
9-11 yr.	1,124 ± 235	97 ± 20	79 ± 33	80 ± 33	131 ± 60	66 ± 30	1,334 ± 254	85 ± 17
12-16 yr.	946 ± 124	82 ± 11	59 ± 20	60 ± 20	148 ± 63	74 ± 32	1,153 ± 169	74 ± 12
Adults	1,158 ± 305	100 ± 26	99 ± 27	100 ± 27	200 ± 61	100 ± 31	1,457 ± 353	100 ± 24

* Values shown above were derived by Drs. E.R. Stiehm and H.H. Fudenberg from measurements made in 296 normal children and 30 adults. Levels were determined by radial diffusion plate method using specific antisera to human immunoglobulins.

Exocrine IgA is so called because it is found in external secretions, such as tears, saliva, colostrum, milk, tracheo-bronchial and intestinal secretions.

Exocrine IgA with a molecular weight of 400,000 consists of two molecules of IgA tied together by a covalently bound peptide chain with a molecular weight 23,000 labelled either as *transport piece* or *secretory piece*. The transport piece functions either to enable the body to secrete the antibody, or, possibly by resisting proteolytic digestion in the external secretions, gives the exocrine IgA great stability.

Many different functions have been attributed to circulating IgA, such as cold agglutinins, iso-agglutinins, bacterial agglutinins, anti-insulins, *etc*. Recent studies indicate that IgA plays an important role in viral immunity.

The occurrence of exocrine IgA in the external secretions suggests that it serves as a protection against invading organisms and as such provides the first line of defense against infection.

IgG

IgG with a molecular weight of about 160,000 and a sedimentation coefficient of 7S comprises between 70 to 80 per cent of the serum immunoglobulins. The supply of IgG in the body is divided equally between the intra- and extravascular compartments. The IgG that is outside the vascular compartment is found beneath the epithelial surfaces.

IgG is secreted by plasma cells.

IgG is the only immunoglobulin capable of passing the placental barrier and by virtue of this characteristic supplies the newborn with maternal IgG which serves it during the early months of life.

There are four subclasses of IgG, namely, IgG_1, IgG_2, IgG_3, and IgG_4. IgG_1 and IgG_3 fix complement well; IgG_2 weakly; IgG_4 not at all.

IgG is concerned with the following functions:

(1) The protection of the body against invading organisms through the neutralization of toxins, and the inactivation and phagocytosis of extracellular bacteria and viruses.

(2) In Intermediate or Arthus type of allergic reaction, IgG provides a precipitating form to develop complexes.

(3) In hyposensitization in reaginic-atopic allergy it provides the blocking antibodies.

(4) In the Rh mechanism it provides the sensitization antibodies.

(5) When body tissues are the target for humoral antibodies, IgG is the commonest source of tissue-specific antibody.

IgD

IgD with a molecular weight of 160,000 and a sedimentation coefficient of about 7S constitutes around 0.2 per cent of the total serum immunoglobulins. Its function has not been established.

IgM

IgM is the largest antibody in size with a molecular weight of 900,000 to 1,000,000 and a sedimentation coefficient of 19S. IgM constitutes between 5 per cent and 10 per cent of the total immunoglobulins. Most of the IgM, about 80 per cent, is intravascular, while the extravascular portion of this antibody is found free beneath the epithelium of the skin, conjunctivae, tracheo-bronchial tree, and intestinal tract. IgM is secreted by small lymphocytes.

IgM does not cross the placental barrier, but it appears early in life, since it is the first antibody produced in the newborn. In most immune responses regardless of the immunogen or the species of animal, the antibodies detected earliest, though usually transiently and in trace amounts are IgM.

Most of the natural antibodies, such as cold agglutinins, and red cell agglutinins belong to this class. IgM seems to play a protective role against microorganisms.

IgM is related to the rheumatoid factor in blood serum.

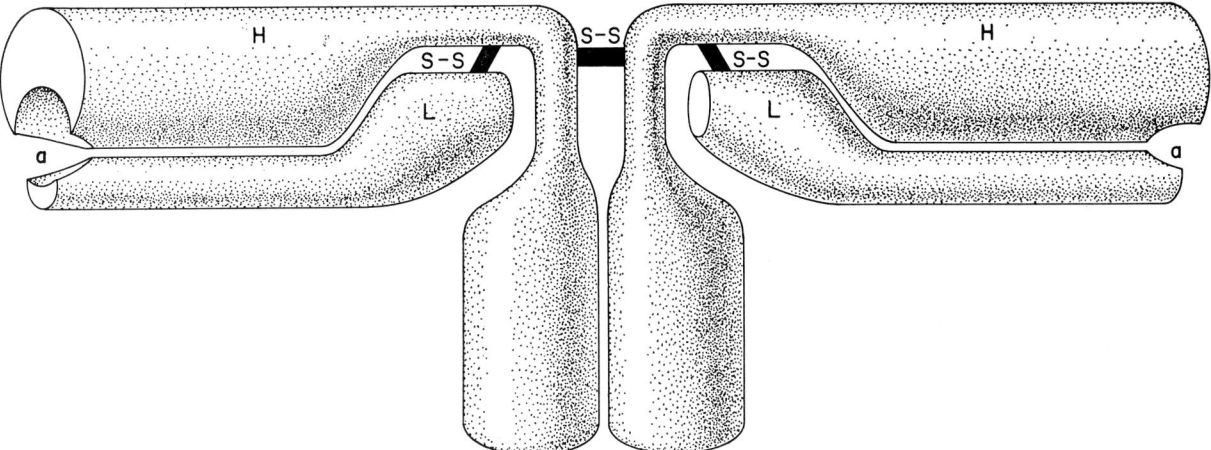

Figure 1-6. Model of IgG antibody molecule. The molecule consists of four chains (ca 150,000):

two identical heavy chains (H)—molecular weight approx. 55,000;
two identical light chains (L)—molecular weight approx. 23,000;
three disulfide bonds (S-S) tie the chains and together with hydrophobic and electrostatic forces hold together the four chains. The antibody combining site (a) receives contributions from both H and L chains. (From Nisonoff, Alfred: Molecules of immunity. In Good, Robert A. and Fisher, David W. (Eds.): *Immunobiology*. Courtesy of Sinauer Associates, Inc.)

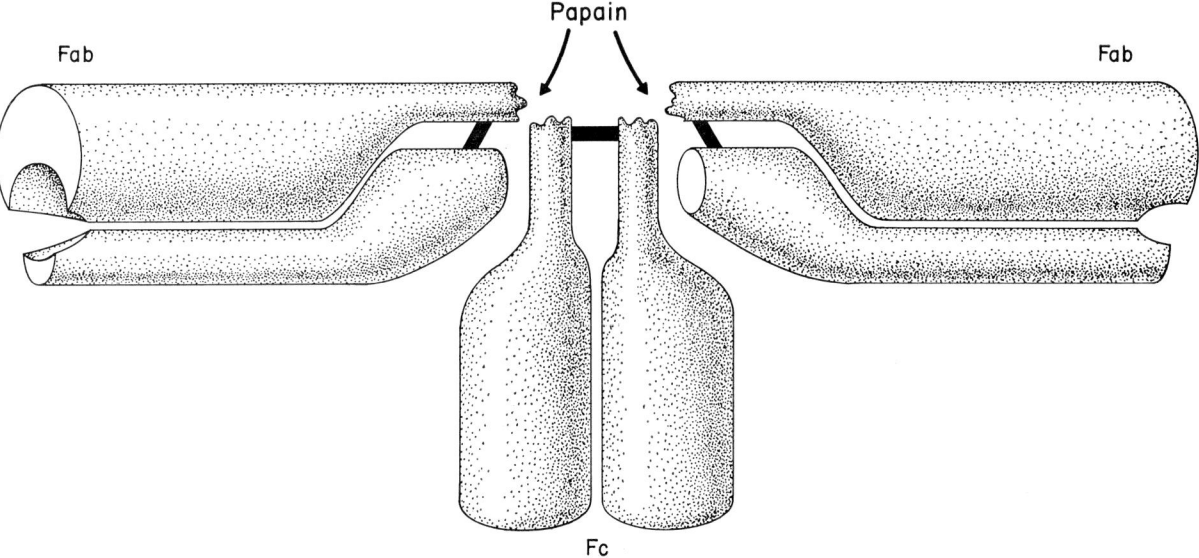

Figure 1-7. Treatment with papain splits the antibody molecule into three parts:
(1) the F_c fraction is crystallizable (homogeneous) and inactive;
(2) and (3) F_{ab} fractions. Each fraction has a portion of an H and L chain. Each F_{ab} fraction has an antibody combining site which is associated with the variable portions of the antibody molecule and therefore determines specificity. (From Nisonoff, Alfred: Molecules of immunity. In Good, Robert A. and Fisher, David W. (Eds.): *Immunobiology*. Courtesy of Sinauer Associates, Inc.)

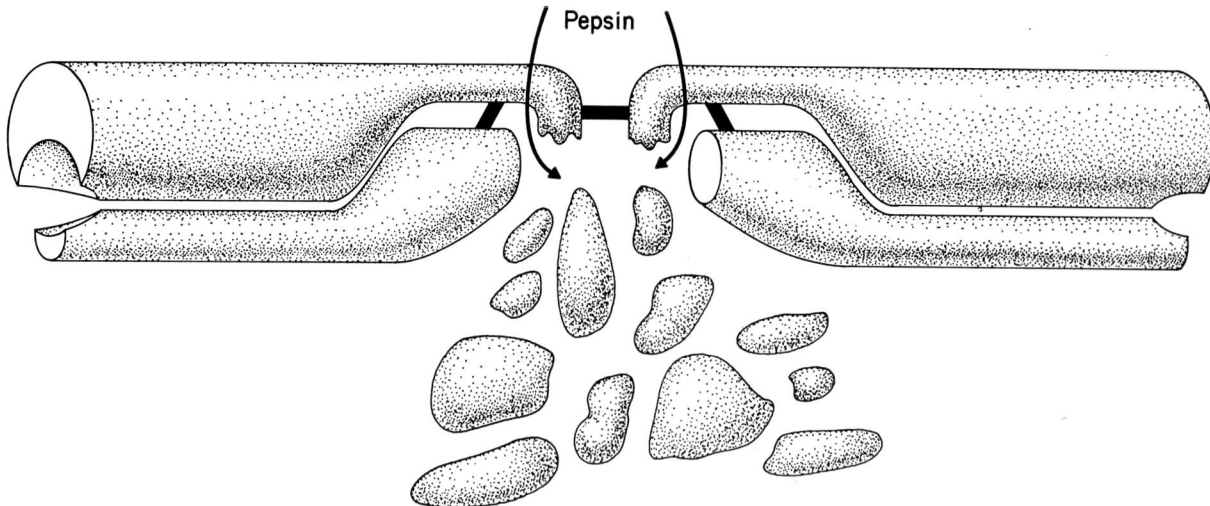

Figure 1–8. Pepsin digestion leaves two F_{ab} fragments joined by a disulfide (–) bond. Both antibody combining sites are attached to this fragment. The F_c fragment is broken up. (From Nisonoff, Alfred: Molecules of immunity. In Good, Robert A. and Fisher, David W. (Eds.): *Immunobiology*. Courtesy of Sinauer Associates, Inc.)

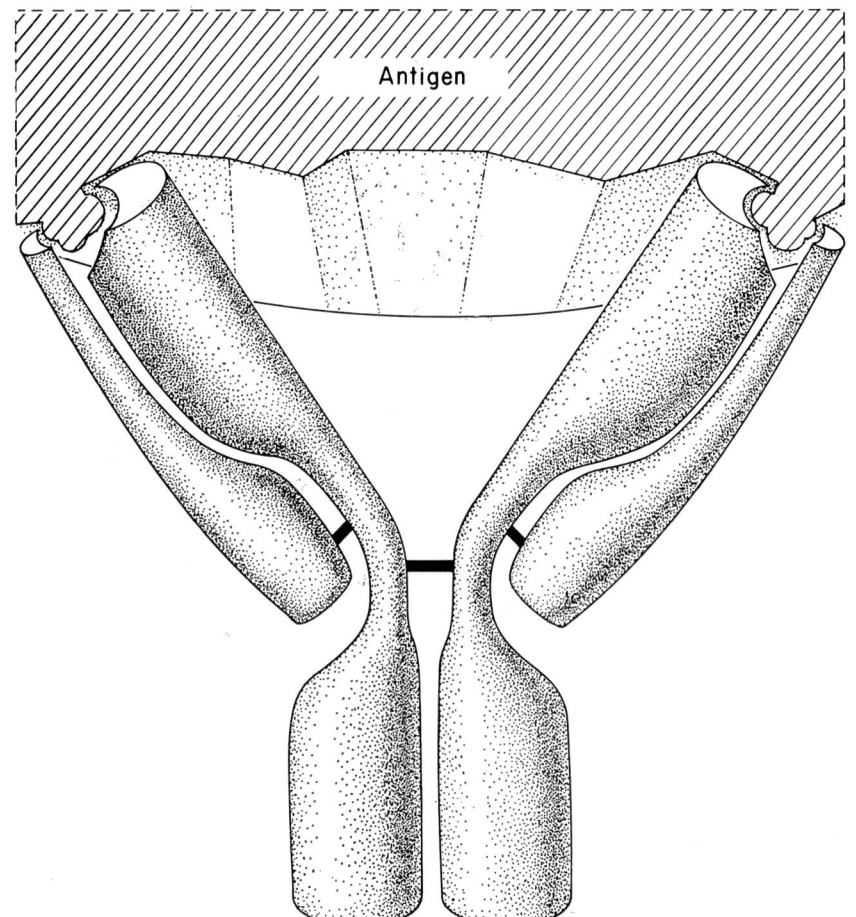

Figure 1-9. Flexibility of the chains permits bivalent combination with a single antigen. See Figure 1-10. (From Nisonoff, Alfred: Molecules of immunity. In Good, Robert A. and Fisher, David W. (Eds.): *Immunobiology*. Courtesy of Sinauer Associates, Inc.)

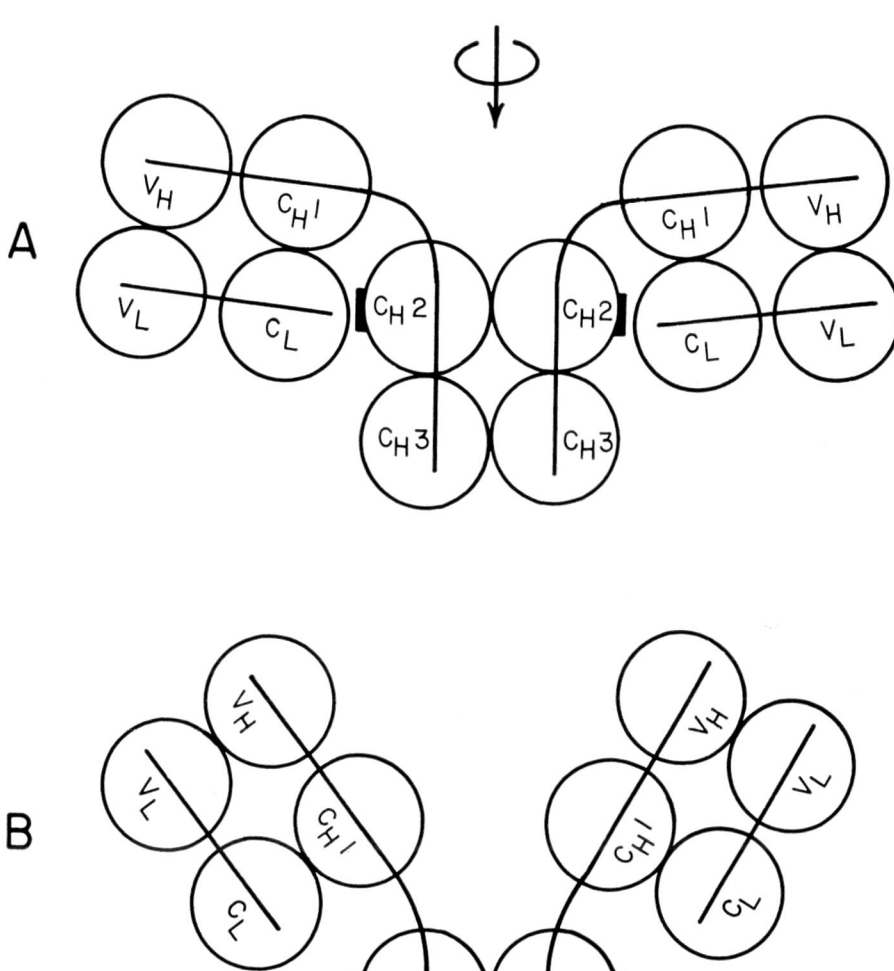

Figure 1-10. V_L, V_H = domain (area) made up of variable homology regions. C_L, C_H1, C_H2, C_H3 = domain made up of constant homology regions. Within each of these groups, domains are assumed to have similar three-dimensional structures and each is assumed to contribute to an active site. The V domain sites contribute to antigen recognition functions and the C domain sites to effector functions. A: Hypothetical arrangement of domains in the free immunoglobulin molecule. The arrow refers to a dyad axis of symmetry. B: Suggested rearrangement after antigen binding. Flexibility of the chains permits bivalent combination with a single antigen (see Fig. 1-9). Complement binding site (**|**). When antibody combines with antigen, the complement binding site is exposed. Compare A with B. (From Edelman, Gerald M.: Antibody structure and molecular immunology. *Ann NY Acad Sci 190:* 5, 1971.)

IgE (Reaginic Antibody)

IgE has recently (1966) been isolated by Ishizaka and Ishizaka and recognized as a separate class of immunoglobulin. IgE is the antibody responsible for the tissue changes in allergic rhinitis, hay fever, bronchial allergy, bronchial asthma, and atopic dermatitis.

Characteristics of IgE antibodies:

(1) QUANTITY: The difficulties encountered in isolating and identifying IgE can be appreciated from the fact that this antibody occurs in very small quantities. IgE constitutes about 0.05 per cent of the total immunoglobulins, or about one out of five thousand molecules in normal individuals. In allergic individuals the concentration is about five or six times greater in the serum plus the cell-bound. The molecular weight of IgE is 200,000, its sedimentation coefficient is 8S, and its carbohydrate content about 10 per cent. IgE is distributed in the epithelial structures of the conjunctivae, the nose, and tracheo-bronchial tree, the intestinal tract, and the skin. Since IgE is present in normal individuals, it must have a function which has not yet been demonstrated.

(2) NON-PRECIPITATING: This antibody *cannot* be demonstrated by precipitation. Other classes of humoral antibodies upon interaction with their specific antigens may form clumps or aggregates which drop out of solution and can be observed *in vitro* as precipitates. Or by attaching them to larger particles (adsorption) they may be brought down from their sera by interaction with their specific antigen (agglutination). IgE does not form precipitates or agglutinins.

(3) HOMOCYTOTROPIC* (Reaginic) Property: IgE antibodies have the capacity to become fixed with greater or lesser persistence to certain cells such as mast cells or basophils. At the site of attachment, they combine with their specific antigen to form complexes which activate enzyme systems that cause the release of mediators which are chiefly histamine† and SRS-A in the human.

The attachment of these antibodies to the skin permits their demonstration by skin testing which is the basis for the term "skin sensitizing," a cardinal feature of IgE, or reaginic-atopic antibodies.

The skin response, induced by released histamine, is characterized by a flare and wheal which appears within seconds or minutes following the introduction of the antigen. The lesion reaches its peak within twenty to thirty minutes and subsides quickly.

Passive Transfer, Prausnitz-Küstner (PK) Reaction: The skin sensitizing property of IgE or reaginic antibody forms the basis of the passive transfer test. Serum from a sensitive individual is injected into the skin of a nonsensitive subject. By this procedure IgE, or reaginic antibodies, are introduced at the site. The IgE antibodies attach themselves to skin components where they remain attached for days. If after twenty-four hours, the time required for complete attachment of antibody to skin, the antigen is injected at the same site, a local reaction characterized by a flare and wheal will be observed. This constitutes a positive passive transfer test.

(4) HEAT LABILE: The skin sensitizing property is heat labile, i.e. heating the serum for four hours at 50° C destroys the ability to sensitize skin.

There are fractions of IgG which also have skin sensitizing properties, but these antibodies *cannot* be demonstrated beyond twenty-four hours after intradermal injection. Unlike IgE antibodies, the skin sensi-

---

* Homocytotropic antibodies (IgE) should be differentiated from cytophilic antibodies (IgG_1 and IgG_3 human). The functional difference is in the kind of cells with which they are capable of binding. Homocytotropic antibodies fix to mast cells and basophils while cytophilic antibodies fix to macrophages and aid in determining the antibody mediated response of this type of cells.

† Histamine is also released by IgG class of antibodies and by all inflammatory reactions, but in these situations the histamine response *does not* dominate the tissue reaction or the clinical pattern.

tizing property of IgG antibodies is not destroyed by heat treatment. The IgG skin sensitizing antibodies play no *known* role in atopic allergic disease.

(5) PLACENTAL TRANSMISSION: IgE antibodies *do not pass* the placenta from mother to child. For this reason specific sensitivity of the reaginic type is not transmitted from mother to child.

(6) IgE antibodies do not pass the choroid plexus and therefore are not found in the cerebrospinal fluid.

THE ANTIGEN-ANTIBODY COMPLEX

The union of the antigen and the antibody is referred to as the Ag-Ab complex. No tissue reaction is induced by either the solitary antigen or the antibody. All the immunological phenomena and the ensuing tissue reactions result from the union of the antigen with its specific antibody.

IgA and *IgD* complexes perform functions still undetermined.

IgE Complexes: Complexes are formed with their specific antigen at the site of their attachment to tissue (mast cells or basophils). The complexes so formed activate enzyme systems which cause the release of chemical mediators which produce tissue changes responsible for this type of allergic response.

IgG Complexes:

(1) Toxins serve as antigens to stimulate antibody formation. These antibodies combine with toxin to neutralize it, (examples: diphtheria, tetanus) and also combine with organisms and blood elements to form complexes (*aggregates*).

(2) IgG provides the blocking antibodies for hyposensitization in reaginic-atopic allergy.

(3) Precipitating IgG forms complexes with specific antigen which activate complement to induce inflammation (Arthus mechanism) (see below).

IgM complexes perform many of the same functions of IgG.

Precipitation Reactions

Antigen molecules usually have multiple determinants and antibodies have multiple combining sites. This multiplicity of antigenic determinants and antibody combining sites presents the opportunity for extensive cross linking of antigen with antibody, resulting in the formation of a three-dimensional lattice work of antigen and antibody which precipitates.

The phenomenon of precipitation has found a variety of applications in the clinical and research laboratories:

(1) The determination of antibody titer through serial dilutions.

(2) Agar diffusion techniques.

(a) Single diffusion in agar: A glass slide is prepared with agar containing antibody. A hole punched in the agar serves as a reservoir for antigen. If positive, after twenty-four hours the antigen will have diffused through the agar to form a ring of precipitate around the hole, indicating an Ag-Ab reaction.

(b) Double diffusion in agar: This technique is usually employed to demonstrate a multiplicity of antigens reacting with a given serum sample. Antibody is placed in a central well of a slide or plate covered with agar.

Different antigens can be placed in various wells, equidistant from the central well. Ag and Ab diffuse toward each other to form a line of precipitate for each Ag-Ab system present. This technique is used for demonstrating the presence of multiple antigens or antibodies, the identification of antigens and antibodies, and to determine their relationship to each other.

Immunoelectrophoresis

Serum proteins can be separated in an electric field depending upon the charge of the protein molecule and to a lesser extent upon the size of the molecule.

Serum placed in a well cut into the agar

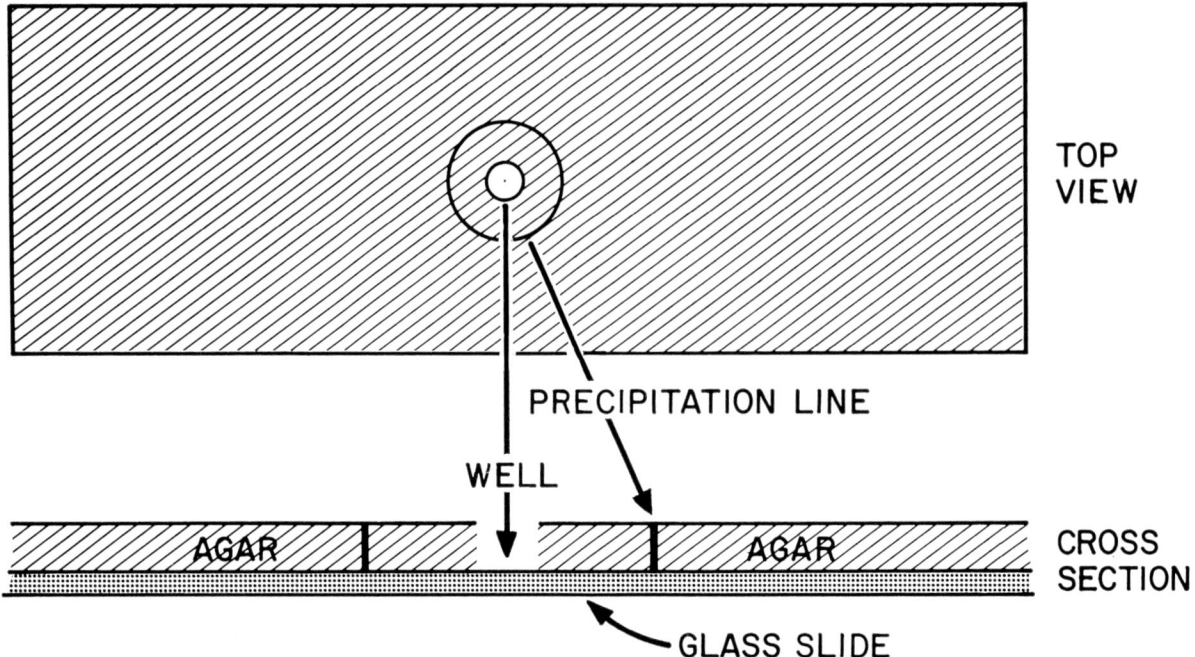

Figure 1-11. Single diffusion in agar. A glass slide is prepared with agar containing antibody. A hole punched in the agar serves as a reservoir for antigen. If positive, after twenty-four hours the antigen will have diffused through the agar to form a ring of precipitate around the hole, indicating an Ag-Ab reaction. (From Gordon, B.L., II and Ford, D.K.: *Essentials of Immunology*. Courtesy of F.A. Davis Co.)

on a slide or plate is electrophoresed. The albumen fraction migrates toward the anode and the IgG migrates toward the cathode.

Parallel to the axis of this electrophoretic separation, a trough is cut and filled with an antiserum against the serum being tested. The fractions separated by electrophoresis and the antiserum in the trough migrate toward each other to produce lines of precipitation. These lines indicate each antigenic protein in the serum tested.

Agglutination Tests

In agglutination reactions the antigens are of particulate size rather than the molecular size of the precipitating phenomenon. Particulate materials, e.g. bacteria, erythro-

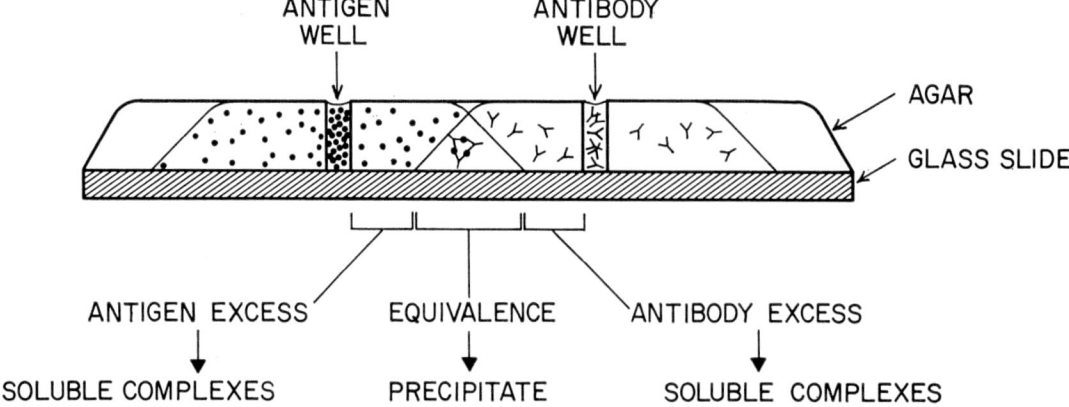

Figure 1-12. Single diffusion in agar. Top view. This procedure is well suited for identification, while the procedure in Figure 1-11 is useful for quantitation.

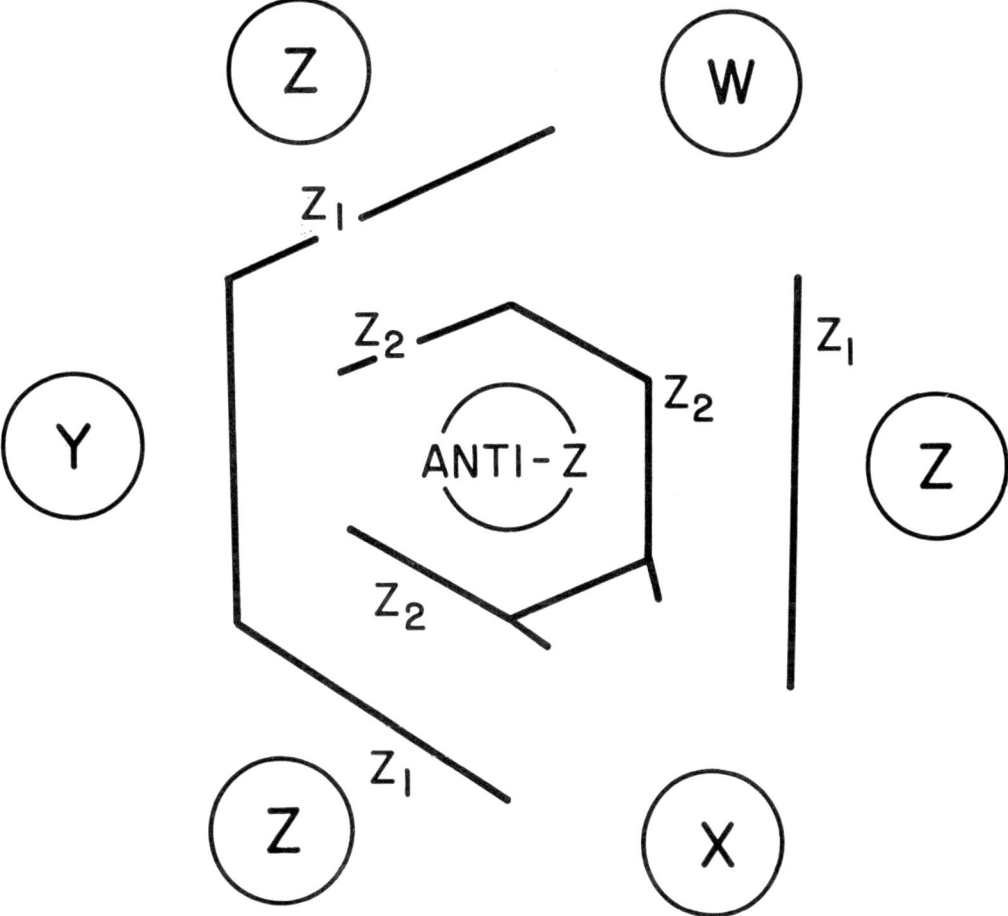

Figure 1-13. Double diffusion in agar. This technique is usually employed to demonstrate a multiplicity of antigens reacting with a given serum sample. Antibody is placed in a central well of a slide or plate covered with agar. Different antigens can be placed in various wells, equidistant from the central well. Ag and Ab diffuse toward each other to form a line of precipitate for each Ag-Ab system present. This technique is used for demonstrating the presence of multiple antigens or antibodies, the identification of antigens and antibodies, and to determine their relationship to each other.

cytes, latex particles, *etc.* can be suspended in saline and mixed with an antiserum. When particulate antigens are mixed with their specific antisera, aggregation of the antigen particles results. The mechanism involved is similar to that which occurs with the precipitation reaction. The multivalent antibodies cross link the antigen particles into complexes of antigen and antibody which, because of their large size, are usually visible to the naked eye. Occasionally, if the particles are small, microscopic examination may be necessary. The phenomenon is called the agglutination reaction.

Agglutination tests can be used for measuring antigens and for assessing antibody titers.

Agglutinating antibody titer is defined as the highest dilution of antiserum that will agglutinate the test antigen under the conditions employed in the test.

Additional techniques for demonstrating antibodies and antigen-antibody complexes include immunofluorescent staining and im-

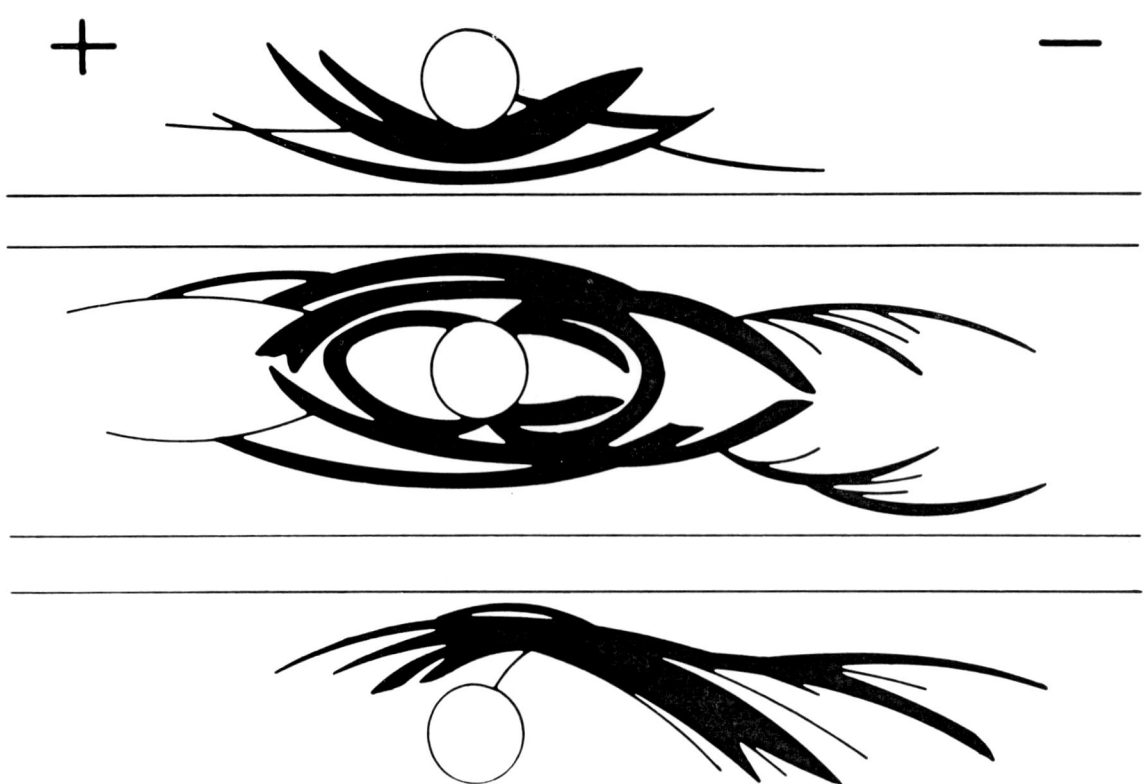

Figure 1-14. Immunoelectrophoresis. The immunoelectrophoretic pattern of bee venom illustrates the multiplicity of antibodies separated in a single sample of serum. Immunoelectrophoresis, a technique depending on both electrophoretic mobility and double diffusion in agar gel, enables high resolution of antigenic components from complex mixtures of antigens (e.g., human plasma proteins). It was the development of immunoelectrophoresis, in fact, that first provided evidence that human immunoglobulins were divisible into major classes, i.e. IgG, IgM, IgA.

muno-autoradiography, which involves radioactive labelling.

For more detailed information concerning the various techniques, the reader is referred to texts on immunological procedures.

CELLULAR ELEMENTS

Immunological competence involves the interaction of a number of highly specialized cells which in some cases act directly upon each other, but more frequently through various mediators produced or released at the time the cell is stimulated by the antigenic material. Each cell has a distinct role which is interrelated with the functions of the various types of cells resulting in an immune response that produces tissue changes manifested as allergic disease.

Current observations in the field of cellular immunology indicate that certain steps in the development of the immune response may be the function of subclasses of cells, as yet unidentified.

The presentation which follows can serve as a guide for the interpretation of more detailed information on function and activity of the various subclasses as it appears in the literature from time to time.

A. Lymphocytes

Lymphocytes constitute a group of cells which are identical in appearance but heterogeneous in function. Although all types of lymphocytes and their various functions have not been fully determined, current studies have identified both short-lived and long-lived lymphocytes in the circulating blood. The short-lived lymphocytes which constitute the major portion of circulating lymphocytes seem to be related to infection, while the long-lived lymphocytes which may persist for months or even years are concerned with delayed hypersensitivity.

Observations seem to support the theories that all lymphocytes are derived from stem cells in the bone marrow. Whether the stem cells are the same for all types or whether each class has its own stem cell is not known. (See also Fig. 19-1.)

In the immune reaction two lines of lymphocytes are involved:

(1) The T-cell which is concerned with cellular immunity
(2) The B-cell which is concerned with the immunity involving humoral antibodies.

The T-cells are derived from stem cells in the bone marrow from where they pass to the thymus to be conditioned and then move on to the various lymphoid structures. It has been observed that neonatal thymectomy prevents cell mediated reactions. Since immunological competence of this strain of cells is in some manner dependent upon an intact thymus at birth, they have been labelled thymus dependent, or T-cells. The various activities of the T-cell will be discussed under delayed hypersensitivity. T-cells produce no antibody and must be differentiated from antibody producing B-cells.

It has been observed that in chickens, the bursa of Fabricius, a pouch which lies behind the cloaca, is associated with the production of humoral antibodies, but not with cell mediated reactions. In mammals no similar structure has been identified, but it is postulated that the analogue is in the gut associated lymphoid tissue (GALT) which is constituted chiefly of the lymphoid structures of the alimentary canal. These include Waldeyer's ring (tonsils, adenoids, and post-pharyngeal structures) which is actually at the proximal end of the gullet; lymphoid structures related to the intestinal tract including Peyer's patches; the cortex and germinal centers of lymph nodes.

In birds, because of the association with the bursa of Fabricius, the cells are termed B-cells (B for bursa), while in man these cells are called either GALT system cells or B-cells (B for bone marrow).

The B-cells remain in the antibody forming centers, where, following stimulation by an antigen, they proliferate and mature into plasma cells which are the chief source of antibody production. Small lymphocytes produce IgM, while plasma cells produce IgG. Following synthesis, antibody is released into the circulation from where it may be delivered into the tissues to serve as extravascular antibody.

It is possible that the antibody forming cells which reside in the subepithelial structures may produce antibody locally which is released into the circulation. This is considered a possibility with IgA and perhaps even IgE and some IgG.

The mechanism by which lymphocytes are instructed by the thymus to behave as T-cells and by the GALT system to behave as antibody producing B-cells is not known. The initial instruction received by the cells is concerned only with their class identification, i.e. whether they behave as T-cells to participate in cellular immunity or B-cells to produce antibody. The exact mechanism for the activation of lymphocytes and the induction of their specificity is not known, except that it is considered necessary for the antigenic material to be processed by macrophages before it is presented to the lymphocytes. Once a cell is activated or sensitized by a specific antigen, it will react only to that antigen and to no other (immunological memory).

The "Helper" T-cell

The T-cells act directly in (1) delayed hypersentitivity, (2) contact dependent cytotoxicity, and (3) graft versus host rejection.

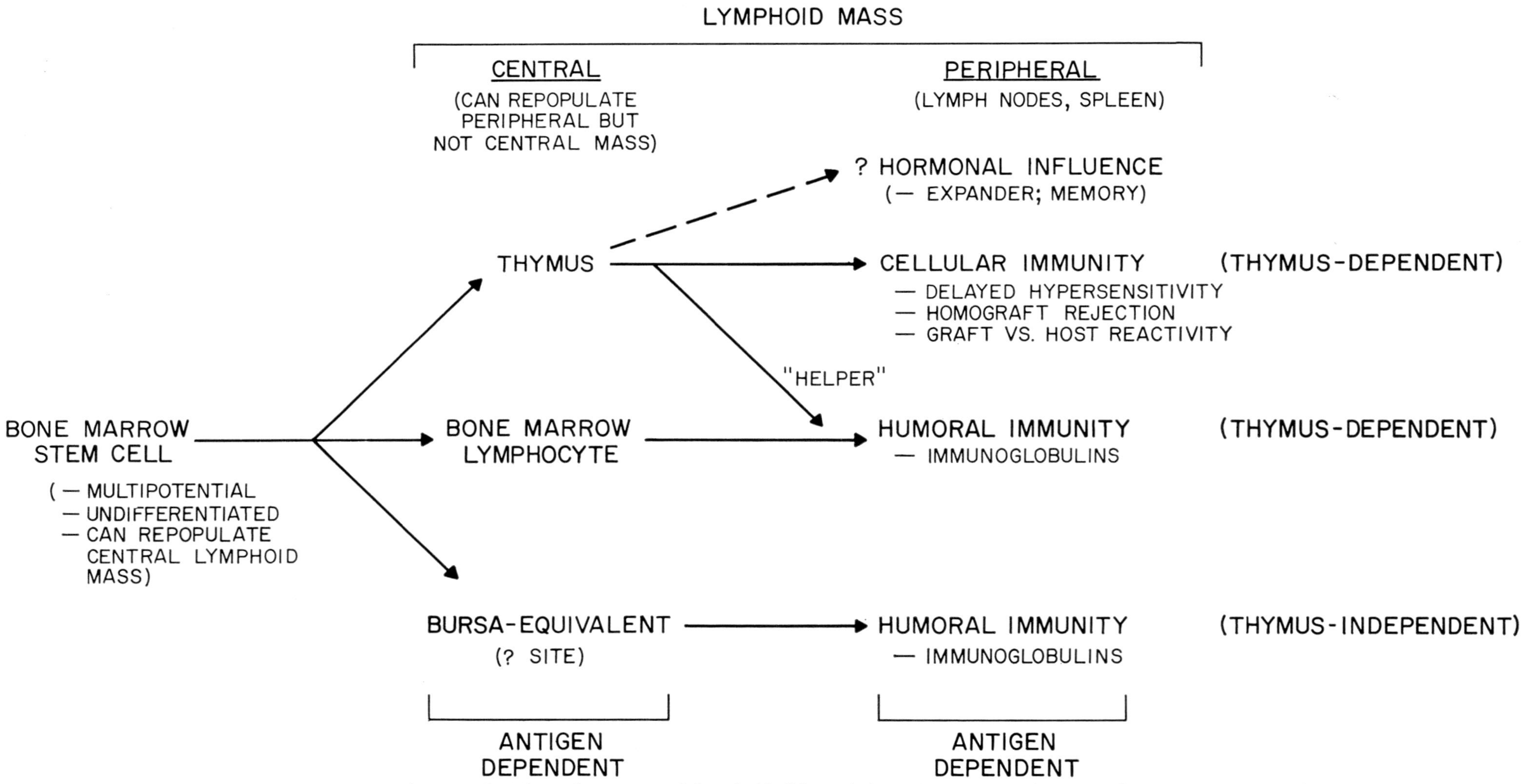

Figure 1-15. Schematic concept of lymphoid differentiation. (From Frenkel, E.P. and Stone, M.J.: The rationale and approach to immunosuppressive therapy. *Adv Intern Med, 17:* 21, 1971.)

B-cells secrete circulating antibodies which are concerned with humoral immunity.

Recent studies seem to indicate that the induction of specific antibodies by B-cells against many antigenic determinants requires the cooperation of T-cells ("helper" cells). The "helper" T-cells that interact with B-cells to induce the secretion of antibody appears to be a different type than the T-cell involved in the various cellular immune responses. The mechanism by which the "helper" T-cells interact with B-cells during the induction of antibody is not clear. However, it has been demonstrated that B-cells may not produce antibody to the haptenic determinants on an immunogen unless the determinants on the carrier portion of the molecule are recognized by T-cells (see Fig. 1-5). But recognition of the determinants on the carrier portion of the molecule does not necessarily lead to antibody production specific for the carrier. Accordingly, T-cells serve as agents of cellular immunity as well as independent "helpers" in humoral immunity.

Thymosin

A lymphocytopoietic factor named *thymosin* has been demonstrated by White and Goldstein in the thymus glands of both animals and man. This product of the thymus is either identical with or closely associated with a protein and has an estimated molecular weight less than 100,000. Purified thymosin does not contain nucleic acid; it is not inactivated with RNase or DNase but is inactivated by inoculation with proteolytic enzymes. Thymosin may influence the rate of maturation of immunological competence in more primitive, potentially competent lymphoid cells.

Current studies on T-cells indicate that there are two and possible three types of T-cells.
  (1) A T-cell that matures solely under the influence of thymosin and functions primarily in cell mediated immune phenomena.
  (2) A T-cell which requires a thymic locus for development and is involved primarily in humoral immune phenomena as a helper cell to B-cells.
  (3) The possibility that the T-cell concerned with graft versus host reactions is a separate class.

B. Mast Cells

Mast cells are of two types:
  (1) Those found in loose, well vascularized connective tissue, especially around the blood vessels.
  (2) Those in the circulating blood labelled as basophils.

Both forms of mast cells store histamine and heparin in their large cytoplasmic granules. Most of the body histamine is stored in these cells. As a result of the antigen-antibody interaction a train of enzymatic reactions is activated which causes the release of both histamine, SRS-A, and heparin from the cells. The mediators are not always released in identical quantities. There is a variety of activators, both qualitatively and quantitatively, which results in differences in the release of these mediators. Such differences in release, especially of histamine, can explain variations in the intensity of the tissue response that may occur.

C. Monocytes

Monocytes constitute between 80 and 90 per cent of the cells mobilized in lesions of delayed hypersensitivity. Monocytes originate in the bone marrow and are transported via the blood stream to the site of involvement. When the monocyte first appears on the scene at the site of reaction, it morphologically resembles a lymphocyte. Immediately following its participation in the action, it may remain lymphocytic in appearance, or may evolve into a typical histiocyte or a macrophage full of phagocytosed material. At different stages of the evolution the cell may be described as a reticulo-endothelial cell, monocyte, histiocyte or macrophage. Even epithelioid and multinuclear giant cells are derived from the same stem. All these terms are synonymous for the same cell at different stages of its evolution.

Monocytic cells are nonspecific and do not produce antibody. Macrophages phagocytize antigen and prepare it for a subclass of lymphocytes, the antigen reactive cells (ARC), which in turn transmit the information to antibody forming lymphocytes (AFC).

D. Eosinophils

It is remarkable that although the origin and function of eosinophils is not known, they are clinically considered as an important diagnostic feature because of their prominence in allergic disease.

It is probable that the newly discovered eosinophil chemotactic factor (ECF) is responsible for much if not all of the eosinophilia which is associated with many of the reaginic (anaphylactic) type reactions.

The presence of eosinophils in nasal and bronchial secretions is presumptive evidence of allergic disease. On the other hand, the absence of eosinophils in respiratory secretions does not rule out a diagnosis of allergic disease. Cases of classical allergic rhinitis or bronchial asthma may fail to demonstrate eosinophils in the secretions.

The presence of a blood eosinophilia is commonly considered a diagnostic indicator of allergic disease. But increased blood eosinophilia should not be relied upon for a diagnosis of allergic disease without other supporting evidence. Some of the highest levels of blood eosinophilia are observed in nonallergic conditions such as parasitic infestations and various dermatological conditions.

MEDIATORS

The chief function of antibody is the recognition of its specific antigen which is accomplished by a union to form the antigen-antibody complex. The tissue changes of the allergic reaction are not a direct response to the Ag-Ab complex, but rather a manifestation of a number of interrelated functions induced by various substances known as mediators, which are either activated, released from cells or synthesized following the formation of the complex. The identity of most of the mediators has not been established but the various activities are well recognized. Since both the mediators and the tissue responses vary with the type of allergic reaction, they will be considered under the discussion of each type of allergic response.

Complement

Complement, one of the most important of all the mediators, is a complex mixture of nine serum proteins which are labelled C_1 through C_9. Actually, there are eleven proteins since C_1 has three subclasses, C_{1q}, C_{1r}, and C_{1s}, which are held together by Ca^{++}. Except for C_{1q} which is a gamma globulin, all the components of complement belong to either alpha or beta globulins. The components C_1, C_2, C_5, C_8 and C_9 are inactivated by heat at 30° C for thirty minutes (heat labile).

The manner in which the various fractions interact and participate in the allergic response is based upon hypotheses which, for the most part, are not confirmed. However, it is generally recognized that complement-binding represents a sequence of events initiated by Ag-Ab complexes involving either IgG or IgM classes of antibody. Neither antigen nor antibody alone can fix complement. IgA and IgE antibodies do not activate complement. Some of the reactions require Ca^{++} or Mg^{++}.

The F_c fraction of the antibody molecule furnishes the effector groupings for activating complement. The manner in which these centers are exposed is illustrated in Figure 1-7.

Complement is associated with the following functions:

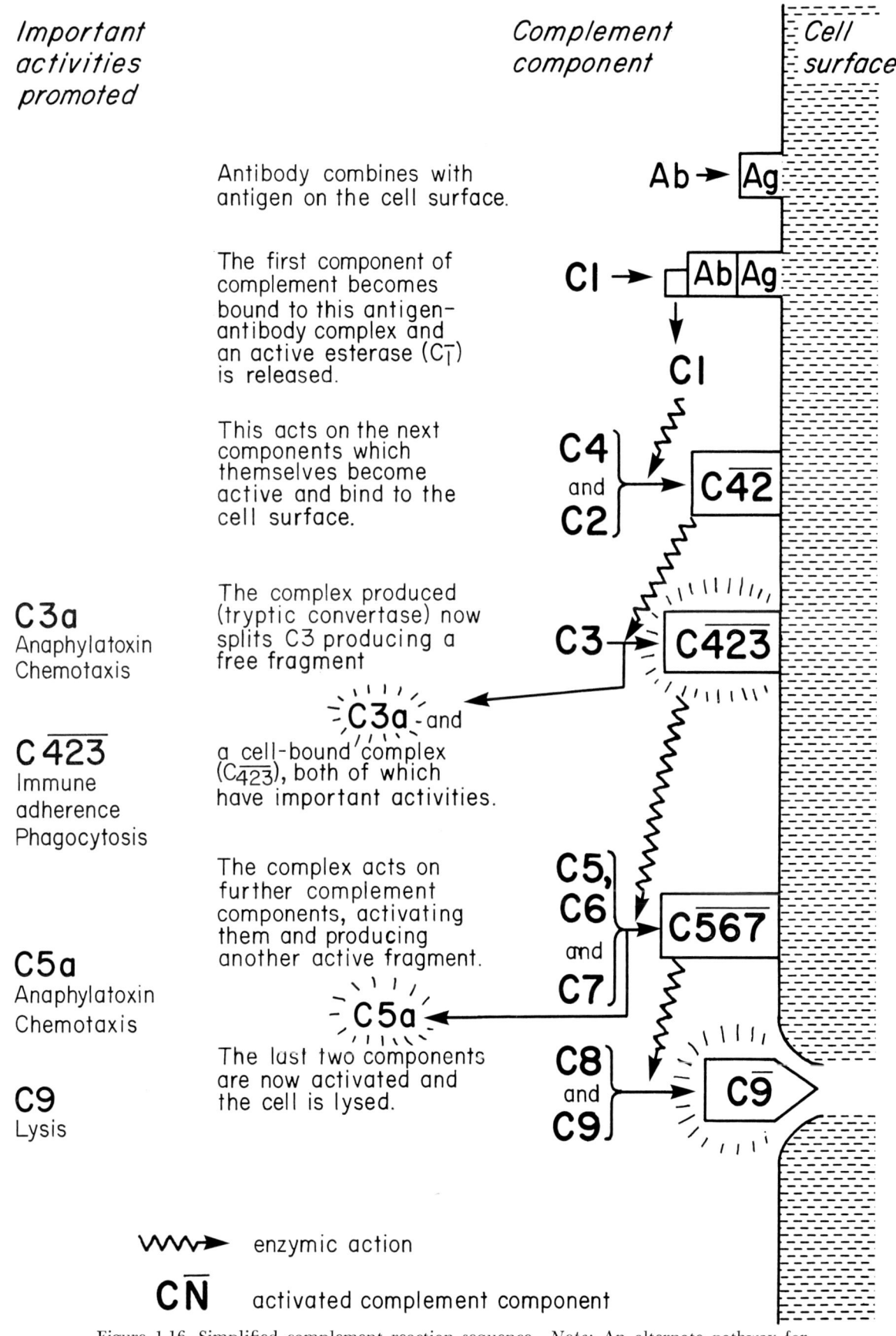

Figure 1-16. Simplified complement reaction sequence. *Note:* An alternate pathway for the activation of the complement sequence via the C_3 component has been reported. This can occur when there are alterations in the steric structure following aggregation of the globulin molecule. The exact mechanism for the steric change has not been defined, but it is considered possible with some infections and perhaps with some drugs. In this system, the tissue reactions induced by the complement system do not require Ag-Ab complexes. (From Herbert, W.J. and Wilkinson, P.C. (Eds.): *A Dictionary of Immunology.* Courtesy of Blackwell Scientific Publications.)

(1) Participation in the parameters of inflammation through
   (a) chemotaxis for PMNLs
   (b) increased phagocytosis of PMNLs
   (c) opsonization*
   (d) increased capillary permeability through anaphylatoxin and histaminic release
(2) Immune adherence†
(3) Bactericidal activity
(4) Viral neutralization
(5) Cytolysis—participation in hemolysis
(6) Mediation of graft rejection

Certain of the functions of complement, such as opsonization, anaphylatoxin, histaminic release, immune adherence and chemotaxis of neutrophils do not require the complete sequence of the enzymatic reaction. (See Fig. 1-16.)

Complement Fixation Reaction (CF)

The complement fixation reaction depends upon the complement hemolytic system which is represented by EAC, in which

E = erythrocyte A = antigen
C = complement

The numerical sequence of complement was governed by the order in which each component of complement was originally identified. Following identification of the components the sequence of reactions was determined to be:

$$C_1-C_4-C_2-C_3-C_5-C_6-C_7-C_8-C_9$$

(see Fig. 1-16)

Procedure: A measured quantity of a known antigen is added to a measured quantity of an unknown serum. If an Ag-Ab reaction occurs, complement will be consumed in proportion to the concentration of Ag-Ab. The remaining complement can be demonstrated by adding a measured quantity of sensitized RBC. The sensitized RBC will be hemolyzed in the presence of free complement. By controlling the quantity of RBC the titer of the amount of complement can be determined.

I. IMMEDIATE HYPERSENSITIVITY

(1) Reaginic Allergy
(2) Atopic Allergy
(3) Anaphylaxis

The immediate type of hypersensitivity (see Fig. 1-15) is so called because the manifestations of the reaction can be observed within seconds or minutes following the administration of the antigen.

When IgE antibody combines with its specific antigen a complex is formed which, activating an enzyme system, releases mediators that induce (1) dilatation of capillaries, (2) increased permeability of small vessels, (3) spasm of smooth muscle and (4) stimulation of exocrine glands. All the tissue responses are reversible so that in the absence of antigen (allergen) there is a complete restitution of tissues to their normal state.

The mediators involved in immediate hypersensitivity are:

(1) Histamine (H-substance)
(2) Slow Reacting Substance—A (SRS-A)
(3) Heparin
(4) Bradykinin

(1) *Histamine:* The richest supply of body histamine is in the granules of mast cells, usually concentrated in connective tissues in proximity to blood vessels and in basophils of the circulating blood. In response to the IgE-antigen complex, histamine is released from cells without destruction of the cell.

The actions induced by histamine are:

(1) contraction of smooth muscle
(2) vasodilatation
(3) increased capillary permeability
(4) stimulation of exocrine glands

---

*Opsonin: A serum substance, usually either antibody or complement, which coats particulate substances such as bacteria, to promote phagocytosis.

†Immune Adherence: The adherence of Ag-Ab-complement complexes to surfaces of nonsensitized particles increases their susceptibility to phagocytosis. The particle may be primate RBC, platelets, starch granules, bacteria or viruses.

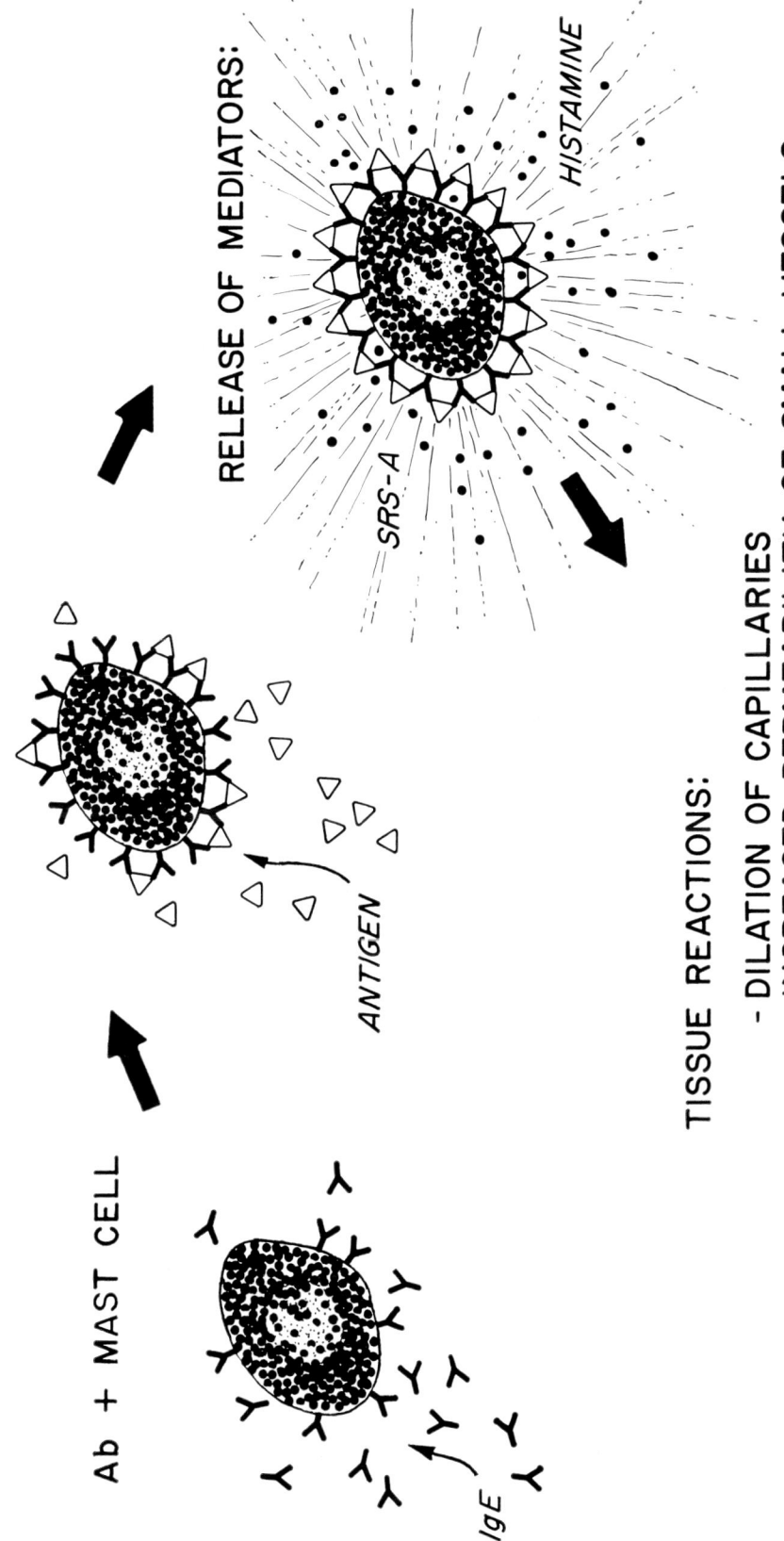

Figure 1-17. Immediate hypersensitivity. The homocytotropic antibody, IgE, attaches to mast cells and basophils. Upon the union of IgE with its specific antigen, an enzyme system is activated which causes the release of mediators. In man, the chief mediators are histamine and SRS-A. Histamine is preformed and released following formation of IgE complexes. SRS-A is synthesized following formation of IgE complexes and subsequently released.

(5) excitant action on cutaneous nerve endings

Note: Although histamine may not stimulate glandular secretion directly, it is possible that an increase in activity of various exocrine glands may be induced secondary to the increase blood supply following dilatation of vessels.

(2) *Slow Reacting Substance—A* (SRS-A): The chemical nature and source of this mediator is not known. Ishizaka has reported the release of SRS-A from monkey lung tissue. Since it can be demonstrated following stimulation of tissue by an Ag-Ab interaction, it is postulated that SRS-A is generated in tissue cells. Apparently, SRS-A must be synthesized after the antibody interacts with its antigen, since its appearance is slower than that of histamine. This slow appearance of the mediator explains the term SRS-A. "A" stands for anaphylaxis, the mechanism with which it is involved.

SRS-A is a strong contractor of smooth muscle which accounts for its importance in the induction of bronchial asthma.

The onset of the action of SRS-A is slower than that of histamine, but once the action is established, its contracting effect upon smooth muscle is equal to that of histamine and its action more prolonged than histamine.

SRS-A is not antagonized by antihistaminic drugs.

(3) *Bradykinin:* Bradykinin is identical with the plasma kinins which are substances that have a powerful action on smooth muscle as well as some vasodilator action. It has been suggested that kinins play a role in the anaphylactic type of Ag-Ab interaction in man.

Bradykinin is considered responsible for the marked hypotension of systemic anaphylaxis, by drawing blood from the pool in the major vessels secondary to marked dilatation of the capillaries.

Because the pharmacologically active mediators are degraded very rapidly, their effect is transient. Their failure to accumulate makes possible the technique of immunotherapy which involves the administration of closely spaced suboptimal injections of antigens (see Chapter 17, Immunotherapy).

Chronic Tissue Changes of Immediate Reactivity

As has been indicated, the tissue changes induced by the immediate type of hypersensitivity are reversible. However, when the irritation of immediate hypersensitivity persists and becomes chronic, the tissue changes resulting are those which are characteristic for any chronic insult, namely, hypertrophy and hyperplasia of tissue.

What constitutes chronicity in allergy is at times difficult to define. In relation to the immediate type of reactivity, it apparently involves uninterrupted irritation of long standing, such as encountered in perennial allergic rhinitis, chronic conjunctivitis, and long standing bronchial allergy.

Short term intermittent insults may induce hypertrophy and hyperplasia, but these, too, are reversible if the episodes are not too long, perhaps several weeks, and if the free periods are long enough for complete reversal of the tissue response, again a matter of weeks. The inherent capacity of most tissues to regenerate and recover is very great. This is observed particularly in the nasal and bronchial mucosa, the conjunctival and corneal tissues, and the skin. Some of these patterns which have been confirmed by biopsies will be discussed below under the various systems.

1. Reaginic Allergy

Before IgE was demonstrated to be a separate class of antibodies, the term reaginic was applied to those antibodies demonstrating all the characteristics of IgE, namely,

(1) humoral, or circulating
(2) skin sensitizing by attachment to skin

(3) inactivation by heat at 50° C for four hours
(4) transferrable by serum—passive transfer
(5) nonprecipitating
(6) non-passage of the placental barrier

2. Atopy

In 1923 Coca maintained that an hereditary or familial predisposition was a prerequisite for the production of the skin sensitizing humoral antibodies known as reagin and now identified as IgE. The hereditary predisposition is presently recognized, but it is related to the individual's ability to produce larger than normal quantities of IgE which predisposes to the immediate type of tissue response. Normally, the concentration of IgE in the serum is about 0.05 per cent or less, while in allergic individuals this is increased by five or six times.

Coca also stated that the reaginic type of reaction was limited to man, but today a similar reaction has been observed in animals, such as cattle, dogs, cats, horses and experimentally in rabbits.

It should be noted that the hereditary constitution entails a propensity to form increased quantities of this class of antibodies and not a specific antibody for a specific allergen. For example, a specific sensitivity for milk, horse dander, or a specific pollen is not inherited, but rather the ability to produce large quantities of the specific antibodies which makes possible tissue reactions that account for the clinical patterns.

3. Anaphylaxis (Greek: *ana*—reverse; *phylaxis*—protection)

In the more recent literature on allergy and immunology the term "anaphylaxis" is used interchangeably with "reaginic" or "atopic." Anaphylaxis is identified with the immediate manifestations of tissue reactions induced by the IgE class of antibodies which have the ability to combine with tissues and induce the release of histamine. Whether antibodies other than those of the class IgE can initiate the same type of tissue response is still not settled. In lower animals non-reaginic antibodies can passively sensitize cells and initiate tissue responses similar to the reaginic or atopic reactions observed in man. For clinical interpretation and evaluation the term "anaphylaxis" can be reserved for the tissue responses induced by IgE or reaginic complexes.

Anaphylaxis occurs in two patterns, of which the cardinal feature is the suddenness and explosiveness of the reaction: (1) local, and (2) systemic.

(1) *Local anaphylaxis:* Limited to a restricted area of skin or a single organ or system. When the skin is involved, it is referred to as "cutaneous anaphylaxis." When a system or organ is involved, the term applied depends upon the part of the body manifesting symptoms, such as hay fever, bronchial asthma.

The wheal and flare reaction induced by skin testing, which is labelled "cutaneous anaphylaxis," is a classical example. Following introduction into the skin of a small amount of antigen, either by the puncture technique or intracutaneous injection, as a result of histamine release, an almost immediate response is observed at the site of the injection. The lesion is characterized by a flare followed very quickly by a wheal extending itself by pseudopodia, much like an amoeba. Within fifteen or twenty minutes the reaction reaches its peak, then starts to subside and is usually absorbed within an hour.

(2) *Systemic Anaphylaxis:* The basic mechanism is the same as in local anaphylaxis except that the reaction is magnified many fold, involving at times all the skin surfaces, the entire capillary network and the smooth muscle of the bronchial tree. Because of the widespread involvement due to the massive release of histamine, the clinical picture is a violent one, starting usually with itching of the scalp, tongue and throat, soon develop-

ing a generalized flushing with very early onset of headache, followed in a few minutes by difficulty in breathing caused by airway obstruction, secondary to either edema of the glottis or involvement of the bronchial tree by muscle spasm and edema. In short order a drop in temperature and a drop in blood pressure is accompanied by shock, followed by loss of consciousness and then death. If early reversal does not set in, the train of events leading to death may occupy a span as brief as fifteen minutes. The reason for the explosive release of histamine is not known.

A similar clinical pattern may be caused by kinins which induce generalized capillary dilatation resulting in transfer of the major blood pool from the vessels to the capillary bed resulting in hypotension and collapse.

The antigens involved in anaphylaxis include:

  pollens
  epidermal factors, such as horse dander
  foods, especially eggs, fish products, and nuts
  chemicals
  drugs, such as penicillin, aspirin
  venoms from stinging insects
  foreign sera, such as diphtheria, tetanus
  virus vaccines

The antibodies resemble IgE in their ability to attach to cell surfaces. In animals these are precipitating antibodies. In man the antibodies can not be precipitated and belong to the class IgE. Because of this difference, the reactions in man are sometimes labelled "anaphylactoid" (like anaphylaxis). Since these antibodies do not involve complement, inflammation is not part of the pathological picture.

Treatment: The mediators in anaphylaxis are short lived. Therefore, if treatment can be instituted immediately, the chances for arresting the process and preventing collapse and death are greatly enhanced.

Immediate emergency treatment consists of administration of 0.5 cc epinephrine-HCl 1-1000 (adrenalin) hypodermically. If the patient starts to complain of any symptoms, such as itching of scalp, tongue or throat, or tightness in the chest, do not wait for further developments, but administer epinephrine immediately. It is preferable to use epinephrine from a brown bottle rather than from an ampoule. *Ampoule epinephrine* at times loses its effectiveness because of the adherence of epinephrine to the white glass. If necessary, within ten to fifteen minutes, repeat the epinephrine.

If the reaction develops during an intravenous injection, withdraw the needle immediately and administer epinephrine 1-1000 subcutaneously. *Do not wait* for clarification of the symptoms. *Time* is of the essence.

Since antihistamines do not control the hypotension and the bronchospasm of anaphylaxis, they are of limited value in the treatment of the vascular component of anaphylaxis.

Antihistamines are of value in controlling edema and itching. Since laryngeal edema is a commonly observed complication of local anaphylaxis, parenteral injection of antihistamines is helpful in the management of this complication of anaphylaxis. (See discussion of antihistamines in Chapter 15.) However, do not give antihistamines first. *Epinephrine has top priority.*

Procedure for Management of Systemic Anaphylaxis

(1) Administer epinephrine-HCl 1-1000 by hypodermic: dose 0.4 to 0.5 cc. If necessary, repeat in ten to fifteen minutes.

(2) Place patient in a recumbent position with the head lowered.

(3) Keep the patient warm—cover with blankets or any available garment.

(4) Place a tourniquet above the site of the injection—if injected material is the cause. Observe the hands and fingers fre-

quently for signs of extreme ischemia. Release the tourniquet intermittently to permit the flow of blood. Releasing the tourniquet may permit the escape of additional damaging antigen, leading to an aggravation of symptoms. Be prepared with additional epinephrine if the reaction increases with the release of the tourniquet.

(5) Make certain that the patient has an adequate airway. If the tongue drops back, grasp the tongue gently and hold forward using a towel for grasping. In the presence of laryngeal edema which is obstructing the airway be prepared for tracheotomy in the event the response to epinephrine fails and cyanosis and stridor become more pronounced. With laryngeal edema intubation is usually unsuccessful.

(6) For hypotension administer intravenous fluids: 5 per cent glucose in water. To the intravenous solution add:

Solu-Cortef®	50 mg
or Prednisone®	100 mg
or dexamethasone	4–20 mg

(7) For cyanosis administer intermittent oxygen.

(8) If respiratory movement fails, administer artificial respiration.

(9) If pharmacologic response to hypodermically administered epinephrine is not observed, intravenous epinephrine may be given. Wet a 2 cc syringe with epinephrine. Withdraw blood in syringe to permit admixture with epinephrine. Inject intravenously very slowly.

(10) To counteract edema and urticaria due to histamine release, administer antihistamines intramuscularly:

diphenhydramine (Benadryl®) HCl
  50 mg
chlorpheniramine (Chlor-Trimeton,®
  Teldrin®) 10 mg

Benadryl injectable in 50 mg doses is the drug of choice for antihistamines.

II. INTERMEDIATE HYPERSENSITIVITY

The Arthus Reaction

The Arthus reaction (see Fig. 1-18) which appears between thirty minutes to a few hours following challenge by the antigen, is intermediate between the immediate, or reaginic-atopic type of allergy which appears within seconds or a few minutes following the challenge, and the delayed type of reactivity which appears about twenty-four hours following challenge. The Arthus lesion is usually absorbed within twenty-four hours except when tissue damage is extreme. The associated hemorrhage and necrosis may lead to a persistence of the lesion for days or even weeks. This contrasts with the response of immediate hypersensitivity which appears almost instantaneously, reaches its peak within about twenty minutes and is usually completely faded within an hour. The delayed lesion which appears after twenty-four hours may persist for days or even weeks.

Recent studies on the mechanisms involved in the Arthus reaction emphasize the importance of this immune response in the interpretation of the pathology observed in a number of clinical conditions, such as drug reactions, including penicillin disease, serum disease, vasculitis, carditis, arthritis, nephritis, extrinsic allergic bronchopneumonia, *etc.*

In the Arthus reaction the antigen is a humoral substance, such as a foreign serum, a drug or a virus. The antibody is always of the precipitating type, usually belonging to the IgG class but at times IgM may be involved. The cardinal feature of the intermediate or Arthus type reaction is the inflammatory tissue response induced by complement (see discussion of complement) which is activated by toxic antigen-antibody complexes formed when antigen is in slight excess over antibody. The interaction between antigen and antibody takes place within the blood vessels which means that basically the

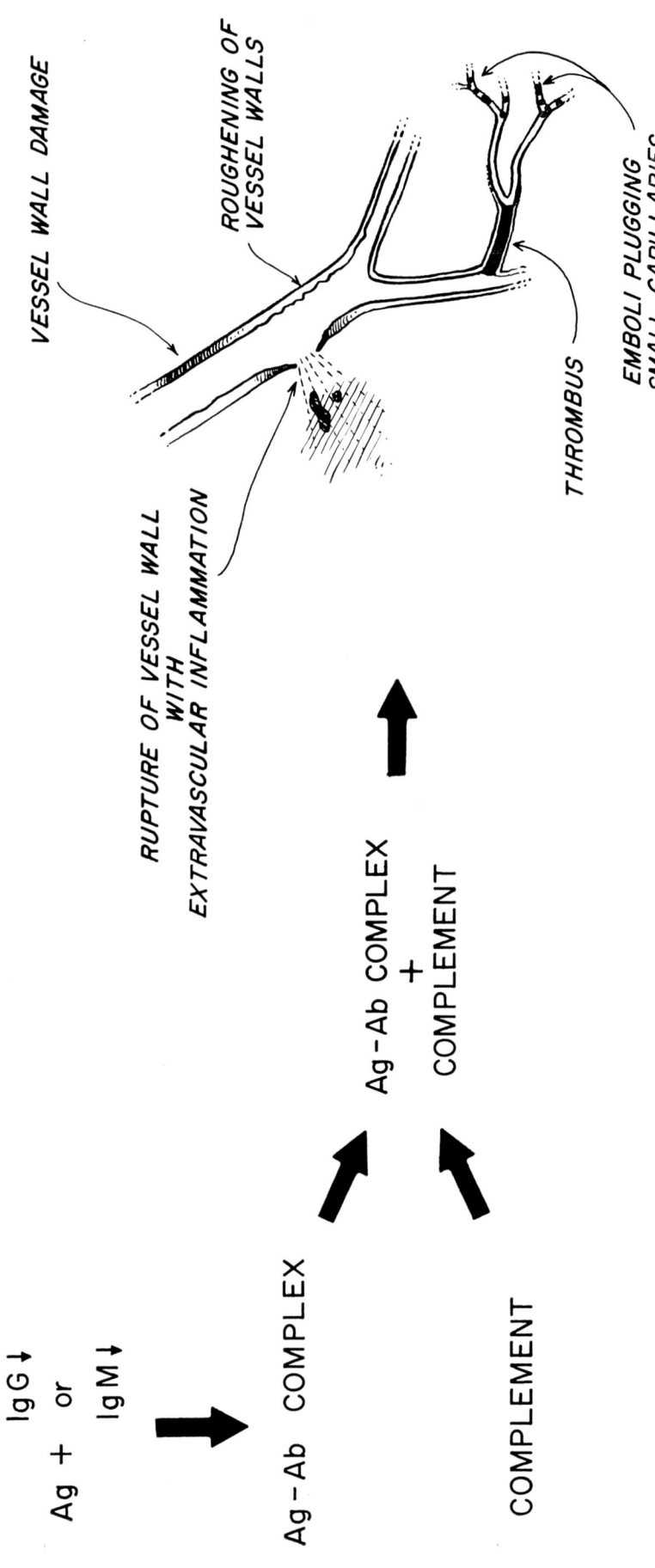

Figure 1-18. The arthus mechanism. The precipitating type of IgG or IgM antibodies form Ag-Ab complexes. When Ag is in slight excess over Ab, the complexes activate complement which initiates the sequence of events indicated in the diagram.

Arthus reaction is an involvement of blood vessels, particularly small capillaries.

The clinical patterns induced by the Arthus reaction vary from a mild innocuous lesion which may heal without causing symptoms, to a generalized vasculitis producing a very complex clinical picture. This broad range of differences in the clinical pattern can be explained by the variables governing the immunological mechanism of the Arthus reaction, the intensity of the inflammatory response, and the distribution of the tissue involvement. At times only a single organ such as the kidney may be the chief target of the reaction.

In a situation when the antibody response is weak and the concentration of antigen is low and in excess of antibody, the process which may involve one of many tissues and organs of the body can smoulder so that long periods may be required before the clinical symptoms are manifested.

The variable factors involved in the immunological mechanism are:

(1) The quantity, the molecular size and the immunogenicity of the antigens. Large antigens are usually more immunogenic.

(2) The concentration of antibody that initially encounters antigen. In the anamnestic* reactions the accelerated production of antibody makes antibody available earlier which results in an accelerated process.

(3) The affinity of the ligand for body proteins as when a low molecular chemical serves as a hapten. The more efficiently the ligand can combine with body tissues the more readily will complete antigens, which are immunogenic, be formed (see Drug Allergy in Chapter 10).

(4) The antigen to antibody ratio which influences the behavioral characteristic of the complexes formed intravascularly.

(a) Complexes formed in extreme excess of antigen are soluble and not toxic because they do not fix complement. When antigen is plentiful and antibody is in small amount, the complexes formed are small and unable to fix complement. They pass through structures and are eliminated.

(b) The complexes formed when antigen is in slight excess over antibody are the most toxic since they activate complement, the chief mediator of the Arthus reaction, with induction of an inflammatory reaction. When antigen is in slight excess over antibody, large complexes are formed that are able to fix complement, are not phagocytized, and do not pass through filtering tissue but are lodged there to cause reactions. Since the large complexes remain in the vascular compartment, they are likely to cause vascular damage.

(c) When antibody is in great excess over antigen, the complexes are very large but are readily phagocytized from the circulation.

The pathological features of the Arthus reaction are as follows:

(1) A roughness of the intima of the vessel walls occurs, with a slowing of the blood stream.

(2) Thrombi develop, which plug small vessels, leading to ischemia and tissue damage.

(3) Release of histamine and serotonin from platelets which aggregate the structures.

(4) Microprecipitates form in the small vessels which serve as emboli to cause occlusion with resulting ischemia and tissue damage.

(5) Complexes deposited in the walls of blood vessels lead to vascular damage with secondary hemorrhage.

(6) Complexes deposited extravascularly activate complement which leads to an inflammatory reaction.

---

* Anamnestic reaction: When antibody levels have decreased after an initial exposure to an antigen, even to the point where serum antibody is no longer detectable, a subsequent stimulation by the antigen will often evoke an increased and an accelerated response called the secondary or anamnestic or memory response.

Since delayed hypersensitivity also has the ability to stimulate an inflammatory response, it is at times difficult to differentiate the lesion of DH from the Arthus reaction on the basis of histopathology.

When the antigen is known, the demonstration of precipitating antibodies can serve as a differential.

III. DELAYED HYPERSENSITIVITY (DH)

The tuberculin reaction has for many years served as the classical example of DH with the result that DH is frequently referred to as the "tuberculin type" of reactivity.

The lesion of DH is usually observed about twenty-four hours after challenge of injection of the antigen into a sensitive individual. It is this characteristic which gives DH its name and distinguishes it from immediate hypersensitivity, which usually appears instantaneously or within minutes, and from the intermediate or Arthus type reaction which appears within five to six hours.

Unlike the immediate or reaginic-atopic form of allergy, DH can be induced in almost all animals including man. Some species of animals and perhaps some humans are more susceptible to the induction of the delayed type of hypersensitivity. In animals this susceptibility varies from strain to strain and at times even in animals within a strain. From this standpoint it must be recognized that in the delayed type of reactivity, as in atopic-reaginic allergy, there is a genetic or hereditary component.

Experimentally, DH can be induced by injecting the antigen in conjunction with Freund's Complete Adjuvant (FCA) which is a water-in-oil emulsion into which mycobacteria or tubercle bacilli are incorporated. How the adjuvant works is not known, but by this procedure sensitivity can be induced experimentally to not only protein substances but also low molecular chemicals.

An individual must have an intact thymus during fetal and neonatal life to have the capacity to react with the DH response. Initially, a limited number of lymphocytes, committed to serve in a general army of defenders with no specific assignment, reside in the reticulo-endothelial centers. It is not until foreign material which serves as the antigen is processed by the macrophages and transported to the committed cells that *specificity* develops. The antigen is usually soluble particulate material such as a bacterial component, a virus, a simple chemical or a drug, and even altered body cell proteins.

Following exposure to a specific antigen, the T-cell proliferates and releases into the circulation a number of sensitized cells which are a part of the constantly circulating pool of lymphocytes that are always on guard against foreign materials.

In the experimental animal an induction or latent period of five days is required following primary exposure to the antigen for sensitivity to be manifested.

The sensitized T-cells are attracted to any site in the tissues where specific antigen is present. Upon contact with its specific antigen the sensitized lymphocyte (1) starts to proliferate (see Fig. 1-20), and (2) recruits for participation in the encounter previously committed but not necessarily specifically sensitized cells, which also proliferate. This development requires about twenty-four hours which therefore is the time required for the appearance of DH. With the persistence of the supply of specific antigen, DH reaction continues; with the exhaustion of antigen the DH response terminates. In the presence of IgE antibody the antigen can be more readily exhausted.

The reaction of DH is more than the expression of a simple encounter between sensitized T-cells and their specific antigens, but rather the response to a complex mechanism involving the participation of a number of mediators. Some of the mediators, such as transfer factor (TF) of Lawrence are present

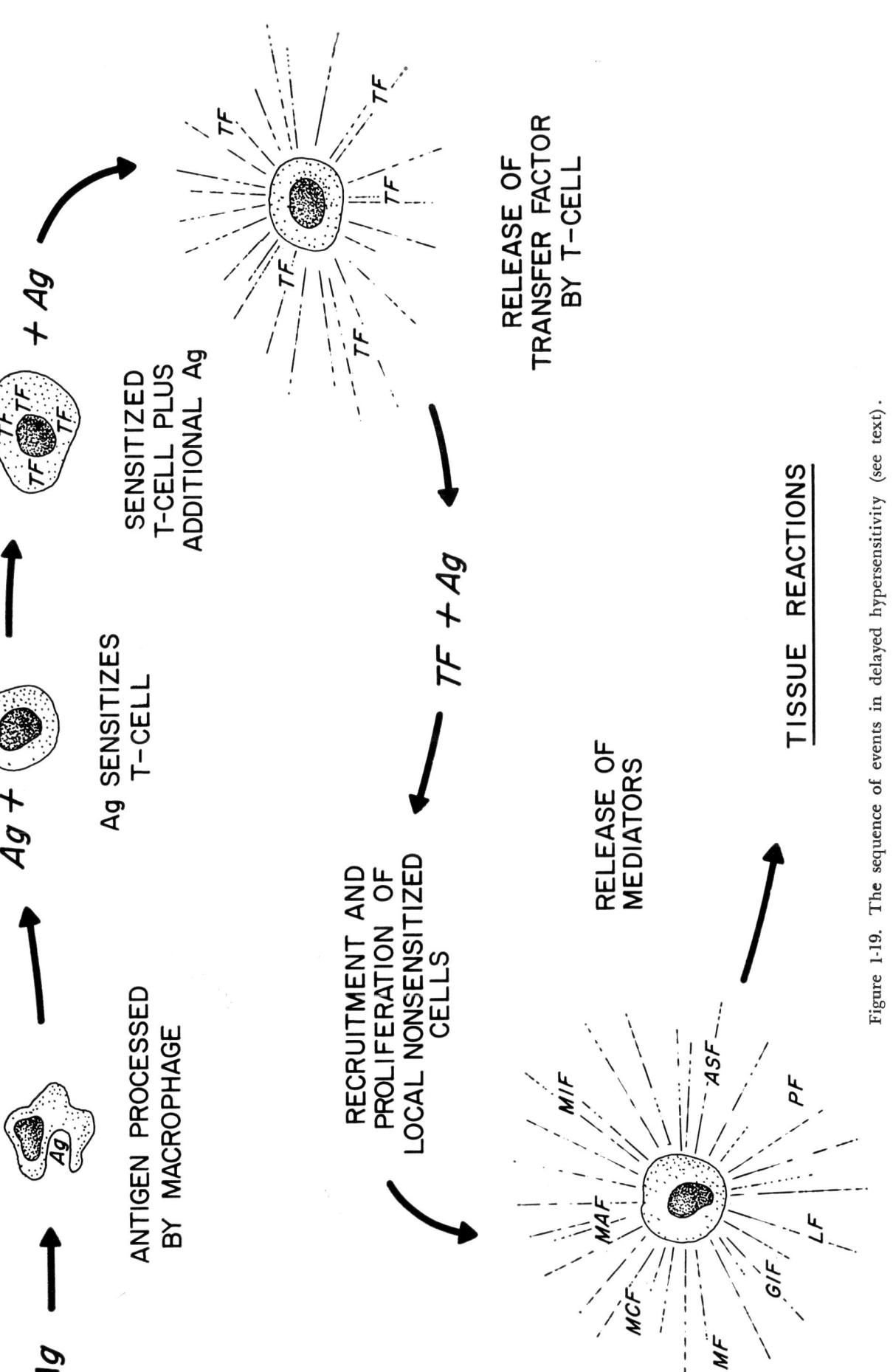

Figure 1-19. The sequence of events in delayed hypersensitivity (see text).

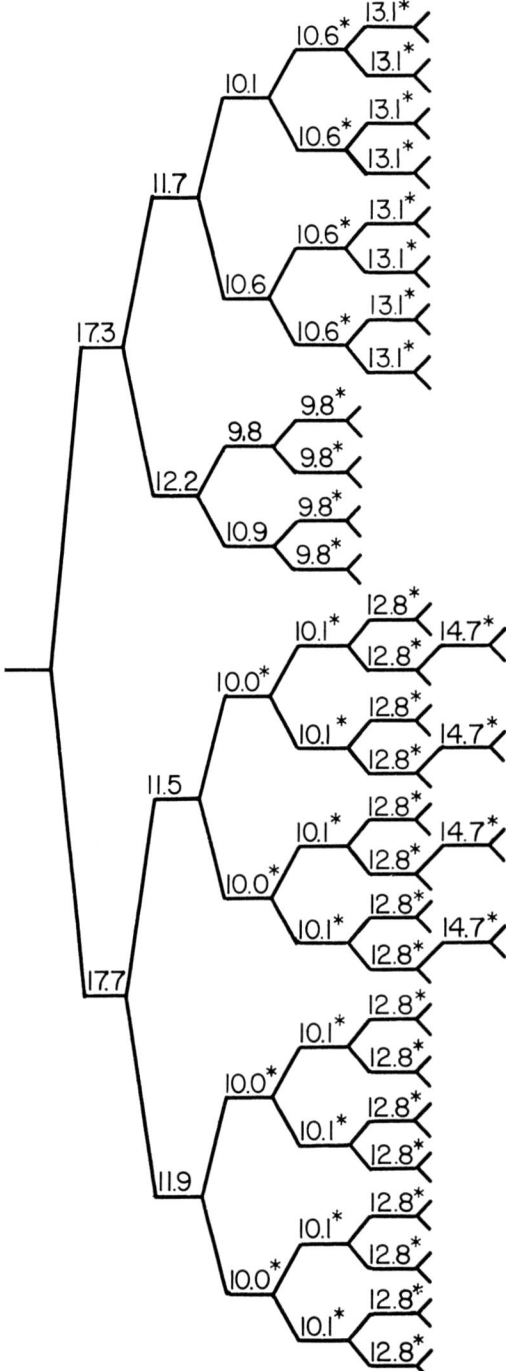

Figure 1-20. Reconstruction of the fate of a single lymphoblast through the sixty-four cell stage after exposure of tuberculin-sensitive human lymphocytes to tuberculin. Generation times shown in hours over appropriate lines; those marked with (*) are average times for a group of cells where it was impossible to follow the fate of a single cell but where the mitoses within the group were clearly seen. (From Marshall, W.H., Valentine, F.T. and Lawrence, H.S.: *J Exp Med, 130:* 327, 1969).

in the cells at the time they encounter antigen, while others are synthesized following the activation of the T-cell by antigen.

Mediators* which participate in DH are:

(1) Transfer Factor of Lawrence (TF)
(2) Migratory Inhibiting Factor (MIF)
 (a) for lymphocytes
 (b) for macrophages
(3) Macrophage Aggregating Factor (MAF)
(4) Macrophage Chemotactic Factor
 Lymphocyte Chemotactic Factor
(5) Mutagenic or Blastogenic Factor
(6) Growth Inhibiting Factor
(7) Lymphotoxic Factor
(8) Permeability Factor
(9) Antibody Stimulating Factor

All the activities indicated have been observed in DH, but to date none of the factors has been characterized. Also unknown is whether each activity represents a separate molecular structure or whether an identical molecule is involved in activities through variations in concentration and environment.

Transfer Factor of Lawrence (TF)

If a specific antigen is incubated with leukocytes obtained from an individual sensitive to the antigen, an interaction between the individual's sensitive cells and the antigen will liberate into the cell-free supernatant solution a material which has been labelled transfer factor (TF) by Lawrence, who originally made the observation.

Transfer factor has the following characteristics:

(1) found in circulating human leukocytes
(2) has a molecular weight less than 10,000
(3) can be lyophilized without impairment of function
(4) is not antigenic
(5) is not an immunoglobulin

---

* The battery of mediators synthesized are called *lymphokines* by Dudley Dumonde.

(6) is immunologically specific, i.e. it carries the identical sensitivities as the donor from whom it is derived.

(a) It confers upon the recipient the identical delayed skin response of the donor, and the recipient is able to serve as the donor for transfer of the sensitivity to a secondary nonsensitive recipient.

(b) If the donor has multiple sensitivities, such as tuberculin and diphtheria toxoid, the multiple sensitivities will be transferred to the recipient.

(c) TF confers upon the recipient's lymphocytes the capacity to respond to the specific antigen or antigens to which the donor is sensitive.

(7) TF may function as a *derepressor* of a select few nonsensitive lymphocytes, committing them to an antigen-responsive state.

(8) Upon conversion by TF the normal lymphocytes, both *in vitro* and *in vivo*, exhibit all the responses to specific antigen of the host, such as:

lymphoblastic transformation
clonal proliferation
migratory inhibitory factor (MIF)
cutaneous reactivity
homograft rejection
lymphotoxin
chemotactic factor (CF)

The clinical application of TF in the management of disseminated intracellular infection is just developing. With increased clinical studies, the importance of TF as a therapeutic agent will receive wider recognition.

In disseminated infection with impaired DH, or anergy, as demonstrated by skin testing, TF has been found to be an effective therapeutic measure.

In the treatment of disseminated vaccinal infection, TF proved effective when high titer specific immunoglobulins failed to halt the progress of the disease.

TF has been reported to be effective in long standing disseminated candidiasis when repeated courses of amphotericin and specific immunoglobulins failed. The patient exhibited an adequate antibody response.

A case of Wiscott-Aldrich syndrome treated successfully with dialyzable transfer factor has recently been reported.

Lawrence states that the only detectable consequences of repeated administration of TF has been an increasing intensity of the transferred DH reaction. Because of this, he recommended the judicious use of dialyzable TF, limiting it to grave intracellular infections in which the outlook is bleak, and when antimicrobial or antiviral therapy is ineffective in eradicating the disease.

Biologic, biochemical and immunologic properties of dialyzable TF are summarized in Figures 1-21 and 1-22.

The interaction between sensitive lymphocytes and specific antigen induces the synthesis of proteins which cause:

(1) The inhibition of normal migration of all types of leukocytes—lymphocytes, macrophages, and PMNLs. One lymphocyte generates sufficient material to effect the migration of about 1,000 macrophages. Migration inhibition factor (MIF)

(2) The aggregation or agglutination of macrophages. Macrophage aggregation factor (MAF)

(3) The attraction to the site of the reaction of lymphocytes and macrophages. Chemotactic factor (CF)

The proteins are heat stable at 56° C for thirty minutes, are nondialyzable and are not immunoglobulins. The proteins have not been characterized. Although they present many characteristics in common, recent studies indicate that MIF and CF are not the same factor.

Lymphocyte Transforming Factor (LTF)

Valentine and Lawrence have demonstrated that when sensitive lymphocytes are incubated *in vitro* with their specific antigen, a nondialyzable, heat stable (56° C) supernatant material is developed which, upon its addition to nonsensitive lymphocytes in the

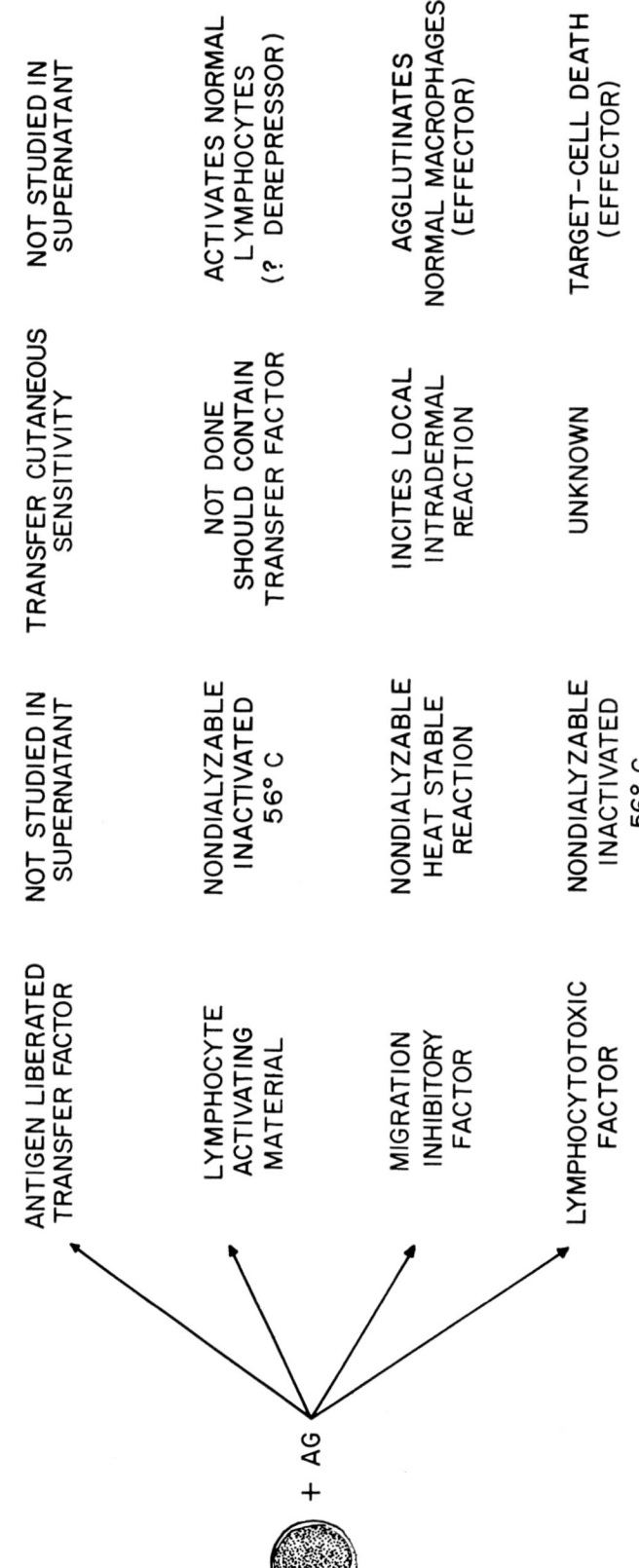

Figure 1-21. Activities produced by or liberated from antigen-responsive human blood lymphocytes after interaction with specific antigen. *Transfer factor:* liberated after one hour incubation with antigen. *Lymphocyte activating material:* produced after twenty-four hours incubation with antigen. *Migration inhibitory factor:* produced after twenty-four hours incubation with antigen—heat stable, MIF is produced by human lymphocytes, some properties listed in this figure were obtained in the guinea pig. *Lymphocytotoxic factor:* produced after thirty-six hours incubation with antigen. (From Lawrence, H.S.: Transfer factor. *Adv Immunol, 11:*195–266, 1969.)

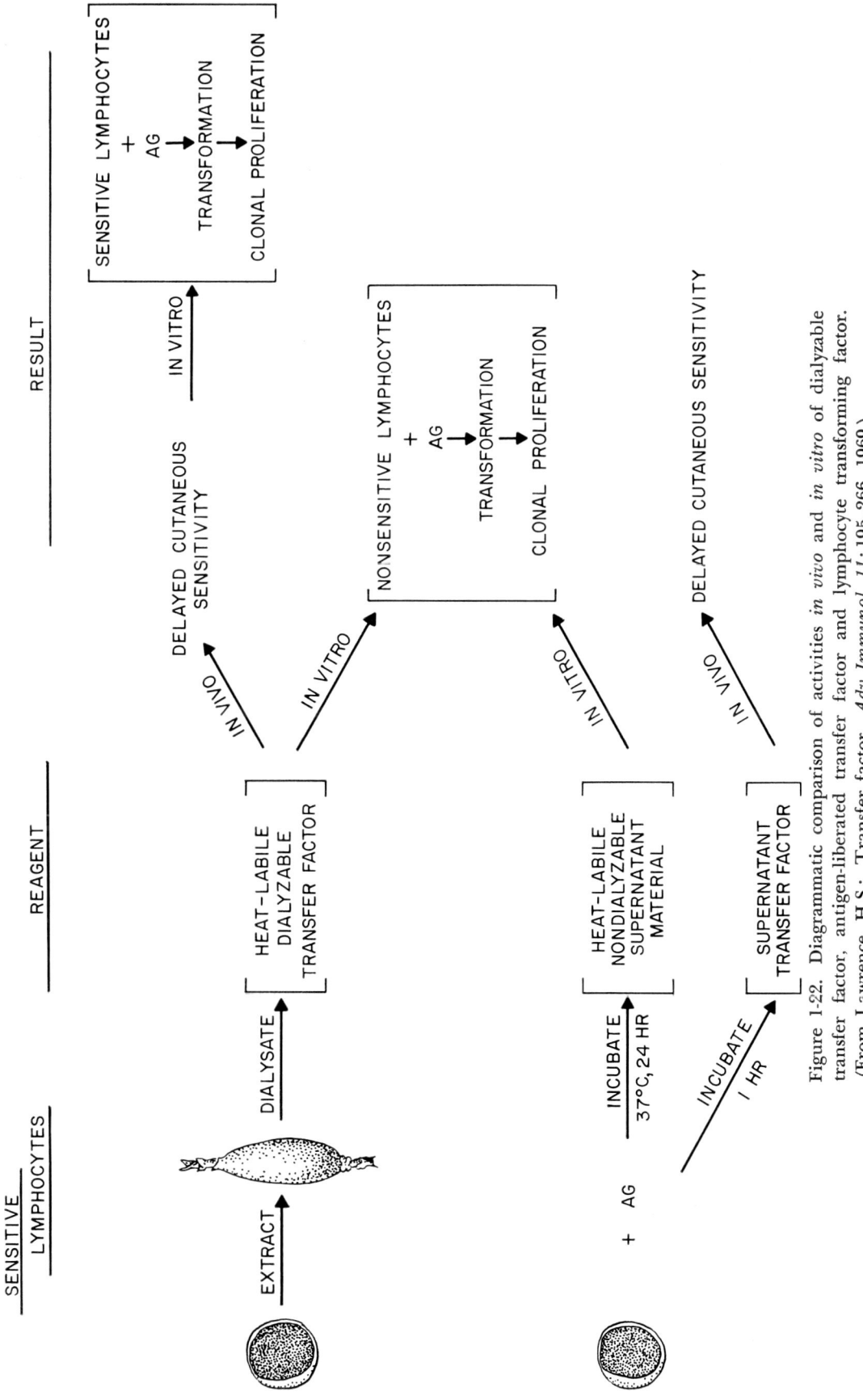

Figure 1-22. Diagrammatic comparison of activities *in vivo* and *in vitro* of dialyzable transfer factor, antigen-liberated transfer factor, and lymphocyte transforming factor. (From Lawrence, H.S.: Transfer factor. *Adv Immunol, 11*: 195–266, 1969.)

presence of specific antigen, causes transformation of the nonsensitive lymphocytes into blast forms and stimulates clonal proliferation. The production of LTF is immunologically specific in its requirements and is *antigen dose dependent*. Dialyzable TF also inhibits some transformation properties, but the relationship between LTF and TF is not established.

It is possible that LTF is responsible for recruiting nonsensitive lymphocytes to participate in the immune reaction.

Lymphotoxin

In vitro studies on a nondialyzable, heat labile (56° C at 30 minutes) extract have demonstrated its ability to round up cells of various types, following which abnormal forms appear with fusion of cells and finally cessation of cell division after a variable number of cycles. It has not yet been demonstrated that antigen-stimulated cells recruited by transfer factor produced lymphotoxins.

Increased Permeability Factor (IPF)

Increased permeability of vessels in association with delayed hypersensitivity has been observed, but the factor responsible has not been identified. It is possible that increased permeability is induced by the associated inflammatory reaction which accompanies DH.

Antibody Stimulating Function (ASF)

The stimulation of B-cells to produce IgG type antibodies has been reported. The association of humoral antibodies with the DH reaction is an extremely important observation, which can explain the presence of antibody in the mechanism of tolerance. The production of humoral antibody and DH have a definite feedback relationship; as one increases, the other decreases. (See Helper T-Cells above).

IV. THE CYTOLYTIC OR CYTOTOXIC RESPONSE

In this classification the body tissues either serve as a target or provide the antigen for a direct encounter with humoral antibody.

Intravascular Reaction (Immunohematology)

(1) The antigen is an integral part of the body cell. Examples:

(a) *Intravascular Transfusion Reaction*: The antigen is an integral part of the RBC, usually of the ABO blood system. The antibody (IgG) is complement fixing. Damage occurs through the hemolytic action of complement.

(b) *Erythroblastosis fetalis and adult hemolytic anemia due to Rh antibody*: The antigen is an integral part of the RBC. In this situation the antibody is *not* complement fixing but is cytophilic, i.e. it has an affinity for macrophages. Hemolytic anemia is secondary to clearing of the RBC by macrophages derived from the reticulo-endothelial system.

(2) Antibody is absorbed by the target cell or chemically combined.
Examples:

(a) *Delayed Post-Transfusion Thrombocytopenia*: Platelets in the transfused blood contain antigenic determinants which are foreign to the recipient's platelets. Antigen provided by the transfused platelets combines with the newly formed antibody to form an Ag-Ab complex. This Ag-Ab complex adsorbs to the recipient's own platelets. Complement activated by the Ag-Ab complex destroys the recipient's platelets producing *delayed* post-transfusion thrombocytopenia.

(b) *Hemolytic anemia following high doses of penicillin over a long period*: Antipenicillin antibodies formed by the patient combine with subsequent doses of penicillin to form an Ag-Ab complex which spontaneously conjugates to RBC membrane resulting in hemolytic anemia.

(c) *Drug Reactions:* Antibody is formed against the drug. The antidrug antibody combines with the drug in the circulation. If IgG type antibody is involved, adsorption of the Ag-Ab complex to platelets proceeds with the activation of complement. The platelets are destroyed by the lytic action of complement or are cleared by the reticulo-endothelial system, leading to thrombocytopenic purpura.

If the antibody involved belongs to the class IgM, the resulting Ag-Ab complex adheres to RBC, leading to activation of complement and action of macrophages of the reticulo-endothelial system. These lead to hemolytic anemia.

In rare patients both IgG and IgM are involved which leads to both thrombocytopenia and anemia. Antibodies may be evoked which react with WBC, resulting in leukopenia. These reactions constitute the "innocent bystander reaction" described by Shulman.

Immunological Tolerance

Tolerance is a very fundamental phenomenon of the immune mechanism characterized by the failure of committed lymphocytes, either T-cells or B-cells or both, to respond to their specific antigenic stimuli. In the literature on immunology this failure to respond is labelled "turning off" because the absence of response is not necessarily a permanent state of the involved cells, since under proper conditions function returns.

The interpretations offered for the possible mechanisms involved in immunological tolerance are still hypothetical, but many relevant observations have been reported, which should be considered.

(1) An antigen that induces tolerance is a *tolerogen.*

(2) Either weak antigens or strong antigens are good tolerogens. The less immunogenic an antigen molecule is, the stronger is its potency to induce tolerance (low zone). The stronger the immunogenic capacity of an antigen, the better is its capacity not only to immunize but to induce tolerance (high zone).

(3) In the newborn, tolerance can be induced for both cell mediated and antibody mediated immunity. In the older individual, tolerance can be induced for either the cellular or the humoral mechanisms, but not both. This suggests that the operation of the mechanism in neonatal life may not be identical with that in the older individual.

(4) When antibody tolerance or antibody suppression is induced, cellular immunity increases, and when cellular immunity is suppressed, antibody response is enhanced. These two systems compete with one another; when one is suppressed, the other is enhanced.

(5) The induction of *low phase* tolerance (weak immunogen) depends upon the presence of antibody.

(6) A critical ratio of antibody to antigen exists in low phase tolerance.

(7) Incomplete "turning off" of cell function is "partial tolerance." Merrill Chase of Rockefeller University states, "There must be a mechanism for restraining an adequate proliferation of recognition cells so that one does not meet ever-ascending responsiveness." (See Chapter 18, Auto-Allergic Disease)

Is Tolerance an Allergic Phenomenon?

If allergy is defined as "altered reactivity" which is any deviation from an individual's baseline (ergy) of immune response, then tolerance which is a variation below the baseline (hypoergy and anergy) must be considered an allergic manifestation, just as the variations above the baseline (hyperergy or hypersensitivity) are considered to be allergy. The recognition of *self* which is the protection of the individual against his own body proteins, is necessary for normal homeostasis (ergy). Any deviation in normal tolerance for the body's tissues is a manifestation of "altered reactivity" or allergic disease (auto-allergic).

SERUM DISEASE

At the turn of the century foreign sera, particularly diphtheria antitoxin, were in common use for treatment. Reactions were observed from two days to even two weeks or more following administration. These reactions were characterized by fever, generalized adenopathy, urticaria, angio-edema and arthralgia, while in severe cases generalized vasculitis, nephritis, carditis and even death occurred. The term "serum sickness" was applied to this syndrome by Pirquet and Schick who studied the condition thoroughly and pointed out that during the course of the disease a "toxic substance" was formed which was responsible for the pathological tissue alterations. This toxic substance is now identified as an antigen-antibody complex.

Serum disease type of reactions are seen less frequently from sera because: (1) sera are administered less frequently, and (2) when administered the product is more highly refined and in much smaller doses. But the incidence of *serum sickness* type of reaction is still quite high because an identical immunologic and clinical pattern is observed with drug allergy, particularly penicillin reactions (see drug allergy in Chapter 10) and also following the inhalation of molds and particulate organic materials, such as grain dust, vegetable dusts, bird droppings, *etc.*

The disease is usually self limited and subsides within a few days, but in some cases it may be protracted because of diffuse vascular and perivascular tissue involvement which leads to organ dysfunction. In a small number of patients death may occur at the height of the reaction.

Mechanism

In serum sickness two types of antibodies are operating simultaneously:

(1) The IgE class of anitbodies as encountered in anaphylaxis or reaginic allergy
(2) The IgG class of antibodies of the precipitating type as encountered in the Arthus reaction.

Serum disease is actually a hybrid of the anaphylactic or reaginic type of reaction and the Arthus reaction.

Reversible tissue responses, characterized by urticaria, angio-edema and even bronchospasm are induced by the release of histamine from mast cells through the action of IgE complexes.

The more severe tissue responses are inflammatory reactions, typical of the Arthus mechanism, which result from the activation of complement induced by complexes formed by the precipitating form of IgG antibody interacting with the specific antigen.

All the inflammatory tissue alterations are governed by the identical factors which operate in the Arthus mechanism (see Arthus reaction), except that in the serum sickness syndrome the offending agent first acts as an immunogen to produce antibodies and then provides the supply of antigen to interact with antibodies to form antigen-antibody complexes.

Very soon following the injection of the serum into the circulation antibodies are produced. At this early stage the amount of antigen is far in excess of the available antibody, so that with the great excess of antigen over antibody only small complexes are formed. The small complexes are soluble, unable to activate complement and are able to be filtered through the kidneys to be excreted without the production of disease. When the volume of serum is small, as occurs today with highly refined products, usually no disease will develop.

As antibody production increases, the serum (antigen) present in the circulation is gradually consumed for complex formation, until, at the level when antigen is in slight excess over antibody, the complexes formed, being very large (over 1,000,000 in mol wt.), are very toxic since they activate complement. These complexes, when they remain in the circulation, cause damage to blood vessel walls with resulting hemorrhage and inflammation. This explains the diffuse vasculitis so frequently observed with serum type disease. When deposited in the various tissues, such as kidneys, heart and joints, inflammatory reactions are produced resulting in signs and symptoms related to the respective organs.

When the supply of serum (antigen) is depleted so that the titer of antibody exceeds the titer of antigen, the complexes formed are very large, are easily phagocytized, and no tissue damage occurs. This is the stage when free antibody is detected in the serum and corresponds to the time when convalescence begins, usually about a week to ten days following the onset of symptoms.

In most cases the disease is usually benign with recovery complete, but with the formation of high titers of toxic antigen-antibody complexes the resulting tissue damage may be irreversible, leading to organ dysfunction, such as renal or cardiac disease, and at times even death. When the disease follows the intramuscular injection of a drug, such as penicillin, the depot may serve as a reservoir for the slow release of antigen which can keep the process active for long periods of time, many weeks or even months. If the antigen released is just sufficient to maintain a slight excess over the amount of antibody produced, the resulting pattern can be very serious, due to the smoldering, irreversible tissue alterations which gradually encroach upon the reserve functional capacity of organs, leading to incapacity of the patient and even death.

Management

Prophylaxis: Before administering sera the patient should be skin tested to determine sensitivity. If a patient offers a history of specific sensitivity, do not try to confirm the sensitivity by skin testing. The procedure is hazardous and can precipitate anaphylaxis.

Technique for testing with sera:

(1) Prepare the volar surface of the arm, preferably with alcohol.

(2) The initial test should be performed with a dilution of at least 1:100,000. Inject intradermally the smallest amount necessary to produce a very small wheal. At no time exceed 0.025 cc. After twenty minutes the test should be read. A positive test is indicated by a flare and wheal reaction. In very young individuals the flare may be very pronounced, while in older individuals, particularly after the sixth decade, no flare may be present, only a whealing reaction. In the aged, pseudopods are not prominent with whealing.

(3) If no reaction is observed after one hour, inject the next concentration—1:10,000 to be followed by 1:1,000; 1:100; 1:10 and then undiluted serum.

The interval between tests may be twenty-four hours, rarely forty-eight hours, but never longer. Longer periods permit the development of antibodies to the testing antigen which can induce a reaction upon subsequent testing.

(4) With a positive test the serum should not be administered. In cases when the administration of the serum is imperative, a program of rapid hyposensitization can be instituted (see hyposensitization for sera and penicillin under management of penicillin reaction).

(5) If skin tests and history are negative, proceed with the administration of the serum. Always inject the serum very slowly, being constantly alert for any untoward symptoms, such as:

(a) feeling of extreme warmth
(b) generalized itching or tingling
(c) localized itching of the scalp, nose, ears, palate, throat
(d) tightness of the chest
(e) coughing

If any of the above symptoms occur, discountinue the injection of the serum immediately and administer epinephrine 1-1000, 0.4 cc by hypodermic.

Do not wait for further symptoms to develop. *Give epinephrine immediately.* Repeat the epinephrine in thirty minutes if symptoms persist.

Treatment of Acute Symptoms of Serum Sickness:

(1) For acute urticaria, angio-edema or bronchospasm administer epinephrine-HCl, 0.4 cc by hypodermic. If necessary, this may be repeated after thirty minutes. Sus-Phrine® (depot epinephrine), 0.25 cc may be administered for a more sustained effect, six to twelve hours.

(2) In many cases the acute symptoms recur as the pharmacological effect of the epinephrine wears off. If the symptoms are those of immediate hypersensitivity, such as urticaria, angio-edema and bronchospasm, *antihistamines* orally may be administered. In some cases intramuscular antihistamines, such as Benadryl® are helpful. The analgesic property of antihistamines is helpful in quieting the patient.

In most cases, particularly those with evidence of organ involvement steroids are the drug of choice.

Since inflammatory tissue reactions are an important feature of the pathology of serum disease, the early administration of steroids for their antiflammatory action is highly recommended (see discussion of steroid therapy in Chapter 15 for schedule of dosage).

REFERENCES

General Texts and Topics in Immunology

1. Aas, Kjell: The biochemistry and immunological basis of bronchial asthma. In Kugelmass, I. Newton (Ed.): *American Lecture Series.* Springfield, Thomas, 1972.
2. Arbesman, C. E., Kantor, S. Z., Rose, N. R. and Witebsky, E.: Serum sickness. *J Allergy, 31:* 257, 1960.
3. Austen, K. F. and Becker, E. L. (Eds.): *Biochemistry of the Acute Allergic Reactions.* Oxford, 1968.
4. Bell, S. D. and Erickson, Z.: Studies in the transmission of sensitization from mother to child in human beings: I. Transfer of skin sensitizing antibodies. *J Immunol, 20:* 447, 1931.
5. Bendixen, G.: Classification of hypersensitivity in relation to clinical disease. *Ann Intern Med, 64:* 668, 1966.
6. Bendixen, G.: Clinical hypersensitivity disorders. In Kugelmass, I. Newton (Ed.): *American Lecture Series.* Springfield, Thomas, 1971.
7. Boyd, W. C.: *Fundamentals of Immunology,* 4th ed. New York, Interscience, 1966.
8. Burnet, Sir Mac Farlane: *Cellular Immunology,* Books 1 and 2 combined. New York, Cambridge U P, 1969.
9. Davis, B. D., Dulbecco, R., Eisen, H., Guisberg, H. S. and Wood, B. W., Jr.: *Microbiology.* New York, Har-Row, 1968.
10. Gell, P. G. H. and Coombs, R. R. A. (Eds.): *Clinical Aspects of Immunology.* Philadelphia, F. A. Davis, 1963.
11. Gitlin, D., Kumate, J., Urrusti, J. and Morales, C.: The selectivity of the human placenta on the transfer of plasma proteins from mother to fetus. *J Clin Invest, 43:* 1938, 1964.
12. Good, R. A., Gabrielsen, A. E., Pollara, B., Gewurz, H. and Finstad, J.: Phylogenetic development of lymphoid tissue. In Cinader, B.: *Regulation of Antibody Response,* 2nd ed. Springfield, Thomas, 1971, pp. 212-231.
13. Good, R. A. and Fisher, D. M. (Eds.): *Immunology.* Stanford, Sinauer Associates, 1971.
14. Humphrey, J. H. and White, R. G.: *Immunology for Students of Medicine.* Philadelphia, F. A. Davis, 1963.
15. Kabat, E. A.: *Structural Concepts in Immunology and Immunochemistry.* New York, H R & W, 1968.
16. Lawrence, S. H. (Ed.): *Cellular and Humoral Aspects of the Hypersensitive States.* New York, Hoeber, 1959.
17. Lichtenstein, L. M. and Norman, P. S.: Human allergic reactions. *Am J Med, 46:* 163, 1969.
18. McKee, W. D.: The incidence and familial occurrence of allergy. *J Allergy, 38:* 226, 1966.
19. Miescher, P. A. and Müller-Eberhard, H. J. (Eds.): *Textbook of Immunopathology.* New York, Grune, 1968.
20. Nisonoff, A. and Thorbecke, G. J.: Immunochemistry. *Annu Rev Biochem, 33:* 355, 1964.
21. Prausnitz, C. and Küstner, H.: Studien über die Uberempfindlichkeit. *Zentralbl Bakteriol (Orig) 1. Abt, 86:* 160, 1921.
22. Reid, R. T., Minden, P. and Farr, R. S.: Biological and chemical differences among proteins having reaginic activity. *J Allergy, 41:* 326, 1968.
23. Samter, M. and Markowitz, S. A.: Nonspecific factors in allergic disease. In Samter, M. and Alexander, H. L. (Eds.): *Immunological Diseases.* Boston, Little, 1965.
24. Samter, M. (Ed.): *Immunological Diseases,* 2nd ed. Boston, Little, 1971.
25. Shaffer, J. H., Logrippo, G. A. and Chase, M. W. (Eds.): *Mechanisms of Hypersensitivity.* Boston, Little, 1959.

26. Tips, R. C.: A study of the inheritance of atopic hypersensitivity in man. *Am J Hum Genet*, 6: 328, 1954.
27. von Pirquet, C. F. and Schick, B.: *Die Serum Krankheit*. Trans. by Schick, B.: Serum Sickness. Baltimore, Williams & Wilkins, 1951.
28. von Pirquet, C. F.: Allergie. *Munch Med Wochenschr*, 53: 1457, 1906.
29. Waldman, T. A. and Strober, W.: Metabolism of immunoglobulins. *Progr Allergy*, 13: 1, 1969.
30. Weir, D. M., (Ed.): *Handbook of Experimental Immunology*. Oxford, Blackwell Scientific Publications, 1967.
31. Weiser, R. S., Myrvik, Q. N. and Pearsall, N. N.: *Fundamentals of Immunology*. Philadelphia, Lea & Febiger, 1969.
32. Williams, C. A. and Chase, M. W.: *Methods in Immunology and Immunochemistry*. New York, Acad Pr, 1971, vols. I, II, III.
33. World Health Organization: Factors regulating the immune response. *Int Arch Allergy Appl Immunol*, 38: 1, 1970.

Cellular Elements

1. Archer, R. K.: Clinical aspects of eosinophilia in atopic disease. *J Allergy*, 42: 109, 1968.
2. Bjorneboe, M., Gormsen, H. and Lundquist, F.: Further experimental studies on the role of plasma cells on antibody production. *J Immunol*, 55: 121, 1947.
3. Blatt, H.: Eosinophilia in allergy. *Rev Allergy*, 20: 650, 1966.
4. Cameron, I. L. (Ed.): Immunoglobulin production by proliferating lymphoid cells. In *Developmental Aspects of the Cell Cycle*. New York, Acad Pr.
5. Ciba Foundation Study Group No. 16: *The Immunologically Competent Cell*. London, Churchill, 1963.
6. Cohn, Z. A.: The structure and function of leukocytes and macrophages. *Adv Immunol*, 9: 163, 1968.
7. Cruikshank, R. and Weir, D. M. (Eds.): *Modern Trends in Immunology*. New York, Appleton, 1967.
8. Dumonde, D. C.: Role of the macrophage in delayed hypersensitivity. *Br Med Bull*, 23: 9, 1967.
9. Dumonde, D. C., Howsens, W. T. and Wolstencroft, R. A.: The role of macrophages and lymphocytes in reactions of delayed hypersensitivity. In Miescher, P. A. and Grabar, P. (Eds.): *Immunopathology*, 5th Int. Sym. Basel, Schwabe, 1968, p. 263.
10. Frei, P. C., Benacerraf, B. and Thorbecke, G. J.: Phagocytosis of the antigen, a crucial step in the induction of primary response. *Proc Natl Acad Sci USA*, 58: 20, 1965.
11. Frenkel, E. and Stone, M. J.: The rationale and approach to immunosuppressive therapy. *Adv Intern Med*, 17: 21, 1971.
12. Galti, R. A., Stutman, O. and Good, R. A.: The lymphoid system. *Annu Rev Physiol*, 32: 529, 1970.
13. Gowans, J. L., McGregor, D. D., Cowen, D. M. and Ford, C. E.: Initiation of immune responses by small lymphocytes. *Nature*, 196: 651, 1962.
14. Gowans, J. L. and McGregor, D. D.: The immunological activities of lymphocytes. *Progr Allergy*, 9: 1, 1965.
15. Gowans, J. L.: Lymphocytes. *Harvey Lect*, 64: 87, 1968–1969.
16. Huber, H., Douglas, S. D. and Fudenberg, H. H.: The IgG receptor: An immunological marker for the characterization of mononuclear cells. *Immunology*, 17: 7, 1969.
17. Keller, R.: Tissue mast cells in immune reactions. *Monogr Allergy*, 2: 1, 1966.
18. Leblond, C. P. and Sainte-Marie, G.: Models for lymphocyte and plasmocyte formation. *Haematopoeisis: Cell production and its regulation*. Ciba Foundation Symposium. London, Churchill, 1960, p. 152.
19. Lowell, F. C.: Clinical aspects of eosinophilia in atopic disease. *JAMA*, 202: 875, 1967.
20. Meuwissen, H. J., Stutman, O. and Good, R. A.: Functions of the lymphocytes. *Semin Hematol*, 6: 28, 1969.
21. Mota, I.: Mast cells and anaphylaxis. *Ann N Y Acad Sci*, 103: 264, 1963.
22. Naterman, H. L.: Clinical aspects of eosinophilia in atopic disease. *JAMA*, 203: 991, 1968.
23. Nossal, G. J. V.: The cellular basis of immunity. *Harvey Lect*, 63: 179, 1968.
24. Pearsall, N. N. and Weisser, R. S.: *The Macrophage*. Philadelphia, Lea & Febiger, 1970.
25. Rebuck, J. W. (Ed.): *The Lymphocyte and Lymphoid Tissue*. New York, Hoeber, 1960.
26. Sell, S. and Asofsky, R. M.: Lymphocytes and immunoglobulins. *Progr Allergy*, 12: 86, 1968.
27. Selye, H.: *The Mast Cells*. Butterworth, 1965.
28. Trowell, O. A.: The lymphocyte. *Int Rev Cytol*, 7: 235, 1958.
29. Unanue, E. R. and Cerottini, J. C.: The function of macrophages in the immune response. *Semin Hematol*, 7: 225, 1970.
30. van Furth, R. (Ed.): *Mononuclear Phagocytes*. Philadelphia, Davis Co, 1970.

Antigens

1. Dumonde, D. C.: Tissue specific antigens. *Adv Immunol*, 5: 245, 1966.
2. Flickinger, R. A.: Embryological development of antigens. *Adv Immunol*, 2: 309, 1962.

3. Kabat, E. A.: Nature of an antigenic determinant. *J Immunol, 97:* 1, 1966.
4. McDevitt, H. O., Askonas, B. A., Humphrey, J. H., Schechter, I. and Sela, M.: The localization of antigen in relation to specific antibody-producing cells. *Immunology, 11:* 337, 1966.
5. Nossal, G. J. V., Austin, C. M. and Ada, G. L.: Antigens in immunity: VII. Analysis of immunological memory. *Immunology, 9:* 333, 1965.
6. Nossal, G. J. V., Austin, C. M., Pye, J. and Mitchell, J.: Antigens in immunity: XII. Antigen trapping in the spleen. *Int Arch Allergy Appl Immunol, 29:* 368, 1966.
7. Sela, M.: Antigenicity: Some molecular aspects. *Science, 166:* 1365, 1969.

Haptens

1. Eisen, H. N., Orris, L. and Belman, S.: Elicitation of delayed allergic skin reactions with haptens: The dependence of elicitation on hapten conjugation with protein. *J Exp Med, 95:* 473, 1952.
2. Eisen, H. N.: Hypersensitivity to simple chemicals. In Lawrence, H. S. (Ed.): *Cellular and Humoral Aspects of Hypersensitive States.* New York, Hoeber-Harper, 1959, pp. 89-122.
3. Landsteiner, K. and Jacobs, J.: Studies on the sensitization of animals with simple chemical compounds. *J Exp Med, 64:* 625, 1936.
4. Landsteiner, K. and Chase, M. W.: Studies on the sensitization of animals with simple chemical compounds. VII. Skin sensitization by intraperitoneal injections. *J Exp Med, 71:* 237, 1940.
5. Plescia, O. J.: The role of carrier in antibody formation. *Curr Top Microbiol Immunol, 50:* 78, 1969.
6. Tarrar, R., Strausbauch, P., Sulica, A. and Sela, M.: The stimulation of anti-hapten antibodies with a protein carrier. *Isr J Med Sci, 7:* 619, 1971.

Specificity

1. Immunochemical specificity: Recent conceptual advances. *Immunochemistry, 6:* 139, 1969.
2. Karush, F.: Immunologic specificity and molecular structure. *Adv Immunol, 2:* 1, 1962.
3. Landsteiner, K.: *The Specificity of Serological Reactions,* 2nd ed. Cambridge, Howard U Pr, 1945.
4. Landsteiner, K.: *The Specificity of Serological Reactions,* Rev. Ed. New York, Dover, 1962.
5. Nisonoff, A. and Inman, F. P.: Structural basis of the specificity of antibodies. Reproduction: Molecular, subcellular and cellular. In Lock, M. (Ed.): *Society for the Study of Developmental Biology.* New York, Acad Pr, 1965.

Immunoglobulins

1. Cohen, S.: General structure and heterogeneity of immunoglobulins. *Proc Roy Soc Lond (Biol), 166:* 114, 1966.
2. Cohen, S. and Milstein, C.: Structure and biological properties of immunoglobulins. *Adv Immunol, 7:* 1, 1967.
3. Cooper, M. D., Peney, D. Y., McKneally, M. F., Gabrielson, A. E., Sutherland, D. E. R. and Good, R. A.: A mammalian equivalent of the avian bursa of Fabricius. *Lancet, 1:* 1388, 1966.
4. Deutsch, H. F. and Fudenberg, H. H.: Immunoglobulin structure and function. *Adv Intern Med, 15:* 377, 1969.
5. Dorrington, K. J. and Tanford, C.: Molecular size and conformation of immunoglobulin. *Adv Immunol, 12:* 333, 1970.
6. Dubiski, S. and Miller, P.: The feed-back mechanism in immunoglobulin synthesis. *Proc Soc Exp Biol Med, 122:* 126, 1966.
7. Fleischman, J. B.: Immunoglobulins. *Annu Rev Biochem, 35:* 835, 1966.
8. Franklin, E. C.: Structure and function of immunoglobulins, relation to allergy. *NY State J Med, 68:* 1, 1968.
9. Gitlin, D.: Current aspects of the structure and function and genetics of the immunoglobulins. *Annu Rev Med, 17:* 1, 1966.
10. Ishizaka, T., Ishizaka, K., Salmon, S. and Fudenberg, H.: Biologic activities of aggregated gammaglobulins. VIII. Aggregated immunoglobulins of different classes. *J Immunol, 99:* 82, 1967.
11. Janeway, C. A., Rosen, F. S., Merler, E. and Alper, C. A.: *The Gamma Globulins.* Boston, Little, 1967.
12. Killander, J. (Ed.): Gamma Globulins. *Nobel Symposium #3,* Uppsala, Sweden. Almquist and Wiksells, Boktryckeri, 1967.
13. Lennox, E. S. and Cohn, M.: Immunoglobulins. *Annu Rev Biochem, 36:* 365, 1967.
14. Merler, E. and Rosen, F. S.: The gamma globulins, I. The structure and synthesis of the immunoglobulins. *N Engl J Med, 275:* 536, 1966.
15. Nomenclature for human immunoglobulins. *Bull WHO, 30:* 477, 1964.
16. Scharff, M. D. and Laskov, R.: Synthesis and assembly of immunoglobulin polypeptide chains. *Progr Allergy, 14:* 37, 1970.
17. Smith, R. T., Good, R. A. and Miescher, P. A.: *Ontogeny of Immunity.* Gainesville, U Florida Pr, 1967.
18. Tiselius, A. and Kabat, E. A.: Electrophoresis of immune serum. *Science, 87:* 416, 1938.

Antibodies

1. Burnet, Sir Mac Farlane: *The Clonal Selection Theory of Acquired Immunity.* Nashville, U Pr, 1958.
2. Cinader, B. (Ed.): *Regulation of the Antibody Response,* 2nd ed. Springfield, Thomas, 1971.
3. Collins-Williams, et al.: Quantitative immunoglobulin level (IgG, IgA, IgM) in children with intractable asthma. *Ann Allergy, 25:* 177, 1967.
4. Cooper, M. D., Pierey, D. Y., McKneally, M. F., Gabrielson, A. E., Sutherland, D. R. and Good, R. A.: Mammalian equivalent of the avian bursa of Fabricius. *Lancet, 1:* 1388, 1966.
5. Edelman, G. M.: Dissociation of gammaglobulin. *J Am Chem Soc, 81:* 3155, 1959.
6. Edelman, G. M. and Gally, J. A.: Antibody structure, diversity and specificity. *Brookhaven Symposium, 21:* 328, 1968.
7. Edelman, G. M. and Gall, W. E.: The antibody problem. *Annu Rev Biochem, 38:* 415, 1969.
8. Edelman, G. M.: Antibody structure: A molecular basis for specificity and control in the immune response. In Wolstenholme, G. E. W. and Knight, J. (Eds.): *Control Processes in Multicellular Organisms.* London, Churchill, 1970, p. 304.
9. Edelman, G. M.: The structure and function of antibodies. *Sci Am, 223:* 34, 1970.
10. Eichwald, H. F. and Shinefield, H. R.: Antibody production by the human fetus. *J Pediatr, 63:* 870, 1963.
11. Eisen, H. N.: The immune response to a single antigenic determinant. *Harvey Lect, 60:* 1, 1966.
12. The evolution of selective and instructive theories of antibody formation. Cold Spring Harbor Symposium. *Quant Biol, 32:* 559, 1967.
13. Frei, P. C., Benacerraf, B. and Thorbecke, C. J.: Phagocytosis of the antigens, a crucial step in the induction of the primary response. *Proc Natl Acad Sci USA, 53:* 20, 1965.
14. Harris, H.: *Human Biochemical Genetics.* London, Cambridge U Pr, 1959.
15. Hood, L. and Talmage, D. W.: Mechanism of antibody diversity: Germ line basis for variability. *Science, 168:* 325, 1970.
16. Lichtenstein, L. M., Holtzman, N. A. and Burnett, L. S.: A quantitative *in vitro* study of the dermatographic distribution and immunoglobulin characteristics of human blocking antibody. *J Immunol, 101:* 317, 1968.
17. *Mechanisms of Antibody Formation.* Proceedings of a symposium held in Prague, May 27–31, 1959. Prague, Publishing House of Czechoslovak Acad of Sciences, 1960.
18. Nisonoff, A., Wissler, F. C. and Lipman, L. N.: Properties of the major component of a peptic digestion of rabbit antibody. *Science, 132:* 1770, 1960.
19. Nossal, G. J. V.: Mechanisms of antibody production. *Annu Rev Med, 18:* 81, 1967.
20. Pink, R. A., Wang, A. and Fudenberg, H.: Antibody variability. *Annu Rev Med, 22:* 145, 1971.
21. Sehon, A. H.: Different types of antibodies produced by allergic individuals depending on route of immunization. In Holub, M. and Jaroskova, L. (Eds.): *Mechanism of Antibody Formation.* Prague, Czechoslovak Acad Sci. New York, Grune and Stratton, 1960, p. 79.
22. Smith, R. T., Miescher, P. A. and Good, R. A. (Eds.): *Phylogeny of Immunity.* Gainesville, U Florida Pr, 1966.
23. Sterzl, J. and Riha, M. (Eds.): *Developmental Aspects of Antibody Formation and Structure.* New York, Acad Pr, 1970.
24. Tada, V. and Ishizaka, K.: Distribution of γ E forming cells in lymphoid tissues of human and monkey. *J Immunol, 104:* 377, 1970.
25. Uhr, J. W. and Möller, G.: Regulatory effect of antibody in the immune response. *Adv Immunol, 8:* 81, 1968.

IgA

1. Allansmith, M. and Buell, D.: The relationship of gamma 1A globulin and reagin in cord sera. *J Allergy, 35:* 339, 1964.
2. Chodirker, W. B. and Tomasi, T. B., Jr.: Gamma globulins: Quantitative relationships in human serum and non-vascular fluids. *Science, 142:* 1080, 1963.
3. Collins-Williams, C., Lamenza, C. and Nizami, R.: Immunoglobulin A. A review of the literature. *Ann Allergy, 27:* 225, 1969.
4. Dayton, D. G., Small, P. A., Chaneck, R. M., Kaufman, H. E. and Tomasi, T. B. (Eds.): *The Secretory Immunologic System.* National Institute of Health, Bethesda, Md.
5. Hansen, L. A. and Johansson, B.: Studies on secretory IgA. In Killander, J. (Ed.): *Gamma Globulins* Nobel Symposium 3. New York, Interscience Publications, 1967, pp. 141–151.
6. Heremans, J. F. and Crabbé, P. A.: *Immunohistochemical studies in exocrine IgA.* Nobel Symposium 3. Sodergam, Sweden, 1967.
7. Smith, M. A., Cooper, M., Wollheim, F., Hong, R. and Good, R.: The IgA system. I. Studies of the transport and immunochemistry of IgA in the saliva. *J Exp Med, 123:* 615, 1966.

8. Svehag, S. E. and Bloth, B.: Ultrastructure of secretory and high polymer serum immunoglobulin A of human and rabbit origin. *Science, 168:* 847, 1970.
9. Tada, V. and Ishizaka, K.: Distribution of γ E forming cells in lymphoid tissues of human and monkey. *J Immunol, 104:* 377, 1970.
10. Tomasi, T. B., Tan, E. M., Solomon, A. and Prendergast, R. A.: Characteristics of an immune system common to certain external secretions. *J Exp Med, 121:* 101, 1965.
11. Tomasi, T. B.: The gamma A globulins: First line of defense. *Hosp Prac 2* (No. 7) : 26, 1967.
12. Tomasi, T. B. and Bienenstock, J.: Secretory immunoglobulins. *Adv Immunol, 9:* 1, 1968.
13. Tomasi, T. B.: *Distribution and synthesis of human secretory components.* Conference on Secretory Immune System, Vero Beach, Fla. Dec. 10–13, 1969.
14. Tourville, D. R., Adler, R. H., Bienenstock, J. and Tomasi, T. B.: The human secretory immunoglobulin system: Immunohistological localization of gamma A, secretory "piece" and lactoferrin in normal human tissues. *J Exp Med, 129:* 411, 1969.
15. Vaerman, J. P.: *Studies of IgA immunoglobulin in man and animals.* Université Catholique de Louvain, 1970.
16. Waldman, R. G.: Respiratory secretion antibody mediates protection in viral respiratory tract infection. *Arch Environ Health, 19:* 1, 1969.
17. Waldman, R. H., Mack, J. P., Stella, M. M. and Rowe, D. S.: Secretory IgA in human serum. *J Immunol, 105:* 43, 1970.

IgD

1. Rogentine, H. N., Rowe, D. S., Bradley, J., Waldman, T. A. and Fahey, J. L.: Metabolism of human immunoglobulin D (IgD). *J Clin Invest, 45:* 1467, 1966.
2. Rowe, D. S. and Fahey, J. L.: A new class of human immunoglobulin. II. Normal serum IgD. *J Exp Med, 121:* 185, 1965.
3. Saha, A., Chowdbury, P., Sandbury, S., Behelak, Y., Heiner, D. and Rose, B.: Studies on human IgD. III. Physiological characterization of human IgD. *J Immunol, 105:* 238, 1970.

IgE

1. Aas, K. and Johansson, S. G. O.: The radioallergo-sorbant test (RAST) in the *in vitro* diagnosis of multiple reaginic allergy. A comparison of diagnostic approaches. *J Allergy,* 1971.
2. Austen, K. F. and Humphrey, J. H.: *In vitro* studies on the mechanism of anaphylaxis. *Adv Immunol, 3:* 1, 1963.
3. Bennich, H., Johansson, S. G. O.: *Studies on a new class of human immunoglobulin.* II. Chemical and physical properties. Nobel symposium 3. Sweden, 1967.
4. Bennich, H. and Johansson, S. G. O.: Structure and biological function of human IgE. *Adv Immunol,* 1971.
5. Berg, T. and Johansson, S. G. O.: IgE concentration in children with atopic disease: A clinical study. *Int Arch Allergy Appl Immunol, 36:* 219, 1969.
6. Bozeral, M., Orgel, H. A. and Hamburger, R. N.: IgE levels in normal infants and mothers and inheritance hypothesis. *J Immunol, 107:* 794, 1971.
7. Gleich, G. J., Averbeck, A. K. and Swedland, H. A.: Concentration of IgE in serum of normal and allergic individuals. *J Allergy, 45:* 108, 1970.
8. Ishizaka, K., Ishizaka, T. and Hornbrook, M. M.: Physiochemical properties of reaginic antibody. V. Correlation of reaginic activity with γ E globulin antibody. *J Immunol, 97:* 840, 1966.
9. Ishizaka, K. and Ishizaka, T.: Physiochemical properties of reaginic antibody. I. Association of reaginic activity with immunoglobulin other than γ A or γ G globulin. *J Allergy, 37:* 169, 1966.
10. Ishizaka, K, Ishizaka, T. and Terry, W. D.: Antigenic structure of γ E globulin and reaginic antibody. *J Immunol, 99:* 849, 1967.
11. Ishizaka, K., Ishizaka, T. and Hornbrook, M. M.: Allergen-binding activity of γ E, γ G, γ A antibodies in sera from atopic patients: *In vitro* measurement of reaginic antibody. *J Immunol, 98:* 490, 1967.
12. Ishizaka, K. and Ishizaka, T.: Identification of gamma E antibodies as a carrier of reaginic activity. *J Immunol, 99:* 1187, 1967.
13. Ishizaka, K., Ishizaka, T. and Menzel, A. E. O.: Physiochemical properties of reaginic antibody. VI. Effect of heat on γ E, γ G and γ A antibodies in the sera of ragweed sensitive patients. *J Immunol, 99:* 610, 1967.
14. Ishizaka, K. and Ishizaka, T.: Human reaginic antibodies and immunoglobulin E. *J Allergy, 42:* 330, 1968.
15. Ishizaka, K., Ishizaka, T., Johansson, S. G. O. and Bennich, H.: Histamine release from human leukocytes by anti-IgE. *J Immunol, 102:* 885, 1969.
16. Ishizaka, K. and Newcomb, R. W.: Presence of γ E in nasal washings and sputum from asthmatic patients. *J Allergy, 46:* 197, 1970.

17. Ishizaka, T., Ishizaka, K., Orange, R. P. *et al.:* The capacity of immunoglobulin E to mediate the release of histamine and slow reacting substance of anaphylaxis (SRS-A) from monkey lung. *J Immunol, 104:* 335, 1970.
18. Ishizaka, K. and Ishizaka, T.: Biologic function of γ E antibodies and mechanisms of reaginic hypersensitivity. *Clin Exp Immunol, 6:* 25, 1970.
19. Ishizaka, T., Ishizaka, K., Bennich, H. and Johansson, S. G. O.: Biologic activities of aggregated immunoglobulin E. *J Immunol, 104:* 854, 1970.
20. Ishizaka, T., Tomioka, H. and Ishizaka, K.: Degranulation of human basophil leukocytes by anti γ E antibody. *J Immunol, 106:* 705, 1971.
21. Johansson, S. G. O., Bennich, H. and Wide, W.: A new class of immunoglobulin in human serum. *J Immunol, 14:* 265, 1968.
22. Johansson, S. G. O., Bennich, H., Berg, T. and Høgman, C.: Some factors influencing the serum IgE levels in atopic diseases. *Clin Exp Immunol, 6:* 43, 1970.
23. Kohler, P. F. and Farr, R. S.: Quantitative comparison of immunoglobulins in atopic (reaginic) and non-atopic (non-reaginic) individuals: Higher D levels in atopic sera. *J Allergy, 39:* 311, 1967.
24. Levy, D. A. and Osler, A. G.: Studies on the mechanism of hypersensitivity phenomena. XVI. *In vitro* assays of reaginic activity in human sera: Effect of therapeutic immunization on seasonal titer changes. *J Immunol, 99:* 1068, 1967.
25. Newcomb, R. W. and Ishizaka, K.: Physiochemical and antigenic studies on human γ E in respiratory fluid. *J Immunol, 105:* 85, 1970.
26. Osler, A. G., Lichtenstein, L. M. and Levy, D. A.: *In vitro* studies of human reaginic allergy. *Adv Immunol, 8:* 183, 1968.
27. Osler, A. G.: Immunology of reaginic allergy: *In vitro* studies. *Clin Exp Immunol, 6:* 13, 1970.
28. Reid, R. T.: Reagin activity associated with immunoglobulins other that IgE. *J Immunol, 104:* 935, 1970.
29. Stanville, D. R.: Reaginic antibodies. *Adv Immunol, 3:* 181, 1963.
30. Stanworth, D. R.: IgE and reaginic antibodies. *Proc R Soc Med, 62:* 33, 1969.
31. Stanworth, D. R.: Immunological mechanisms of immediate type hypersensitivity reactions. *Clin Exp Immunol, 6:* 1, 1970.
32. Tada, V. and Ishizaka, K.: Distribution of γ E forming cells in lymphoid tissues of human and monkey. *J Immunol, 104:* 377, 1970.

Mediators

1. Beall, G. N.: Histamine: The view today. *Calif Med, 106:* 296, 1967.
2. Bergstrom, S. and Samuelson, B. (Eds.): *Prostaglandins.* Nobel Symposium 2. New York, Interscience, 1966.
3. Brockelhurst, W. E.: *Histamine and other mediators in hypersensitivity reactions.* Proc III Intern Congr Allergol, 1958, pp. 361–371.
4. Brockelhurst, W. E.: The release of histamine and formation of a slow-reacting substance (SRS-A) during anaphylactic shock. *J Physiol (London), 151:* 416, 1960.
5. Brockelhurst, W. E.: Slow-reacting substance and related compounds. *Progr Allergy, 6:* 539, 1962.
6. Brockelhurst, W. E.: Pharmacological mediators of hypersensitivity reactions. In Gell, P. G. H. and Coombs, R. R. A. (Eds.): *Clinical Aspects of Immunology.* Oxford, Blackwell, 1968, pp. 611–632.
7. Brockelhurst, W. E.: Kinin and kinin-forming enzymes in anaphylaxis. In Austen, K. F. and Becker, E. L.: *Biochemistry of the Acute Allergic Reaction.* Oxford, Blackwell, 1968, pp. 297–302.
8. Brockelhurst, W. E. and Lahiri, S. C.: Formation and destruction of bradykinin during anaphylaxis. *J Physiol (London), 165:* 39, 1962.
9. Cochrane, C. G.: Mediators of the Arthus and related reactions. *Progr Allergy, 11:* 135, 1967.
10. Doeglass, H. M. G. and Nater, J. P.: Histamine in foods causing false positive scratch tests. *J Allergy, 42:* 164, 1968.
11. Dumonde, D. C.: Lymphokines: Molecular mediators of cellular immune responses in animals and man. *Proc R Soc Med, 63:* 899, 1970.
12. Dumonde, D. C.: Lymphokines: Mediators and regulators of cellular immunity. In Miescher, P. A. (Ed.): *VIth Int Sym on Immunopathology.* Schwabe, Basel, 1971.
13. Dumonde, D. C. and Maini, R. N.: The clinical significance of mediators of cellular immunity. *Clin Allergy, 1:* 123, 1971.
14. Editorial. Anaphylactic reactions to tetracyclines. *JAMA, 192:* 150, 1965.
15. Frick, O. L.: Mediators of atopic and anaphylactic reactions. *Pediat Clin North Am, 16:* 95, 1969.
16. Humphrey, J. H.: Biochemical mediators of antigen-antibody reactions. In Brown, E. A. (Ed.): *Allergology.* Oxford, Pergamon, 1962, pp. 71–83.
17. Ishizaka, T., Ishizaka, K., Orange, R. P. *et al:* Release of histamine and slow reacting substance

of anaphylaxis (SRS-A) by γ E system from sensitized monkey lung. *J Allergy, 43:* 168, 1969.
18. Kahlson, G. and Rosengren, E.: Histamine. *Annu Rev Pharmacol, 5:* 305, 1965.
19. Kellermeyer, R. W. and Graham, R. C.: Kinins, possible physiologic and pathologic roles in man. *N Engl J Med, 279:* 754, 1968.
20. *Ibid.,* p. 802.
21. *Ibid.,* p. 859.
22. Kolb, W. P. and Granger, C. A.: Lymphocyte *in vitro* cytotoxicity: Characterization of human lymphotoxin. *Proc Natl Acad Sci USA, 61:* 1250, 1968.
23. Lawrence, H. S. and Landy, M. (Eds.): *Mediators of cellular immunity.* Proceeding of an international conference, Augusta, Mich. New York, Acad Pr, 1969.
24. Levy, D. A. and Osler, A. G.: Studies on the mechanism of hypersensitivity phenomenon. IX. Histamine release from human leukocytes by ragweed pollen antigen. *J Immunol, 97:* 203, 1966.
25. Lichtenstein, L. M. and Osler, A. G.: Studies on the mechanism of hypersensitivity phenomenon. IX. Histamine release from human leukocytes by ragweed pollen antigen. *J Exp Med, 120:* 507, 1964.
26. Maini, R. N., Bryceson, A. D. M., Wolstencroft, R. A. and Dumonde, D. C.: Lymphocyte mutagenic factor in man. *Nature, 224:* 43, 1969.
27. Melam, H., Pruzansky, J. J. and Patterson, R.: Histamine release from leukocytes with antigen E and whole ragweed extract. *J Allergy, 45:* 43, 1970.
28. Melmon, K. L. and Cline, M. J.: Kinins. *Am J Med, 43:* 153, 1967.
29. Nelson, D. S.: Immune adherence. *Adv Immunol, 3:* 131, 1963.
30. Noah, J. W. and Brand, A.: Release of histamine in the blood of ragweed-sensitive individuals. *J Allergy, 25:* 210, 1954.
31. Page, I. H.: *Serotonin. Year Bk Med,* Chicago, 1968.
32. Schachter, M.: Introduction to kinins: A group of vasoactive peptides. *Fed Proc, 27:* 49, 1968.
33. Wolstencroft, R. A., Matthew, M., Oates, C. M., Maini, R. N. and Dumonde, D. C.: Lymphocyte mitogenic factor in cell mediated immunity. In Dumonde, D. C. (Ed.): *The role of lymphocytes and macrophages in the immunological response.* Symp XIII Intl Cong Haemot. Berlin, Springer, 1970.
34. Wolstenholme, G. E. W. and O'Connor, C. M. (Eds.): *Ciba Foundation Symposium on Histamine.* London, Churchill, 1956.

Ag-Ab Complex

1. Barkin, G. D. and McGovern, J. P.: Anaphylaxis and serum sickness allergy statistics. *Ann Allergy, 24:* 602, 1966.
2. Cannon, P. R. and Marshall, C. E.: Studies on the mechanism of Arthus phenomenon. *J Immunol, 40:* 127, 1941.
3. Cochrane, C. G. and Koppler, D.: Immune complex in disease. *Adv Immunol, 14,* 1971.
4. Cochrane, C. G. and Hawkins, D.: Studies on circulating immune complexes. III. Factors governing the ability of circulating complexes to localize in blood vessels. *J Exp Med, 127:* 137, 1968.
5. Cochrane, C. G.: The role of immune complexes and complement in tissue injury. *J Allergy, 42:* 113, 1968.
6. Dixon, F. J., Vasquez, J. J., Weigle, W. O. and Cochrane, C. G.: Pathogenesis of serum sickness. *Arch Pathol, 65:* 18, 1958.
7. Dixon, F. J.: The role of antigen-antibody complexes in disease. *Harvey Lect, 58:* 21, 1962–63.
8. Dixon, F. J.: The role of antigen-antibody complexes in disease. *Harvey Lect, 58:* 21, 1968.
9. Eisen, H. N.: The immune response to a single antigenic determinant. *Harvey Lect, 60:* 1, 1966.
10. Feinstein, A. and Rowe, A. J.: Molecular mechanism of formation of an antigen-antibody complex. *Nature, 205:* 147, 1965.
11. Kabat, E. A.: The nature of an antigenic determinant. *J Immunol, 97:* 1, 1966.
12. Sela, M.: Structure and specificity of synthetic polypeptide antigens. *Ann N Y Acad Sci, 169:* 23, 1970.
13. Weigle, W. O.: Fate and biological action of antigen-antibody complexes. *Adv Immunol, 1:* 283, 1961.
14. Weigle, W. O. and Dixon, F. J.: Relationship of circulating antigen-antibody complexes, antigen elimination and complement in serum sickness. *Proc Soc Exp Biol Med, 99:* 226, 1958.

Complement

1. Austen, K. F.: Inborn errors of the complement system of man. *N Engl J Med, 276:* 1363, 1967.
2. Cochrane, C. G.: The role of immune complexes and complement in tissue injury. *J Allergy, 42:* 113, 1968.
3. Complement workshop: Nomenclature of complement. *Immunochemistry, 3:* 495, 1966.
4. Gewurz, H., Pickering, R. J., Clark, D. S. *et al:* The complement system in prevention, mediation and diagnosis of disease and its useful-

ness in the determination of immunopathogenetic mechanisms. Immunologic deficiency diseases in man. In Bergsma, D. and Good, R. A. (Eds.): *Birth Defects Original Articles Series.* New York, The National Foundation, 1968, p. 596.
5. Humphrey, J. H. and Dourmashkin, R. R.: The lesions in cell membranes caused by complement. *Adv Immunol, 11:* 75, 1969.
6. Mayer, M.: Mechanism of hemolysis by complement. In Wolstenholme, G. E. W. and Knight, J. (Eds.): *Ciba Foundation Symposium on Complement.* Boston, Little, 1965, p. 4.
7. Müller-Eberhard, H. J.: Chemistry and reaction mechanisms of complement. *Adv Immunol, 8:* 1, 1968.
8. Müller-Eberhard, H. J.: Complement. *Annu Rev Biochem, 38:* 389, 1969.
9. Nelson, R. A., Jr.: The role of complement in immune phenomena. In Zweibach, B. W. *et al.: The Inflammatory Process.* New York, Acad Pr, 1965, p. 819.
10. Osler, A. G.: Functions of the complement system. *Adv Immunol, 1:* 131, 1961.
11. Yachnin, S.: Functions and mechanisms of action of complement. *N Engl J Med, 274:* 140, 1966.

Thymus

1. Archer, O. K. and Pierce, J. C.: Role of thymus in development of immune response. *Fed Proc, 20:* 26, 1961.
2. Arnason, B. G., Jankovic, B. D. and Waksman, B. H.: A survey of the thymus and its relation to lymphocytes and immune reactions. *Blood, 20:* 617, 1962.
3. Arnason, B. G., Jankovic, B. D. and Waksman, B. H.: Effect of thymectomy on delayed hypersensitivity reactions. *Nature, 194:* 99, 1962.
4. Burnet, Sir MacFarlane: The immunological significance of the thymus. *Aust Ann Med, 11:* 79, 1962.
5. Ciba Foundation Symposium: *The Thymus: Experimental and clinical studies.* London Churchill, 1966, pp. 360–380.
6. Claman, H. N., Chaperon, E. A. and Selner, J. C.: Thymus-marrow immunocompetence. II. The requirement for living thymus cells. *Proc Soc Exp Biol Med, 127:* 462, 1968.
7. Claman, H. N. and Chaperon, E. A.: Immunological complementation between thymus and marrow cells: A model for the two-cell theory of immunocompetence. *Transplant Rev, 1:3,* 1969.

8. Davies, A. J. S.: The thymus and the cellular basis of immunity. *Transplant Rev, 1:* 43, 1969.
9. Gershon, R. K., Wallis, V., Davies, A. J. S. and Leuchars, E.: Inactivation of thymus cells by antigen. *Nature 218:* 380, 1968.
10. Good, R. A. and Gabrielson, A. E. (Eds.): *The Thymus in Immunobiology.* New York, Harper & Row, 1964.
11. Good, R. A. and Papermaster, B. W.: Ontogeny and phylogeny of adaptive immunity. *Adv Immunol, 4:* 1, 1964.
12. Miller, J. F. A. P., Marshall, A. H. E. and White, R. G.: Immunological significance of the thymus. *Adv Immunol, 2:* 111, 1962.
13. Miller, J. F. A. P. and Osoba, D.: Role of the thymus in the origin of immunological competence. In Wolstenholme, G. E. W. and Knight, J. (Eds.): *The Immunologically Competent Cell: Its Nature and Origin.* Ciba Foundation Study Group No. 16. London, Churchill, 1963, p. 62.
14. Miller, J. F. A. P. and Osoba, D.: Current concepts of the imunological function of the thymus. *Physiol Rev, 47:* 437, 1967.
15. Miller, J. F. A. P.: The thymus yesterday, today and tomorrow. *Lancet, 2:* 1299, 1967.
16. Wolstenholme, G. E. W. and Knight, J. (Eds.): *Hormones and the Immune Response.* Ciba Foundation Study Group No. 36. London, Churchill, 1970.

Delayed Hypersensitivity (DH)

1. Benacerraf, B. and Green, I.: Cellular hypersensitivity. *Annu Rev Med, 20:* 141, 1969.
2. Benacerraf, B. and Gell, P. G. H.: Immunological specificity of delayed and immediate hypersensitivity reactions. In Grabar, P. and Miescher, P. A. (Eds.): *Mechanism of Cell and Tissue Damage Produced by Immune Reactions.* Basel, Schwabe, 1962, pp. 136–145.
3. Bloom, B. R. and Chase, M. W.: Transfer of delayed-type hypersensitivity: A critical review and experimental study on the guinea pig. *Progr Allergy, 10:* 131, 1967.
4. Brostoff, J., Greaves, M. E. and Roitl, T. M.: Cellular hypersensitivity in patients with summer hay fever. *Lancet, 1:* 803, 1969.
5. Crowle, A. J.: *Delayed Hypersensitivity in Health and Disease.* Springfield, Thomas, 1962.
6. David, J. R., Lawrence, H. S. and Thomas, L.: Delayed hypersensitivity *in vitro:* II. Effect of sensitive cells on normal cells in the presence of antigen. *J Immunol, 93:* 274, 1964.

7. David, J. R.: Delayed hypersensitivity *in vitro* and its mediation by cell-free substances formed by lymphoid cell-antigen interaction. *Proc Natl Acad Sci USA, 56:* 72, 1966.
8. Flax, M. H. and Caulfield, J. B.: Cellular and vascular components of allergic contact dermatitis. *Am J Pathol, 43:* 1031, 1963.
9. Gell, P. G. H. and Benacerraf, B.: Delayed hypersensitivity to simple protein antigens. *Adv Immunol, 1:* 332, 1961.
10. Mackness, G. B. and Blanden, R. V.: Cellular immunity. *Progr Allergy, 11:* 89, 1967.
11. Turk, J. L.: Delayed hypersensitivity: Specific cell-mediated immunity. *Br Med Bull, 23:* 1, 1967.
12. Uhr, J. W.: Delayed hypersensitivity. *Physiol Rev, 46:* 359, 1966.
13. Wolstenholme, G. E. W. and Knight, J. (Eds.): *Hormones and the Immune Response.* Ciba Foundation Study Group No. 36. London, Churchill, 1970.

Tolerance

1. Ada, G. L.: Antigen binding cells in tolerance and immunity. *Transplant Rev, 5:* 105, 1970.
2. DeWeck, A. L. and Frey, J. R.: *Immunotolerance to simple chemicals:* Hypersensitivity to simple chemicals as a model for the study of immunological tolerance. Monographs in Allergy, No. 1 American Elsevier, New York, 1966.
3. Diener, E. and Armstrong, W. D.: The induction of immunity and tolerance *in vitro*. *Lancet, 16:* 1281, 1967.
4. Diener, E., Shortman, K. and Russell, P.: Induction of immunity and tolerance *in vitro* in absence of phagocytic cells. *Nature, 225:* 731, 1970.
5. Diener, E. and Feldman, M.: Antibody mediated suppression of the immune response *in vitro*. II. A new approach to the phenomenon of immunological tolerance. *J Exp Med, 132:* 31, 1970.
6. Diener, E., Feldman, M. and Armstrong, W. D.: Induction *in vitro* of immunological tolerance to the H-antigens of Salmonella adelaide in immunological tolerance to microbial antigens. *Ann N Y Acad Sci, 181:* 119, 1971.
7. Dresser, D. W. and Mitchison, N. A.: The mechanism of immunological paralysis. *Adv Immunol, 8:* 129, 1968.
8. Feldman, M. and Diener, E.: Antibody-mediated inhibition of the immune response *in vitro*. I. Evidence for a central effect. *J Exp Med, 131:* 247, 1970.
9. Immunological tolerance to microbial antigens. *Ann N Y Acad Sci, 181,* 1971.
10. Landy, M. and Brown, W. (Eds.): Immunological tolerance. *Perspectives in Immunology: Series of Publications Based on Symposia.* New York, Acad Pr, 1969.
11. Miescher, P. A. and Müller-Eberhard, H. J. (Eds.): Immunologic unresponsiveness. In *Textbook of Immunology.* New York, Grune, 1968.
12. Mitchison, N. A.: Immunological paralysis as a dosage phenomenon. In Proc Sym: *Regulation of the Antibody Response.* Springfield, Thomas, 1967.
13. Mitchison, N. A.: The ability of T and B lymphocytes to see protein antigens. In Cross, A. (Ed.): *Third Sigrid Juselius Foundation Symposium on Cell Cooperation in the Immune Response.* New York, Acad Pr, 1970.
14. Nossal, G. J. V.: Immunological tolerance: A new model system for low zone induction. *Ann N Y Acad Sci, 129:* 822, 1966.
15. Nossal, G. J. V. and Mitchell, J.: The thymus in relation to immunological tolerance. In *Thymus, Experimental and Clinical Studies.* Ciba Foundation Symposium. London, Churchill, 1966.
16. Rowley, D. A., Fitch, F. W., Axelrad, M. A. and Pierce, C. W.: The immune response suppressed by specific antibody. *Immunology, 16:* 549, 1969.
17. Shellam, G. R. and Nossal, G. J. V.: Mechanism of induction of immunological tolerance. IV. The effects of ultra-low doses of flagellin. *Immunology, 14:* 273, 1968.
18. Triplett, E. L.: On the mechanism of immunologic self recognition. *J Immunol, 89:* 505, 1962.

Transfer Factor

1. Kempe, C. H.: Studies in smallpox and complications of smallpox vaccination. *Pediatrics, 26:* 176, 1960.
2. Lawrence, H. S.: Transfer factor. *Adv Immunol, 11:* 195, 1969.
3. Lawrence, H. S. and Valentine, F. T.: Transfer factor and other mediators of cellular immunity. *Am J. Pathol, 60:* 437, 1970.
4. Lawrence, H. S.: Transfer factor and cellular immune deficiency disease. *N Engl J Med, 283:* 411, 1970.
5. Levin, A. S., Stites, D. P., Spitler, L. E. *et al.:* Induction of "delayed hypersensitivity" in a Wiscott-Aldrich patient by transfer factor. *Clin Res, 18:* 428, 1970.
6. Paque, R. E., Kniskern, P. J., Dray, S. and Baram, P.: *In vitro* studies with transfer factor: Transfer of the cell migration inhibition correlate of delayed hypersensitivity in humans with cell lysates from humans sensitized to histoplasmin, coccidioidin or PPD. *J Immunol, 103:* 1014, 1969.

Chapter 2

ALLERGIC DISEASES OF THE UPPER RESPIRATORY TRACT

ALLERGIC DISEASE of the upper respiratory tract is rarely, if ever an involvement of a single structure such as the nose, the throat, the sinuses, *etc.* Involvement is usually all inclusive for the region, so that an evaluation of the signs and symptoms for purposes of diagnosis and treatment should consider all of the following structures:

(1) the nose
(2) the throat—including Waldeyer's ring of lymphoid tissue; and palate and uvula
(3) the sinuses
(4) the eustachian tubes
(5) the middle ear
(6) the eyes (see Chapter 3, Allergic Diseases of the Eye).

Each of these structures will be discussed briefly before considering the signs, symptoms, diagnosis and treatment of the anatomical region, which will be treated collectively as a unit.

The Nose

Allergic Rhinitis
Hay Fever
Polyps

Histology of the Nose

The nasal mucosa presents the following histological divisions:
(1) the epithelium
(2) the basement membrane
(3) the tunica propria or subepithelial layer.

(1) The epithelial layer consists of ciliated, columnar, supporting columnar and goblet cells which rest upon a basement membrane.

(2) The basement membrane is a collagenous layer with fine openings (canaliculi) which permit the passage of leukocytes and tissue fluids into the epithelial layer.

(3) The tunica propria or subepithelial layer has a dense network of capillaries immediately below the basement membrane. Below this capillary layer are mucus and seromucus glands, and then a layer carrying the larger vessels and the cavernous sinuses which form the erectile tissue. A network of connective tissue supports these structures. Scattered throughout the connective tissue and paricularly near the vessels and seromucus glands are cellular elements, such as lymphocytes, plasma cells, polymorphonuclear leukocytes and mast cells.

Under normal conditions mucus is produced, chiefly by the seromucus glands. The goblet cells contribute only a fraction of the mucus.

The Pathology of Nasal Allergic Disease (Allergic Rhinitis and Hay Fever)

In the allergic individual, IgE or reaginic antibody is attached to the mast cells distributed throughout the connective tissue of the tunica propria. The interaction of reaginic antibody with its specific allergen causes histamine to be released from the mast cells. The histamine acts upon the capillary network to produce dilatation and increased permeability. Since the dense network lies immediately below the basement membrane in the tunica propria, their dilatation causes an erythema which may be observed as a blushing or redness of the mucosa. However, the erythema is very transitory as it is blotted out by the pallor produced by the edema resulting from the increased transudation of plasma fluids into the tissue spaces. Edema may be very slight and barely perceptible, or very marked, producing a high degree of swelling with resulting obstruction of the airways. Edema is most pronounced in the turbinates which may entirely fill the air passages and press upon the septum.

In extreme involvement, the tissue fluids pass through the canaliculi in the basement membrane to the epithelial cells which become very swollen. At this stage the nasal mucosa has a bluish pallor. At times the turbinates may appear violaceous or almost blue. Very rarely, edema may be so severe as to cause blanching of the turbinates.

The stimulation of glands produces a liberal quantity of seromucoid exudate which drops posteriorly as "postnasal drip" and anteriorly as nasal discharge.

In the very acute allergic reaction, such as occurs with the seasonal symptoms of hay fever which is induced by pollens, the exudate is predominantly serous and therefore thin and less viscid than with the chronic involvement. The profuse serous exudate causes redness of the nares and frequently excoriation.

Intense itching of the nose, the palate and the throat, accompanied by paroxysms of sneezing and conjunctival involvement form the basic pattern of complaints for hay fever. At times itching is referred to the ear canals and the eustachian tube.

On microscopic examination of the nasal secretions, eosinophils are frequently but *not* consistently observed.

The above pattern constitutes the basic response in uncomplicated nasal allergy. When the allergic episode is of short duration, several days or several weeks, as is encountered in seasonal hay fever, there is reversal of the nasal pathology with a complete restitution of the tissues.

Variations in the basic pattern of allergic rhinitis may occur because of alterations in the mucosa induced by:

(1) climatic factors
(2) perennial allergic edema either intermittent or constant
(3) inhalation of irritating vapors, chemicals, dust or tobacco smoke
(4) recurrent chronic infection
(5) the persistent use of topical medications or nasal sprays
(6) infection.

Any of the above factors may produce histologic changes of variable degrees, characterized by epithelial hypertrophy and hyperplasia; distention of the goblet cells which are greatly increased in number, and fibrosis of the submucosa. The regenerative capacity of the nasal mucosa is comparable to that observed in the skin. As a result, after removal of the irritant following brief periods of exposure, there is complete restitution of the mucosa. With chronic persistent irritation, the mucosa becomes thickened and appears reddened. Because of the thickened mucosa, edema is not apparent but may be replaced by a reddened, thickened mucosa which in longstanding cases may even appear atrophic.

With persistent irritation the greatly increased number of goblet cells remains as a source of copious mucoid discharge. With infection the discharge is purulent; crusts representing dried secretion may be present. With marked atrophy very little discharge may be present.

Nasal Obstruction in Allergic Rhinitis and Hay Fever

Obstruction is not necessarily an index to the degree of edema. Anatomical factors such as the size of the nose, deviation of the septum, or septal spurs may contribute to obstruction.

Noses differ greatly in size. A small nose has a relatively narrow airway, so that even a slight increment of edema or a small amount of discharge may produce annoying obstruction. This is particularly true in young children. An infant may experience considerable difficulty breathing through its nose with only a slight allergic reaction. As the child grows older and the nasal passages become larger, the same degree of allergic response may cause less discomfort. At times, this is misinterpreted as "growing out" of the allergy.

A markedly deviated septum or a spur may impinge upon an airway so that only a slight increment of edema will cause obstruction.

At times obstruction may shift or alter with a change in position. Such changes are usually secondary to a shift of edema fluid. Not infrequently upon arising in the morning a patient may experience a feeling of nasal obstruction. This may be secondary to a hydrostatic shift or a change in body temperature which may serve as a nonspecific excitant to trigger mucosal edema.

The deepest level of the tunica propria contains the large blood vessels and the cavernous sinuses which constitute the erectile tissue. Engorgement of these tissues may explain the obstruction frequently experienced with nonallergic conditions, such as emotional states, the menses and pregnancy. In this situation the fullness of the nose is accompanied by the reddish color of engorgement rather than the pallor of allergic edema. Antihistamine drugs are ineffective in these cases.

Nasal Polyps

The exact cause of nasal polyps is not known, although it is generally recognized that nasal polyps are more frequently associated with allergy, while infection is the agent of second importance. However, recent studies implicate a nonallergic mechanism as a common cause of nasal polyposis.

Aspirin, indomethacin and tartrazine (FD&C yellow #5) have been implicated as nonallergic factors (see discussion on aspirin sensitivity, Chapter 10).

Polyps seem to arise from edema secondary to permeability of the capillaries in the submucosal capillary network. The tissue spaces between the individual connective tissue fibers become filled with fluid to such a degree that the stroma can no longer resist the pressure of the edema fluid, resulting in prolapse and polyp formation.

Usually only the connective tissue stroma of the capillary layer is involved, with the result that the polyp is made up of an epithelial covered sac of myxomatous tissue with edema fluid. In these cases the polyps have a grayish or slightly amber, glistening appearance.

At times the glandular layer or even the lower vascular layer may be involved in the prolapse, so that the polyp may have a more mucoid content, or even appear vascular.

When infection is a concomitant factor in the inflammatory reaction, the polyp may gain a reddened, crinkled, granular surface which is frequently coated with muco-pus or pus.

Although edema is an important factor in the development of polyps, there is no correlation between degree or persistence of edema and the development of polyps. Individuals with only moderate edematous reaction of the mucosa may develop polyps while some with severe mucosal edema show no incidence of polyposis. The development of polyps also shows no relation with the persistence of edema.

The development of polyps seems to bear a great relationship to histological variations in the mucosa and to infection. In some individuals the mucosa may be thinner, and rather loosely attached, predisposing to greater distention and prolapse by edema fluid. This loose characteristic of the mucosa as a predisposing factor perhaps explains the high incidence of polyposis in the middle meatus and in the ethmoid regions where the mucosa is usually thinner and more loosely attached.

Infection may produce mucosal changes which predispose to polyp formation.

Diagnosis: Polyps are usually visible on nasal inspection. It may be necessary at times to shrink the mucosa to permit adequate visualization. At times only multiple cysts may be observed involving the tips of the turbinates.

The Throat

I. *The Pharyngeal Lymphoid Structures (Waldeyer's Ring)*

The pharyngeal lymphatic ring of Waldeyer, which is situated at the proximal end of the gullet, represents the uppermost portion of the Gut Associated Lymphoid Tissue (GALT) System. This group of lymphoid tissue is involved in the formation of antibody.

Waldeyer's ring includes:

(1) The lateral pharyngeal bands
(2) the pharyngeal granulations
(3) the lingual tonsils
(4) the palatine tonsils
(5) the adenoids or pharyngeal tonsil.

(1) The lateral pharyngeal bands occupy the angles formed by the tonsils and the post-pharyngeal wall. They can be seen on direct examination of the throat. These structures are frequently mistaken for the *adenoid*.

(2) The pharyngeal granulations are clusters of lymphoid tissue situated on the post-pharyngeal wall between the two lateral pharyngeal bands. The other lymphoid structures are collections of dense masses of lymphoid cells.

(3) The lingual tonsils are situated on either side of the base of the tongue.

(4) The tonsils are oval masses occupying the fossae formed by the anterior and posterior pillars. They are made up of masses of lymphoid cells with actively mitotic germinal centers. The mesial surface is covered with stratified epithelium which convolutes into deep folds in order to cover the deep crypts usually present in the tonsil.

(5) The adenoid or pharyngeal tonsil occupies a variable area of the roof and posterior wall of the nasopharynx. Unless it is considerably enlarged, it is visible only with a laryngoscopic mirror. The adenoid is formed of three or more masses of lymphoid tissue, but the most common pattern is that of a central body and two lateral lymphoid groupings separated by vertical clefts which correspond to tonsilar crypts.

All the lymphoid structures are prominent from birth until puberty at which time they begin to involute, so that in adult life they do not present the conspicuous lymphoid pattern of childhood. The involvement of the pharyngeal lymphoid masses contributes an important part to the pattern of allergic disease of the upper respiratory tract.

The activity of the immunological response induces hyperplasia and hypertrophy of the tissues, but the edema resulting from the antigen-antibody interaction is the most important feature of lymphoid involvement.

Edema can cause a marked increase in size of the tonsil, which at times may project into the fauces often meeting in the midline to produce obstruction and interference with deglutition. With edema the tonsils lose their deep cryptic character, appear pale, boggy, with a crinkled surface coated with glistening mucus.

The edematous adenoid may be large enough to fill the entire nasopharyngeal space, causing nasal obstruction which induces mouth breathing. At times the adenoid can be enlarged sufficiently to protrude below the margin of the soft palate. When this happens the adenoid is readily seen upon examination of the throat.

Obstruction by the edematous adenoid in the child is responsible for the so-called adenoid facies characterized by pallor, pinching of the nose, staring of the eyes, shortening of the upper lip and the open fish-like mouth. Many clinicians attribute the high arched palate resulting in dental malocclusion to adenoid obstruction. Orthodontists do not agree with this explanation for the dental malocclusion.

After puberty and particularly in the adult, the marked edema of the tonsils and the adenoid with the ensuing obstructive features are not observed as commonly. At this stage the tonsils may be small and atrophic. Because of chronic fibrosis and scarring, they are unable to respond with edema. As a result they do not present the characteristic pallor observed with allergic involvement in childhood.

At all ages the lateral pharyngeal bands are involved. Hypertrophy and edema may result in increased size, so that at times these structures are mistaken for extensions of the adenoid. They have special importance when they impinge upon the eustachian ostiae to produce ear symptoms.

The pharyngeal granulations are also involved in the allergic reactions at all ages. Their increase in size is variable, but very commonly they produce the hobnail appearance of the post-pharyngeal wall which is particularly characteristic of acute and chronic allergic involvement. At times these granulations may appear confluent to resemble an adenoid mass in the posterior wall of the oropharynx.

Following adeno-tonsillectomy, granulations of the pharyngeal wall become particularly prominent, perhaps manifesting a compensatory response of the immune reaction for lost lymphoid tissue.

II. The Palate and Fauces

The hard palate, as has been mentioned, is frequently high arched and narrowed. Most pediatricians consider this to be secondary to nasal obstruction usually of allergic origin.

The soft palate is frequently pale and covered with glistening mucus.

The fauces are commonly edematous. In chronic involvement the margins of the fauces may appear thickened and reddened.

The uvula is very frequently edematous and elongated. A long, tapered, pale uvula is highly suggestive of chronic postnasal drip. It suggests the appearance of an icicle which becomes elongated with the constant drip of water frozen at the tip.

The Sinuses

The sinus mucosal lining is a continuation of the nasal mucosa. In the sinuses the mucosa is thinner and more loosely attached than in the nose. Glands in the sinuses are fewer than in the nose except at the ostiae where there is a greater distribution of glands in a very loosely attached mucosa. This is a very important feature in the production of symptoms in sinus involvement. The anatomical structure at the ostiae predisposes to edema which leads to obstruction of the ostiae which in turn is manifested either as localized pain or headache or both (see Symptomatology).

In children the degree of sinus development will influence the clinical pattern. At birth only the maxillary and ethmoidal sinuses are developed, while the frontal pneumatizes during the first or second year of life. At three years of age the sphenoid begins to develop.

Eustachian Tube and Middle Ear

Since allergic involvement of the eustachian tubes and middle ears is rarely an isolated manifestation, the discussion of these organs is included with Allergic Diseases of the Upper Respiratory Tract.

Eustachian Tube

The eustachian tube serves as the communication between the middle ear and the naso-pharynx for the entrance of air into the middle ear, an essential for normal hearing function.

The mucosa of the cartilaginous portion of the eustachian tube is a continuation of the nasal mucosa. It has identical pseudostratified ciliated columnar epithelium with numerous goblet cells. The substantia propria at the pharyngeal end is loose and complex, containing a capillary network, seromucus glands and numerous lymphocytes. As the tube approaches the tympanic cavity the mucosa becomes thinner so that in the long portion, the epithelium is a single layer of cuboidal cells with a thin fibrous substantia propria which is very intimately attached to the periosteum. At times the fibrous layer is indistinguishable from the periosteum.

The thickness of the mucosa, as well as the number of mucus glands, goblet cells and lymphocytes varies from individual to individual, which may contribute to the variation in the allergic patterns observed.

Lymphoid tissue is distributed freely at the pharyngeal orifice, at times forming the tubal tonsil.

These structural characteristics of the pharyngeal end of the auditory canal, i.e. the thick loose mucosa and the lymphoid tissue, are susceptible to hyperplasia and edema induced by the allergic reaction with resulting obstruction of the ostiae. By virtue of the anatomy, it is understandable that the obstruction of the eustachian orifice with resulting tubal dysfunction is a common complication of allergic involvement of the nasopharynx. *This* occurs particularly in children, and most commonly between the ages of four to six years.

Eustachian dysfunction is responsible for two important conditions:

(1) impaired hearing
(2) serous otitis.

Eustachian obstruction is an important cause of hearing impairment. In children the hearing impairment, which is often overlooked may be responsible for delayed development of speech, poor performance at school, short attention span and at times even misinterpreted as mental retardation.

Although the etiology of serous otitis remains unproven, recent experimental evidence supports the contention that the condition arises secondary to obstruction of the eustachian orifice. Recent studies indicate that over 20 per cent of allergic children suffer from eustachian dysfunction. With such a high incidence it is important that the condition be ruled out in all allergic children.

The Middle Ear

Middle ear involvement is a common accompaniment of allergic tubo-tympanitis, which in turn is very frequently associated with allergic involvement of the upper respiratory tract.

The Tympanic Cavity (Middle Ear)

The tympanic cavity is lined with simple squamous epithelium except near the membrane tympanicum, the opening of the auditory tube, where it is cuboidal in character. The mucosa, like that of the long portion of the eustachian tube of which it is a continuation, is firmly attached to the bone. There are no glands reported in the tympanic cavity. It may be because of these anatomical features that no primary allergic involvement of the tympanic cavity has been reported. Secondary implication of the tympanic cavity is a common observation in upper respiratory allergic disease. This usually follows obstruction of the eustachian tube at its ostiae. Because of the prevalence of lymphoid tissue about the eustachian ostiae in allergic children, disease of the tympanic cavity such as otitis media and serous otitis occur quite frequently. Obstruction of the eustachian tube restricts drainage which predisposes to infection of the middle ear.

Obstruction also causes a decrease in air pressure within the middle ear, resulting in the flow of plasma elements from the vessels to the tympanic cavity to be manifested as *serous otitis*.

Anatomy of the Tympanic Membrane (Ear Drum) (MT)

The tympanic membrane consists of two layers of collagenous fibers and fibroblasts except for Shrapnell's membrane which is a flaccid portion of the tympani in the anterior superior quadrant, which contains no collagen.

The inner surface of the MT is covered by the mucus membrane of the tympanic cavity. It consists of simple squamous epithelium which lies upon a lamina propria of sparse collagen fibers and capillaries. The mucosa is firmly attached to the submucosa.

The external surface of the MT is covered by a thin layer of skin devoid of hair and other appendages. The external epithelial layer, as compared with the internal mucosal lining is loosely attached so that any involvement of the MT results in its separation from the submucosa.

Although primary allergic involvement of the MT has not been reported, vesicular and bullous lesions of the external surface are not an unusual accompaniment of allergic disease of the ear. It is likely that instead of the wheal formation of urticaria, the edema fluid of the allergic reaction causes a separation of the loosely attached epithelial layer which is viewed either as vesicles or bullae on otoscopic examination. The sudden development of such lesions is accompanied by excrutiating pain, while in cases with a gradual onset, the patient may experience no symptoms. In this case, the lesions are detected during a routine ear examination.

The vesicles and bullae are difficult to differentiate from those observed with viral infections. In most cases the content of the lesions is straw color and serous, while in viral infection they are more commonly violaceous in hue or hemorrhagic with dilated vessels on the surface. In those accompanying the allergic reaction, pain may be the only complaint; there is no fever or other evidence of infection. However, examination of the nose and throat is usually typical of allergic involvement.

In chronic allergic involvement of the eustachian tube, the MT may lose its normal luster, appear retracted, have a disturbed light reflex, and manifest thickening from scarring. Calcareous deposits may be present, particularly in adults with longstanding tubo-tympanitis. Such changes in the MT should suggest chronic tubo-tympanitis on an allergic basis.

Allergic Laryngitis

See discussion of the Allergic Patient, Chapter 13.

Diagnosis

The diagnosis of allergic disease of the upper respiratory tract is made upon the patient's history and the physical findings.

The history should attempt to establish that the patient is an allergic individual (see Chapter 13, The Allergic Patient). It is important to determine whether symptoms are perennial, perennial with seasonal exacerbations or purely seasonal. When seasonal, the date of onset and duration of symptoms are important.

When symptoms are acute the physical findings are commonly those of classical allergic rhinitis or hay fever, characterized by pallor and edema of the mucosa with turgescence of the turbinates. Serous or seromucoid discharge is usually present.

When symptoms are of long standing, even acute exacerbations may not manifest the classical pattern of pallor and edema. In such cases very often the mucosa is reddened and at times even thickened with only slight to moderate enlargement of the turbinates. In these patients examination of the throat can be helpful in establishing a diagnosis. In children and in younger individuals, involvement of the lymphoid structures of Waldeyer's ring by edema and pallor are suggestive of allergic involvement. In older individuals the lymphoid hyperplasia is usually not quite as prominent.

The fauces are usually edematous and glistening, while the uvula is most often succulent. The uvula may be elongated and tapered or normal in length with a nob-like hypertrophic tip. Both patterns are suggestive of irritation induced by chronic postnasal drip.

The presence of mucoid strands bridging the airways of the nose, in the absence of infection, is suggestive of allergic involvement. The presence of copious mucoid discharge over the post-pharyngeal wall is supportive evidence for allergic involvement, while muco-purulent postnasal secretions indicate the presence of infection either primarily or as a complicating factor.

A complaint of a profuse watery nasal discharge which fails to respond to treatment with antihistamines and at times even to moderate doses of corticosteroids is suggestive of a reaction to (1) aspirin or other salicylates, (2) indomethacin, and (3) tartrazine (FD&C yellow #5). The patient complains that the nose seems like a drippy faucet. Usually there is no accompanying paroxysmal sneezing and no excoriation as observed with hay fever. Investigation for the offending agents and their elimination can lead to a dramatic response. Since the mechanism is not allergic, skin testing is of no diagnostic value for the identification of these factors. (See discussion of Aspirin Sensitivity and Food Colorings.)

The presence of enlarged cervical lymph nodes, particularly at the angles of the jaw, usually indicates infection.

Both the history and the physical examination should not be limited to an isolated segment of the upper respiratory tract but should include the entire region, even the findings in the ears and the eyes.

Skin testing can offer supportive evidence for the diagnosis, but on the basis of skin testing alone a diagnosis of allergic disease is hazardous.

Laboratory Tests: Nasal smears for eosinophils are not reliable; a negative nasal smear for eosinophils does not exclude allergic rhinitis.

Roentgenograms of the sinuses may show chronic thickening of the mucosa which is presumptive but not positive evidence of allergic involvement.

Treatment

Treatment of acute symptoms involves control of offending factors when they can be identified and medication with antihistamines and nasal decongestants (see Chapter 15, Drugs Used In Treatment of Allergic Disease).

Nasal sprays or topical therapy to the nose is not recommended. The irritation and rebound may aggravate the condition.

For patients with very acute symptoms, such as encountered with seasonal hay fever, a short course with corticosteroids may be indicated when (1) the patient can not be controlled with antihistamines, and (2) when the patient with acute symptoms presents himself during the pollinating season which does not permit complete evaluation and specific immunotherapy. See discussion of steroids in Chapter 15 for schedule of dosage and treatment pattern.

During the period of intermission patients with acute exacerbations and hay fever should be investigated thoroughly to determine the causative factors. When indicated, immunotherapy should be instituted. A similar program of study should be applied to patients with perennial symptoms.

REFERENCES

1. Ash, J. E. and Baum, Muriel.: *An Atlas of Otolaryngic Pathology*. Published under joint sponsorship of The Academy of Ophthalmology and Otolaryngology; The American Registry of Pathology; The Armed Forces Institute of Pathology. Washington, D.C., 1956.
2. Ballenger, J. J.: *Diseases of the Nose, Throat and Ears*. Philadelphia, Lea & Febiger, 1969.
3. Baxter, J. D. and Rose, B.: The histaminic content of allergic and nonallergic human nasal membrane with simultaneous observations on eosinophils. *J Allergy* 24: 18, 1953.
4. Becker, Walter: *Atlas of Otorhinolaryngology and Bronchoesophagology*. Philadelphia, Saunders, 1969.

5. Bloom, W. and Fawcett, D. W.: Textbook of Histology, 8th ed. Philadelphia, Saunders, 1962.
6. Cocoa, Arthur F., Walzer, Matthew and Thommen, August A.: *Asthma and Hay Fever in Theory and Practice.* Springfield, Thomas, 1931.
7. Connell, J. T.: Quantitative intranasal pollen challenge II. Effect of daily pollen challenge, environmental pollen exposure and placebo challenge on the nasal membrane. *J Allergy, 41:* 123, 1968.
8. Connell, J. T.: Quantitative intranasal pollen challenge III. The priming effect in allergic rhinitis. *J Allergy, 43:* 33, 1969.
9. DeWeese, D. D. and Saunders, W. H.: *Textbook of Otolaryngology,* 2nd ed. St. Louis, Mosby, 1964.
10. Dolovitch, J., Back, N. and Arbesman, C. E.: Kinin-like activity in nasal secretions of allergic patients. *Int Arch Allergy Appl Immunol, 38:* 337, 1970.
11. Eggston, A. and Wolff, D.: *Histopathology of the Ear, Nose and Throat.* Baltimore, Williams and Wilkins, 1947.
12. Frankland, A. W.: Seasonal hay fever and asthma treated with pollen extracts. *Int Arch Allergy Appl Immunol, 6:* 45, 1955.
13. Grove, R. C. and Farrier, J. B.: Chronic hyperplastic sinusitis in allergic patients: A bacteriologic study of two hundred operative cases. *J Allergy, 11:* 271, 1939.
14. Hansel, F. K.: Clinical and histopathologic studies of the nose and sinuses in allergy. *J Allergy, 1:* 43, 1929.
15. Hansel, F. K.: *Allergy of the Nose and Paranasal Sinuses.* St. Louis, Mosby, 1936.
16. Heetderks, D. R.: Reaction of normal nasal mucus membrane. *Am J Med Sci, 174:* 231, 1927.
17. Hilding, A. C.: The respiratory epithelium as a vital organ and some pathological changes in it due to common diseases. *Acta Otolaryngology, 37:* 138, 1949.
18. Holmes, T. H., Trenting, T. and Wolff, H. G.: *The Nose.* Springfield, Thomas, 1950.
19. Marks, M. B.: Physical signs of allergy of the respiratory tract in children. *Ann Allergy, 25:* 310, 1967.
20. Marks, M. B.: Allergic shiners: Dark circles under the eyes in children. *Clin Pediatr, 5:* 655, 1965.
21. McGovern, J. P., Haywood, T. J. and Fernandez, A. A.: Allergy and secretory otitis media: An analysis of 512 cases. *JAMA, 200:* 124, 1967.
22. Proetz, A. W.: *Essays on Applied Physiology of the Nose.* St. Louis, Annals, 1943.
23. Rappaport, B. Z.: Antigen antibody reactions in allergic human tissues: III. Immunofluorescent study of allergic nasal mucosa. *J Immunol, 93:* 792, 1964.
24. Remmington, J., Vosti, K., Lietze, A. and Zimmerman, A.: Serum proteins and antibody activity in human nasal secretions. *J Clin Invest, 43:* 1613, 1964.
25. Rossen, R. D., Alford, R. H., Butler, W. T. and Vannier, W. E.: The separation and characterization of proteins intrinsic to nasal secretion. *J Immunol, 97:* 369, 1966.
26. Rossen, R. D., Schade, A., Butler, W. T. and Kasl, J. A.: The proteins in nasal secretions: A longitudinal study of the γ A globulin, γ G globulin, albumins, siderophilia and total protein concentrations in nasal washings from adult male volunteers. *J Clin Invest, 45:* 768, 1966.
27. Said, S. I., Maddox, Y. T., Muren, O. and Kirby, B. J.: Mast cells in the lung: Distribution and possible role in histamine release and uptake. *Clin Res, 16:* 374, 1968.
28. Salvaggio, J. E., Cavanaugh, J. J. A., Lowell, F. and Leskowitz, S.: A comparison of the immunologic responses of normal and atopic individuals to intranasally administered antigen. *J Allergy, 35:* 62, 1964.
29. Semenov, H.: Pathology of nose and paranasal sinuses in relation to allergy. *Trans Am Acad Ophthalmol Otolaryngol 56:* 121, 1952.
30. Semenov, H.: The surgical pathology of nasal sinusitis. *JAMA, 111:* 2189, 1938.
31. Sherman, W. B., Stull, A., and Cook, R. A.: Serolgic changes in hay fever cases treated over a period of years. *J Allergy, 11:* 225, 1940.
32. Spain, W. C.: Allergic rhinitis. In Cooke, R. E. (Ed.): *Allergy in Theory and Practice.* Philadelphia, Saunders, 1947.
33. Vaughn, W. T. and Black, J. H. (Eds.): *Practice of Allergy.* St. Louis, Mosby, 1954.
34. Zimmerman, A. L.: Serum proteins and antibody activity in human nasal secretions. *J Clin Invest, 43:* 1613, 1964.

Chapter 3

ALLERGIC DISEASES OF THE EYE

THE MOST FREQUENTLY encountered allergic disease of the eyes and eyelids include:

Reaginic-atopic conjunctivitis
Contact allergy of the dermal surface of the lid
Contact allergy of the conjunctival surface of the lid
Contact allergy of the skin and conjunctivae (dermato-conjunctivitis)
Vernal conjunctivitis

The following allergic diseases occur less frequently but because of the hazard to vision they present very important clinical problems:

The cornea
    Diffuse and punctate keratitis
    Marginal infiltration
    Phlyctenular keratitis
    Combined involvement of the cornea and conjunctiva (kerato-conjunctivitis)
Allergic involvement of the sclera
Uveitis including choroiditis-iritis-cyclitis and irido-cyclitis
Allergic involvement of the lens (cataract), retina, and optic nerve

ALLERGIC REAGINIC CONJUNCTIVITIS

Allergic reaginic conjunctivitis is one of the most common forms of eye allergy. The allergens inducing the immediate response are the same as those encountered in immediate hypersensitivity elsewhere in the body, namely, pollens, epidermal factors, foods and molds. The airborne allergens with ready access to the conjunctivae, upon contact with the sensitized tissue, induce the immediate type of reactivity. When foods are involved which is less frequent than with the airborne allergens, the response may be delayed for several hours, which suggests that the immediate or reaginic type of allergy may not be involved but rather the Arthus type of reaction. It is not unusual for two mechanisms to operate simultaneously to produce a clinical pattern.

Allergic conjunctivitis occurs in two forms: (1) acute, and (2) chronic.

Acute Reaginic-Atopic Conjunctivitis

The signs and symptoms of acute reaginic-atopic conjunctivitis include marked injection and redness of the conjunctivae, edema, and a profuse watery discharge accompanied by intense itching, burning, scratchiness and occasionally pain of varying degrees. The classical example of this involvement is hay fever.

Injection and redness are caused by the marked dilatation of the very dense capillary network which shows through the very thin epithelial layer. Dilatation of vessels, producing hyperemia, is most marked in the palpebral conjunctivae, but not infrequently the injected small vessels are contrasted prominently against the white scleral background.

Edema, resulting from increased permeability of the capillaries, involves both the palpebral and bulbar conjunctivae. The conjunctiva is more loosely attached as it recedes from the lid margin toward the eye to form the transitional fold. It is in the areas of loosely bound tissues that edema is most pronounced, expecially along the lower transitional fold from where it may be reflected onto the lower bulbar conjunctivae. This is readily observed by retracting the lower lid.

Discharge, which is usually profuse and watery, is supplied mostly by the lacrimal glands. The function of the lacrimal secretions (tears) is to moisten, lubricate and flush the ocular and palpebral surfaces. With the recent demonstration of antibodies in external secretions, and particularly IgA in tears, it is very likely that the tears represent the first line of defense against invading organisms of the eye. The profuse lacrimation of conjunctivitis is an exaggeration of the normal response of the glands in an endeavor to wash away an offending agent.

With more intense reactions the discharge may have a more viscid and at times a ropy consistency due to mucus supplied by the mucus glands situated along the lid margins and the goblet cells interspersed throughout the palpebral conjunctival epithelium.

Intense itching is the most common subjective symptom. Burning, a sense of scratching, and more rarely varying degrees of pain may be the complaint. The liberal distribution of nerve endings in the conjunctiva explains the frequency and the intensity of the subjective symptoms.

Diagnosis: When acute conjunctivitis occurs with the hay fever syndrome, diagnosis usually presents no problem. When hay fever is not part of the pattern, the first prerequisite is the determination that the patient is an allergic individual (see Chapter 13, The Allergic Patient). The identification of the allergen either through history or skin testing helps to support the diagnosis.

Reaginic-atopic conjunctivitis rarely occurs as an isolated complaint. In most cases there is accompanying nasal involvement. The classical findings of edema and pallor of the nasal mucosa will help to substantiate the diagnosis of reaginic-atopic conjunctivitis.

Inorganic materials such as lime and lye, which may serve as nonallergic irritants, are usually reported by the patient.

Viral infection particularly in the form of epidemic kerato-conjunctivitis presents the most challenging problem in differential diagnoses. A preauricular adenopathy usually accompanies the infection. Scrapings of the eye will reveal mononuclear leukocytes rather than eosinophils, which support a diagnosis of allergy. Failure to respond to antihistamines also suggests a diagnosis of infection.

Chronic Reaginic-Atopic Conjunctivitis

In all chronic cases, the subjective symptoms of itching, burning, photophobia and dryness are present. In some patients there are no objective findings to explain their severe complaints. In such cases, a history confirming that the individual is allergic will suggest the diagnosis, while confirmation of the diagnosis will be supported by the presence of allergic disease elsewhere, most commonly in the nose. The pale, boggy nasal mucosa with turgescent turbinates obstructing the airways is strong positive evidence of allergy. A swab of the eye scrapings will show eosinophils, but this need not be pathognomonic.

The objective findings may vary with the duration of the illness. With chronicity both hyperplasia and hypertrophy develop. In patients offering a history of moderate duration—several weeks or even several months—injection and edema are observed but only to a moderate degree. Even in longstanding chronic forms edema may be observed in the loosely attached tissues, especially at the lower transitional fold where, upon retraction of the lid, it appears glassy and succulent. The thickening of the epithelium with chronicity masks the underlying congestion, imparting a pallor to the conjunctiva.

With chronicity the goblet cells of the palpebral conjunctivae increase in number to provide greater quantities of mucus which make the discharge more viscid than watery.

As in all forms of allergic conjunctivitis, eosinophils are present in the scrapings.

Treatment of Reaginic-Atopic Conjuctivitis

Treatment is the same for both the acute and uncomplicated chronic forms of atopic conjunctivitis.

For specific therapy, see Chapter 17, Immunotherapy.

For relief of acute symptoms various eye-drop preparations are effective, such as:

Neo-Synephrine® Hydrochloride Ophthalmic 0.125% in 15 ml container

Vasocon-A® Ophthalmic (see Chapter 15, Drugs Used in Treatment of Allergic Disease)

Local treatment should be limited to several days. With prolonged topical medication the risk of inducing reactions is very great. The reaction may be a simple irritation from the medication, but very infrequently an allergic reaction to the drug develops. Not infrequently the reaction is induced by preservatives or other excipients in the product. A change to a product from a different manufacturer may clear the irritation.

Oral treatment with antihistamines or if indicated with corticosteroids is preferable to topical treatment. There is no oral antihistamine that displays greater effectiveness in the management of allergic conjunctivitis. The choice of antihistamine must be governed by the tolerance and the response of the patient (see Chapter 15, Drugs Used in Treatment of Allergic Disease). When antihistamines are found ineffective, oral steroids should be considered, but only for short term therapy (see discussion on steroid therapy in Chapter 15).

FOLLICULAR CONJUNCTIVITIS

In the substantia propria of the conjunctiva, a very thin layer of lymphoid tissue (the conjunctival adenoid) is present immediately beneath the epithelial surface. This lymphoid structure makes its first appearance about the third month of life, becomes prominent throughout childhood and involutes in adult life. In young adults as well as children in whom the lymphoid structures of Waldeyer's ring are well developed, the conjunctival lymphoid tissue may be quite prominent. The parallel course displayed by the conjunctival and upper respiratory lymphoid structures which is characterized by prominence in childhood and involution in adult life, suggests an identical role in the immune response. With hyperplasia of Waldeyer's ring in the allergic child, it is not unusual to observe a similar response of the conjunctival lymphoid tissue (follicular conjunctivitis).

In response to any irritant—infectious, noninfectious or allergic—the conjunctival lymphoid structures hypertrophy and gather into follicles. The follicles, which are pinhead sized and either round or oval in shape, produce a slight elevation of the thin overlying epithelium. These slight elevations are most prominent along the inferior fornix, but may extend into the tarsal plate. The surface of the conjunctiva appears granular (follicular conjunctivitis).

Follicular conjunctivitis, which is not an unusual observation in childhood, is readily recognized upon retraction of the lower lid. The diagnosis of allergic follicular conjunctivitis can usually be supported by the findings of allergic disease elsewhere, especially allergic rhinitis. Isolated allergic conjunctivitis, without other organ involvement, occurs very rarely.

Hypertrophy of the papillae, which are finger-like extensions of the substantia propria, are observed at the corneal limbus and the lid margins. Near the cornea they rarely exceed four or five in number and can readily be differentiated from the granular folliculitis which involves the fornix.

VERNAL CONJUNCTIVITIS

Vernal conjunctivitis is a very complex and enigmatic disease of unknown etiology. The disease is commonly included in discussions of reaginic-atopic conjunctivitis because of the following features:

(1) A familial and personal history of allergic disease is positive in about 50 per cent of the cases.

(2) The disease recurs periodically during warm weather, usually during the spring and summer season. The condition usually clears during the winter months.

(3) Patients frequently have positive skin reactions for pollens.

(4) Eosinophils are usually found in the conjunctival secretions.

Upon analyzing these points, many inconsistencies are revealed:

(a) A history of allergic disease is not essential. Many cases of vernal conjunctivitis offer no such history.

(b) & (c) The occurrence during warm weather and the occurrence of positive skin reactivity infers a sensitivity to pollen. No correlation between positive reactions and symptomatology can be demonstrated.

Many patients continue their symptoms beyond the time when both pollens and molds are cleared from the atmosphere. Avoidance of the factors to which the patient reacts has no influence upon the course of the disease.

(d) The presence of eosinophils as an isolated feature is not sufficient to support a diagnosis of atopic allergy.

In support of an endocrine disturbance as the etiological factor the following features are mentioned:

(1) The disease has a high incidence in children with a predisposition in boys. Hpogonadism is a frequent observation in the boys afflicted. Most of the cases clear spontaneously after puberty.

(2) Thyroidism is frequently observed.

Signs and Symptoms

Itching, lacrimation and photophobia are dominant symptoms. Two forms of tissue reaction are observed: (1) the palpebral, and (2) the limbal.

In the palpebral form the characteristic fully developed lesion consists of flat papillae of varying sizes and shapes which become polygonal in configuration, producing the readily recognizable "cobblestone" appearance. The lesions are usually limited to the tarsal plate of the upper lid. In more severe reactions the lower lid may be involved.

The limbal form is characterized by either focal or general opacities at the corneal limbus which, as the disease progresses, develop discrete yellow or grayish elevations.

The discharge in both types is thick, ropy, creamy white, forming a pseudo-membrane which can be stripped easily from the conjuctiva without bleeding.

Injection of the conjunctiva usually is present.

The inconsistencies in the history, and the evolution of the unusual "cobblestone" lesions are difficult to reconcile with reaginic-atopic allergic disease. In any event the cause is still very elusive.

Although the condition usually clears spontaneously, and the acute symptoms respond to systemic corticosteroids, supervision by a trained ophthalmologist is usually advisable.

PHLYCTENULES

Until recently phlyctenules were considered, almost exclusively, as a manifestation of tuberculous involvement. They are now recognized as an allergic response induced by a variety of antigenic materials including the products of bacteria and viruses.

The typical phlyctenule consists of an accumulation of lymphocytes which appears as a small pinkish-white elevation or nodule accompanied by an engorgement of the conjunctival vessels which cluster around the base of the elevations. The remainder of the conjunctiva is usually clear, but a mild degree of hyperemia may be present. The apex or peak of the nodule ulcerates and then heals during a ten to fourteen day period, when the phlyctenule gradually shrinks to the level of the conjunctiva.

The lesions may occur in the conjunctiva when the condition is known as phlyctenular conjunctivitis, or extend to the cornea when it is called phlyctenular keratitis, or more frequently it involves the limbus when both the conjunctiva and cornea are involved, to be designated as phlyctenular keratoconjunctivitis.

The symptoms are blepharospasm and photophobia, especially when the cornea is involved.

Treatment

In most cases the cause of the disease is benign and self-limited. Corticosteroid therapy is recommended for its anti-inflammatory action.

Cool pads to the eyes frequently gives relief. At times one per cent atropine is useful for resting the iris and ciliary body.

THE EYELIDS

Reaginic-atopic involvement of the eyelids may be manifested as edema or atopic dermatitis.

Edema may occur in varying degrees, ranging from barely perceptible puffiness to extreme swelling as encountered in angioedema.

The dermal and conjunctival layers of the lid are attached very loosely to the underlying stroma. The fascial attachment of the lids is very firm, forming a closed compartment which prevents the spread of fluids to the adjacent parts such as the cheek or the forehead. As a result even a slight amount of edema fluid restricted to the confines of the lid is noticeable and may be the first manifestation of a more generalized reaction. With extensive edema, peri-orbital swelling becomes pronounced.

Edema of the lids occurs very frequently with allergic conjunctivitis and also as a manifestation of generalized allergic involvements, such as urticaria, angio-edema and serum disease.

INVOLVEMENT OF THE LID MARGINS (BLEPHARITIS)

With chronic involvement of the conjunctiva, changes in the lid margins may develop giving them a thickened, reddened, scaly appearance labelled as blepharitis. Itching is a dominant symptom, which leads to considerable local trauma from rubbing of the eyes. Secondary infection is a common complication. Marked changes of the lid margin are rarely observed without infection. When infection is present, it is possible that sensitivity to the organism or a component of the organism may develop. In such cases the delayed type of allergy would be induced, which is characterized by cellular infiltration. It is possible that various types of the allergic response operate in the chronic changes of blepharitis. When the antigen is one of the common allergens such as pollen and epidermals and molds, the immediate type of reactivity would be present. When foods are involved, an Arthus type of inflammatory response must be suspected while with organisms the delayed response would be observed. It is possible that in some cases more than one type of allergic response may be involved.

The best prognosis can be anticipated in the reaginic-atopic reaction. Identification of the allergen and hyposensitization would offer the most promising control.

For symptomatic treatment short courses of corticosteroids are recommended (see Chapter 15, Drugs Used in Treatment of Allergic Disease). With an Arthus type reaction, if the antigen is identified and eliminated, the response should be very good, with a complete restitution of tissues.

Involvement with delayed hypersensitivity reactions offers the poorest prognosis. Since there are no recognized techniques for hyposensitization against delayed hypersensitivity, the *only* prospect is in symptomatic treatment with oral corticosteroids with the hope that the antigen will exhaust itself with a resolution of the process.

It is always advisable to avoid topical treatment of any kind.

CONTACT DERMATITIS AND CONJUNCTIVITIS

Contact dermatitis involving the skin of

the lids is the most common allergic involvement of the eye. Frequently both the skin and conjunctivae are involved, when the condition is known as dermato-conjunctivitis.

Various contactants induce the delayed type of allergic response (see contact dermatitis).

Any contactant may serve as the etiologic agent, but cosmetics and drugs are by far the commonest offenders.

With primary involvement of the skin the commonest contacts are the cosmetics, such as:

    nail polish
    mascara
    eye shadow
    hair dyes and tints
    hair sprays
    basic conditioners and shampoos

When cosmetics cause the reaction, there is usually no conjunctival involvement. With severe reactions both the skin of the lids and the conjunctivae are involved.

When the conjunctiva is primarily involved, it is usually induced by topical medication, such as drops, ointments or creams. If the medication washes over the lids, channels of dermatitis following the flow of the liquid may be present. In reactions to topical medications, not infrequently the preservatives contained in the medications, such as a mercurial product, may be the offender rather than the pharmacologically active principle of the drug. Following the initial exposure to the offending agent, seven to eight days may elapse before the onset of the reaction. In patients previously sensitized, the reaction usually appears after twenty-four to thirty-six hours.

With acute involvement the subjective symptoms of itching and burning are intense. The skin is swollen, intensely red and weeping. The dried exudate forms crusts.

With prolonged involvement itching and burning are still present, but the acute weeping reaction is replaced by thickening of the skin with dryness and scaling.

Diagnosis: A history that identifies the contactant is important both for diagnosis and management. Since contact dermatitis may occur in nonatopic as well as atopic individuals, a history of allergy is of no assistance. A history reporting the use of a cosmetic for long periods, even years without a reaction does not exclude the chemical as an offender. Not infrequently, a patient may report the use of the same brand of fingernail polish or some other cosmetic for many years with no adverse reaction, but suddenly sensitivity may develop and contact dermatitis will develop. Failure to recognize these features frequently leads to a failure in diagnosis and control of the disease.

ALLERGIC DISEASE OF THE CORNEA

There are a number of corneal diseases identified on the basis of morphology, such as

    superficial keratitis
    punctate keratitis
    isolated ulcers
    ring ulcers
    interstitial or parenchymatous keratitis
    kerato-conjunctivitis

Although these diseases are attributed to an allergic mechanism, the nature of that tissue reaction is not clarified.

Some forms of keratitis are attributed to a reaginic-atopic mechanism since the offending allergen is demonstrated to be either a pollen or a food. In the absence of mast cells as a source of the mediator histamine and the lack of blood vessels to furnish edema fluid, it is difficult to correlate the lesions of keratitis with a reaginic-atopic tissue response. The fact that corneal involvement occurs during the course of atopic diseases does not necessarily imply that the immune mechanism is identical. It is possible that more than one type of tissue reaction is operating simultaneously. This is commonly observed in serum type disease.

The cornea responds to injections of antigens in a unique manner depending upon the type of antigen, its concentration, previous sensitization and the mode of administration. The fact that the cornea is exposed to both exogenous and endogenous antigens is an important determining factor in the tissue response.

Some recent studies by Sery, Nagy and Barber help clarify some of the complex corneal responses. These investigators observed two distinct immune phenomena in the corneal response to the injection of foreign protein. One was the classical Wessely phenomenon and the other a local immune corneal reaction.

The Wessely phenomenon is a keratoconjunctivitis accompanied by the development at the corneal-scleral junction of immune precipitates and cellular infiltrates forming a ring or ring segments. This response is very suggestive of an Arthus type reaction.

The local immune reaction develops as a faint ring enclosing a disc opacity within fifteen minutes to two hours and intensified in twenty-four to forty-eight hours into a sharp, well-defined ring and disc with very little expression beyond the marginal limits of the injection site. Since antibody must be present in the cornea for the reaction to occur, the investigators postulate that following a Wessely limbal reaction antibodies migrate into the cornea and remain fixed for long periods; or that during the Wessely reaction cells capable of producing antibodies (immunocytes) wandered into the cornea and remained fixed in the corneal tissue for indefinite periods. IgG and IgA antibodies have been demonstrated in the cornea by Alansmith and Herman. Upon challenge with the specific antigen a local reaction characterized by the ring and disc occur.

It is conceivable that with exogenous antigens such as pollen, molds or even bacteria, local reactions involving the superficial corneal layer produce the pattern of *punctate* keratitis upon reaction with migrated antibody or immunocytes in the corneal tissue.

The diagnosis of these complex tissue reactions should be reserved for the ophthalmologist who has sophisticated equipment to assist him.

Symptoms

The symptoms of corneal involvement are pain, photophobia, blepharospasm, lacrimation, and impaired vision.

Signs

The changes in the cornea will depend upon the location of the tissue reaction and the degree of the tissue response.

Types of Involvement

(1) Isolated or multiple circumscribed superficial lesions involving the epithelium.
(2) Stromal infiltration with dulling of the caudal surface, impaired transparency.
(3) Complete absorption of the stromal involvement with restitution of the cornea.
(4) Incomplete absorption with organization and fibrosis leading to opacities.
(5) Suppuration with ulcer formation.
(6) Scar formation.
(7) Circumcorneal injection with conjunctivitis and involvement of the neighboring parts.

ALLERGIC DISEASES OF THE UVEA

In allergic involvement of the uveal tract the reaction may be limited to one segment, such as iritis, cyclitis, iridocyclitis and choroiditis, or in more severe reactions the entire uvea may participate (uveitis).

Unlike the cornea, the uvea is a compartment closed to the exterior which excludes the possibility of exogenous antigens operating directly upon the tissues. The highly vascular nature of the organ makes it very susceptible to allergic reactions involving blood vessels such as in the Arthus mechanism. But vascularity alone is not sufficient to explain the unique tissue reactions observed in uveal tract allergic disease. Current observations indicate that the eye behaves much like a lymph node in manifesting immunological memory. In other words, once a cell capable of producing antibody in response to its specific stimulus enters the interstitial spaces in the uveal tract, these cells will remain for indefinite periods and the eye will retain an immunological memory as long as the cells are present in its tissues.

As in the cornea, deposits of immunoglobulins have been demonstrated in the limbus and in the choroid.

In addition to the role of both humoral and tissue antibodies in allergic eye disease two other mechanisms must be recognized:

(1) The delayed type of allergic response induced by the tubercle bacilli, the streptococci and other organisms, viral agents and haptenic conjugates with body proteins.

(2) The very liberal supply of collagen in all structures of the eye can serve as an important factor in the auto-immune mechanism. Experimentally, opacity has been induced in rat cornea following the injection of anti-rat collagen antibodies.

SIGNS AND SYMPTOMS OF IRIDOCYCLITIS

circumcorneal injection
tenderness in the ciliary region
swelling of the upper lid
reduced vision
impaired opacity of the lens

More deep-seated changes can be detected upon examination by the ophthalmologist.

The diagnosis of choroditis (scleritis and retinal and optic nerve) usually requires the skill of the ophthalmologist.

GENERAL MANAGEMENT

Except for the more common and benign conditions such as involvement of the eyelids and conjunctiva, it is advisable to consult with an ophthalmologist in the management and treatment of allergic eye diseases. The ophthalmologist will be able to diagnose more accurately the nature of the involvement as well as determine the degree of tissue reaction and the progress of the disease. Although many cases will respond to therapy with corticosteroids, such therapy offers no assurance that the condition will not recur upon withdrawal of the medication. The attending physician can play an important role in identifying the etiologic agent such as a food factor—including the various food aditives (see Chapter 8, Adverse Reactions to Foods and Food Chemicals)—infection, drugs, chemicals—such as encountered in cosmetics—and at times unusual *environmental factors*.

Scleritis, retinitis and optic nerve involvement by the allergic process is governed by the same immunological problems encountered in corneal and uveal allergic diseases. The problem is one for the trained ophthalmologist.

REFERENCES

1. Allansmith, M. and Hutchinson, D.: Immunoglobulins in the conjunctiva. *Immunology, 12:* 225, 1967.
2. Allansmith, M. and McClellan, B.: Immunoglobulin levels in human tears. (Abstract). *Invest Ophthalmol, 8:* 240, 1969.
3. Allansmith, M. and O'Connor, R.: Immunoglobulins: Structure, function and relation to the eye. *Survey of Ophthalmol, 14:* 367, 1970.
4. Claman, H., Merrill, D. and Hartley, T.: Salivary immunoglobulins: Normal adult values and dissociation between serum and salivary levels. *J Allergy, 40:* 151, 1967.
5. Doggart, J. H.: *Diseases of Children's Eyes.* St. Louis, Mosby, 1947.
6. Duke-Elder, S.: *System of Ophthalmology.* St. Louis, Mosby, 1965, vols. 8 and 9.
7. Goldman, H. and Witmer, R.: Antikörper in Kammerwasser. *Ophthalmologica (Basel), 127:* 323, 1954.
8. Greer, C. H.: *Ocular Pathology.* Oxford, Blackwell, 1963.
9. Hogan, M. J. and Zimmerman, L. E.: *Ophthalmic Pathology,* 2nd ed. Philadelphia, Saunders, 1962.
10. Holt, L. B.: *Pediatric Ophthalmology.* Philadelphia, Lea & Febiger, 1964.
11. Isa, A. M., Hanna, L., Linscott, W. D. and Jawetz,

E.: Experimental inclusion conjunctivitis in man. IV. The nature of the antibody response. *J Immunol, 101:* 1154, 1968.
12. Josephson, A. S. and Lockwood, D. W.: Immunoelectrophoretic studies of the protein component of normal tears. *J Immunol, 93:* 532, 1964.
13. Liebman, S. D. and Gillis, S. S.: *The Pediatricians Ophthalmology.* St. Louis, Mosby, 1966.
14. Little, J. M., Centifanto, Y. M. and Kaufman, H. E.: Immunoglobulins in tears. *Am. J Ophthalmol, 68:* 898, 1969.
15. Maumenee, A. E. and Silverstein, A. M. (Eds.): *Immunopathology of Uveitis.* Baltimore, Williams and Wilkins, 1964.
16. Maurice, D.: The structure and transparency of the cornea. *J Physiol, 136:* 263, 1957.
17. Neuman, E.: A review of four hundred cases of vernal conjunctivitis. *Am J Ophthalmol, 47:* 166, 1959.
18. Peretz, W. I. and Tomasi, T. B.: Aqueous humor proteins in uveitis. *Arch Ophthalmol, 65:* 20, 1961.
19. Proctor, D. F.: *The Nose, Paranasal Sinuses and Ears in Childhood.* Springfield, Thomas, 1963.
20. Ruedermann, A. D.: Ocular manifestations of allergy. In Thomas, J. W. (Ed.): *Allergy in Clinical Practice.* Philadelphia, Lippincott, 1961, pp. 256-274.
21. Salzman, M.: *Anatomy and Histology of the Human Eyeball in the Normal State.* Chicago, Chicago University Press, 1912.
22. Scobee, R. G.: *A Child's Eye.* St. Louis, Mosby, 1952.
23. Sery, T. W., Nagy, M. R., and Barber, G. W.: Corneal hypersensitivity: I. Escape kinetics of antigen from sensitized corneas. *J Immunol, 106:* 217, 1971.
24. Sery, T. W. and Nagy, M. R.: Corneal hypersensitivity: II. Specific binding of antigen in sensitized cornea. *J Immunol, 106:* 226, 1971.
25. Settipane, G. A., Connell, J. T. and Sherman, W. B.: Reagin in tears. *J Allergy, 36:* 92, 1965.
26. Sherman, H., Feldman, L. and Walzer, M.: Studies in atopic hypersensitiveness of the ophthalmic mucus membrane. *J Allergy 4:* 437, 1933.
27. Silverstein, A. M.: In Gell, P. G. H. and Coombs, R. R. A. (Eds.): *Clinical Aspects of Immunology.* Philadelphia, Davis Co, 1963, pp. 555-569.
28. Sloan, P. G.: External diseases of the eye. (Annual review) *Am J Optomol, 47:* 629, 1970.
29. Smelser, G. K.: *The Structure of the Eye.* Intl Cong of Anatomists, 7th. New York, 1960.
30. Theodore, F. H. and Schlossman, A.: *Ocular Allergy.* Baltimore, Williams and Wilkins, 1958.
31. Wolf, E.: *Anatomy of the Eye and Orbit.* London, Lewis, 1968.

Chapter 4

ALLERGIC DISEASES OF THE LOWER RESPIRATORY TRACT

Anatomical Features and Pathophysiology

OVER THE PAST FEW YEARS excellent studies have reported on the finer anatomical structure of the lung. Many well documented structural features have added to the understanding of the complex operation of the lung which in turn assists in the interpretation of both the mechanical (respiratory movements) and chemical (gas exchange) dysfunctions secondary to allergic tissue reactions.

On the basis of both anatomy and function, the lung can be divided into three segments:

(1) The cartilaginous segment of the conducting portion of the lung which includes the trachea (2.5 cm in diameter) and the bronchi which decrease in size to 1.0 mm in diameter.

(2) The transitional fibromuscular, mechanical portion of the conducting segment includes the bronchioles and the terminal bronchioles, which are concerned with regulating the flow of gas to and from the lung.

(3) The acini, which are the gas exchange units of the lung, include the respiratory bronchioles, the alveolar ducts, the alveolar sacs, and the alveoli. The respiratory bronchioles and the alveolar ducts have alveoli apposed to their walls which results in a dual function, conduction and exchange of gas.

Recognition of the three segments of the lung is helpful in the interpretation of the signs and symptoms of allergic pulmonary disease.

1. CARTILAGINOUS PORTION: Cartilage is present to the level of the bronchioles which are approximately 1.0 mm in diameter. In the trachea and larger bronchi the cartilage occurs as C-shaped rings with the open ends of the C lying posteriorly. Fibroelastic bands tie together the open ends of the cartilage. As the bronchi become smaller, the cartilage loses its configuration to occur as plaques which are bound together in a strong layer of collagen and elastic fibers. The fibroelastic bands give this portion of the bronchial tree a degree of rigidity but no absolute fixation. Since the cartilaginous portion of the airway lies outside the lung proper, it has no extrinsic support, but depends upon the fibroelastic cartilaginous structure. This structure prevents collapse of the tube during the drop in pressure that occurs as air flows from the alveoli to the mouth during expiration, as well as overexpansion during inspiration.

The mucosa of the trachea and larger bronchi is similar to that found in the nose, which is ciliated pseudostratified epithelium with numerous goblet cells interspersed. The epithelium rests upon a basement membrane, beneath which lies the tunica propria. Immediately beneath the basement membrane is a capillary network which is less dense in the larger airways but becomes more dense as it approaches the fibroelastic portion of the bronchial tree.

The dense fibroelastic network of the submucosa has free cellular elements consisting of lymphocytes, plasma cells, histiocytes and mast cells. Seromucus glands and goblet cells are present throughout the tunica propria.

The normal sheet of mucus covering the mucosa is produced primarily by the seromucus glands. This sheet of mucus is moved toward the mouth by ciliary action. In response to the allergic reaction or any other irritant, there is a considerable increase in the number of goblet cells which become major contributors of mucus, whereas under normal conditions their contribution of mucus is only a minor one. The ciliary action is readily damaged by dry air. In the allergic reaction with the production of large quantities of mucus, humidified air is very essential to maintain ciliary action to clear the passages of excess mucus.

In the trachea and in the larger bronchi with C-shaped cartilaginous rings, smooth muscle is distributed as a longitudinal band along the apertures of the C-rings. Spasm of the longitudinal muscle bundle occurs frequently in allergic reactions involving the trachea and the larger bronchi, resulting in rigidity but no contraction of these airways. The expansile and contractile movements of these larger airways which occur with the normal respiratory cycle are restricted by the muscle spasm and produce difficulty in breathing. The patient reports a sense of tightness high up in the chest rather than true dyspnea.

In spite of the terms "bronchial allergy" and "bronchial asthma," the cartilaginous segment of the bronchial tree, which includes the airways above the bronchioles, does not contribute appreciably to the signs and symptoms of these diseases.

2. THE TRANSITIONAL, FIBROMUSCULAR OR MECHANICAL SEGMENT: This segment of the bronchial tree which is non-cartilaginous is constituted of the terminal bronchioles, several generations of respiratory bronchioles and the alveolar ducts. Since the walls of the respiratory bronchioles and the alveolar ducts have a variable number of alveoli apposed to their walls, they are actually a mixture of the transitional and gas exchanging zones. The diameters of this portion of the bronchial tree range from 0.65 mm for the terminal bronchioles to 0.45 mm and 0.40 mm for the respiratory bronchioles (See Table 4-I and Fig. 4-1.)

In the non-cartilaginous segment, the epithelium is cuboidal in character which becomes thinner as the airways become smaller. As the mucosa becomes thinner, it loses the goblet cells, the seromucus glands and the cilia so that in the terminal bronchioles (0.65 mm) and below none of the accessory structures are present.

In the respiratory bronchioles the mucosal lining is interrupted by the openings into the alveolar sacs. In the alveolar ducts the mucosa is absent and is replaced by numerous openings into the alveolar sacs where the epithelium is continuous with that of the ducts.

The fibromuscular segment of the bronchial tree lies embedded within the lung so that the surrounding structures offer extrinsic support. In the bronchioles the fibrous layer is very thin but smooth muscle is thick and prominent.

In the smaller bronchi and bronchioles the fibroelastic bands and smooth muscle form a criss-cross, spiral geodesic network continuous with the interlobar septa of the lung proper.

At the level of the alveolar ducts the entire wall which is occupied by alveolar openings consists of only a fine meshwork of elastic and thin collagenous fibers with a few single

Table 4-I

	No.	Diameter of Individual Structures	Total Cross Section of Area
Trachea	1	2.5 cm	5.0 sq cm
Main bronchus	2	11–19 mm	3.2 sq cm
Lobar bronchi	5	4.5–13.5 mm	2.7 sq cm
Bronchi	variable	variable	variable
Terminal bronchi	1,000	1.0 mm	7.9 sq cm
Bronchioles	variable	variable	variable
Terminal bronchioles	35,000	0.65 mm	116 sq cm
Respiratory bronchioles	variable	variable	variable
Terminal respiratory bronchioles	630,000	0.45 mm	1,000 sq cm
Alveolar ducts and sacs	14×10^6	0.4 mm	1.76 sq meters
Alveoli	300×10^6	0.25–0.30 mm	70 sq meters

Total cross sectional area rapidly increases which is responsible for the very low resistance in airflow in the small airways of the lungs.

Total alveolar surface area is related to body length and varies from 40 to 100 sq meters.

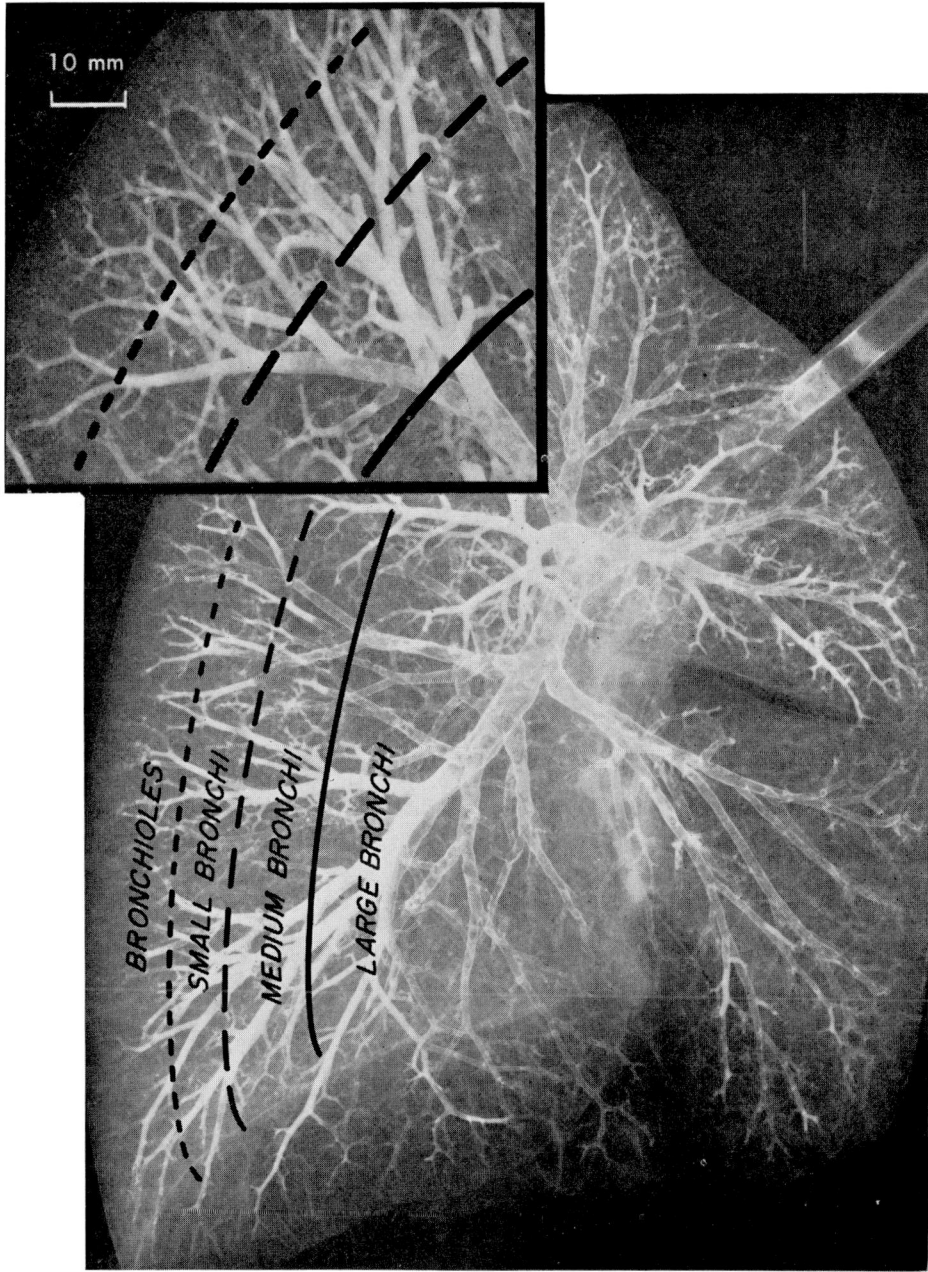

Figure 4-1. Micro-opaque barium insufflation of bronchial tree in fresh air inflated lung; x-rayed with industrial film. Insert is actual size of adult lung. *Bronchioles* are 2 cm from lung margin. Small bronchioles, next 2 cm. Intermediate (medium), first bifurcation of insert. Diameters are given in Table 4-1. (Courtesy of Robert Wright, M.D., Professor Pathology, University of California Medical Center, San Francisco, California.)

muscle fibers. This network of the alveolar ducts forms the entrance way to the alveoli.

The fibroelastic strands of the geodesic network of the transitional segment are continuous with fibroelastic bands in the interlobar septa and the lung parenchyma. With expansion of the lung on inspiration the continuous fibroelastic fibers pull outward upon the walls of the small airways to keep them patent. With expiration the bands which act as guy-wires relax to produce a narrowing of the bronchioles but not sufficiently to cause complete collapse. In bronchial allergy and particularly in bronchial asthma there is an exaggeration of this mechanism. Edema, muscle spasm and mucus cause obstruction which leads to air trapping, resulting in increased residual air in the lungs, causing hyperaeration with expansion of the lungs. The expanded lung causes a pull upon the fibromuscular bronchioles embedded in the lung. As a result, hyperaeration, a pathological condition, helps to compensate for the obstruction of the smaller air passages produced in bronchial allergic disease.

The transitional portion of the bronchial tree serves as a safety valve to help regulate the flow of air to and from the lung. By virtue of this function the fibromuscular segment of the bronchial tree is responsible for most of the signs and symptoms of bronchial asthma.

In addition to the mechanical factors, the tonus of the highly developed smooth muscle in the walls of the bronchioles plays a very important role in their patency.

Smooth muscle tonus is governed by several factors:

(1) The bronchi and bronchioles are innervated by sympathetic and parasympathetic fibers. How impulses from these nerves influence muscle tone is not understood.

(2) Chemical mediators, such as histamine, SRS-A and perhaps kinins act upon receptor sites to influence muscle tone.

(3) CO_2 tension in expired air influences muscle tone of the bronchioles.

When the CO_2 tension of expired air drops below 30 mm Hg, the smooth muscle contracts which results in narrowing of the airways, leading to increased airway resistance that impairs the flow of air.

The air trapping of bronchial asthma leads to a lowered CO_2 tension in the expired air that induces muscle spasm which causes narrowing of the bronchioles.

The tethering effect of the fibroelastic fibers is not sufficient to overcome the contraction of the smooth muscle. As a result, the narrowing, which interferes with the flow of air, causes bronchiolar obstruction heard on auscultation as fine inspiratory or expiratory wheezes, but particularly the latter.

In addition to the obstruction caused by a disturbance of the mechanical regulatory mechanism of the transitional segment, the allergic tissue reaction contributes to the obstruction by (1) smooth muscle spasm, (2) edema, and (3) increased production of mucus and the inflammatory reaction when the Arthus mechanism operates.

(1) Smooth muscle spasm induced by the action of either histamine or SRS-A or both is the most important cause of airway obstruction in bronchial asthma. It is possible that the small ring of smooth muscle at the entrance of the alveolar ducts into the alveoli play a very important role in the pathology of asthma. Some anatomists feel that the function of the sphincters is to turn on and turn off the reserve alveolar units. During normal respiration, contraction of the sphincters shuts off the reserve units so that they lie dormant, while during increased respiratory demands, by relaxation of the sphincters, the reserve alveoli are brought into action.

(2) The edema induced by the release of histamine in the allergic response can produce a high degree of obstruction with a picture of severe respiratory distress. A small increment of edema can induce a considerable obstruction in the tiny airways with diameters ranging between 0.4 mm and 0.65 mm. Unquestionably, edema is an important factor and particularly in serious clinical patterns, while the obstruction secondary to the muscle spasm is caused by SRS-A, the dominant mediator in less severe clinical patterns. This situation is observed clinically in asthmatic patients with dry wheezes that respond very quickly to sympathomimetic drugs with no residual adventitious breath sounds.

(3) Mucus and particularly inspissated mucus plugs can play an important role in causing the obstruction of allergic bronchial

disease and bronchial asthma. Clinically, it appears that mucus is a more consistent finding in bronchial allergy, while in bronchial asthma the component of muscle spasm is the dominant factor in causing obstruction. However, the combination of muscle spasm with inspissated mucus plugs produces the most serious clinical patterns which frequently lead to status asthmaticus.

The transitional portion of the bronchial tree has no goblet cells, no mucus glands and no cilia. Evidence seems to indicate that the seromucoid secretions observed in those structures with bronchial asthma do not originate proximally from the airways containing goblet cells and seromucus glands. The source of mucus in this segment of the bronchial tree is attributed to the Clara cells. The Clara cells are derived from normal cuboidal cells in response to any irritation.

Mucus-producing Clara cells, which project into the lumen of the tubules, may be a response to the irritation of the allergic reaction. On the other hand, recent studies seem to implicate the Clara cells in the excretion of surfactants rather than mucus. Because of these differences in opinion the exact function of the Clara cells is not known nor is the source of mucus in the transitional zone determined.

3. THE GAS EXCHANGE SEGMENT: The acinus which is the basic ventilatory unit of the lung is constituted of respiratory bronchioles, alveolar ducts, atria and alveolar sacs. There are between two to nine respiratory bronchioles in an acinus. About eighteen last order terminal bronchioles arise from one terminal bronchus which gives rise to about four hundred alveolar ducts and sacs in an acinus. The small terminal airways do not permit the passage of particles greater than six microns in diameter into the alveolar sacs. As a result the allergens responsible for bronchial allergy and bronchial asthma, such as pollens, epidermal factors and some molds which have diameters of ten microns or greater, do not gain access to the alveolar

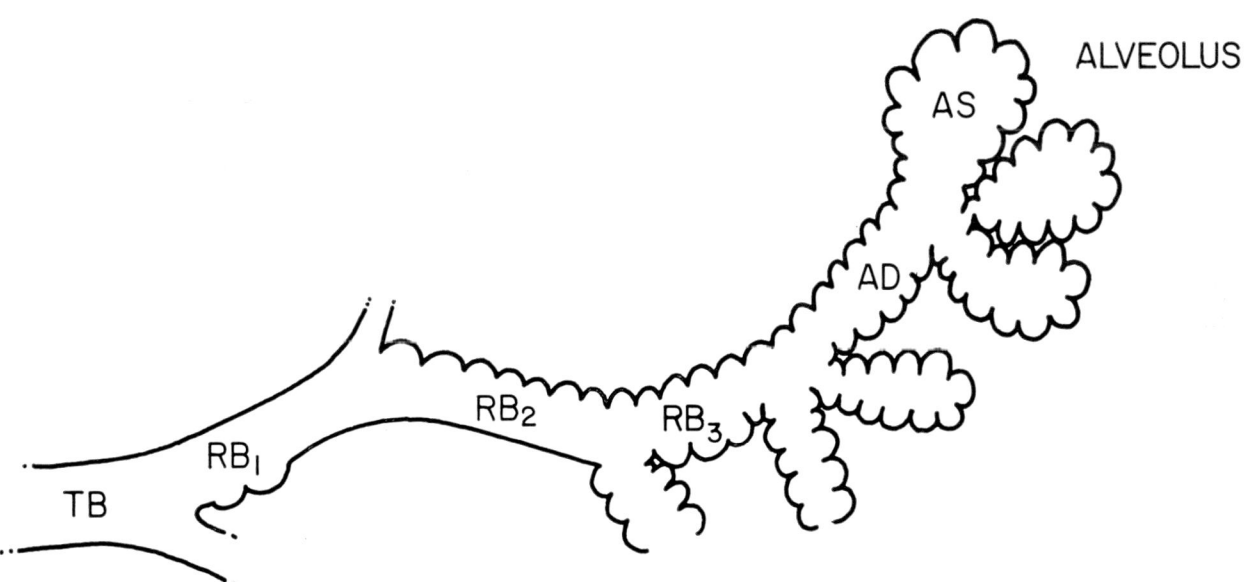

Figure 4-2. Component parts of an acinus. Diagram of the acinus or gas exchanging portion of the lung. There are three orders of respiratory bronchioles (RB) with progressively more alveoli on their walls. A third order respiratory bronchiole (RB_3) is followed by an alveolar duct (AD) whose wall is formed by alveoli. An alveolar sac (AS) succeeds the alveolar duct and represents the blind end of the respiratory passage. (From Thurlbeck, W.M.: Chronic obstructive lung disease. In Sommers, Sheldon C. (Ed.): *Pathology Annual.* Courtesy of Appleton-Century-Crofts, Inc.)

spaces to induce reaginic type allergic reactions. On the other hand, particles of six microns or less, provided by organic dusts, spores and some molds, do gain access to the alveolar spaces where they interact with the sparsely distributed mast cells to produce reaginic type tissue responses. This, undoubtedly, explains the migratory infiltrations observed in some diseases, such as allergic pulmonary aspergillosis (see discussion of extrinsic allergic bronchopneumonia below).

The necessary conditions for the development of the intermediate or Arthus type mechanism are present. Particulate antigens, provided by spores and organic dusts gain access to antibodies in the rich network of capillaries. In many parts of the lung parenchyma the alveolar epithelium and the capillary epithelium are adjacent to each other. At times even the epithelium is lacking, which provides a simple situation that permits the passage of antigen through the capillary wall to form complexes with precipitating types of IgG antibody. In the presence of antigen excess, complement is activated to induce the Arthus type of inflammatory response in the vessel walls, in the alveolar interstitial tissue and in the walls of the bronchioles (see extrinsic allergic bronchopneumonia below).

The inflammatory reaction of the Arthus mechanism releases histamine which can induce increased capillary permeability, resulting in localized patches of edema.

The delayed type of hypersensitivity can produce primary parenchymal involvement. Delayed hypersensitivity explains the granulomatous lesion observed in some pulmonary conditions, such as tuberculosis and farmer's lung. Histopathologically, it is often difficult to differentiate the inflammatory infiltration of an Arthus type reaction from the pattern observed with delayed hypersensitivity. In the Arthus reaction, when the specific antigen can be identified, the demonstration of precipitins in the patient's serum will support the diagnosis of an Arthus reaction.

The involvement of the lung by dual immune mechanisms can occur. In atopic individuals infected with aspergillus, both IgE and IgG antibodies are produced, while in patients with farmer's lung or similar diseases both the delayed hypersensitivity and Arthus mechanisms operate.

ALLERGIC DISEASE OF THE BRONCHIAL TREE

Patterns of Uncomplicated Bronchial Allergy and Bronchial Asthma

Interaction of IgE with its specific allergen (antigen) induces the release of histamine and SRS-A.

Histamine causes dilatation and increased permeability of vessels, resulting in edema; stimulation of glands which causes increased production of mucus or seromucus secretions; and smooth muscle spasm which causes bronchospasm.

SRS-A induces only muscle spasm which is usually more sustained than that induced by histamine.

In uncomplicated bronchial allergy all the tissue changes induced by edema and muscle spasm are reversible. Following an attack, the tissues return to normal with no evidence of pathology. Variations in the intensity of edema, glandular secretions and muscle spasm determine the clinical pattern observed.

I. Mild Involvement

A slight degree of edema with a slight or even moderate production of mucus or seromucus exudate may cause no symptoms except *cough*. The cough is usually productive of seromucoid exudate which is clear or slightly grayish in color but not purulent. *Dyspnea* if present is very mild, since the seromucoid exudate of low viscosity produces no obstruction of the airways. Since there is no obstruction, wheezing is usually absent. When present, the wheezes are very fine in quality suggesting some obstruction of the finer bronchioles.

Coarse bubbling rhonchi produced by air

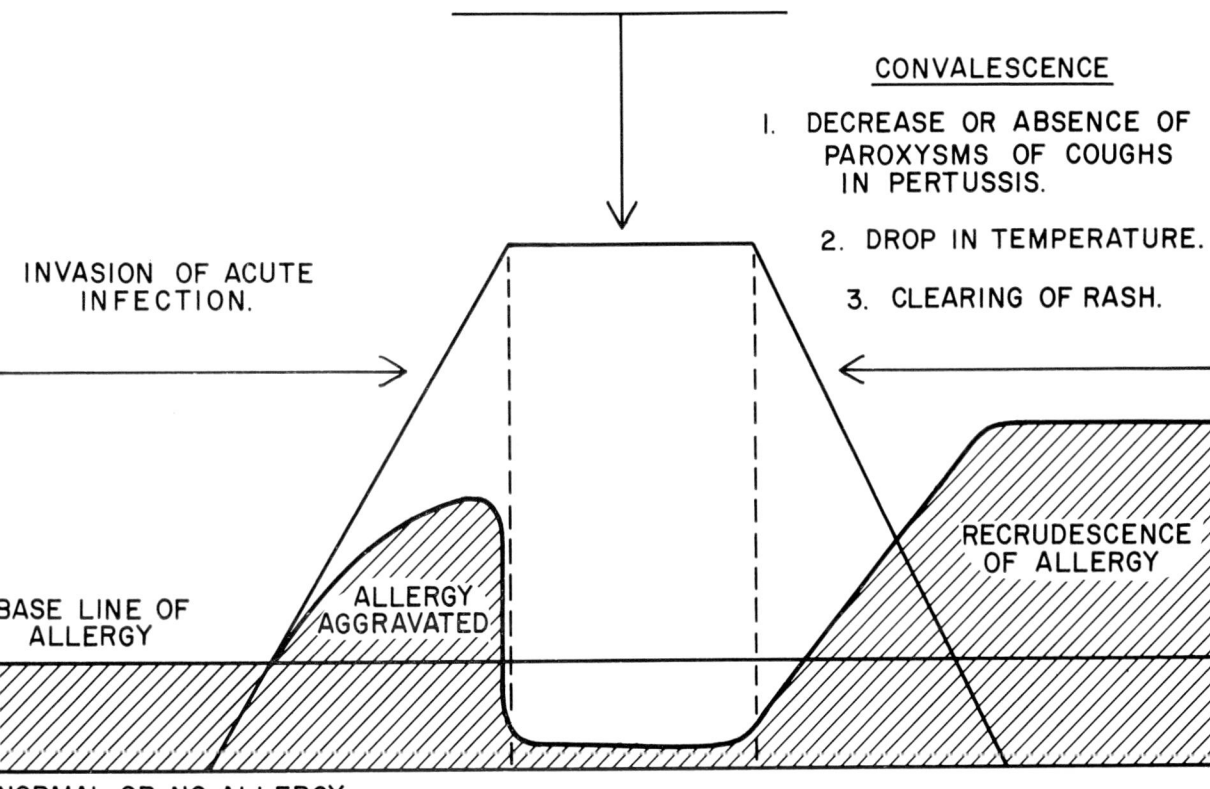

Figure 4-3. Schematic presentation of the influence of acute infectious diseases upon the clinical course of allergy.

rash of the eczematous individual will clear until convalescence.

The second pattern (see Fig. 4-4) is observed very commonly in association with bacterial infections of the upper or lower respiratory tract. In the upper respiratory tract, clinical conditions, such as rhinopharyngitis, acute tonsillitis with or without adenitis, adenoiditis, sinusitis, acute otitis or any combination of these clinical patterns may precipitate symptoms of allergy in the allergic individual.

The interaction of infection and allergy with lower respiratory tract involvement is a common observation at all ages. In pediatric practice it is very frequently observed as the child experiencing recurrent episodes of bronchial symptoms (allergic bronchitis), precipitated by an upper respiratory infection. In the adult, in addition to upper respiratory infection, there are lower respiratory conditions, such as chronic bronchitis, bronchiectasis, and emphysema that serve to complicate the allergic tissue response and provide a bacterial flora for triggering the mechanism, causing symptoms of asthma.

EXTRINSIC AND INTRINSIC ASTHMA: Asthma is frequently classified as extrinsic and intrinsic.

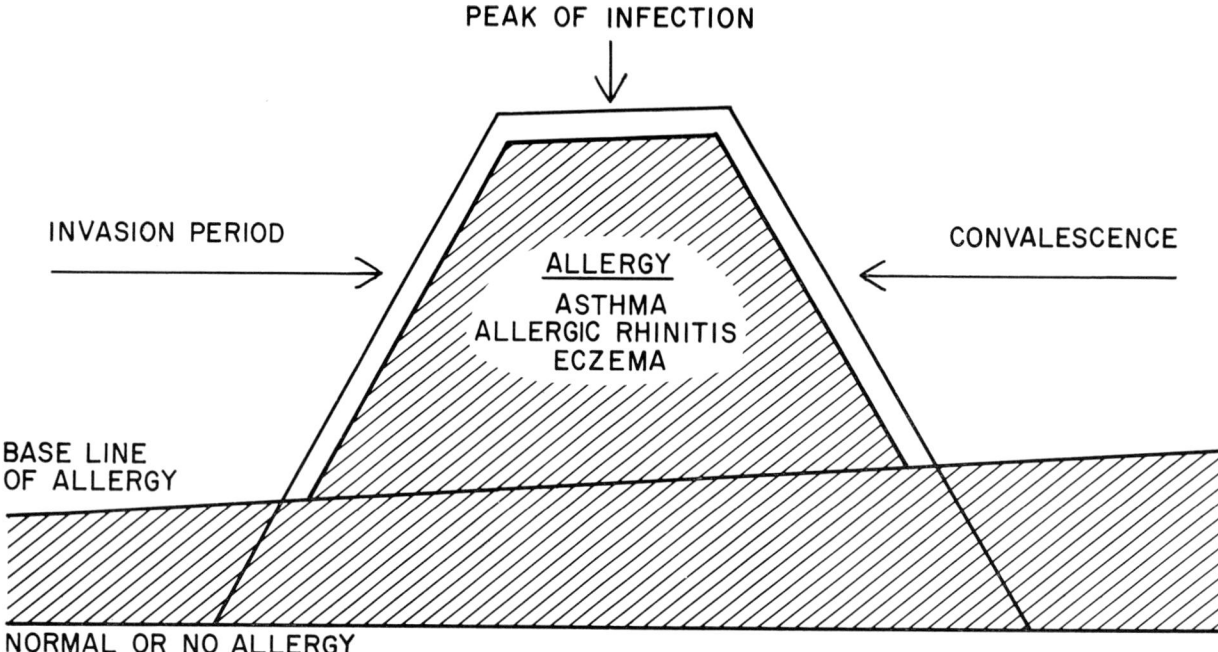

Figure 4-4. Schematic presentation of the influence of an acute upper respiratory infection (bacterial) upon the clinical course of allergy.

Extrinsic Asthma: The term extrinsic asthma is applied to the cases of bronchial allergy and bronchial asthma when an exogenous etiologic agent is identified either by history or a positive skin test. Reliance upon a positive skin test is not sufficient to identify an exogenous agent. Not infrequently, haptenic factors, such as drugs, chemicals and foods which cannot be identified by skin testing may be at fault. The extrinsic asthmas occur more frequently in younger individuals, usually under forty years of age.

Intrinsic Asthma: When an exogenous factor cannot be identified, and an infectious component participates in the clinical pattern, the syndrome is frequently labelled as intrinsic asthma. The implication in most instances is that bacteria are the causative agents. But there are no immunological features to support bacterial sensitivity.

(1) The bacteria or bacterial products when implicated by skin tests show delayed reactivity rather than immediate.

(2) The disease in any given case cannot be correlated with one specific type or organism.

(3) Bacteria or bacterial products induce the delayed type of reactivity. The tissue response observed is the reversible tissue reaction of reaginic allergy which cannot be correlated with the cellular infiltration induced by the delayed type of response *provoked* by bacteria or bacterial products.

(4) The provocation of symptoms with small doses of vaccine is mentioned as supporting evidence for bacterial sensitivity. The reactions following such injections are not of the immediate type but usually delayed for days or weeks. This does not correlate with immediate type of allergy.

(5) A provocative challenge with various bacterial agents resulting in the precipitation of symptoms is offered as supportive evidence for bacterial sensitivity. In most cases the provocative agent cannot be correlated with a specific organism. In addition, in most instances the challenge is performed on patients who recently recovered from an attack of asthma. In individuals who have not experienced asthma for several years the response is identical to that of a normal individual. This observation would suggest that many of the subjects challenged with pro-

vocative tests were clinically free of asthmatic symptoms, but were experiencing a smoldering allergic tissue involvement without clinical symptoms. In such a state the patient will respond to any nonspecific irritant. With *absolute* control of the allergic tissue reaction the patient will manifest the same response as a normal individual.

(6) The proponents of the bacterial concept of intrinsic asthma report that the condition occurs most frequently after the age of forty years, while the onset of asthma in younger individuals is usually extrinsic in type. The older age group is more commonly afflicted with chronic pulmonary diseases, such as chronic bronchitis, bronchiectasis and emphysema in which bacterial infection plays an important role. The presence of bacteria should not necessarily implicate them as a cause of allergy.

(7) Cases of so-called intrinsic asthma do not demonstrate an increased IgE serum titer.

Infections unquestionably influence the allergic reaction. The exact mechanism is not known. It is possible that bacteria, bacterial products and toxins may exert their effects through a pharmacological action upon cell receptors, in which case no allergic mechanism would be involved, although the symptoms may be identical with those induced by reaginic allergy. For example, in pertussis it is postulated that the adrenergic beta receptor system is inhibited, which induces hypersensitivity to histamine in mice. In a similar manner it is possible that bacteria and bacterial products can have some effect upon the various receptors, predisposing those individuals to clinical reactions with a pattern of asthma.

II. Noninfectious Agents

The noninfectious agents include:

cold air
air pollutants
irritating gases and vapors
smoke (including tobacco)
physical exertion of any type, such as running, jumping, exercising
emotional disturbances of any type including laughing and crying

The secondary factors are superimposed upon conditions provided by the primary factors. Unless the primary factors are operating, the secondary factors are ineffectual. The allergic tissue response in some patients may be so slight that no clinical symptoms are observed. The only evidence that the allergic reaction is operating may be an increased irritability of the bronchial tree, which upon provocation by any of the secondary factors induces wheezing of various degrees. At times the wheezing can only be detected on auscultation. Whether the mechanism is increased irritability of nerve endings or a local involvement of the bronchioles has not been determined, but in either case, the clinical response is identical.

The presence of increased irritability has been demonstrated by various provocative inhalant tests. Here again, in many studies the time elapsed since an attack of asthma was not considered. In patients who had been free of asthmatic symptoms for several years, the response to the provocative tests was the same as observed in normal non-asthmatic individuals.

The Beta-Adrenergic Blockade Hypothesis*

The beta-adrenergic blockage hypothesis offered by Szentivanyi proposes that bronchial asthma is induced by an imbalance of β-adrenergic receptors. (See Chapter 15 for discussion of adrenergic receptors.) This theory stipulates that bronchial asthma is a unique pattern of local hyperactivity to a broad spectrum of stimuli. According to this concept, the allergic mechanism is only one of many nonspecific stimuli that are capable of disturbing the homeostatic balance of various cells in the bronchial tissue, which leads to β-adrenergic receptor blockade with resulting bronchial asthma.

---

* Szentivanyi, A.: The beta-adrenergic theory of the atopic abnormality of bronchial asthma. *J Allergy* 42: 203, 1968.

The hypothesis is constructed upon experimental observations made on pertussis-treated mice. The principal feature of the treated mice that relates to human bronchial asthma is their hyperactivity to histamine, bradykinin, serotonin and acetylcholine as well as to nonspecific respiratory irritants. Mice injected with *B. pertussis* plus egg albumen develop two types of homocytotropic antibodies: (1) a heat labile skin sensitizing antibody quite similar in behavior to human IgE and (2) a labile IgG type of antibody which remains fixed to skin for only a few hours.

Attempts are made to draw analogies between the observations in mice and human bronchial asthma and to unify the many diverse factors involved in bronchial asthma into a single mechanism based upon a defect of the beta—adrenergic receptor system. It is stimulating to attempt to interpret bronchial asthma on the basis of homeostatic disturbances at the cellular level; however, any valid conclusions must await a better understanding of the cascade of enzyme systems operating on the cell membrane as well as increased knowledge concerning the intracellular biochemical reactions.[†]

THE COMPLICATIONS OF BRONCHIAL ALLERGIC DISEASE

Status Asthmaticus

If the obstructive features of bronchial asthma in a patient who has been experiencing symptoms for twenty-four hours are not relieved by repeated injections of epinephrine administered over a period of thirty to sixty minutes, the condition is commonly referred to as status asthmaticus.

In status, the patient's anxiety is greatly increased. *Cough* is very persistent, harassing and usually nonproductive. *Dyspnea* is labored and accompanied by marked inspiratory retractions coupled with participation of the accessory respiratory muscles of the neck. The chest is expanded and elevated, and in spite of the great inspiratory effort, thoracic excursions are minimal, which explains the faintly audible wheezing and breath sounds on auscultation. On percussion the note is hyperresonant. Cyanosis may be present.

The patient gets no rest; he is unable to sleep, which leads to extreme fatigue and at times exhaustion. Disorientation of the patient is an important sign of impending status asthmaticus. Exhaustion diminishes the voluntary breathing effort, resulting in diminished expansion of the lung which contributes to the inability to ventilate the lungs because of increased narrowing of the bronchioles and the alveolar ducts. Dehydration is usually pronounced.

The sequence of events in status asthmaticus involves dehydration, ventilatory failure with hypoxemia, progressive hypercapnia, worsening hydrogen ion accumulation, lactic acidosis, extreme fatigue and exhaustion which may be followed by death.

At times death is sudden with no premonitory warning. The patient may appear improved with a good response to bronchodilators. Carbon dioxide tension may be normal or only slightly elevated; however, arterial pCO_2 can be markedly depressed. It is for this reason that patients in status require constant monitoring of blood gases and pH until recovery is almost complete.

The cause of death varies in asthma and in status. Cardiac arrest following persistent hypoxemia over a period of days and at times hours has been reported. Hypercapnia is not a dependable index, since increased CO_2 may not develop until late in the illness and at times too late to reverse the process. In the presence of infection or when asthma is complicated by chronic pulmonary pathology, inspissated mucus plugs may be a cause of death.

An increased number of deaths from asthma has been reported, particularly by observers in Great Britain and Australia where the cause is attributed to increased use and

---

[†] Green, David E. (Ed.): Membrane structure and its biological applications. *N Y Acad Sci, 195;* 1972.

abuse of aerosols medicated with sympathomimetic drugs, such as isoproterenol and epinephrine.

Treatment of Bronchial Allergy*†

The basic principle of treatment in all forms of bronchial allergy involves the relief of obstruction induced by edema, bronchospasm, inspissated mucus and mucus plugs.

Mild and Moderate Involvement:

(1) The first prerequisite is an adequate fluid intake. Water not only counteracts dehydration but is the best of all expectorants. For the average adult a minimum of 2,000 cc in twenty-four hours and for children, proportionately lesser quantities.

(2) For counteracting bronchospasm and edema the sympathomimetic drugs and the methyl xanthines are usually effective. Drug mixtures, such as ephedrine, theophylline and Atarax® (Marax®), or ephedrine, theophylline and phenobarbital (Tedral®) are usually efficacious. For patients requiring continued medication or a repetition of the drug for frequently repeated episodes, because of the risk of dependency, the mixtures containing Atarax are preferred to any compounds containing barbiturates in any form. When the patient reports a preference for a product containing barbiturates, dependency should be suspected.

(3) For expectorant action potassium iodide (KI) is the most reliable preparation. Iodides incorporated into mixtures are not recommended, since the dosage cannot be adjusted to the patient's requirements and tolerance. When iodides cannot be tolerated, the guaicol expectorant drugs may be prescribed.

(4) Infection is usually not a complicating factor in the milder forms of bronchial allergy. However, the patient should be carefully observed at frequent intervals since within a matter of hours infection can become a very important complicating factor. This is particularly observed in children.

If the symptoms fail to respond with conservative management, infection must be considered a factor, even in patients with mild symptoms of the disease. Treatment for infection with antibiotics should be instituted.

Infection as a complicating agent may not necessarily involve the lung. Infection of the upper respiratory tract or a focus of infection elsewhere in the body can be an activating agent and require management accordingly.

(5) Except for the antiasthmatic mixtures indicated above, mixtures of drugs are not recommended. It is not advisable to prescribe cough mixtures of any type and particularly the preparations that contain sedatives, antitussives and antihistamines. Sedatives are undesirable since they suppress the upper respiratory center. Antitussives suppress cough which is contraindicated in bronchial allergic disease. Antihistamines have a drying effect upon the respiratory mucosa which may aggravate the condition and even predispose to pneumonitis. The objective of treatment is to correct obstruction which cannot be achieved by suppressing the respiratory center and the cough reflex or by drying the mucosa.

(6) Corticosteroids are usually not indicated in the milder forms of bronchial allergy.

(7) With bronchial allergy of any degree it is always important to determine if possible the exciting agent or agents. The patient's environment should be carefully checked for possible offenders, such as hairy animals, feathers, felt or jute carpet pads, spray materials of various types (see discussion on environmental control, Chapter 17). Has the patient visited an uncontrolled environment? A visit to the zoo, the circus, an animal pet shop, a barn or a stable may be

---

* More detailed discussion regarding the various medications will be found in Chapter 15, Drugs Used in Treatment of Allergic Disease.

† For management in infancy, see Chapter 14, The Allergic Infant.

the fault. Has the patient ingested any food, beverage or drug that can serve as a trigger?

For patients with a known sensitivity to pollens, it is advisable to diminish as much as possible the exposure to pollens. Windows should always be closed, especially at night when precipitation of pollens may be greatest. If the patient is a city dweller, trips to the open country should be avoided. Car windows should always be closed.

For some patients air conditioning and electronic precipitators are helpful.

(8) Definitive management is discussed in Chapter 17, Immunotherapy.

Bronchial Asthma (Severe Involvement): The treatment of the patient with bronchial asthma is the same as that outlined for less severe forms of bronchial allergy except for the management of the acute paroxysmal episode and the use of corticosteroids.

Epinephrine-HCl 1-1000 by hypodermic in doses of 0.4 cc is the initial drug of choice for treatment of the acute paroxysm of bronchial asthma. The initial dose of epinephrine can be followed with 15 ml of Elixophyllin® which is usually a helpful adjunct. If the patient fails to respond, the dose of epinephrine may be repeated within fifteen minutes. The patient may experience a pharmacological response to the drug as evidenced by pallor, tachycardia and at times vomiting, with no relief of symptoms. If the patient fails to respond, the regimen for status asthmaticus outlined below should be considered.

In many patients the administration of intravenous fluids (water with 5 per cent glucose) is followed very early by a marked improvement in the patient's condition.

The patient suffering an acute paroxysm of bronchial asthma with physical findings suggestive of a dry lung, e.g. sibilant and sonorous rhonchi with no moist bubbling rhonchi, will usually respond to epinephrine without the necessity of further medication. In these cases the administration of Sus-Phrine (as a depot) is a good precautionary measure to carry the patient for a short period following the exhaustion of the effects of the epinephrine-HCl 1-1000.

The patient with diffusely scattered coarse rhonchi in addition to the sibilant and sonorous rhonchi, will usually have a residual of physical findings following control of the acute paroxysmal episodes with epinephrine. These patients require further medication, in the form of corticosteroids and bronchodilators. Sus-Phrine can be administered following the epinephrine-HCl to control the symptoms until corticosteroids and antiasthmatic medication becomes effective.

Corticosteroids are usually the drug of choice for these patients (see discussion on corticosteroids in Chapter 15, Drugs Used in Treatment of Allergic Disease).

The concomitant administration of antiasthmatic preparations usually reduces the dose of corticosteroids required for control and also permits a more rapid phasing out of corticosteroid therapy.

For cyanosis, the carefully regulated administration of oxygen is helpful (see Oxygen Therapy under Treatment of Status Asthmaticus). In the presence of cyanosis, if the patient fails to show an adequate response to epinephrine-HCl and methyl xanthines and oxygen, the procedure for management of status asthmaticus should be instituted immediately.

Following the administration of epinephrine, the patient may experience some improvement, but on physical examination rhonchi and wheezes are still present. In this situation infection should be considered as a possible complicating factor, requiring the administration of antibiotics as early as possible. As a general rule, if the question of infection is doubtful, the safer procedure is always to administer antibiotics very early without waiting for a worsening of the clinical pattern. Early control of infection can frequently abort status asthmaticus.

The definitive management for bronchial asthma is discussed under Immunotherapy (Chapter 17).

Treatment of Status Asthmaticus

Status asthmaticus is usually an emergency situation, requiring immediate and at times heroic procedures to prevent deepening of all the pathological states which may lead to loss of consciousness and even death of the patient. It is important that the physician be cool and restrain his concern, to avoid adding to the patient's *anxiety* state.

When possible, the patient should be hospitalized immediately to have readily accessible all procedures not available in either the home or the office.

The initial procedure should always be the administration of epinephrine-HCl 1-1000 by hypodermic in doses of 0.4 to 0.5 cc. This may be repeated within thirty minutes if necessary.

Drugs given by mouth act too slowly to be beneficial.

When epinephrine-HCl fails to induce desired relief from symptoms, it is commonly referred to as "adrenalin fastness." There are many theories offered to explain adrenalin fastness. In most instances adrenalin fastness is usually due to dehydration. With dehydration the patient will show lack of signs of the pharmacological activity of the epinephrine, such as pallor, tremor and accelerated heartbeat; no influence upon the asthmatic symptoms is observed. This *lack of response* in the asthmatic symptoms may be attributed to the failure to dislodge the mucus plugs from the airways narrowed by edema and muscle spasm. Not infrequently the plugs are purulent from secondary infection. The breakdown of bronchial mucosa and the impairment of ciliary action serve to complicate the obstruction.

The effects of dehydration may operate even when a patient offers a history of taking what seems to be adequate fluids by mouth. If adrenalin offers relief, intravenous fluids may not be necessary, but if adrenalin fails to show a response, intravenous fluids should be administered immediately. In some patients epinephrine will offer only temporary relief; symptoms recur within a few hours. This occurs frequently when infection is present. Intravenous therapy should be considered in such situations. *Delay* may predispose to a persistence of symptoms or even an aggravation of symptoms.

In the dry form of asthma, when no coarse rhonchi but only sonorous and sibilant rales are present, status asthmaticus occurs very rarely. Apparently this type of asthma is secondary to smooth muscle spasm induced by SRS-A. Response to epinephrine-HCl is excellent.

Since status asthmaticus is induced by obstruction of bronchioles with damming back of secretions, secondary infection occurs very frequently. Specific therapy for the infection must be instituted very early.

Procedure for Treatment of Status Asthmaticus

(1) When possible the patient should be admitted to a medical center or to a hospital equipped with an intensive respiratory unit. If the center is remote, treatment should be started immediately before transporting the patient.

The environment should always be controlled for factors which can serve as allergens, such as feather pillows, hairy animals, felt carpet pads, *etc.*

(2) Intravenous Therapy

IV therapy with 5 per cent glucose in water can usually be started immediately before the laboratory studies are available. Most patients in status are severely dehydrated, even when offering a history of large quantities of fluids by mouth. Oral fluids are not a substitute for intravenous fluids which should be administered regardless of the quantity of fluids taken by mouth. Following the initial 500 cc, the patient will frequently manifest an improved response to epinephrine.

(3) The following laboratory procedures should be ordered routinely: complete blood count, urinalysis, arterial blood (brachial or

radial) for measurement of p_aO_2, p_aCO_2, and pH.

(4) Chest roentgenograms in A-P, lateral and oblique positions.

(5) Antibiotics.*

Most patients in status have a complicating component of infection. Antibiotics can be administered even in the absence of a hemogram. The choice of drug is governed by the tolerance of the patient.

(6) Corticosteroids*

It is important to determine if the patient had been receiving corticosteroids. With a history of previous corticosteroids, the continued administration of the drug is mandatory.

The dose and choice of corticosteroids for intravenous therapy should be governed by the needs of the patient. Corticosteroids can be added to the intravenous fluids.

Do not administer depot corticosteroids.

(7) Expectorants

Sodium iodide 0.5 gm to 1.0 gm can be added to the intravenous fluids. Iodides are frequently helpful in decreasing the viscosity of the bronchial secretions.

(8) Aminophylline

Twenty-five mg in 20 ml can be administered over a fifteen to twenty minute period by "piggy back."

(9) Sodium Bicarbonate

For the correction of acidosis as indicated by the pH, bicarbonate in a dose of 88 mEq can be administered intravenously over a period of five minutes. This can be followed by intravenous drip as indicated. The indications are governed by serial pH measurements.

(10) Oxygen

Oxygen should not be administered unless controlled by serial measurements for p_aO_2. When administered by nasal catheter, the rate is three liters per minute. When administered by the Venturi mask, the concentration is 24 to 28 per cent. Uncontrolled administration of oxygen can precipitate CO_2 narcosis.

(11) Bronchodilator by aerosol

In most cases when the usual procedures for management of the patient in status have been carried out, it is not necessary to resort to aerosol bronchodilators. When aerosols are administered they can be given by air compressor or by an intermittent positive pressure apparatus.

For isoproterenol 1:200 the dose is seven drops in 2 ml of normal saline for ten minutes out of the hour. At times it is administered for five minutes every fifteen minutes.

(12) Sedatives

Because of the anxiety and apprehension of the patient the temptation to resort to sedatives is very great. Since these symptoms are a response to defects in ventilation and gas exchange, they are usually uncontrollable until the deficiencies are corrected. In addition, sedatives can mask the clinical pattern and prejudice the judgment of the physician.

With hypoxemia sedatives should never be administered, even when p_aCO_2 is normal.

Do not administer morphine or opiates to any asthmatic; *do not* give barbiturates. Both opiates and barbiturates depress the respiratory center and may aggravate the condition.

Do not give antihistamines. These drugs cause drying of the bronchial mucosa. Antihistamines are ineffective in any form of asthma.

(13) Occasionally, ether-in-oil rectally may be helpful for an extremely restless patient: ether 5 cc in 30 cc of a vegetable oil (olive, sesame). Peanut oil and cottonseed oil are not recommended.

Bronchitis

Bronchitis and bronchial allergy occur together very frequently. Since both are pulmonary obstructive diseases involving the mucosa of the airways, the clinical patterns are identical. Depending upon the degree of mucosal involvement, the clinical patterns

---

* See Chapter 15, Drugs Used in Treatment of Allergic Disease.

may range from mild to very severe. In the mild form there may be no complaints, not even cough. The only finding is the occurrence of a few coarse and sibilant rhonchi. In the more severe forms productive cough and shortness of breath are prominent. Coarse rhonchi and wheezes are present throughout the chest, indicating the presence of obstruction. The mucosa is highly irritable, subjecting the patient to frequent exacerbations of acute symptoms induced by either infectious or noninfectious irritants.

The irritants can precipitate recurrent and even paroxysmal episodes, presenting signs and symptoms identical with bronchial asthma. In the adult with persistent mucosal changes such episodes are observed very frequently. These are difficult to differentiate from true allergic disease.

In the child, and particularly since the advent of antibiotics, chronic bronchitis is observed infrequently. What is labelled chronic bronchitis may be recurrent episodes of bronchial allergy (allergic bronchitis, asthmatic bronchitis), usually precipitated by upper respiratory infections.

When infection is present, the sputum is purulent. With upper respiratory infection the patient may experience a purulent post nasal drip, which also induces coughing. The patient frequently reports this condition as a purulent productive cough which he attributes to lower respiratory involvement. Physical examination will readily determine the source of the discharge as a post nasal drip. In these cases pulmonary findings may be very slight.

Only a history of atopic allergy with or without positive skin tests can support the presence of an allergic component. When allergy is present, instituting allergy management may succeed in improving the condition. This is particularly true in children in whom persistent chronic mucosal changes have not yet developed. In the adult with persistent, irreversible mucosal changes, controlling the allergy will prevent acute episodes but may not effect a complete cure.

The question is frequently raised whether allergy can cause chronic bronchitis. Chronic changes in the bronchi, even to the degree of saccular bronchiectasis, are well documented as a sequel to Arthus type reactions as observed with extrinsic allergic bronchopneumonia. The role of reaginic type allergy in the development of chronic bronchitis is not quite as clear. Uncomplicated bronchial allergy, even in its severest form, such as bronchial asthma, induces reversible tissue changes which have been confirmed by biopsy. Most of the pathological studies in asthma have been made on chronic cases, in whom it is difficult to differentiate the tissue changes induced by the reaginic allergic reaction from those caused by the chronic bronchitis, which are usually complicated with infection. Although the evidence is not absolute, it is conceivable that chronic reaginic allergic states may induce pathological changes similar to those observed in chronic bronchitis. Chronic reaginic allergic involvement of the nasal mucosa induces hypertrophy and hyperplasia with increased numbers of goblet cells, plus thickening of the basement membrane and fibrosis of the submucosa. It is reasonable to expect that the mucosa of the bronchial tree which is actually an extension of the nasal mucosa may respond in a similar manner to persistent insults by reaginic allergy to produce chronic changes.

Atelectasis

Atelectasis results from complete obstruction of an airway usually induced by edema, mucus plugs, and muscle spasm. Since these are characteristic of reaginic allergic tissue reactions, atelectasis is a frequent complication of bronchial allergy.

Obstruction of a large airway is the result of combined edema and viscid mucus which forms a plug. With obstruction of a bronchus an entire lobe may become atelectatic as in middle lobe disease.

Sudden plugging occurs when viscid mucus serves as a tamponade in a bronchus with marked edema. Symptoms develop very suddenly. Dyspnea is intense, respirations are very rapid, *cough is severe* and harassing, and temperature is suddenly elevated to 104 or 105 degrees. The physical findings are those typical of atelectasis. Roentgenogram is positive for atelectasis.

In some cases the plug may be dislodged spontaneously with coughing followed by a sudden relief from symptoms. More commonly, epinephrine-HCl 1-1000 is necessary to reduce the edema which permits release of the plug and subsequent clearing of symptoms.

Plugging of a bronchus may develop very gradually in which event onset of symptoms will be less dramatic. Physical findings and roentgenograms are the same as with the sudden onset.

This syndrome may occasionally be encountered in children with bronchial allergy.

The small bronchioles which are below the level of cartilage are very readily obstructed by muscle spasm, edema and mucus, acting either in combination or separately. Such obstruction may produce small patches of atelectasis which cannot be diagnosed either by physical examination or roentgenogram, since they are masked by the surrounding aerated alveoli. Obstruction occurs very readily in children, especially under the age of seven years in whom the diameters of even the larger airways are relatively small.

Thin seromucoid secretions rarely produce obstruction, as they are readily propelled by the cilia and easily dislodged by the coughing reflex. Thick, viscid mucus readily causes obstruction.

If obstruction due to plugging is not relieved, the resulting atelectatic area may soon become involved by infection leading to pneumonitis. In some cases of longstanding collapse due to obstruction, fibrosis may produce irreversible tissue changes.

Emphysema

Emphysema is a chronic obstructive pulmonary disease for which the cause is frequently not known.

Studies of the histopathology implicate bronchiolar and alveolar duct obstruction, resulting in air trapping with secondary alveolar rupture. The bronchiolar and alveolar ducts, embedded in parenchymal tissue, are surrounded by fibroelastic bands which are continuous with the elastic fibers of the surrounding lung. These fibers serve to maintain the patency of these ducts during expiration. With involvement of the fibroelastic fibers, the bronchioles and alveolar ducts collapse, inducing air retention, followed by alveolar disruption.

Clinically, the condition is manifested as hyperaeration, marked expansion of the chest with increased A-P diameter, wheezing and progressively increasing exertional dyspnea.

Since bronchial allergy is also an obstructive disease, its occurrence with emphysema aggravates the clinical pattern.

The pathological changes involved in emphysema are not reversible, so that complete relief cannot be had from sympathomimetic drugs or any other form of medication. The tissue changes induced by the allergic component when present are reversible, so a degree of relief can be expected by controlling the allergy through routine allergy management. The failure to obtain relief with sympathomimetic drugs is an important differential between chronic obstructive disease and the reversible bronchial involvement of allergic disease.

PULMONARY FUNCTION

The principal function of the lung is the delivery of adequate supplies of oxygen to meet the metabolic requirement of cells and the removal of CO_2, the waste product of cellular metabolism. This is achieved through: (1) the mechanics of respiration, and (2) the diffusion of gases through the ventilatory portion of the lung.

I. The Mechanics of Respiration

The requirement of oxygen at rest ranges from 200 to 250 ml/minute. Upon extreme exertion this may be increased twentyfold. These great differences in the demand for oxygen induce both direct and indirect stimuli upon the respiratory centers and the airways to produce variations in the volume of gas passing into and out of the lungs. At the same time the blood transport system accommodates to the variations in the supply of gas by an increase in both stroke volume and rate, which during exercise can raise cardiac output from 5 liters/minute to 25 to 30 liters/minute.

The volume of gas entering and leaving the lung is governed by the respiratory movements of inspiration and expiration.

Inspiration is accomplished by the contraction of the diaphragm, the intercostal muscles, and in cases of extreme demand, by the accessory muscles of the neck and at times the abdominal muscles. Muscular contraction creates a positive pressure which overcomes the "elastic" recoil of the lungs and the thoracic cage, the resistance of the airways, and the functional resistance of the pulmonary tissues and the chest wall.

Expiration occurs passively upon relaxation of the muscles at the end of inspiration and by the elastic recoil of the parenchyma.

Elastic Recoil

The helical structure of the collagen and elastic fibers of the lung give this organ a spring-like quality which together with *surface tension* is responsible for *elastic recoil* (rebound of the lung), an important function in expiration.

The pressure required to overcome elastic recoil is related to the movement of a given volume of air, which is known as *static compliance* (C_{st}). Any condition that reduces the elasticity of the lung, e.g. fibrosis, edema or granulomatous infiltrates, will reduce compliance.

Surface Tension and Pulmonary Surfactants

Since the studies of von Neergaard in 1929, it has been generally recognized that surface tension is concerned with the retractive forces of the lung. Recent studies have demonstrated the presence of surfactants which play a role in the interrelationship between structure, mechanical forces and surface tension in the lung.

Pulmonary Surfactants

Surfactants are materials that lower surface tension of the medium in which they reside. In the mammalian lung these materials consist of proteins, carbohydrates, and lipids including particularly the phospholipids (dipalmitoyl, lecithin, sphingomyelin, phosphatidyldimethylethanolamine, and others). All these materials reside in the ultramicroscopically thin acellular lining layer that covers the alveolar cells. The origin of the surfactants is not known.

The importance of pulmonary surfactants has been assumed from *in vitro* measurements or estimates of surface tension, from which studies several theories have evolved.

1. The "zero surface tension, anti-edema" concept of Pattle based upon the following observations:

(a) The major force that tends to *move liquid into the capillaries*, i.e. promote alveolar dryness, is plasma colloid osmotic pressure which is approximately 22 mm Hg in the dog.

(b) The major force that tends to *drive liquid out of the capillaries*, i.e. promote pulmonary edema, includes:

(1) capillary hydrostatic pressure	7 mm Hg
(2) interstitial colloid osmotic pressure	5 mm Hg (dog)
(3) interstitial negative pressure	10 mm Hg (dog)
Total	22 mm Hg

Accordingy, the forces that tend to move liquid out of the capillaries (22 mm Hg) and the forces that tend to move liquid into the capillaries (22 mm Hg) are balanced, resulting in a maintenance of liquid flux without a net gain or loss between capillaries and alveoli.

2. The concept of Clements which states that as an area decreases, e.g. during deflation of the lung, surface tension falls toward zero, so that at small volumes tension is a negligible force. This theory assumes that tension varies directly with area, so that the net surface force which tends to promote alveolar collapse (the same inward force that promotes the movement of liquids out of the capillaries) is similar among alveoli of different sizes and thus prevents the tendency of small alveoli to empty into larger ones.

3. Colacicco and Scarpelli have unified the "zero surface tension, anti-edema" theory of Pattle and the "variable surface tension" theory of Clements. The studies of these investigators on the surface properties of pulmonary dipalmitoyl lecithin (DPL) in unbuffered 0.15 M NaCl showed that zero surface tension is produced and maintained upon relatively slight compression of the surface film. On the basis of this observation they suggest that alveolar surface tension is at or near zero dynes per centimeter throughout the respiratory cycle. Thus the anti-edema and anti-atelectasis function of pulmonary surfactants is nearly constant throughout the normal life span of the lung. Any disruption of the surfactant system will lead to liquid accumulation in the alveoli and a tendency of the alveoli to collapse spontaneously.

Resistance

Airway Resistance: The cartilage-containing airways are not imbedded in the lung, and as a result they are more affected by transpulmonary pressure (the difference between pressure at the mouth and intrapleural pressure) than by changes in lung volume.

Below the level of cartilage, resistance varies with lung volume. The fibroelastic bands of the transitional airways (bronchioles and below) are continuous with those of the lung. As a result, expansion of the lung exerts a pull upon the walls of these airways, causing an increase in their diameters, which decreases their resistance. Peribronchial pressure is equal to or more negative than pleural pressure. Changes in the resistance are not only related to elastic recoil at high lung volumes, but also depend upon bronchomotor tone. In the absence of such tone, the resistance of the tracheo-bronchial tree changes markedly at low lung volumes, remains relatively constant over the mid-lung volume, and then actually increases somewhat at high lung volumes.

Airway resistance contributes approximately 80 per cent to the total resistance.

Obstruction of the airways in bronchial asthma by muscle spasm and mucus plugs causes a sudden increase in resistance, which prolongs expiration and prevents complete emptying of the acinar unit. The next inspiration causes more air-trapping with enlargement of the acinar unit, which means an increase in functional reserve capacity. The increased lung volume augments the elastic recoil which provides greater expiratory force.

Tissue resistance is caused by displacement of lung tissue itself, the rib cage, the diaphragm and the abdominal muscles.

Terms in Respiratory Physiology

The terms listed below are those commonly encountered in the clinical management of respiratory problems. The definitions are concise and intended as a guide for supplemental reading.

Subdivisions of Lung Volume

(VC) *Vital Capacity*: the maximal volume of air that can be expelled from the lungs by a forceful effort following a maximal inspiration. VC can easily be measured with a spirometer.

(TLC) *Total Lung Capacity*: volume of gas in the lungs at the end of a maximum inspiration.

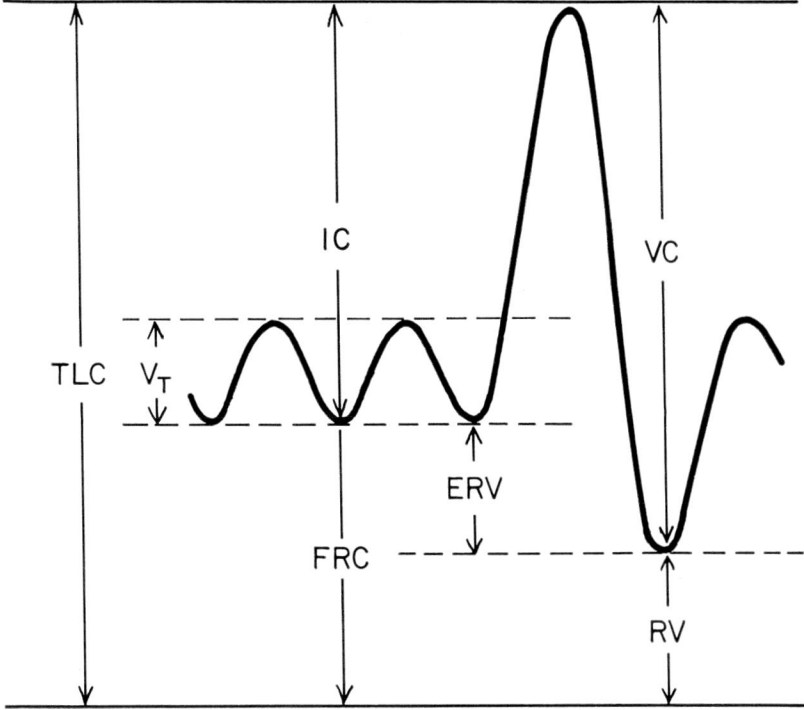

Figure 4-5. Subdivisions of lung volume: TLC = Total lung capacity, FRC = Functional residual capacity, VC = Vital capacity, ERV = Expiratory reserve volume, RV = Residual volume, IC = Inspiratory capacity, V_T = Tidal volume. (From Bates, D.V., Macklem, P.T. and Christie, R.V.: *Respiratory Function in Disease.* Courtesy of Saunders.)

(ERV) *Expiratory Reserve Volume:* maximal volume that can be expired from resting expiratory level.

(RV) *Residual Volume:* volume of gas in lungs at the end of maximal expiration.

(FRC) *Functional Residual Capacity:* volume of gas in the lungs at the resting end-expiratory level.

(IC) *Inspiratory Capacity:* maximal volume that can be inspired from the resting expiratory level.

(V_T) *Tidal Volume:* the volume of gas expired with each breath.

Ventilation Measurements

(V_E) *Resting minute ventilation:* the quantity of air expired per minute, measured with a recording spirometer.

(V_D) *Anatomical dead space:* the volume of all non-gas exchanging passages in the lung usually comprising the upper airway and bronchial tree as far as the respiratory bronchioles.

(V_A) *Alveolar ventilation* is the fraction of total ventilation (V_E) that enters the gas exchanging surface of the alveoli.

$$V_E - fV_D \text{ anatomical} = V_A$$
$$f = \text{respiratory rate}$$

Table 4-II: NORMAL VALUES*

Tension. pO_2 arterial:	Adults = 75–100 mm Hg
	Children = 75–100 mm Hg
pH, arterial, blood:	Adults = 7.35–7.45
	Children = 7.37–7.44
Carbon dioxide tension (pCO_2), arterial blood:	Adults = 35–45 mm Hg
	Children = 32–40 mm Hg
Base excess (by Astrup):	Adults = −2.3 to +2.3 mEq per liter
	Children = −4.0 to +4.0 mEq per liter

FEV_1 expressed as a percentage of predicted normal value (% pred FEV_1) based on the age, sex, and height of the patient.

* Berglund, E. *et al.*: Spirometric studies in normal subjects. In Forced expirograms in subjects between 7 and 70 years of age. *Acta Med Scand, 173:* 185–192, 1963.

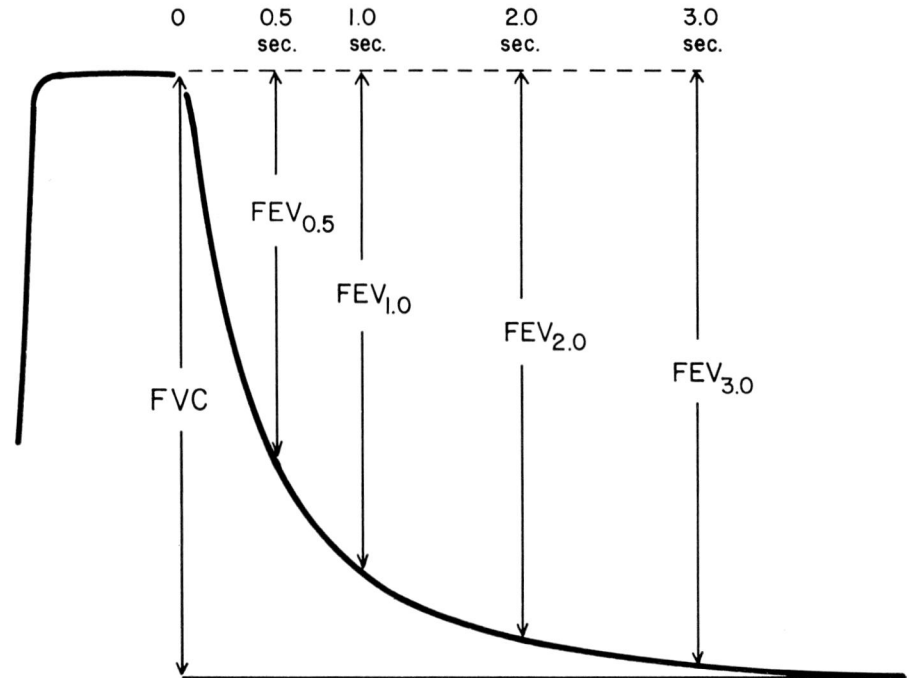

Figure 4-6. The forced expiratory spirogram is here diagrammed to show the forced vital capacity (FVC) and the 0.5 second, 1.0 second, 2.0 second, and 3.0 second forced expiratory volumes ($FEV_{0.5}$, $FEV_{1.0}$, $FEV_{2.0}$ and $FEV_{3.0}$). From Baum, Gerold: *Textbook of Pulmonary Disease*. Courtesy of Little, Brown & Co.)

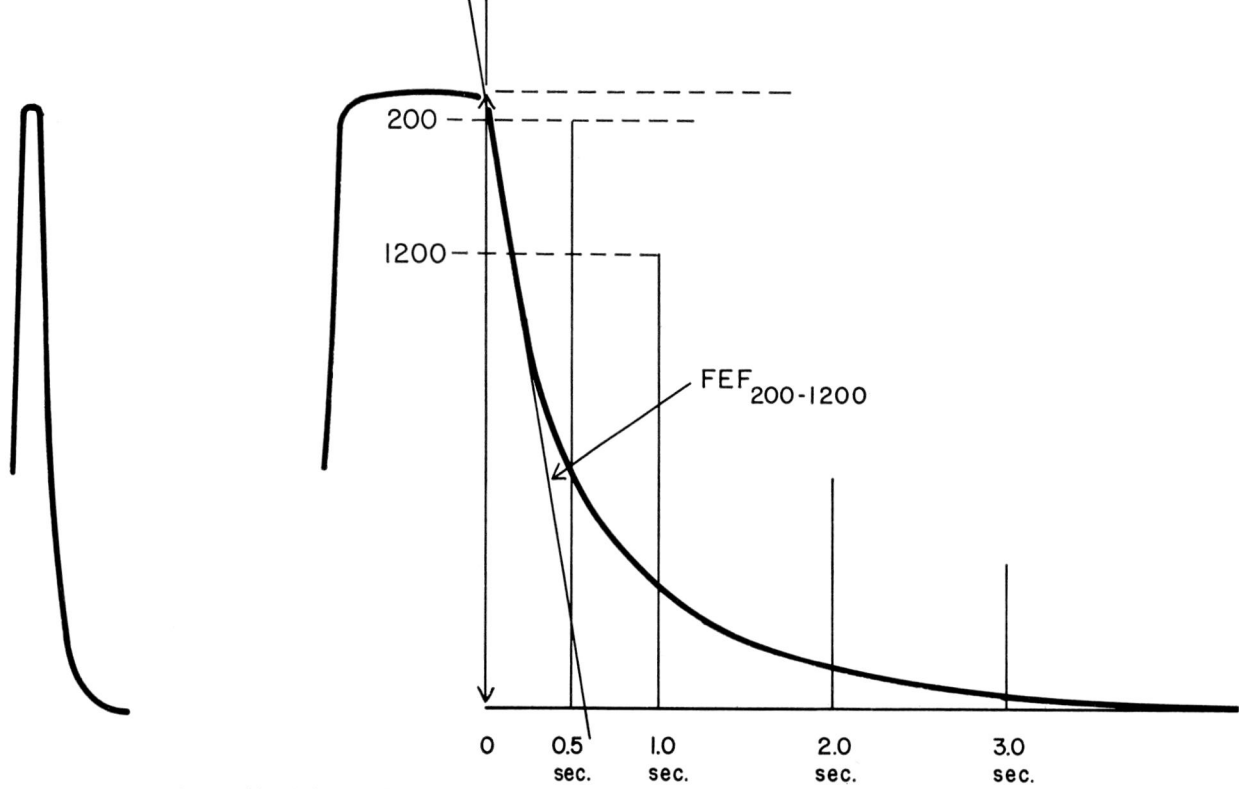

Figure 4-7. The $FEF_{200-1200}$ (previously called the MEFR) is shown here as the slope obtained by connecting the intersections of the forced expiratory spirogram (FES) with horizontal lines representing 200 ml and 1,200 ml below maximal inspiration. (From Baum, Gerold: *Textbook of Pulmonary Disease*. Courtesy of Little, Brown & Co.)

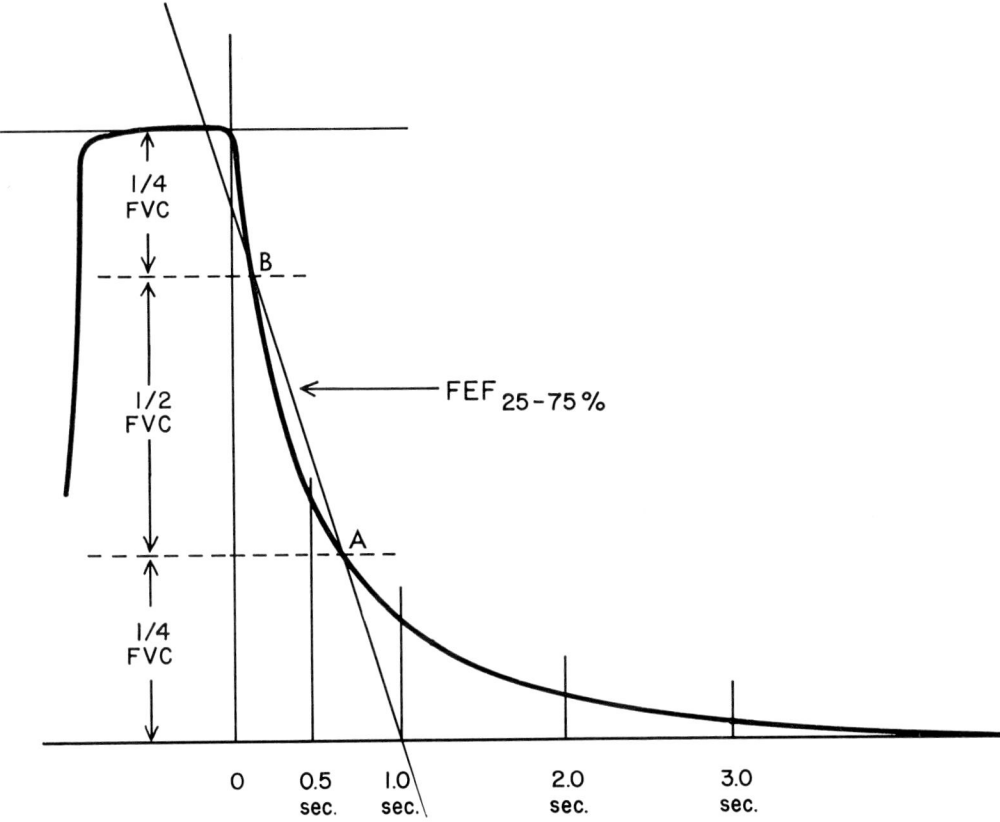

Figure 4-8. The forced expiratory spirogram (FES) here shows the forced mid-expiratory flow measurement (FEF$_{25\%-75\%}$). *A* represents the intersection of the FES with the line between the first and second quarter of the forced vital capacity volume (25%). *B* represents the intersection of the FES with the line between the third and fourth quarter of the forced vital capacity volume (75%). The slope of the line connecting *A* and *B* is the forced mid-expiratory flow (FEF$_{25\%-75\%}$). (From Baum, Gerold: *Textbook of Pulmonary Disease.* Courtesy of Little, Brown & Co.)

(MBC) *Maximal Breathing Capacity*: the maximal volume of air that a subject can breathe per minute.

Because of the many deficiencies and variables involved in the performance of this test, it has been replaced by a single breath measurement of ventilation ability.

Single Breath Measurements

This measurement can be made on a recording spirometer. The forced expiratory spirogram (FES) measurements are:

1. (FVC) FORCED VITAL CAPACITY: For the forced vital capacity (FVC) the subject exhales rapidly as well as forcefully. In normal individuals, for practical purposes, FVC = VC.

In obstructive pulmonary disease, as in bronchial asthma, chronic bronchitis and emphysema, VC is greater than FVC.

The measurements are:

(1) Forced vital capacity (FVC)
(2) Forced expiratory volume at 0.5 seconds (FEV$_{0.5}$), at 0.75 seconds (FEV$_{0.75}$) and at 1.0 second (FEV$_{1.0}$).

The most valid prediction formulas currently available for the normal adult values for FVC, FEV$_{0.5}$ and FEV$_{1.0}$ are indicated in Figures 4–9 and 4–10.

2. (RV) RESIDUAL VOLUME: the volume of

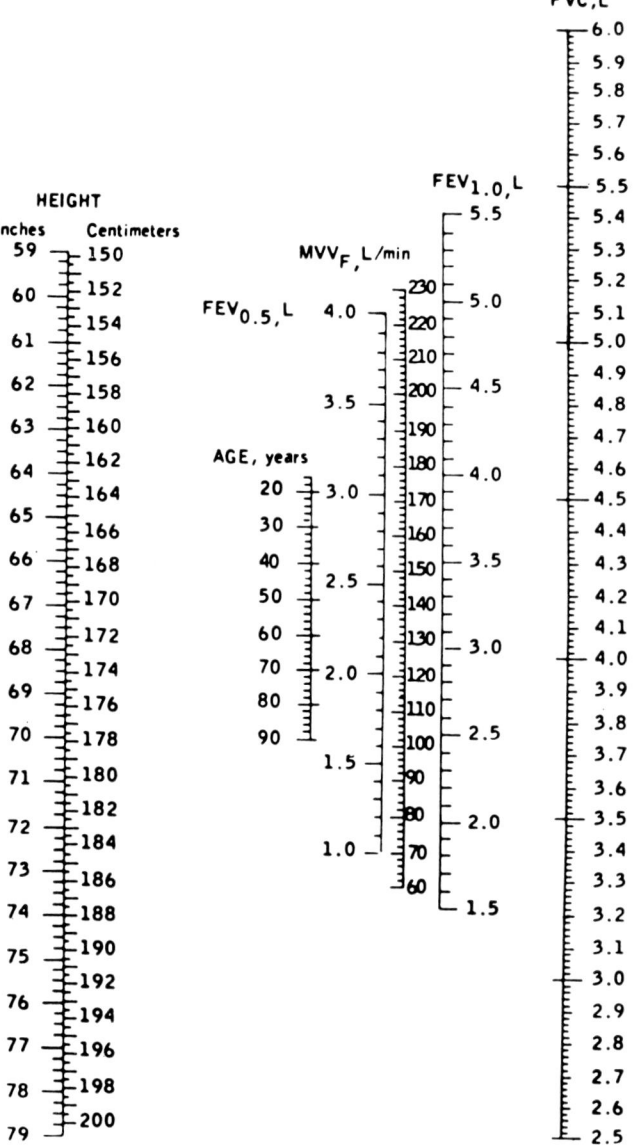

Figure 4-9. Nomogram for prediction of FVC, $FEV_{0.5}$, $FEV_{1.0}$, and MVV_F from age and height in adult men.

To Use Nomogram: Lay a straight edge between the patient's height as read on the *height* scale and his age as read on the *age* scale. Predicted normal values can be read directly from the points where the straight edge crosses the $FEV_{0.5}$, the MVV_F, the $FEV_{1.0}$, and the FVC scales.

$$FVC, L = 0.133H - 0.022A - 3.60. \quad (SEE = 0.58 \text{ L})$$
$$MVV_F, L/min. = 3.39H - 1.26A - 21.4. \quad (SEE = 29.0 \text{ L/min.})$$
$$FEV_{0.5}, L = 0.050H - 0.24A + 0.24. \quad (SEE = 0.51 \text{ L})$$
$$FEV_{1.0}, L = 0.094H - 0.028A - 1.59. \quad (SEE = 0.52 \text{ L})$$

Key:
H = Height in inches
A = Age in years
SEE = Standard error of estimate
FVC = Forced vital capacity
MVV_F = Maximal voluntary ventilation (free)
$FEV_{0.5}$ = 0.5 second forced expiratory volume
$FEV_{1.0}$ = 1.0 second forced expiratory volume

(From Kory, Ross C.: Laboratory aids in investigating pulmonary diseases. In Baum, Gerold (Ed.): *Textbook of Pulmonary Disease.* Courtesy of Little, Brown & Co.)

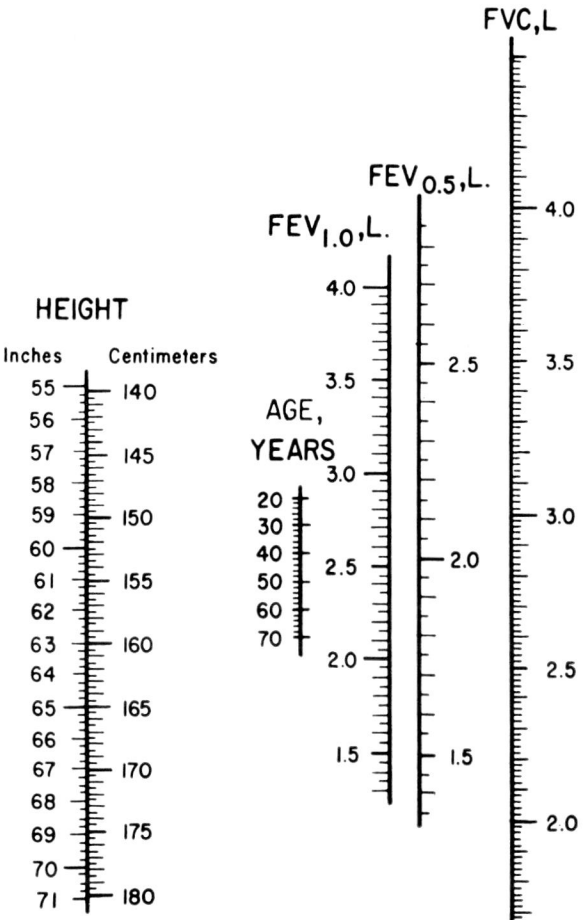

Figure 4-10. Nomogram for prediction of FVC, $FEV_{0.5}$, and $FEV_{1.0}$ in women based on studies of 450 normal women ranging in age from 20 to 70 years.

To use Nomogram: Lay a straight edge between the patient's height as read on the *height* scale and his age as read on the *age* scale. Predicted normal values can be read directly from the points where the straight edge crosses the $FEV_{1.0}$, the $FEV_{0.5}$, and the FVC scales.

$$FVC = 0.041H - 0.018A - 2.689 \quad (SEE = 0.371 \text{ L})$$
$$FEV_{0.5} = 0.018H - 0.011A - 0.297 \quad (SEE = 0.306 \text{ L})$$
$$FEV_{1.0} = 0.028H - 0.021A - 0.867 \quad (SEE = 0.330 \text{ L})$$

Key:
H = Height in cm
See key to Figure 4-9 for other abbreviations.
(From Kory, Ross, C.: Laboratory aids in investigating pulmonary diseases. In Baum, Gerold (Ed.): *Textbook of Pulmonary Disease*. Courtesy of Little, Brown & Co.)

gas in the lungs at the end of maximal expiration.

This compartment of the lung usually requires techniques and equipment available in pulmonary physiology laboratories.

(1) *Closed circuit helium dilution method:* The subject is switched into a closed circuit containing a suitable percentage of helium in the air and breathes quietly until no further fall in helium takes place. This procedure is applicable for clinical use. There are several reports in the literature describing the technique and the application of this procedure.

(2) *The open circuit nitrogen clearance method*: This method involves the displacement of nitrogen from the lungs by oxygen breathing and calculation of the volume of nitrogen expired by analysis of the nitrogen content of expired air.

(3) *The body plethysmograph method*: The patient is placed in an airtight chamber in which volume changes in the intrathoracic gas can be calculated from the simultaneous rarefaction of the surrounding gas in the plethysmograph.

(4) *Radiological method*: The volume of the heart and both domes of the diaphragm and of the pulmonary blood and lung tissue are subtracted from the volume of the thorax as determined by planimetry from a P-A chest roentgenogram. These determinations have been correlated with plethysmographic determinations with a high degree of agreement. The overall coefficient is 0.966.

II. The Ventilatory Portion of the Lung

The acinus which is constituted of respiratory bronchioles, alveolar ducts, atria and alveolar sacs is the basic unit of the gas exchanging portion of the lung. There are between two to nine respiratory bronchioles in an acinus. About eighteen last order terminal bronchioles arise from one terminal bronchus which gives rise to about four hundred alveolar ducts and sacs in an acinus (see Fig. 4-2).

The dense network of capillaries actually forms a pool of blood. The span between capillaries is usually less than the diameter of a capillary. The capillaries may be separated from the alveoli by a very fine interstitial layer, which frequently is absent, permitting direct apposition between the capillary endothelium and the alveolar epithelium. In some places even the alveolar epithelium is absent, permitting the capillary to have direct contact with the alveolar air space. This anatomical arrangement allows free diffusion of gases from the alveoli to the capillaries (O_2) and from the capillaries to the alveoli (CO_2).

At sea level air contains approximately 21 per cent oxygen and 79 per cent nitrogen with an atmospheric pressure of 760 mm Hg. The concentration of CO_2 and other gases is negligible.

The partial pressure of oxygen (pO_2) at sea level is calculated as follows:

Atmospheric oxygen = 21 per cent or 21/100

Atmospheric pressure = 760 mm Hg
21/100 × 760 = 159 mm Hg

As air passes through the upper respiratory tract, it becomes fully saturated with water vapor which has a partial pressure of 47 mm Hg. This reduces the oxygen pressure to 149 mm Hg.

760 mm Hg (atmos) − 47 Hg (aq. tension) × 21/100 = 149

The amount of air entering the acini for ventilation equals the amount of air moved with each breath (Tidal Air, V_T) minus the air in the dead space. Therefore, an individual breathing 450 ml with a dead space of 150 ml will ventilate 300 ml with each breath. If the respiratory rate is 15 per minute, then the total volume of air ventilated will be 15 × 300 ml = 4,500 ml/minute.

At rest every 100 ml of blood permits 5.56 ml of CO_2 to diffuse into the alveolar spaces, and 7 ml of oxygen is carried away from the acinus by 100 ml of blood.

The partial pressure of CO_2 in the acinus is 713 × 5.6/100 = 40 mm Hg.
The partial pressure of O_2 in the acinus is 713 × (21% − 7%) = pO_2 100 mm Hg.

The requirement of oxygen at rest ranges from 200 to 250 ml per minute. Upon extreme exertion this may be increased twentyfold, which indicates the tremendous reserve capacity of the lung. The utilization of the great reserve pulmonary capacity to meet variations in demand ranging from rest to extreme exertion is probably governed by the "turning off" and "turning on" (variations in ventilation) of the supply of gas to selected atria by the contraction of the few muscle fibers present in the terminal air passages. With the "turning off" and "turning on" of atria to adjust to the varying demands for oxygen, a mechanism must be present to direct the blood flow from nonfunctioning (nonaerated) atria to functioning (aerated) atria to prevent improper gas exchange. The mechanism for this control is suggested by Vane* who postulates,

It has been known for a long time that when a portion of a lung collapses or is not properly perfused with air, blood is diverted from that area, the purpose presumably being to ensure that all blood passing through the lung receives the maximum feasible increment of oxygen. Prostaglandins seem to be excellent candidates for the role of local controller of pulmonary circulation. PGE_2 is released by distended lung tissue (as both we and Wylie have demonstrated) and its release is probably proportional to the degree of stretch; thus the greater the inflation (stretch) of a particular lung region, the greater the vasodilation and blood flow to that same area, and the lower the proportion of blood passing through the inadequately aerated regions.

---

* Vane, John R.: Prostaglandins and the aspirin-like drugs. *Hospital Practice*, New York, H-P Publishing Co., 1972.

Blood Oxygen and Blood Oxygen Tension (pO_2)

In a simple solution the relationship between the gas concentration and gas tension forms a straight line at any given temperature. However, when the solution contains buffer systems such as in the blood or special methods for transporting the gas, such as RBC, the relationship is not linear. This is illustrated in Figure 4-11.

One gram of hemoglobin combines chemically with 1.34 ml of O_2. With a normal he-

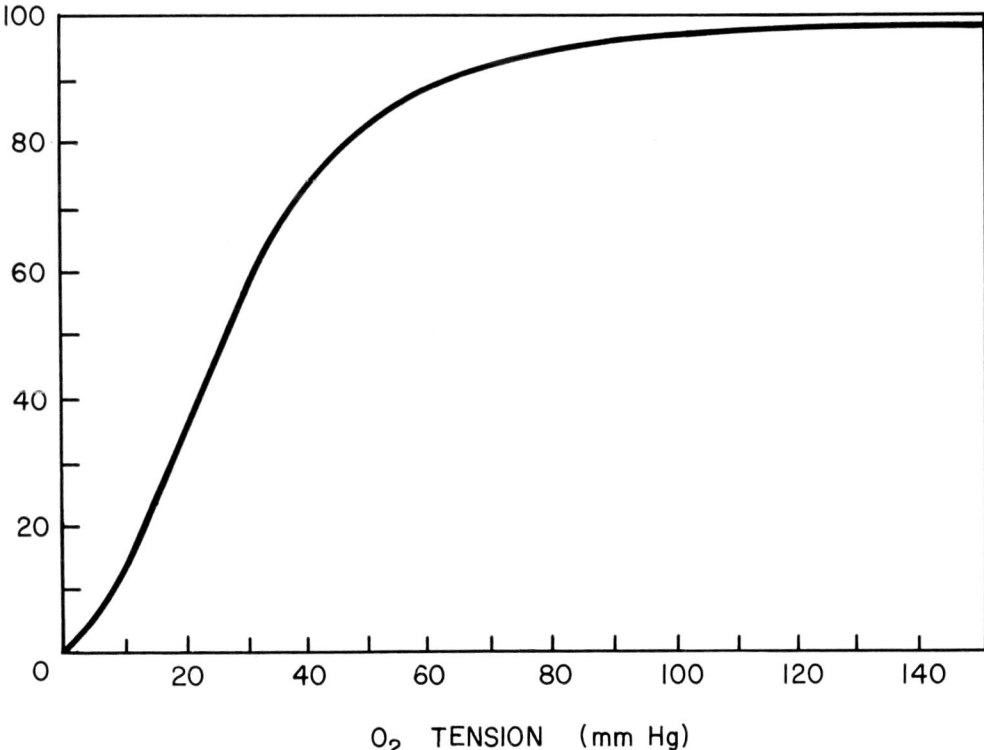

Figure 4-11. The oxyhemoglobin dissociation curve. This normal dissociation curve illustrates the relationship between oxygen saturation and oxygen tension for whole blood of normal hematocrit and at a pH of 7.4.

moglobin value of 15 gm the oxyhemoglobin (HbO_2) capacity of a normal individual is 15×1.34 ml O_2/100 ml blood.

The amount of O_2 in solution is very small but the small amount accounts for the partial pressure of oxygen (pO_2) in blood. Normally, the partial pressure of O_2 in blood is slightly less than the partial pressure of O_2 in the acinus, where it is approximately 100 mm Hg. This difference permits the diffusion of O_2 from the alveoli to the capillaries where O_2 is equivalent to 0.3 volume per cent (ml/100 ml of blood) dissolved in arterial blood.

The amount of O_2 in combination with hemoglobin at any time depends upon the partial pressure of O_2 in the blood or in the air that is in equilibrium with the blood. When pO_2 increases, more oxygen is taken up by the red cells. When pO_2 decreases, oxygen is given off by the red cells.

The maximum amount of oxygen that can be carried by a unit volume of blood is called its oxygen capacity (S_{O_2}). Oxygen capacity depends upon the quantity of hemoglobin the blood contains (normally 15 mg) and the partial pressure of O_2.

Carbon Dioxide Content (pCO_2) and Acid Base Balance (pH)

Carbon dioxide (CO_2) in blood occurs in four states:

(1) In simple solution in plasma (approximately 5%),
(2) In bound form as bicarbonate (H_2CO_3) (85–90%),
(3) In bound form with plasma proteins (less than 2%),
(4) In bound form with hemoglobin (between 2 and 10%).

The basic formulae involved in CO_2 transport in blood are:

(1) $H_2O + CO_2 = H_2CO_3$ (carbonic acid)
(2) $H_2CO_3 \xleftrightarrow{\text{dissociates}} H^+ + HCO_3^-$ (bicarbonate ion)
(3) $H^+ + HCO_3 \xleftrightarrow{\text{dissociates}} H_2CO_3 \xleftrightarrow{\text{dissociates}} CO_2 = H_2O$

The CO_2 diffuses through the capillary-alveolar membrane and is exhaled.

CO_2 combines with hemoglobin to form carbamide compounds. Although the RBC carries only a small percentage of the total CO_2 in the blood, they play an essential role in the transport of CO_2 to the lungs. Red blood cells contain the enzyme carbonic anhydrase which rapidly hydrates the CO_2 as it passes through the RBC membrane and converts it into carbonic acid (formula #1).

Carbonic acid dissociates rapidly into H^+ ions and bicarbonate ions (formula #2).

The bicarbonate ions (HCO_3) quickly penetrate the RBC membrane and enter the plasma in exchange for chloride ions. By means of this reaction most of the CO_2 produced by cellular metabolism is carried by the blood as bicarbonate.

The CO_2 combined with plasma proteins is also catalyzed through the action of carbonic anhydrase.

Acid-Base Balance

When CO_2 goes into solution in water, it forms a weak acid (H_2CO_3) which acts as a buffer. Through this chemical reaction CO_2 plays a very important role in the regulation of acid-base balance or pH of the blood.

The normal pH of arterial blood equals 7.40 ± 0.02.

CO_2 content of normal arterial blood equals 56 ml/100 ml of blood.

As the blood passes through the systemic capillary bed, it picks up CO_2 which is removed as it passes through the pulmonary bed.

The relationship of CO_2 to pH operates according to the Henderson-Hasselbach equation:

$$pH = pK + \log \frac{HCO_3^- \text{ (bicarbonate } CO_2\text{)}}{H_2CO_3 \text{ (dissoved } CO_2\text{)}}$$

constant $pK = 6.11$ normal blood $pH = 7.41$

Substituting:

$$7.41 = 6.11 + \log \frac{HCO_3^-}{H_2CO_3}$$

$\log HCO_3/H_2CO_3$ would be 1.30, the logarithm of 20.

Therefore, normal pH 7.41, the ratio $\frac{HCO_3}{H_2CO_3}$ must equal 20:1.

Pulmonary Function in Allergic Bronchial Disease

The broad range of clinical patterns encountered in allergic bronchial disease, which vary from mild asymptomatic pulmonary involvement to life threatening status asthmaticus, explains the great differences in the values of measurements of both pulmonary mechanics and ventilation.

The Asymptomatic Patient

The asymptomatic patient with allergic bronchial disease may have smoldering pathology as evidenced by several criteria. Not infrequently, these patients, because of a lowered threshold of irritability, are more prone to respond with wheezing following exposure to irritants, such as cold, dust, chemicals, histamine and mecholyl. Following exercise, these patients may experience varying degrees of wheezing and at times pulmonary hypertension may be induced by physical activity. In addition, a significant fall in FEV may be recorded following exercise. The response to exercise in the asymptomatic patient can serve as a useful diagnostic aid when bronchial asthma is suspected.

During the asymptomatic interval between acute episodes, the patient may have disturbances of compliance with pulmonary over-inflation as measured by the functional reserve capacity. Regional variations in ventilation and perfusion of the lungs may be present with no symptoms.

BRONCHIAL ASTHMA: The chief mechanical difficulty in bronchial asthma is the increased flow resistance secondary to bronchospasm. As a result of increased airway resistance, the work of breathing in asthma may be increased from five to ten times that of the normal. Obstruction caused by edema and mucus are also important contributing factors as a cause of airway resistance. Although obstruction due to muscle spasm occurs to some degree in the larger airways, the main site of involvement appears to be in the valve-like fibromuscular transitional segment of the bronchial tree. The maximal mid-expiratory flow rate (MMEF) and FEV are sensitive indicators of the obstructive changes. The MBC, FEV, MMEF and peak flow rates have all been reported in different studies. McFadden and Lyons classified the severity of airway obstruction in asthmatics by expressing the one second forced expiratory volume (FEV_1) as a percentage of predicted normal value (% of predicted FEV_1) based on age, sex, and height of the patient.

The patients were classified as follows:

Degree of Airway Obstruction	% of Predicted Values
severe	25
moderate	26–50
mild	51–85

In asthmatic subjects FEV correlates better with lung compliance than with airway resistance. In emphysema the correlation between airway resistance and FEV_1 is very close.

The vital capacity (VC) has been used to follow patients with asthma, but this indicator is much less sensitive than studies of dynamic lung volume. The VC is usually decreased in patients with asthma, but with moderate hyperinflation and slight decrease in MMEF, the VC may be relatively normal.

Obstruction of airways leads to overinflation of the lungs, resulting in a decreased elastic recoil of the lung which is manifested as a decrease in compliance. The dynamic compliance is usually decreased in asthma.

By use of plethysmography major increases in TLC and FRC were noted in asthmatic patients, whereas when measured by gas dilution these increased values were not observed.

In the uncomplicated asthmatic patient all the abnormal measurements of function return to normal values following the administration of bronchodilators, such as isoproterenol and epinephrine-HCl.

HYPOXEMIA: In the discussion regarding the pulmonary reserve capacity it was pointed out that parts of the lung are "turned on" and "turned off" in order to meet the varying demands of pulmonary ventilation. Recent studies on prostaglandins indicate that they may play a role in shunting capillary flow from poorly aerated or nonaerated alveoli to distended and well aerated alveoli. The nonuniformity in gas distribution which is normally present in the lung is also present in patients with asthma. These differences in aeration in the normal and asthmatic lung have been demonstrated by various studies of pulmonary function but particularly the more recent techniques utilizing radioactive xenon and macroaggregated radioalbumen.

These studies have demonstrated that the asthmatic lung can reduce perfusion to zones that are poorly ventilated. This also occurs in the normal lung. Apparently the shunting mechanism involved in the asthmatic patient does not differ from that which occurs in the normal lung except that in the asthmatic, the system does not operate efficiently and permits blood transport through poorly aerated parts of the lung which results in inadequate oxygenation of the blood or lowered pO_2. This is supported by recent studies that demonstrated lowered arterial oxygen saturation in patients with only moderately severe degrees of bronchospasm. In more severe cases of bronchial asthma and particularly in status asthmaticus, pO_2 can be lowered to very critical levels, even as low as 50 per cent of normal.

In the management of the severe asthmatic patient it is important to recognize that pO_2 can be lowered to a dangerous level (as low as 50% for patients in status) without a concomitant elevation in pCO_2. This critical lowering of oxygen tension can occur without radiological evidence of atelectasis and what is even more serious, without any warning by the appearance of the patient suggesting the critical level of the hypoxemia.

Recent studies on severe asthmatics have shown that a rise in arterial pCO_2 occurs late and may be a terminal event following days or hours of hypoxemia without hypercapnia.

RESPIRATORY ACIDOSIS AND ALKALOSIS: Following a report by an *ad hoc* committee of the New York Academy of Sciences Conference in 1965, it was agreed that the terms "acidosis" and "alkalosis" in reference to respiratory physiology should designate a physiological disturbance rather than a chemical disturbance. Accordingly, the terms are used to designate a disturbance of mechanism whatever the resultant pH. (See discussion of Acid-Base Balance in this chapter.)

An increase in pCO_2 as in alveolar hypoventilation will decrease arterial pH (respiratory acidosis) providing there is no change in the bicarbonate concentration of body fluids. An elevated pH (respiratory alkalosis) results from lowering pCO_2 as in hyperventilation. Since varying degrees of alveolar hyperventilation and hypoventilation are observed in patients with bronchial asthma, the arterial blood may be alkalotic, acidotic or even normal, depending upon the state of ventilation present.

Asthmatic patients with either mild or moderate obstruction of the airways will have either a normal or an alkalotic arterial blood pH, while with severe obstruction or in status asthmaticus the arterial pH will be acidotic.

Carbon dioxide retention can vary from low (hypocapnia) to high (hypercapnia) and at times normal (normocapnia). These variations in CO_2 retention are observed from patient to patient and at times for the same patient depending upon changes in the clinical pattern of the patient.

CYANOSIS: The normal individual has 15 mg of Hb/100 ml of blood. As blood passes through the pulmonary capillary network, it becomes oxygenated so that arterial blood contains practically no unoxygenated Hb. However, as blood passes through the systemic capillaries, it releases approximately 5 to 6 per cent of oxygen by volume which results in 3.75 gm of unoxygenated Hb. The critical level for the appearance of cyanosis is 5.0 gm or more of unoxygenated Hb. Since 3.75 gm, which is the normal level of unoxygenated Hb, is below the critical level of 5.0 gm, cyanosis is not a feature of normal gaseous exchange.

Cyanosis is not observed in uncomplicated bronchial allergy or bronchial asthma. When complicated by infection, cyanosis may appear particularly in young children.

Cyanosis occurs frequently with status asthmaticus when it is indicative of a critical, life threatening state of the patient.

Allergic Bronchopulmonary Disease
Allergic Alveolitis
Extrinsic Allergic Bronchopneumonia

When involvement of the lung parenchyma is associated with atopic diseases of the bronchial tree, the alterations in the lung are secondary to airway obstruction which leads to air trapping, hyperaeration, impairment of compliance, disturbances of gas exchange and atelectasis with superimposed pneumonia.

Most of the allergens that induce reaginic type of allergic response are 10 microns in diameter or greater and therefore cannot gain access to the alveolar spaces.

Primary involvement of the parenchyma or the alveoli of the lung is caused by particles six microns or less, which include a number of molds, spores and various organic dusts. Various antigenic materials have been incriminated as the cause of pulmonary parenchymal involvement. Although different names have been applied to the same clinical pattern depending upon the source of the antigen involved, they are actually the same disease with identical immunologic responses and identical pathologic changes. Accordingly, the same immunopathologic response has been reported as allergic aspergillosis, pigeon breeders disease or bird fanciers disease, while farmer's lung, bagassosis, bird fanciers disease, *etc.* (see Table 4-III) may be the identical syndrome induced by an antigen derived from a different source.

On the basis of the immune response bronchopulmonary allergic disease falls into two classes: (1) patients with evidence of delayed hypersensitivity (DH) with concomitant precipitating type IgG antibodies for which farmer's lung is the prototype, and (2) atopic individuals with immediate hypersensitivity reactions, induced by IgE antibodies with concomitant precipitating IgG antibodies for which allergic aspergillosis is the prototype.

Farmer's Lung

The clinical description of farmer's lung by Campbell in 1932 was the first docu-

Table 4-III: ALLERGIC BRONCHOPULMONARY DISEASE

Disease	Source of Material	Antigenic Agent
Farmer's lung	Moldy hay	
Bagassosis	Moldy bagasse	Thermophilic *Actinomyces*
Mushroom workers lung	Mushroom compost	
Suberosis	Cork bark	
Malt workers lung	Moldy barley	*Aspergillus fumigatus*
	Malt dust	*Aspergillus clavatus*
Maple bark strippers disease	Moldy bark	*Cryptostroma (Coniosporium) corticale*
Sequoiosis	Moldy sawdust	*Graphium* and *Aureobasidium pullulans*
Cheese workers lung	Cheese manufacture	Penicillin species
Wheat weevil disease	Infested wheat flour	*Sitophilus granarius*
Laundry detergent workers lung	Detergents with enzymes	Enzymes of *B. subtiles*
Bird fanciers disease	Budgerigar (parakeet)	Bird droppings
Pigeon breeders lung	Pigeons	Sera
	Duck and turkey feathers	*Aspergillus fumigatus*
	Hens	Hen droppings
Allergic aspergillosis	Moldy hay	*Aspergillus fumigatus* and others
	Moldy vegetables	
	Organic dusts	
	Bird droppings	Sera or molds

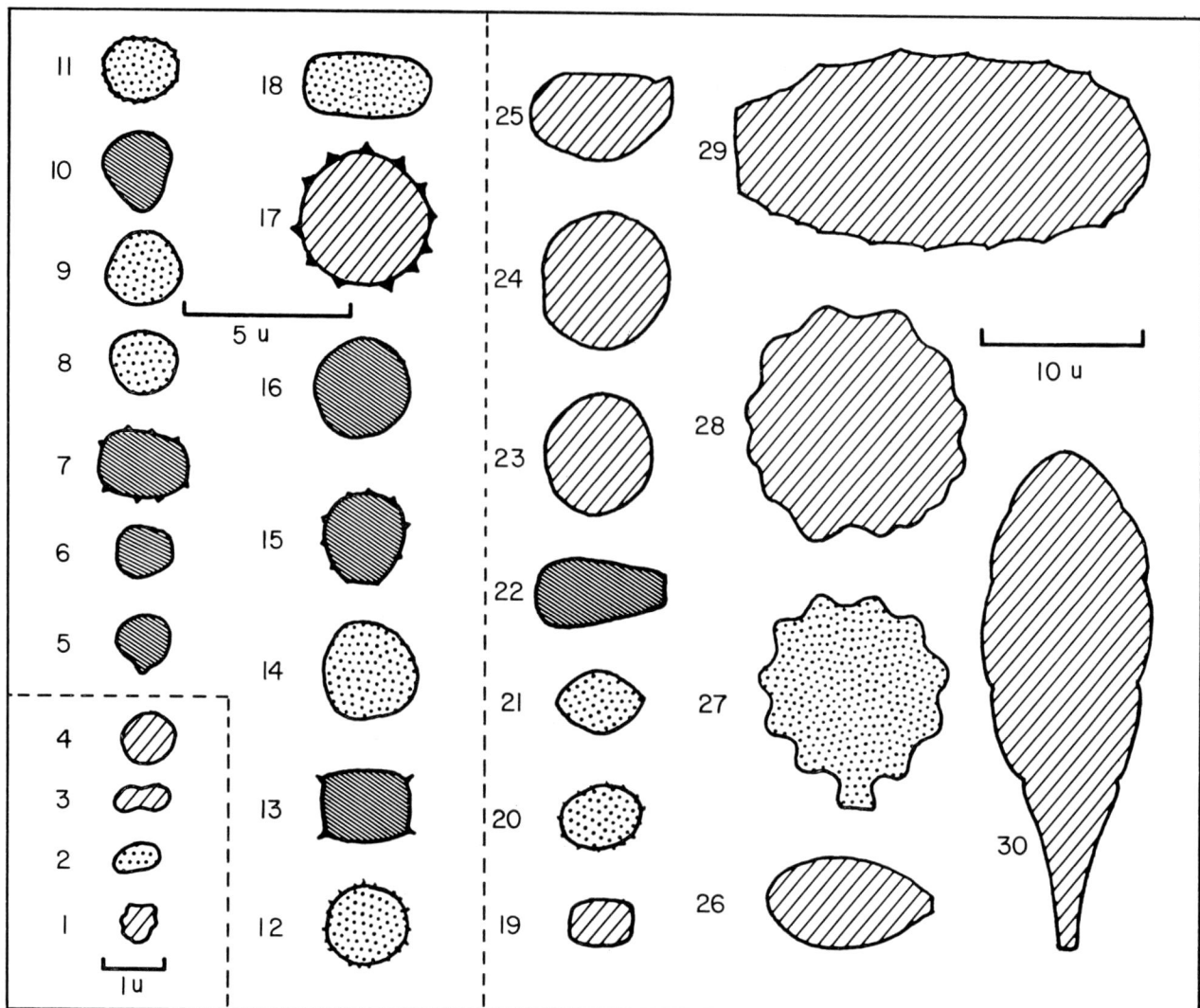

Figure 4-12. Spores in allergies and mycoses of man and animals. Outlines of the airborne spores of Fungi and Actinomyces causing allergies and mycoses. The species are arranged in order of the minimum recorded diameter or length of their spores. Directly pathogenic species—dark shading; allergenic species—light shading; species isolated from animal lungs—dotted.

1. *Thermoactinomyces vulgaris* Tsiklinsky.
2. *Streptomyces fradiae* (Waksman and Curtis) Waksman and Henrici.
3. *Thermomonospora viridis* (Schuurmans *et al.*) Küster and Locci.
4. *Micropolyspora* sp.
5. *Histoplasma capsulatum* Darling.
6. *Aspergillus terreus* Thom.
7. *Aspergillus fumigatus* Fresenius.
8. *Mucor pusillus* Lindt.
9. *Absidia corymbifera* (Cohn) Saccardo and Trot.
10. *Blastomyces dermatitidis* Gilchrist and Stokes.
11. *Penicillium piceum* Raper and Fennell.

mented report for any of this group of syndromes. Following the initial reports on farmer's lung, the association with the handling of moldy hay was recognized, but for several years the disease was attributed to a fungal infection. In 1963 Pepys demonstrated that the growth of the thermophilic Actinomyces, *Micropolyspora faeni* (formerly *Thermopolyspora polyspora*) in hay is the major source of antigen which induces an immune response responsible for the disease. Another strain of thermophilic Actinomyces, *Microspora vulgaris,* has been shown to cause farmer's lung, perhaps more commonly in the United States than in England from which country the majority of the reports on this disease has originated. There may be other organisms as yet unidentified, that develop in hay which produce a similar pattern.

Clinical Patterns: Farmer's lung occurs in both acute and chronic forms depending upon the intensity and the frequency of exposure to the offending antigen. The condition has not been reported in children under ten years of age.

The *acute phase* usually occurs within hours following exposure to the moldy hay and is characterized by a "flu"-like pattern with anorexia, headache, fever, slight cough usually productive of clear mucus but at times the mucus may be blood tinged. Progressive exertional dyspnea is the most prominent complaint. In some patients cyanosis may be present. On physical examination of the lungs crepitations are heard, especially over the lower lobes. On roentgenogram a disseminated miliary involvement is observed. In some cases "soft," poorly defined opacities become confluent in places, especially in the middle and lower lung fields. The normal sharp definition of the pulmonary vessels is reduced.

Respiratory function studies early in the acute phase usually show a decrease in the following measurements: FEV_1, vital capacity, diffusing capacity, and compliance. All

---

12. *Trichoderma viride* Fries.
13. *Coccidiodides immitis* Rixford and Gilchrist.
14. *Aspergillus candidus* Link.
15. *Emmonsia rescens* Emmons and Jellison.
16. *Aspergillus flavus* Link.
17. *Aspergillus niger* Van Tieghem.
18. *Absidia ramosa* (Lindt) Lender.
19. *Cryptostroma corticale* (Ellis and Everhart) Gregory and Waller.
20. *Aspergillus repens* (Corda) de Bary.
21. *Chaetomium funicola* Cooke (ascospore).
22. *Allescheria boydii* Shear (conidium).
23. *Ustilago maydis* (de Candolle) Tulasne.
24. *Papularia sphaerosperma* (Persoon ex Fries) von Höhnel.
25. *Sepula lacrymans* (Wulfen ex Fries) Karsten.
26. *Cladosporium herbarum* Fries.
27. *Humicola lanuginosa* (Griffon and Maublanc) Bunce.
28. *Epicoccum nigrum* Link.
29. *Puccinia graminis* Persoon (uredospore).
30. *Alternaria* sp. (after *Austwick,* 1966).

(From Pepys, J.: *Hypersensitivity Diseases of the Lungs due to Fungi and Organic Dusts.* Courtesy of S. Karger.)

measurements return to normal with resolution of the acute attack except for compliance which may remain reduced at 60 per cent to 80 per cent of predicted values. Therapy will induce an improvement of all measurements, except when corticosteroids are discontinued compliance may remain reduced.

Early in the acute phase oxygen saturation of arterial blood at rest may be near cyanosis level (82 to 85 %); pCO_2 is usually low in all patients during the acute phase.

In the *chronic* phase patients complain of weakness, especially of the thigh muscles, noticeable on exertion. Cough is persistent and not necessarily productive. Progressive exertional dyspnea is again the dominant complaint. In some patients orthopnea develops. Cyanosis is a more frequent observation in the chronic phase, while pulmonary hypertension with cor pulmonale and clubbing of the fingers are not unusual complications. The crepitations heard at the base of the lungs in the acute phase are usually absent during the chronic phase.

The roentgenogram of the chronic patient usually shows diffuse fibrotic changes which develop following the acute stage. In some patients the miliary nodular infiltrations observed in the acute cases may persist in the chronic phase and appear together with fibrosis. Contraction of the upper lobes is frequently observed at this stage.

Pulmonary function tests may show deficits in measurements of function at rest, similar to those observed in the acute phase.

In patients with chronic disease with mild impairment, the pulmonary function tests at rest may be normal but during exercise the deficiencies become manifest.

Histopathology: The tissue reactions of the acute phase manifest sarcoid-like granulomata, interstitial inflammatory changes (pneumonitis), bronchiolar involvement, vascular lesions and foreign body giant cells.

Sarcoid-like granulomata are a feature of the early acute stage, appearing within three weeks following the onset of symptoms and slowly resolving over a period of twelve months. The granulomata are tubercles consisting of epithelioid cells, giant cells of Langhans and foreign body-type cells with a number of lymphocytes around the periphery. Central necrosis of the granulomata is observed at times. With chronicity the granulomata absorb, to be replaced by fibrosis. Not infrequently granulomata persist and are present together with fibrosis; however, in most cases the granulomata are gradually replaced.

Interstitial Inflammatory Changes (Interstitial Pneumonitis)

A constant finding of the acute phase is the cellular infiltration of the interalveolar septa which resembles an interstitial pneumonic process that is usually in close relationship to a respiratory bronchiole. The reaction forms a nodule which consists of plump proliferating alveolar epithelial cells with prominent groups of lymphocytes, and with a few acute inflammatory cells, neutrophils and eosinophils. A few plasma cells are present. In the center of the alveolus dense masses of fresh reticulin are present.

Bronchiolar Lesions: Obstructive lesions of the bronchioles occur in all acute cases due to a disintegration of a segment of the bronchiolar wall which is replaced by a mass of mixed cells, fibrin and debris which completely fills the lumen. Neutrophils and mononuclear cells are common.

The bronchopneumonic process of the acute state, suggested by the interstitial cellular infiltration and the bronchiolar involvement would support the recommendation of Seal, Hapke and Thomas that farmer's lung and all similar clinical conditions be labelled as "extrinsic allergic pneumonitis or bronchopneumonia" rather than "extrinsic allergic alveolitis" as proposed by Pepys, since the latter terminology implies limitation of the process to the alveoli.

Vascular Lesions: Very early in the acute phase there is present an acute vasculitis affecting the alveolar capillaries and some small arterioles. Platelets and fibrin deposition together with thrombi and neutrophils infiltrate the affected vessel wall. This reaction is suggestive of the tissue response observed with an Arthus type reaction (see discussion of Arthus Reaction in Chapter 1). No arteritis of a severity comparable to the vasculitis seen in the capillaries occurs. Foreign body giant cells are frequently observed in the tissue reactions, but their significance is not explained.

The chronic phase of farmer's lung is characterized by diffuse interstitial fibrosis, focal peribronchial confluent areas of fibrosis, cellular infiltration, "honeycomb" or cystic and emphysematous changes. Involvement is predominantly of the upper lobes. Cor pulmonale is a frequent complication of the chronic phase. Granulomatous lesions may be present in some chronic cases, but they are not characteristic of this phase.

Immunology: Precipitating IgG antibodies, specific for the thermophilic Actinomyces, can be demonstrated in the sera from patients with farmer's lung. In allied conditions as listed in Table 4-III, precipitins for the specific organism of each clinical pattern can be demonstrated.

The presence of specific IgG antibodies in the patient's serum, and also in the tissues as demonstrated by the immunofluorescent technique, together with the histopathological changes characteristic for the Arthus type reaction support the concept that farmer's lung and allied clinical patterns are manifestions of the intermediate or Arthus type of immune response.

The question of associated delayed hypersensitivity (DH) is not conclusive but highly suggestive. It is conceivable that following the individual's initial encounter with the specific antigen, a delayed type of hypersensitivity develops. It has been demonstrated that when DH is induced, humoral antibodies are evoked at the same time. These antibodies could be responsible for the Arthus type reaction of farmer's lung.

It is possible that following the induction of sensitivity any subsequent encounter with the specific antigen will evoke both DH and the Arthus type reaction, but the predominance of the Arthus component masks the presence of a DH response, except when the patient is observed very early in the acute phase of the disease. This concept is supported by the histological appearance of farmer's lung very early in the acute stage, which has much in common with the histology of segmental lesions of childhood tuberculosis. In this case, an intra-alveolar edema with macrophages and interstitial pneumonitis plus an increase in reticulin in the alveolar septa is associated with noncaseating tubercles.

Diagnosis: The diagnosis of the acute phase of farmer's lung is dependent upon a history of exposure to the dust of moldy hay, moldy vegetables or other organic dusts and bird droppings, followed within a few hours with the acute "flu"-like pattern. On physical examination crepitations are usually heard at the base of the lungs. The roentgenogram shows the characteristic miliary involvement. The diagnosis is supported by demonstrating precipitating IgG antibodies in the patient's serum specific for the incriminated dusts.

The chronic phase usually offers a history of previous acute episodes. Exertional dyspnea is very pronounced. The chest roentgenogram shows the diffuse fibrosis with the major involvement in the upper lobes. The demonstration of precipitating antibodies in the patient's serum specific for the suspected dust is conclusive support for the diagnosis.

Treatment: The most important aspect of treatment is removal of the patient from contact with the offending dust. Continued exposure prevents resolution of the acute reaction and risks induction of the chronic phase with irreversible tissue changes and aggravation of symptoms.

For acute symptoms, corticosteroids are recommended.

Pulmonary Aspergillosis

The clinical patterns of pulmonary aspergillosis are dependent upon a dual immune mechanism, involving IgE antibodies produced in atopic individuals with subsequent tissue reactions, and precipitating IgG antibodies which induce the Arthus type reaction.

Etiology: The disease is caused by various species of the genus *Aspergillus,* of which *Aspergillus fumigatus* is the most frequent offender. Although the organism has a wide distribution, the induction of disease is usually subsequent to the exposure to high concentrations of the Aspergillus as may be encountered in moldy hay, moldy vegetables, moldy grain, vegetable dusts and in bird droppings and feathers. In this respect the epidemiology of pulmonary aspergillosis is quite similar to that of farmer's lung.

The capacity of Aspergillus to evoke IgE antibodies in atopic individuals differentiates it from the thermophilic Actinomyces of farmer's lung in which disease precipitating IgG antibodies are the only antibodies involved. The Aspergillus antigen has the capacity to evoke IgE antibodies, but only if the individual is atopic, which means, the inherent capacity to respond with increased IgE titers, when properly stimulated. In nonatopic individuals Aspergillus antigen does not evoke the IgE response.

Pepys classifies the responses to Aspergillus in two ways.

I. In Atopic Individuals

(1) *Patients with uncomplicated asthma*: This group is constituted of atopic individuals who manifest an immediate whealing skin reaction on testing with Aspergillus extracts, as well as with the extracts of the common allergens, such as pollens and epidermal factors. Some patients of this group may manifest a dual reaction on testing with Aspergillus extracts: the immediate whealing reaction followed by an "early delayed" response of the Arthus type.

(2) *Asthma with Pulmonary Eosinophilia (APE)*: The patients in this group usually present a history of asthma of variable duration in some cases dating to early childhood. The antecedent asthmatic attacks may not necessarily be due to the Aspergillus, but may be a response to one or more of the common allergens to which the patient is sensitive and to which the patient reacts upon skin testing. To explain the uncomplicated bronchial asthma on the basis of Aspergillus sensitivity depends upon the ability of the Aspergillus antigen to evoke IgE antibodies in an atopic individual without the concomitant production of IgG antibodies. This is a point that requires clarification. On the other hand, if the isolated production of IgE by the Aspergillus does not occur, it is reasonable to believe that the uncomplicated asthma reported in the patients in group (1) was an expression of the response to common allergens, such as pollens, environmental factors and foods to which the patient is sensitive and to which positive skin reactions can be elicited.

There is invariably a history of exposure to larger than ordinary quantities of mold, spores, organic dusts or bird droppings.

At the onset symptoms include generalized aches and pains, fever, rapid weight loss, progressive dyspnea, intermittent cough which may be productive of mucus plugs and at times hemoptysis.

Transitory pulmonary infiltrations which may be present for days or even weeks occupy different portions of the lung which are observed in roentgenograms as opaque shadows. The infiltrations, which are usually in the region of the medium sized bronchi, may represent a peribronchial process or collapse of a segment, a lobe or an entire lung. Episodic airway obstruction accompanies these changing infiltrations of the lung and are evidenced by a reduction in the forced expiratory volume to 70 per cent or less of vital capacity.

Saccular bronchiectasis may be present at the site of the infiltrations, which are usually around the medium sized bronchi. The conditions that produce the bronchiectatic changes may also contribute to the development of pulmonary infiltrations. The Aspergillus is capable of growing within the lumen of the bronchus where it establishes colonies which serve as foci for the constant discharge of antigen. This liberal supply of antigen provides an excess of antigen over antibody which leads to an Arthus type of inflammatory reaction that destroys a segment of the bronchial wall which is recognized as saccular bronchiectasis. The growing fungus can be identified in mucus plugs coughed up in the sputum.

Fibrosis of the upper lobes with contraction is a frequent complication in allergic Aspergillosis with pulmonary eosinophilia.

Blood eosinophilia is always above $500/mm^3$ with a usual range between $1,000/mm^3$ and $4,000/mm^3$. Eosinophilia persists between acute episodes, but values are reduced on steroid therapy.

Sputum: In most cases upon repeated examination of the sputum the Aspergillus can be demonstrated, even in the absence of pulmonary infiltrations. The organism can invariably be recovered from mucus plugs.

Skin Tests: The skin tests show a dual response, the immediate whealing reaction of reaginic (IgE) allergy observed in atopic individuals and the "early delayed" response of the Arthus type. A positive skin test indicates that the patient has been sensitized to Aspergillus antigens but does not mean active disease. Without a positive skin test a diagnosis of allergic aspergillosis cannot be made, since prior sensitization is essential for the development of tissue reactions. Skin test reactions without clinical symptoms are a common observation in clinical allergy.

Precipitins: Precipitins of variable titers can be demonstrated in the sera of all patients with allergic aspergillosis. Generally, precipitin titers are higher with active growth of the organism but the development of acute episodes and the presence of lung shadows do not necessarily correlate with precipitin titers. This would indicate that precipitin titer is not the critical determining factor for the development of pulmonary tissue reactions. The histopathology of the diseased lung in allergic aspergillosis with pulmonary eosinophilia is that of the Arthus type reaction. This is supported by lung biopsies and immunofluorescent studies that demonstrate IgG, IgM, IgA antibodies and components of complement which are the essential ingredients for initiating the Arthus mechanism. The Arthus mechanism requires an excess of antigen over antibody which, in this group of patients with allergic aspergillosis, is provided by the exposure to larger than usual concentrations of the antigen. This is supported by the consistent history of exposure to large supplies of antigen in every patient with acute episodes. In some patients the growth of the fungus within the bronchi provides foci for the supply of antigen. It is not essential that the titer of precipitins be high. Case reports in the literature indicate that patients with either high or low precipitin titers may experience acute reactions with infiltrations.

Precipitins may be present in a patient's serum, at either high or low titers with no active disease. Patients in group one may in some cases manifest serum precipitins without pulmonary reactions. The difference between group one patients and group two patients is the excess of antigen over antibody which initiates an Arthus type tissue reaction. Both antigen and antibody may be present, but unless the critical balance between antigen and antibody concentration is disturbed in the direction of antigen excess, as occurs with exposure to rich supplies of antigen in moldy hay, moldy grain, moldy vegetables, organic dust, bird droppings or foci of fungal growth within the airways, no acute tissue reaction develops because the Arthus reaction is not initiated.

With exhaustion of the antigen, precipitins are not demonstrable in the serum; however, the immediate whealing reaction persists.

II. Nonatopic Subjects

The production of IgE antibodies which can be demonstrated by immediate skin reactivity is contingent upon (1) the capacity of the antigen or allergen to evoke IgE antibodies, and (2) the ability of the individual to respond to the specific stimulus with IgE antibodies, which means an atopic individual.

In the nonatopic patient, Aspergillus can induce the production of precipitating IgG antibodies, but no IgE antibodies, because the nonatopic individual does not have the capacity to respond in this manner.

The nonatopic individual who has been sensitized to Aspergillus will upon subsequent challenge with the specific antigen manifest allergic bronchopneumonia which involves both bronchi and alveoli in an Arthus type response but without evidence of eosinophilia.

Although *Aspergillus fumigatus* is the most common species of Aspergillus involved in human reactions, other strains of Aspergillus can produce similar reactions. Aspergillus has been shown to cross react with various strains of fungi which makes it possible for an individual to manifest the clinical pattern of Aspergillus sensitivity following an initial encounter with this organism. The cross reactivity with other molds may explain the adverse response reported in treating aspergillosis patients with penicillin.

Invasive Form: In patients with impaired resistance or with immunologic deficiencies, the Aspergillus may become invasive of tissue and produce systemic disease.

Treatment: Treatment involves removal of the patient from contact with sources of the fungi, such as moldy hay, moldy grain, moldy organic dusts and bird droppings. When the source of the antigen is an aspergilloma, surgical removal may be necessary.

Aggravation of the disease following the administration of penicillin has been reported.

Response to corticosteroids is usually dramatic, particularly when treatment is instituted early in the course of the disease. The dose of steroids should be adequate to arrest symptoms and if possible stop the progress of the disease. Not infrequently, under such management the sputum becomes free of organisms, infiltrations cease to develop, the FEV_1 is restored to normal, and the patient recovers fully.

With a history of repeated episodes that have resulted in pulmonary fibrosis, considerable atelectasis and lobar collapse, the response to steroids is not as favorable.

No adverse responses to corticosteroids have been reported in the management of cases of allergic aspergillosis. In these conditions corticosteroids do not predispose to the dissemination of infection.

Course of the Disease: In patients with a mild degree of sensitivity whose exposure to the antigen has not been extreme, the pulmonary damage is slight and the course is usually benign. In this group of patients both time and corticosteroids are the great healers. After several years the manifestations of the lesions die out, so that episodes of asthma do not occur, pulmonary eosinophilia does not appear, and the patient is restored to normal health. As the asthma is relieved, the nidus of infection may be expectorated. No precipitins are demonstrable in the serum, and the patient recovers.

When lung damage is permanent, colonization of the involved areas by the Aspergillus may persist. If the lesions are not too severe, they may remain occult but more frequently chronic lung disease develops with contraction, secondary to bronchial occlusion, or continued damage to parenchymal tissues is caused by either the Arthus tissue reaction or endotoxins of the fungus. Contractions and lobar collapse occurs more frequently in the upper lobes, perhaps due to decreased ventilation, a situation that is observed with tuberculosis.

Aspergilloma

In chronic cases damaged tissue or cavities in the lung may be colonized by the organism to form a tumor-like mass called an aspergilloma. On the roentgenogram the aspergilloma appears as an opaque, ball-like opacity surrounded by an aerated zone.

The precipitin test is not always positive with an aspergilloma. In some patients surgical removal of the tumor-like mass is necessary for control of the disease.

Bird Fanciers Disease

The clinical pattern known as bird fanciers disease has been so named because the antigenic materials responsible for the allergic reactions are derived from various bird droppings, such as the Budgerigar (parakeet), parrot, pigeon and hen.

Precipitins against bird droppings can be demonstrated in the sera of the birds. It is thought that the serum proteins are excreted through the gut of the birds and appear in the droppings to serve as antigens. In addition, birds are susceptible to fungal infections, particularly the *Aspergillus fumigatus*. The fungi appear in the droppings to serve as a source of antigenic material which induces extrinsic allergic bronchopneumonia in humans.

Depending upon the antigen, the patterns may resemble serum sickness with pulmonary involvement when induced by serum proteins; pulmonary aspergillosis when the Aspergillus is involved or farmer's lung when other fungi are the cause.

Treatment consists of avoidance of the source of the antigen and corticosteroids for the acute stage.

REFERENCES
Anatomy of the Lung

1. Avery, M. E.: *The Lung and Its Disorders in the Newborn Infant,* 2nd ed. Philadelphia, Saunders, 1968.
2. Aviado, D. M.: *The Lung Circulation.* 2 vols. New York, Pergamon Press, 1965.
3. Bensch, K. G.: Electron microscopy in the study of the lung. In Liebow, A. and Smith, D. E. (Eds.): *The Lung.* Baltimore, Williams & Wilkins, 1968, pp. 323–331.
4. Bloom, W. and Fawcett, D. W.: *Textbook of Histology.* Philadelphia, Saunders, 1968.
5. Blumenthal, B. J. and Boren, H. G.: Lung structure in three dimensions after inhalation and fume fixation. *Rev Tuber, 79:* 764, 1959.
6. Brown, E. S.: Chemical identification of a pulmonary surface-active agent. *Fed Proc, 21:* 438, 1962.
7. Campbell, E. J. M., Agostoni, E. and Davis, J. N.: *The Respiratory Muscles: Mechanics and Neural Control.* Philadelphia, Saunders, 1970.
8. Conference on Ciliary Function. *Am. Rev Resp Dis, 93* (no. 3), 1966.
9. Cumming, G. and Hunt, L. B. (Eds.): A model of lung elasticity and some of its implications. In: *Form and Function of the Human Lung.* Proc. of symposium on breathlessness. Edinburgh, Livingston, 1968.
10. Cumming, G. and Hunt, L. B. (Eds.): *Form and Function in the Human Lung.* Baltimore, Williams & Wilkins, 1968.
11. Dunnill, M. S.: Postnatal growth of the lung. *Thorax, 17:* 329, 1962.
12. Dunnill, M. S., Massarella, G. R. and Anderson, J. A.: A comparison of the quantitative anatomy of the bronchi in normal subjects, in status asthmaticus, in chronic bronchitis and in emphysema. *Thorax, 24:* 176, 1969.
13. Elektronoptische Beobachtungen im Alveolarbereich der Lunge. *Beitr Pathol Anat, 116:* 177, 1956.
14. Florey, H., Carleton, H. M. and Wells, A. O.: Mucus secretion in trachea. *Br J Exp Pathol, 13:* 269, 1932.
15. Fung, Y. C. and Sobin, S. S.: Theory of sheet flow in lung alveoli. *J Appl Physiol, 26:* 472, 1969.
16. Green, M.: How big are the bronchioles? *St. Thomas' Hosp Gaz, 63:* 136, 1964.
17. Heinemann, H. O.: Surfactant of the lung. *Adv Intern Med, 14,* 1968. Chicago, Year Bk Med.
18. Hentel, W. and Longfield, A. N.: Stereoscopic study of the inflated lung. *Dis Chest, 38:* 357, 1960.
19. Horsfield, K. and Cumming, G.: Morphology of the bronchial tree in man. *J Appl Physiol, 24:* 373, 1968.
20. Jeanloz, R. W.: Some observations on the present day needs of research on mucus. *Ann N Y Acad Sci, 130:* 965, 1966.
21. Kleinerman, J. and Cowdrey, C. R.: The use of cinematography of serial sections in the study of lung pathology. *Am Rev Resp Dis, 89:* 200, 1964.

22. Liebow, A. A., and Smith, D. E.: *The Lung*. Baltimore, Williams & Wilkins, 1968.
23. Liebow, A. A. and Smith, D. E. (Eds.): *Studies on the Lung*. International Acad of Patho Monograms. Baltimore, Williams & Wilkins, 1968.
24. Macklem, P. T., Proctor, D. F. and Hogg, J. C.: The stability of the peripheral airways. *Resp Physiol, 8:* 191, 1970.
25. Marchand, P., Gilroy, J. C. and Wilson, V. H.: An anatomical study of the bronchial vascular system and its variations in disease. *Thorax, 5:* 207, 1950.
26. McFadden, E. R. and Lyons, H. A.: Airway resistance and uneven ventilation in bronchial asthma. *J Appl Physiol, 25:* 365, 1968.
27. Mead, J., Takeshima, T. and Leith, D.: Mechanical interdependence of distensible units in the lungs. *Fed Proc, 26:* 551, 1967.
28. Miller, W. S.: *The Lung*. Springfield, Thomas, 1937.
29. Oderr, C.: Architecture of the lung parenchyma; studies with a specially designed x-ray microscope. *Am Rev Resp Dis, 90:* 401, 1964.
30. Pattle, R. E.: Properties, function and origin of the alveolar lining layer. *Nature, 175:* 1125, 1955.
31. Pattle, R. E.: The lining layer of the lung alveoli. *Br Med Bull, 19:* 41, 1963.
32. Reid, L.: Bronchial mucus production in health and disease. In Liebow, A. A. and Smith, D. E.: *The Lung*. Baltimore, Williams & Wilkins, 1968, pp. 87–108.
33. Rosenzweig, D. Y. and Filley, G. F.: Postmortem lung studies. Mechanical and bronchographic properties. *Am Rev Resp Dis, 88:* 6, 1963.
34. Scarpelli, E. M.: *The Surfactant System of the Lung*. Philadelphia, Lea & Febiger, 1968.
35. Simpson, H., Forfar, J. O. and Grubb, D. J.: Arterial blood gas tensions and pH in acute asthma in childhood. *Br Med J, 3:* 460, 1968.
36. Spencer, H.: *Pathology of the Lung*. 2nd ed. New York, Pergamon Press, 1968.
37. Staut, Norman C.: The interdependence of pulmonary structure and function. *Anaesthesiology, 24:* 831, 1963.
38. Sturgess, J. A., Palfrey, A. J. and Reid, L.: The viscosity of bronchial secretions. *Clin Sci, 38:* 145, 1970.
39. Tappan, V. and Zalar, V.: The pathophysiology of bronchial mucus. *Ann N Y Acad Sci, 106:* 157, 1963.
40. von Hayek, H.: *The Human Lung*, trans. by V. E. Krahl. New York, Hafner, 1960.
41. von Hayek, H.: Cellular structure and mucus activity in the bronchial tree and alveoli. In de Reuck, A V. S. and O'Connor, M. (Eds.): *Ciba Foundation Symposium on Pulmonary Structure and Function*. London, Churchill, 1962, p. 100.
42. Wang, N. S. and Thurbecke, W. M.: Scanning electron microscopy of the lung. *Human Pathol, 1:* 227, 1970.
43. Weibel, E. R. and Gomez, D.: Geometry and dimensions of human airways. *Fed Proc, 21:* 439, 1962.
44. Weibel, E. R. and Gomez, D. M.: Architecture of the human lung. *Science, 137:* 577, 1962.
45. Weibel, E. R.: *Morphometry of the Human Lung*. New York, Acad Pr, 1963.

Bronchial Asthma

1. Aas, K.: Allergic asthma in childhood. *Arch Dis Child, 44:* 1, 1969.
2. Aas, K.: The biochemical and immunological basis of bronchial asthma. In Kugelmass, I. Newton (Ed.): *American Lecture Series*. Springfield, Thomas, 1972.
3. American Thoracic Society: Definition and classification of chronic bronchitis, asthma and pulmonary emphysema. Statement by Committee on Diagnostic Standards for Non-tuberculous Respiratory Diseases. *Am Rev Resp Dis, 85:* 762, 1962.
4. Backlund, L. and Irnell, L.: Compliance in bronchial asthma. *Acta Med Scand, 183:* 281, 1968.
5. Bates, D. V.: *Pulmonary Function in Spasmodic Asthma*.
6. Bates, D. V.: Impairment of respiratory function in bronchial asthma. *Clin Sci, 11:* 203, 1952.
7. Beale, H. D., Fowler, U. S. and Comroe, J. H., Jr.: Pulmonary function studies in 20 asthmatic patients in the symptom free interval. *J Allergy 23:* 1, 1952.
8. Boyd, E. M.: Expectorants and respiratory tract fluid. *Pharmacol Rev, 6:* 521, 1954.
9. Briscoe, W. A. and McLemore, G. A., Jr.: Ventilatory function in bronchial asthma. *Thorax, 7:* 66, 1952.
10. Busey, J. F., Fenger, E. P. K., Hepper, N. G., Kent, D. C., Kilburn, K. H., Matthews, L. W., Simpson, D. G. and Grzybowski, S.: Management of status asthmaticus. *Am Rev Resp Dis, 97:* 735, 1968.
11. Cardell, B. S. and Bruce-Pearson, R. C.: Death in asthmatics. *Thorax, 14:* 341, 1959.
12. Death from asthma. *Lancet, 1:* 1412, 1968.
13. Dunnill, M. S.: The pathology of asthma with special reference to changes in bronchial mucosa. *J Clin Pathol, 13:* 27, 1960.
14. Dunnill, M. S.: The pathology of asthma. *Transactions of World Asthma Conference*, 1965.
15. Fraser, R. G. and Paré, J. A. P.: *Diagnosis of Diseases of the Chest*, 2 vols. Philadelphia, Saunders, 1970.
16. Gandevia, B.: The changing pattern of mortality

from asthma in Australia. II. Mortality and modern therapy. *Med J Aust, 1:* 884, 1968.
17. Glynn, A. A. and Michaels, L.: Bronchial biopsy in chronic bronchitis and asthma. *Thorax, 15:* 142, 1960.
18. Gold, W. M., Kaufman, H. S. and Nadel, J. A.: Elastic recoil of the lungs in chronic asthmatic patients before and after therapy. *J Appl Physiol, 23:* 433, 1967.
19. Houston, J. C., deNevasquez, S. and Trounce, J. R.: A clinical and pathological study of fatal cases of status asthmaticus. *Thorax, 8:* 207, 1953.
20. Johnstone, D. E.: A study of the natural history of bronchial asthma in children. *Am J Dis Child, 115:* 213, 1968.
21. Kirkpatrick, C. H. and Keller, C.: Impaired responsiveness to epinephrine in asthma. *Am Rev Resp Dis, 96:* 692, 1967.
22. Kraepelieu, S.: Respiratory studies in asthmatic children during symptom-free periods. *Acta Paediatr Scand, 46:* 277, 1956.
23. Lecks, H. I., Wood, D. W. and Dorens, J.: Segmental atelectasis and pulmonary shunting in acute bronchial asthma and status asthmaticus. *Ann Allergy, 23:* 636, 1965.
24. Levine, G., Hanley, E., MacLeod, P. and Macklem, P. T.: Gas exchange abnormalities in mild bronchitis and asymptomatic asthma. *N Engl J Med, 282:* 1277, 1970.
25. Lowell, F. C., Schiller, I. W. and Lynch, M. T.: Estimation of daily changes in the severity of bronchial asthma. *J Allergy, 26:* 113, 1955.
26. McCarter, J. H. and Vasquez, J. J.: The bronchial basement membrane in asthma. Immunohistochemical and ultrastructural observations. *Arch Pathol, 82:* 328, 1966.
27. McFadden, E. R., Jr. and Lyons, H. A.: Airway resistance and uneven ventilation in bronchial asthma. *J Appl Physiol, 25:* 365, 1968.
28. McFadden, E. R., Jr. and Lyons, H. A.: Arterial blood gas tension in asthma. *N Engl Med, 278:* 1027, 1968.
29. McNeil, R. S., Nairn, J. R., Millar, J. S. and Ingram, C. G.: Exercise-induced asthma. *Q J Med, 35:* 55, 1966.
30. Meisner, P. and Hugh-Jones, P.: Pulmonary function in bronchial asthma. *Br Med J, 1:* 470, 1968.
31. Mellin, R. B., Lord, G. P. and Fishman, A. P.: Dynamic behavior of the lung in acute asthma. *Med Thorac, 24:* 81, 1967.
32. Meneely, G. R., Renzetti, A. D., Steele, J. D., Wyatt, J. P. and Harris, H. W.: Chronic bronchitis, asthma and pulmonary emphysema. Definition and classification of chronic bronchitis, asthma and pulmonary emphysema. *Am Rev Resp Dis, 85:* 762, 1962.
33. Messer, J. W., Peters, G. A. and Bennet, W. A.: Causes of death and pathologic findings in 304 cases of bronchial asthma. *Dis Chest, 38:* 616, 1960.
34. Middleton, E.: The anatomical and biochemical basis of bronchial obstruction in asthma. *Ann Intern Med, 63:* 695, 1959.
35. Mishkin, F. and Wagner, H. N., Jr.: Regional blood flow during acute asthmatic attacks. *Radiology, 88:* 142, 1967.
36. Mithoefer, J. C., Porter, W. F. and Karetsky, M. S.: Indications for the use of sodium bicarbonate in the treatment of intractable asthma. *Respiration, 25:* 201, 1968.
37. Neder, G. A., Jr., Derbes, V. J., Carpenter, C. L., Jr. and Ziskind, M. M.: Death in status asthmaticus: Role of sedation. *Dis Chest, 44:* 263, 1963.
38. Overholt, R. H.: Trigger mechanism in asthma. *Dis Chest, 35:* 587, 1959.
39. Palmer, K. N. V. and Diament, M. L.: Effect of salbutanol in spirometry and blood gas tensions in bronchial asthma. *Br Med J, 1:* 31, 1969.
40. Palmer, K. N. V. and Diament, M. L.: Hyperemia in bronchial asthma. *Lancet, II:* 318, 1968.
41. Pasternack, B.: The prediction of asthma in infantile eczema: A statistical approach. *J Pediatr, 66:* 164, 1965.
42. Rebuck, A. S. and Read, J.: Assessment and managment of severe asthma. *Am J Med, 51:* 788, 1971.
43. Rebuck, A. S. and Read, J.: Exercise-induced asthma. *Lancet, II:* 429, 1968.
44. Rees, H. A., Millar, J. S. and Donald, K. W.: Adrenalin in bronchial asthma. *Lancet, II:* 1164, 1967.
45. Rees, H. A., Borthwick, R. C., Millar, J. S. and Donald, K. W.: Aminophylline in bronchial asthma. *Lancet, II:* 1167, 1967.
46. Rees, H. A., Millar, J. S. and Donald, K. W.: A study of the chemical cause and arterial blood gas tensions of patients in status asthmaticus. *Q Med J, 37:* 541, 1968.
47. Rowe, A. H. and Rowe, A. H., Jr.: *Bronchial Asthma, Its Diagnosis and Treatment.* Springfield, Thomas, 1963.
48. Roy, E. C., Seabury, J. H. and Johns, L. E.: Spirometric evaluation of orthoxine in bronchial asthma. *J Allergy, 20:* 364, 1949.
49. Schiller, I. W., Beale, H. D., Franklin, W., Lowell, F. C. and Halperin, M. H.: The potential danger of oxygen therapy in severe bronchial asthma. *J Allergy, 22:* 423, 1951.
50. Shapiro, J. B. and Tate, C. F.: Death in status asthmaticus: A clinical analysis of eighteen cases. *Dis Chest, 48:* 484, 1965.
51. Sonne, L. M. and Georg, J.: The respiratory changes during attacks of bronchial asthma. *Acta Med Scand, 138:* 33, 1950.

52. Speizer, F. E., Doll, R. and Heaf, P.: Observations on recent increase in mortality from asthma. *Br Med J, 1:* 335, 1968.
53. Speizer, F. E., Doll, R., Heaf, P. and Strang, L. B.: Investigation into use of drugs preceding death from asthma. *Br Med J, 1:* 339, 1968.
54. Swineford, O., Jr.: Asthma and hay fever. In McGovern, J. P. (Ed.): *American Lecture Series.* Springfield, Thomas, 1971.
55. Szentivanyi, A.: The beta-adrenergic theory of atopic abnormality of bronchial asthma. *J Allergy, 42:* 203, 1968.
56. Tai, E. and Read, J.: Blood gas tensions in bronchial asthma. *Lancet, I:* 644, 1967.
57. Tow, D. E., Mishkin, F. S. and Wagner, H. N., Jr.: Regional distribution of pulmonary arterial blood flow in acute asthma. *JAMA, 203:* 1019, 1968.
58. Tromp, S. W.: Influence of weather and climate on asthma and bronchitis. *Rev Allergy, 22:* 1027, 1968.
59. Waddell, J. A., Emerson, P. A. and Gunstone, R. F.: Hypoxia in bronchial asthma. *Br Med J, 2:* 402, 1967.
60. Williams, D. A.: Deaths from asthma in England and Wales. *Thorax, 8:* 137, 1953.
61. Williams, D. A. and Leopold, J. G.: Death from bronchial asthma. *Acta Allergol, 14:* 83, 1959.
62. Williams, M. Henry, Jr. and Levin, M.: Sudden death from asthma. *Resp Dis, 94:* 608, 1966.
63. Woolcock, A. J. and Read, J.: Lung volumes in exacerbations of asthma. *Am J Med, 41:* 259, 1966.
64. Woolcock, A. J. and Mead, J.: The static elastic properties of the lungs in asthma. *Am Rev Resp Dis, 98:* 788, 1968.

Pulmonary Function

1. American College of Chest Physicians, Committee on Pulmonary Physiology: Clinical spirometry. Recommendation of section on pulmonary function testing. *Dis Chest, 43:* 2, 1963.
2. Barry, C. T.: The Snider match test. *Lancet, II:* 964, 1962.
3. Bartels, H., Bucherl, E., Hertz, C. W., Rodewald, G. and Schwab, M.: *Methods in Pulmonary Physiology,* trans. by J. M. Workman. New York, Hafner, 1963.
4. Bates, D. V., Ball, W. C., Jr. and Bryan, A. C.: Use of xenon[133] in studying the ventilation and perfusion of the lung. In *Dynamic Clinical Studies and Radioisotopes.* U.S. Atomic Energy Commission, 1964.
5. Bates, D. V., Macklem, P. T. and Christie, R. V.: *Respiratory Function in Disease.* Philadelphia, Saunders, 1971.
6. Bernstein, I. L. and Kreindler, A.: Lung compliance and pulmonary flow resistance. I. Clinical studies in symptomatic and asymptomatic asthmatic children. *J Allergy, 34:* 127, 1963.
7. Berglund, E., Birath, G., Byiere, J., Grunsky, G., Kjellmer, O., Sandquist, I., and Söderholm, B.: Spirometric studies in normal subjects. I. Forced expirograms in subjects between 7 and 70 years of age. *Acta Med Scand, 173:* 185, 1963.
8. Bjune, J.: Spirometric studies in normal subjects. IV. Ventilatory capacities in healthy children 7 to 17 years of age. *Acta Pediatr, 52:* 232, 1963.
9. Butter, J., Caro, C. G., Alcala, R. and DuBois, A. B.: Physiological factors affecting airway resistance in normal subjects and in patients with obstructive respiratory disease. *J Clin Invest, 39:* 584, 1960.
10. Comroe, J. H. and Nadel, J. A.: Screening tests of pulmonary function. *N Engl J Med, 282:* 1249, 1970.
11. Cook, C. S. and Hamman, J. F.: Relation of lung volumes to height of healthy persons between the ages of 5 and 38 years. *J Pediatr, 59:* 710, 1961.
12. Cotes, J. E., Rossiter, C. E., Higgins, I. T. T. and Gibson, J. T.: Average normal values for the forced expiratory volume in white Caucasian males. *Br Med J, 1:* 1016, 1966.
13. Cunningham, D. J. C. and Lloyd, B. B. (Eds.): *The Regulation of Human Respiration.* Proceedings of the J. S. Haldane Centenary Symposium. Oxford, Blackwell, 1963.
14. Current concepts of acid-base measurement. *Ann NY Acad Sci, 133,* 1966.
15. Dawson, A.: Reproducibility of spirometric measurement in normal subjects. *Am Rev Resp Dis, 93:* 264, 1966.
16. Dayman, H.: The expiratory spirogram. *Am Rev Resp Dis, 83:* 842, 1961.
17. De Reuck, A. V. S. and O'Connor, M.: *Pulmonary Structure and Function.* Ciba Foundation Symposium. London, Churchill, 1962.
18. Ferris, B. G., Jr. and Smith, C. W.: Maximum breathing capacity and vital capacity in female children and adolescents. *Pediatrics, 12:* 341, 1953.
19. Fraser, R. G. and Paré, J. A. P.: *Diagnosis of Disseases of the Chest.* 2 vols. Philadelphia, Saunders, 1970.
20. Fraser, R. G. and Paré, J. A. P.: *Organ Physiology, Structure and Function of Lung.* Philadelphia, Saunders, 1971.
21. Gaensler, E. A.: Evaluation of pulmonary function: Methods. *Annu Rev Med, 12:* 385, 1961.
22. Gandevia, B. and Hugh-Jones, P.: Terminology for measurements of ventilatory capacity. *Thorax, 12:* 290, 1957.

23. Gilson, J. C. and Hugh-Jones, P.: The measurement of total lung volume and breathing capacity. *Clin Sci, 7:* 185, 1949.
24. Guleria, J. R., Talwar, J. R., Malhotra, O. P. and Pande, J. N.: Effect of breathing cold air on pulmonary mechanics in normal man. *J Appl Physiol, 27:* 320, 1969.
25. Guyatt, A. R. and Alpers, J. H.: Factors affecting airway conductance: A study of 752 working men. *J Appl Physiol, 24:* 310, 1968.
26. Guyatt, A. R., Alpers, J. H., Hill, I. D. and Bramley, A. C.: Variability of plethysmographic measurememnts of airway resistance in man. *J Appl Physiol, 22:* 283, 1967.
27. Harbord, R. P. and Woolner, R. (Eds.): *Symposium on Pulmonary Ventilation.* Altwickam, England, John Sherratt & Son, 1959.
28. Heaf, P. J., and Prime, F. J.: The compliance of the thorax in normal human subjects. *Clin Sci, 15:* 319, 1956.
29. Hugh-Jones, P. and Campbell, E. J. M.: Respiratory physiology. *Br Med Bull, 19:* 1963.
30. Kazemi, H.: Pulmonary function tests. *JAMA, 206:* 2302, 1968.
31. Kennedy, M. C. S., Thorsby-Pellman, D. C. and Oldham, P. D.: Pulmonary function studies in normal boys. *Arch Dis Child, 32:* 347, 1957.
32. Leith, D. E. and Mead, J.: Mechanisms determining residual volume of lungs in normal subjects. *J Appl Physiol, 2:* 221, 1967.
33. LeRoy, N. B. and Guerrant, J. L.: Breathing mechanics in asthma. *Ann Intern Med, 63:* 572, 1965.
34. Lloyd, B. B.: The chemical stimulus to breathing. *Br Med Bull, 19:* 10, 1963.
35. *The Lung: Clinical Physiology and Pulmonary Function Tests,* 2nd ed. Chicago Year Bk, 1962.
36. Macklem, P. T.: Airway obstruction and collateral ventilation. *Physiol Rev,* in press.
37. Mead, J., Turner, J. M., Macklem, P. T. and Little, J. B.: Significance of the relationship between lung recoil and maximum expiratory flow. *J Appl Physiol, 22:* 95, 1967.
38. Meakin, J. C. and Davies, H. W.: *Respiratory Function in Disease.* Edinburgh, Oliver & Boyd, 1925.
39. Morehouse, L. E. and Miller, A. T.: *Physiology of Exercise.* (Harvard University Monograph No. 11). St. Louis, Mosby, 1948.
40. Murray, A. and Cook, C. D.: Measurement of peak expiratory flow rates in 220 normal children from 4.5 to 18.5 years of age. *J Pediatr, 62:* 186, 1963.
41. Palmer, K. N. V. and Diament, M. L.: A comparison of pulmonary function in bronchial asthma and chronic obstructive bronchitis. *Thorax, 25:* 101, 1970.
42. Pilcher, J. M. (Ed.): Monograph on the behavior of aerosols. *Ann NY Acad Sci, 105:* 25, 1963.
43. Porter, R. (Ed.): *Breathing.* Hering-Breuer Centenary Symposium. Ciba Foundation Symposium. London, Churchill, 1970.
44. Priban, I. P.: An analysis of some short term patterns of breathing in man at rest. *J Physiol (Lond), 166:* 425, 1963.
45. Regional lung function. *Scandinavian Journal of Respiratory Diseases,* Supplement 62. Copenhagen, Munskgaard, 1966.
46. Rosenblatt, G., Alkalay, I., McCann, P. D., and Stein, M.: The correlation of peak flow rate with maximal expiratory flow rate and one-second forced expiratory volume and maximum breathing capacity. *Am Rev Resp Dis, 87:* 589, 1963.
47. Shapiro, W., Johnson, C. E., Dameron, R. A., Jr. and Patterson, J. L., Jr.: Maximum ventilatory performance and its limiting factors. *J Appl Physiol, 19:* 199, 1964.
48. Simonson, B. G., Jacobs, F. M. and Nadel, J. A.: Mechanism of changes in airway size during inhalation of various substances in asthmatics. Role of autonomic nervous system. *Am Rev Resp Dis, 95:* 873, 1967.
49. Smith, C. A.: *The Physiology of the New Born Infant,* 3rd ed. Oxford Blackwell Scientific Publications. Springfield, Thomas, 1959.
50. Stein, M., Tanabe, G., Rege, V. and Khan, M.: Evaluation of spirometric methods used to assess abnormalities in airway resistance. *Am Rev Resp Dis, 93:* 257, 1966.
51. Strang, L. B.: The ventilatory capacity of normal children. *Thorax, 14:* 305, 1959.
52. Wade, O. I. and Bishop, J. M.: *Cardiac Output and Regional Blood Flow.* Oxford, Blackwell Scientific Publications, 1962.
53. West, J. B.: *Lung Function: Assessment and Application in Medicine.* Oxford, Blackwell Scientific Publications, 1968.

Acid-Base Balance

1. Acid-base terminology. Report by an *ad hoc* committee of the New York Academy of Sciences Conference. *Lancet II:* 1010, 1965.
2. Astrup, P.: Apparatus for the determination of carbon dioxide tension in blood and plasma, total content of carbon dioxide in plasma and bicarbonate content in "separated" plasma at a fixed carbon dioxide tension (40 mm. Hg). *Scand J Clin Lab Invest, 8:* 33, 1956.
3. Astrup, P.: Ultramicro methods for determining pH, pCO_2 and standard bicarbonate in capillary blood. Lecture delivered at the Ciba Founda-

tion *Research Forum* on "Acid Base Balance." London, 1958.
4. Astrup, P., Jørgensen, W., Siggaard, A. O. and Engel, K.: Acid-base metabolism: A new approach. *Lancet, I:* 1035, 1960.
5. Cumming, G.: Gas mixing efficiency in the human lung. *Resp Physiol, 2:* 213, 1967.
6. Cumming, G., Horsefield, K., Jones, J. G., and Muir, D. C. F.: Gaseous diffusion in the airways of the human lung. *Resp Physiol, 2:* 386, 1967.
7. Kappagoda, C. T., Linden, R. J. and Snow, H. M.: An approach to the problems of acid-base balance. *Clin Sci, 39:* 169, 1970.
8. Mellengaard, K.: Alveolar-arterial oxygen difference: Size and components in normal man. *Acta Physiol Scand, 67:* 10, 1966.
9. Michel, C. C., Lloyd, B. B. and Cunningham, D. J. C.: The *in vivo* carbon dioxide dissociation curve of the plasma. *Resp Physiol, 1:* 121, 1966.
10. Platts, M. M. and Greaves, M. S.: The composition of the blood in respiratory acidosis. *Clin Sci, 16:* 695, 1957.
11. Power, G. G.: Gaseous diffusion between airways and alveoli in the human lung. *J Appl Physiol, 27:* 701, 1969.
12. Rahn and Fenn: A graphic analysis of the respiratory gas exchange. The O_2-CO_2 diagram. *American Physiological Society,* Washington, D.C., 1955.
13. Stone, D. J.: Respiration in man during metabolic alkalosis. *J Appl Physiol, 17:* 33, 1962.
14. Wolstenholme, G. E. W. and Knight, J. (Eds.): *Circulatory and Respiratory Mass Transport.* A Ciba Foundation Symposium. London, Churchill, 1969.
15. Weisberg, H. F.: *Water, Electrolyte and Acid-Base Balance. Normal and Pathological Physiology as a Basis for Therapy,* 2nd ed. Baltimore, Williams and Wilkins, 1962.

Extrinsic Allergic Bronchopneumonia

1. Azuma, J. *et al.*: Skin testing and precipitation antigen from *Aspergillus fumigatus* for diagnosis of aspergillosis. *Am Rev Resp Dis, 95:* 305, 1967.
2. Baldus, W. P. and Peter, J. B.: Farmer's lung: Report of two cases. *N Engl J Med, 262:* 700, 1960.
3. Barrowcliff, D. F. and Arblaster, P. G.: Farmer's lung: A study of an early acute fatal case. *Thorax, 23:* 490, 1968.
4. Bishop, J. M., Melnick, S. C. and Raine, J.: Farmer's lung studies of pulmonary function and etiology. *Q J Med, 32:* 257, 1963.
5. Bradford, J. K., Blalock, J. B. and Wascom, C. M.: Bagasse disease of the lung: Early histopathologic changes demonstrated by lung biopsy. *Am Rev Resp Dis, 84:* 582, 1961.
6. Buechner, H., Prevatt, A. L., Thomson, J. and Blitz, O.: Bagassosis. A review with further historical data, studies of pulmonary function and results of adrenal steroid therapy. *Am J Med, 25:* 234, 1958.
7. Bunghurst, L. S., Byrne, R. N. and Gershon-Cohen, J.: Respiratory disease of mushroom workers. *JAMA, 171:* 15, 1959.
8. Bush, A. M. and Anzimet, D. J.: Precipitating antibodies in asthma. A preliminary communication. *NZ Med J, 72:* 28, 1970.
9. Cadham, F. T.: Asthma due to grain rusts. *JAMA, 83:* 27, 1924.
10. Campbell, J. M.: Acute symptoms following work with hay. *Br Med J, 2:* 1143, 1932.
11. Chan-Yeung, M. *et al.*: Allergic bronchopulmonary aspergillosis: Clinical and pathologic study of three cases. *Chest, 59:* 33, 1971.
12. Cohen, I. H. *et al.*: Sequoiosis: Granulomatous pneumonitis associated with redwood sawdust inhalation. *Am J Med, 43:* 785, 1967.
13. Davies, G., and Reid, L.: Growth of alveoli and pulmonary arteries in childhood. *Thorax, 25:* 669, 1970.
14. Dickie, H. A. and Rankin, J.: An acute granulomatous interstitial pneumonitis occurring in agricultural workers. *JAMA, 167:* 1069, 1958.
15. Emanuel, D. A., Wenzel, F. I., Bowerman, C. I. and Lawton, B. R.: Farmer's lung. Clinical, pathologic and immunologic study of twenty-four patients. *Am J. Med, 37:* 392, 1964.
16. Farmer's lung. Thermophilic Actinomyces as a source of "farmer's lung hay" antigen. *Lancet, II:* 607, 1963.
17. Finegold, S. M., Will, D. and Murray, J. F.: Aspergillosis. A review and report of twelve cases. *Am J Med, 27:* 463, 1959.
18. Fink, J. N., Barborian, J. J. and Sosman, A. J.: Immunologic studies of pigeon breeder's disease. *J. Allergy, 39:* 214, 1967.
19. Fink, J. N., Sosman, A. J., Barborian, J. J., Schleuter, D. P. and Holmes, R. A.: Pigeon breeder's disease. A clinical study of hypersensitivity pneumonitis. *Ann Intern Med, 68:* 1205, 1968.
20. Fuller, C. J.: Farmer's lung. *Dis Chest, 42:* 176, 1962.
21. Gregory, P. H., Festenstein, G. N., Lacey, M. E. and Skinner, F. A.: Farmer's lung disease; The development of antigens in molding hay. *J Gen Microbiol, 36:* 429, 1964.
22. Hapke, E. J., Seal, R. M. E., Thomas, G. O., Hayes, M. and Meek, J. C.: Farmer's lung. *Thorax, 23:* 451, 1968.

23. Hargreave, F. E., Pepys, J., Longbottom, J. L. and Wraith, D. C.: Bird breeder's (fancier's) lung. *Lancet, 1:* 445, 1966.
24. Hargreave, F. E., Pepys, J. and Holford-Strevens, V.: Bagassosis. *Lancet, 1:* 619, 1968.
25. Henderson, A. H., English, M. P. and Vecht, R. J.: Pulmonary aspergillosis. *Thorax, 23:* 513, 1968.
26. Henderson, A. H. and Pearson, J. E. G.: Treatment of bronchopulmonary aspergillosis in the observations in the use of natamycin.
27. Hughes, W. F.: Hypersensitivity pneumonitis. I. A discussion of farmer's lung. *Ohio State Med J,* 1971, p. 730.
28. Laubach, C.: Farmer's lung: Disease in eastern Pennsylvania. *NY State J Med, 65:* 3020, 1965.
29. Longbottom, J. L. and Pepys, J.: Pulmonary aspergillosis: Diagnostic and immunologic significance of antigen and C-substance in *Aspergillus fumigatus. J Pathol, 88:* 141, 1964.
30. Lumm, J. A.: Millworker's asthma: Allergic response to the brain weevil (*Sitophilus granarium*). *Br J Ind Med, 23:* 149, 1966.
31. Mearns, M., Young, W. and Batten, J.: Transient pulmonary infiltrations in cystic fibrosis due to allergic aspergillosis. *Thorax, 20:* 385, 1965.
32. Page, M. and Van Zandt, H. C.: Farmer's lung: Report of a case with lung biopsy. *Am Rev Resp Dis, 87:* 576, 1963.
33. Parish, W. E.: Farmer's lung. Part. I. An immunological study of some antigenic components of moldy foodstuffs. *Thorax, 18:* 83, 1963.
34. Pepsy, J.: *Hypersensitivity Diseases of the Lungs due to Fungi and Organic Dusts.* Basel, S. Karger, 1969.
35. Pepys, J. and Jenkins, P. A.: Precipitin (F.L.H.) test in farmer's lung. *Thorax, 20:* 21, 1965.
36. Pepys, J.: Hypersensitivity to inhaled organic antigens. *J R Coll Phys, 2:* 42, 1967.
37. Pepys, J. et al.: *Candida albicans* precipitins in respiratory disease in man. *J Allergy, 41:* 305, 1968.
38. Pilat, L., Stanescu, I. and Teculescu, D.: Weaver's asthma. *Acta Allergol, 22:* 39, 1967.
39. Pimentel, J. C.: Furrier's lung. *Thorax, 25:* 387, 1970.
40. Pirie, H. M., Dawson, C. O., Breeze, R. G., Sehman, I. E. and Wiseman, A.: Precipitins to *Micropolyspora faeni* in adult cattle of selected herds in Scotland and northwest England.
41. Rankin, J., Kobayashi, M., Barbee, R. A. and Dickie, H. A.: Pulmonary granulomatoses due to inhaled organic antigens. *Med Clin North Am, 51:* 459, 1957.
42. Rankin, J., Jaschke, W. H., Collier, O. C. and Dickie, H. A.: Physiopathologic features of the acute interstitial granulomatous pneumonitis of agricultural workers. *Ann Intern Med, 57:* 606, 1962.
43. Reed, C. E., Sosman, A. and Barbee, R. A.: Pigeon breeder's lung. A newly discovered interstitial pulmonary disease. *JAMA, 193:* 261, 1965.
44. Sakula, A.: Mushroom worker's lung. *Br Med J, 3:* 708, 1967.
45. Salvaggio, J. E., Buechner, H. A., Seabury, J. H. and Arquenburg, P.: Bagassosis: I. Precipitins against extracts of crude bagasse in the serum of patients. *Ann Intern Med, 64:* 748, 1966.
46. Salvaggio, J. E., Seabury, J. H., Buechner, H. A. and Kundur, V. G.: Bagassosis: Demonstration of precipitins against extracts of thermophilic Actinomycetes in the sera of affected individuals. *J Allergy, 39:* 106, 1967.
47. Seal, R. M. E., Hapke, E. J., Thomas, G. O., Meek, J. C. and Hayes, M.: The pathology of the acute and chronic states of farmer's lung. *Thorax, 23:* 469, 1968.
48. Staines, F. H. and Forman, J. A.: A survey of "farmer's lung." *J R Coll Gen Pract, 4:* 351, 1961.
49. Totten, R. S., Reid, D. H. S. and David, H.: Farmer's lung. Report of two cases in which lung biopsies were performed. *Am J Med, 25:* 803, 1958.
50. van Toorn, D. W.: Coffee worker's lung. *Thorax, 25:* 399, 1970.
51. Weill, H., Buechner, H. A., Gonzales, E., Herbert, S. J., Ancoin, E. and Ziskind, M. M.: Bagassosis: A study of pulmonary function in 20 cases. *Ann Intern Med, 64:* 737, 1966.
52. Wenzel, F. J., Emanuel, D. A., Lawton, B. R. and Magnin, G. E.: Isolation of the causative agent of farmer's lung. *Ann Allergy, 22:* 533, 1964.
53. Williams, J. V.: Pulmonary function studies in patients with farmer's lung. *Thorax 18:* 255, 1963.

Chapter 5

GASTROINTESTINAL ALLERGY

Immunological Considerations

IN BIRDS THE Bursa of Fabricus is associated with the production of humoral antibodies. To determine the counterpart of the bursa in man, considerable investigation is centered about the gut associated lymphoid tissues (GALT). These include Waldeyer's ring, the aggregated lymphoid tissues which are represented by the appendix and Peyer's patches, and the nonaggregated lymphocytes of the intestinal epithelium and the lamina propria.

It is generally recognized that the GALT system participates in the immune response of both the entire body and the local immune reactions of the gastrointestinal tissues, yet little is known regarding the contributions of the gut to the mechanisms of the body's immune response.

The demonstration of all five classes of immunoglobulins, IgA, IgD, IgE, IgG, and IgM in the intestinal tissues would suggest that the gastrointestinal tract may serve as an immunological target, participating in all types of immune tissue reactions. The responses may be cellular, as observed in delayed hypersensitivity; Ag-Ab complexes, as occur in Arthus mechanism; localized or systemic anaphylaxis involving IgE or reaginic antibody; and cytotoxic, as observed in some of the auto-allergic reactions.

IgA, particularly in the secretory form, is the predominant immunoglobulin of the gastrointestinal tract. From studies by Ishizaka, it seems that IgA is produced locally in the tissues, but although IgA is considered to be the first line of defense against infection, the exact role played by this immunoglobulin is unsettled.

IgD has been demonstrated in the rectal mucosa but not in the external secretions. The function of IgD is not known.

IgE: Tada and Ishizaka have demonstrated a predominant distribution of IgE plasma cells in both the respiratory and gastrointestinal tissues. Although direct evidence for local IgE antibody formation is lacking, the presence of these cells in great numbers is suggestive that IgE antibody is produced locally and participates in allergic tissue reactions. In the interstices of the rectal mucosa IgE-containing cells approximate IgM cells in number, but both IgE and IgM cells are more numerous than IgG and IgD lymphoid cells.

IgG and IgM lymphocytes are distributed throughout the gastrointestinal mucosa.

The association of gastrointestinal disturbance, such as diarrhea and malabsorption, with immune deficiency states is generally recognized, but the relationship between the defects in the immune system and gastrointestinal symptoms is uncertain in view of the inconstant histological pattern and the unpredictable response to therapy.

Clinical Considerations

Incidence

In the absence of allergic involvement in other systems of the body, it is usually difficult to confirm a diagnosis of gastrointestinal allergic disease. There are no symptoms specific for gastrointestinal allergy: all the signs and symptoms may be caused by nonallergic mechanisms such as enzyme deficiency, or disturbances of receptor sites by chemicals such as drugs or food additives. Complaints attributed to a single food item, whether allergic or nonallergic, are very often controlled by the patient through the elimination of the suspected food. Such complaints rarely come to the attention of the physician. The incidence of primary gastrointestinal disease is difficult to determine, since clinical patterns cannot always be specifically related to any of the allergic mechanisms.

Gastrointestinal disorders as a primary complaint come to the attention of the practicing allergist rather infrequently. In an unpublished survey of one thousand case histories of patients attending the Allergy Department of the Kaiser Foundation Hospitals, only 0.5 per cent reported primarily for gastrointestinal symptoms, while 22 per cent of all patients with allergic disease of other systems also had gastrointestinal symptoms as a secondary complaint.

It is possible that many unresolved gastrointestinal complaints due to obscure factors such as pollens, food additives and drugs pass unrecognized as potential allergic diseases.

Etiologic Agents

The common allergens, pollens, environmentals, foods and molds, may cause gastrointestinal allergic disease. In addition, drugs and other chemicals can serve as causative agents.

Pollens

Very rarely, pollens may produce primary gastrointestinal disease. Symptoms are seasonal and coincide with the pollinating season. Symptoms may range from simple gastric upsets to severe abdominal distress which can simulate an acute appendix. In the cases observed, the clinical pattern could be related to positive skin tests.

It is not unusual for gastrointestinal symptoms to be associated with seasonal respiratory allergic disease induced by pollens.

Environmentals and Molds

Although there are no cases reported of primary allergic gastrointestinal disease induced by environmental factors and molds, theoretically, it is conceivable that such clinical patterns could occur.

Foods

Although all symptoms induced by foods are not on the basis of an allergic mechanism, foods are undoubtedly the commonest causes of allergic gastrointestinal disturbances. When foods cause allergic disease, the pattern may either appear immediately or be delayed.

In the immediate response, the symptoms of gastrointestinal allergy may appear almost instantaneously or within a few minutes following ingestion of the food. Included in this group are:

>   tingling of the lips
>   itching of the palate
>   canker sores
>   macroglossia
>   nausea
>   vomiting
>   pylorospasm with gastric distress
>   eructations and distention
>   diarrhea, cramping and at times pain
>   allergic rhinitis
>   asthma

Generalized urticaria may accompany the acute symptoms or at times appear following the development of the acute symptoms.

Although skin tests are frequently positive when the symptoms are immediate, such testing is usually not necessary since in most cases the patient can identify the offending food.

Testing is contraindicated when very antigenic substances, such as egg white, fish or shellfish are involved because of the risk of precipitating constitutional reactions.

In the delayed response, symptoms may appear hours or even a few days following the ingestion of the offending food. The symptoms of the delayed response do not differ materially from those induced by acute reactions, but, in addition, fatigue, lassitude, nervousness and constipation may be complaints. The delayed symptoms are usually less severe but tend to be more persistent. The persistence may be attributed to the prolonged action of the food following ingestion.

The mechanism of the delayed form is undetermined. It is possible that through the process of digestion, peptides, polypeptides and small chemical structures serving as haptens may be released. These products of digestion could induce any type of allergic reaction, but the most likely seem to be the immediate or reaginic and the intermediate or Arthus type. When the lips are involved (cheilitis) such as induced by lipsticks or chapsticks, and in some cases of oral cankers, the delayed type of hypersensitivity is involved. Elimination of the offender is followed by rapid clearing.

For acute discomfort of cankers, a solution of 50 per cent peroxide for mouth washes is often helpful, while touching the canker base with 0.5 per cent of 1.0 per cent $AgNO_3$ solution often relieves the pain.

Serum disease type of reaction is not infrequently observed with food sensitivity.

Since the antigens involved are the products of digestion, they are not identified. This may explain the unreliability of most food tests in allergy.

Drugs and Chemicals (see Chapter 10, Adverse Reactions to Drugs).

Diagnosis and Management

In most acute cases the identification of the offending agent usually presents no problem. Elimination of the offending factor in most cases is followed very quickly by a clearing of the reaction. When necessary for acute discomfort, antihistamines or oral steroids may be administered.

In the delayed form the first prerequisite is the awareness that allergic reactions can produce the clinical patterns and the identification of the patient as an allergic individual. A history of allergic involvement is strong presumptive evidence that the gastrointestinal complaints may be caused by an allergic mechanism.

A carefully developed history is the most important diagnostic procedure in the diagnosis of gastrointestinal allergic disease. Skin tests for food are not reliable (see discussion on Skin Testing, Chapter 17). Elimination diets may be helpful in both diagnosis and management of the patient.

For persistent symptoms antihistamines are recommended. Occasionally a short program with corticosteroid therapy may be advisable to temporarily control severe symptoms.

REFERENCES

1. Bull, D. M., Bienenstock, J. and Tomasi, T. B., Jr.: Studies on human intestinal immunoglobulin A. *Gastroenterology, 60:* 370, 1971.
2. Cornes, J. S.: Number, size and distribution of Peyer's patches in human small intestine. *Gut, 6:* 225, 1965.
3. Crabbé, P. A., Carbonara, A. O. and Heremans, J. F.: The normal human intestinal mucosa as a major source of plasma cells containing gamma A immunoglobulins. *Lab Invest, 14:* 235, 1965.
4. Crabbé, P. A. and Heremans, J. F.: The distribution of immunoglobulin-containing cells along the human gastrointestinal tract. *Gastroenterology, 51:* 305, 1966.
5. Crabbé, P. A. and Heremans, J. F.: Selective IgA deficiency with steatorrhea: A new syndrome. *Am J Med, 42:* 319, 1967.
6. Felser, F., Blum, N., Sandberg, D. and Kaiser, M. H.: Adult allergic gastroenteropathy with protein losing enteropathy. *Gastroenterology, 54:* 1233, 1968.
7. Fichtelius, K. E.: The gut epithelium: A first level lymphoid organ? *Exp Cell Res, 49:* 87, 1968.
8. Freter, R.: Detection of coproantibody and its formation after parenteral and oral immunization of human volunteers. *J Infect Dis, 111:* 37, 1962.

9. Freter, R. and Gangarosa, E. S.: Oral immunization and production of coproantibody in human volunteers. *J Immunol, 91:* 724, 1963.
10. Gruskay, F. L. and Cook, R. E.: The gastrointestinal absorption of unaltered protein in normal infants recovering from diarrhea. *Pediatrics, 16:* 76, 1955.
11. Ingelfinger, F. J., Lowell, F. C. and Franklin, W.: Gastrointestinal allergy. *N Engl J Med, 241:* 303, 1949.
12. Kraft, Summer C. and Kirsner, Joseph B.: Immunological apparatus of the gut and inflammatory bowel disease. *Gastroenterology, 60:* 922.
13. Perey, D. Y. E., Cooper, M. D. and Good, R. A.: Lymphoepithelial tissue of the intestine and differentiation of antibody production. *Science, 161:* 765, 1968.
14. Taylor, K. B.: Immunological mechanisms of the gastrointestinal tract. *Gastroenterology, 51:* 1058, 1964.
15. Taylor, K. B.: Immune mechanisms in gastroenterology. In Badenoch, J. and Brooke, B. N. (Eds.): *Recent Advances in Gastroenterology*. London, Churchill, 1965, pp. 24–48.
16. Tomasi, T. B. and De Coteau, E.: Mucosal antibodies in respiratory and gastrointestinal disease. *Adv. Intern Med, 16:* 401, 1970.
17. Waldner, T. A. *et al.*: Allergic gastroenteropathy, a cause of excessive gastrointestinal protein loss. *N Engl J Med, 276:* 761, 1967.
18. Walzer, M.: Allergy of the abdominal organs. *J Lab Clin Med, 26:* 1867, 1961.
19. Watson, David W.: Immune responses in the gut. *Gastroenterology, 56:* 944, 1969.

Chapter 6

ALLERGIC DISEASES OF THE SKIN

ANATOMY

THE SKIN VARIES BOTH histologically and physiologically over different regions of the body. On the average the skin is about 2 mm in thickness, but this varies from the very thin skin of the eyelids which is less than 2 mm to the thicker skin over the hands, feet and buttocks where it may measure 3 to 4 mm in thickness. The skin also varies in its attachment over different parts of the body, such as the very loose skin of the eyelids to the taut and firmly attached skin of the anterior tibial regions. The distribution of the hair and the various glands also differ with body regions.

Skin structure varies greatly with age. At birth, over most parts of the body the skin is about one millimeter in thickness, a dimension it retains through most of early childhood. During infancy the skin is loose and delicate, in striking contrast to the inelastic, wrinkled skin of the aged.

Structure of the Skin

The skin consists of two main layers: (1) the epidermis, and (2) the corium.

(1) The Epidermis

The *epidermis* is a thin cellular membrane that contains no blood vessels, no lymphatics, and no connective tissue. The epidermis consists of two main layers—the stratum germinativum which is constituted of living cells and the stratum corneum which is entirely dead cells. The innermost layer of the stratum germinativum provides the growth cells for the epidermis. All the cells of the epidermis are derived from this basal layer. As the cells reproduce, they are pushed outward. In their migration toward the surface, they gradually become flatter and their nuclei less pronounced. As the viable cells pass through the transitional zone toward the surface, they lose their nuclei to form very flattened, interlaced, cornified cells, which form the several layers of the stratum corneum.

In infancy the stratum corneum is very thin, consisting of only a few layers of cornified cells.

(2) The Corium

The *corium* is almost entirely connective tissue which is about 90 per cent collagen with a limited distribution of elastin. Between the bundles of collagen and elastin there is a small amount of matrix with sparsely distributed cellular elements.

The highly vascular, superficially situated stratum papillare, or papillary body, nourishes the epithelium. The surface of this layer has a well-defined papillary structure which impresses its pattern of ridges and furrows upon the undersurface of the epidermis. The sculpturing of the papillary ridges in the finger pads constitutes the "finger prints."

The reticular layer, which is the innermost portion of the corium, consists of a dense network of collagen and elastin fibers in a small amount of matrix. This layer in contrast to the papillary layer which has a rich capillary network contains few capillaries. The reticular layer, which is the main source of tensile strength of the skin, has embedded within it the hair and the various glands.

The cellular elements of the corium which include fibrocytes, histiocytes and mast cells are derived from a single stem—the reticulum cell.

(1) The fibrocytes produce collagen, elastin and matrix.

(2) The histiocytes which are tissue wandering cells are phagocytes, and as such play a role in processing materials that serve as *antigens*.

(3) The mast cells release histamine and heparin. Heparin is considered to be involved in the production of collagen.

The matrix or ground substance of the corium, occupying the spaces between the bundles of collagen and elastin, is a mucoid material composed of muco-polysaccharides. The matrix decreases with age. In *infancy* it is prominent in relation to the fibrous elements, which gives the infant's skin a loose and delicate structure. With advancing age the matrix decreases in quantity so that in the normal adult the matrix or ground substance appears to be absent histologically. This variation in the relative amount of ground substance to collagen and elastin fibers is an important factor governing the response in cutaneous reactions.

Nonmedullated nerve fibers are distributed freely throughout the corium and to a lesser degree reach into the epidermis.

THE HYGROSCOPIC NATURE OF THE STRATUM CORNEUM: Although the stratum corneum is a multiple layer of dead cells and appears dry, it contains about 15 per cent water. When the water content drops below a critical level which is about 10 per cent, the structure of the stratum corneum is disturbed. Fissures and cracks develop which disrupt the protective function of this layer, exposing the underlying epidermis to various irritants, either physical or chemical. Dryness of the skin indicates a lack of water, not a lack of oil, so that frequently a dry skin can be improved by soaking.

DERMATITIS

Definition: As used in this text, the term dermatitis applies to all types of skin involvement regardless of etiology, characterized by a combination of cutaneous reactions, such as erythema, edema, oozing vesiculation and crusting in the acute forms; dryness, scaling, hyperkeratosis and lichenification in the chronic forms. Itching is a common symptom in all forms.

By this definition, allergic dermatitis is only one form of dermatitis.

Eczema

Eczema is a descriptive term of many etiologies, and accordingly has a variety of interpretations that defy classification.

In its earliest application, the term "eczema" designated the weeping, vesicular dermatoses as observed in "infantile eczema" or contact dermatitis. Today there is great confusion in the application of the term, since some dermatologists designate any chronic dermatitis, regardless of etiology, as "eczema," while others restrict the term to mean any allergic dermatitis, either acute or chronic, but more frequently the latter.

Allergic Dermatitis

  I. Infantile Atopic Dermatitis
 II. Atopic Dermatitis
III. Contact Dermatitis

Foreword: In considering allergic dermatitis one is confronted with the confusion that arises from the varied application of the term "eczema." In this discussion eczema is used as a descriptive term with multiple etiologies, among which are included the various forms of "allergic dermatitis."

Specific and Nonspecific Factors in Allergic Skin Disease

In the interpretation of allergic skin disease it is important to recognize that the response of the skin is governed by specific and nonspecific factors.

The specific factors relate to the type of allergic reaction provoking the train of events which lead to cutaneous manifestations. These vary with each type of allergic response.

(1) In the *immediate* or *reaginic-atopic* type of allergy the tissue response may vary from no *visible* tissue change to extreme erythema, edema, vesiculation and oozing. When no tissue response is apparent, *itching* may be the only indication of an allergic reaction. In atopic allergy the itching may be secondary to the release of either histamine or lysozyme from mast cells.

(2) In the *intermediate* type of allergy the skin lesions are manifestations of the inflammatory response induced by the Arthus mechanism. These may vary from small, slightly indurated papules to extensive areas of inflammatory involvement which at times may be hemorrhagic, ecchymotic and even necrotic, as in drug allergy.

(3) In the *delayed* type of allergy the tissue reaction is characterized by a cellular response accompanied by inflammation. These lesions may range from small, slightly indurated papules, with and without central necrosis as seen in drug allergy, to extensive areas of involvement characterized by erythema, edema, vesiculation and oozing as observed in contact dermatitis. The edema, vesiculation and oozing associated with the delayed type of reactivity may be induced by the permeability factor released by the T-cells of delayed hypersensitivity.

The nonspecific factors include (1) the histological variations in the skin, and (2) the response to irritants.

(1) The histological variations of the skin associated with body regions and age differences are factors influencing the ultimate patterns observed in response to the allergic tissue reaction, e.g. the distribution of edema fluids in loose and taut skin, or the decreased or absence of reaction in hairy parts as compared with non-hairy parts.

The loose corium of the infant permits the dissipation of edema fluids, while the thin epidermis with its thin stratum corneum permits edema fluids to reach the surface where it is manifested as weeping, oozing and vesiculation.

(2) Response to Irritants: All epithelial structures, including not only the skin but also the mucosal linings of the nose and the respiratory tract respond to irritants with hyperplasia and hypertrophy.

The irritant may be intrinsic as induced by any inflammatory or allergic reaction or extrinsic as induced by any chemical or a mechanical agent—such as scratching.

In the skin the response to irritation differs in the infant as compared with the individual beyond two years of age. In the infant the response to an external irritant such as scratching and rubbing is erythema and edema fluid which is dissipated throughout the loose corium and extends into the epidermis to produce cellular edema which appears on the surface as microscopic vesicles and free fluid recognized as weeping and oozing.

In infancy the epidermis does not respond to irritation with hyperplasia and hypertrophy. As a result the stratum corneum in infancy does not manifest hyperkeratosis* and lichenification.†

The exceptions to this acute response are observed in seborrheic dermatitis, Leiner's disease and congenital ichthyosis. None of these conditions is an allergic disease. Their etiologies are undetermined.

In individuals beyond infancy, the response to irritation of the skin is characterized by increased activity of the keratinocytes. The keratinocytes which constitute the majority of the epidermal cells are very responsive to irritants of any type and any degree. The increased activity results in increased numbers and size of the cells which move toward the epithelial surface to pro-

---

* Hyperkeratosis: thickening of the keratinized layer, the stratum corneum.

† Lichenification: thickening of the skin with exaggeration of its normal markings so that striae form a criss-cross pattern.

duce a thickened horny layer recognized as hyperkeratosis and lichenification.

In response to irritation the corium also manifests hyperplasia and hypertrophy which is not apparent macroscopically.

Pruritus (Itching)

Pruritus or itching which leads to mechanical irritation by either scratching or rubbing is the most important single nonspecific factor that leads to histopathologic changes in the skin.

Recent observations on the mechanism of itching have demonstrated that the symptom accompanies those irritations of the skin in which proteolytic enzymes are released. These involve all inflammatory processes including allergic skin reactions. The small unmyelinated nerves distributed in both the corium and the epidermis are stimulated by the proteolytic enzymes which may be present in only trace amounts; dilutions as high as 1:1,000,000 may be effective. The antigen-antibody reaction may be inadequate to produce perceptible tissue reactions, but sufficient to release the minute quantity of enzymes necessary to activate the nerve endings responsible for the sensation of itching. Allergic itching without skin lesions is not an unusual clinical observation.

Itching provokes scratching which serves as an external irritant to activate keratinocytes which eventually results in hyperkeratosis, acanthosis and lichenification. The degree of response is proportional to both the intensity and duration of the itching. As has been pointed out, the infant's skin does not respond to scratching and rubbing with hyperkeratosis and hyperplasia.

Itching varies from individual to individual. Some persons seem to have a low threshold of tolerance for itching, so that even a mild degree of intrinsic irritation may provoke intense scratching, resulting in trauma to the skin as evidenced by scratch marks and eventually pronounced activation of keratinocytes leading to hypertrophy, acanthosis and lichenification. In other patients, the intensity of the itching may vary from time to time depending upon the degree of inflammation, the intensity of the allergic reaction or even the emotional state of the individual.

On the basis of this interpretation, it readily becomes apparent that the manifestations of allergic skin disease may not necessarily be a primary response to the allergic reaction, but rather a secondary manifestation induced by the mechanism of scratching provoked by itching.

Onset and Course of Atopic Dermatitis *In Infancy*

Infantile atopic dermatitis (infantile eczema) rarely appears before six weeks of age but more often after two months. The initial lesion is usually a small, erythematous papular patch over one or both cheeks. Since the initial lesion presents nothing distinctive to support a diagnosis of atopic dermatitis, the diagnosis is usually established as the disease evolves. The initial erythematous-papular lesions are soon followed by an intensification of the redness, with coalescence of the lesions which very early manifest minute vesicles that give the skin a ground glass appearance with a transparent quality. Oozing and weeping become pronounced while drying of the exudate forms honey-colored crusts. To complete the pattern, scratching and rubbing produces excoriations which appear as denuded, raw, bleeding patches.

The face and forehead are the sites of predilection in infancy, but very early in the course of the disease, the involvement may extend to the neck, the postauricular areas, and particularly to the bends of the arms and legs, which are the classical sites of involvement in *atopic* dermatitis at any age. When the reaction is more severe, the torso or entire body may show involvement. The circumoral and peri-orbital regions are usually free.

The disease may continue without remission throughout the first two years of life, or it may wax and wane with brief periods of clearing of the skin followed by exacerbations. As the infant approaches the second year of life the disease usually clears spontaneously. When the disease persists beyond infancy the cutaneous lesions may lose their acute character and for a period of months or even a year enter a subacute phase constituted of a mixture of both acute and chronic efflorescences.

Atopic Dermatitis

The term atopic dermatitis is usually reserved for the period beyond infancy when the lesions have a chronic character.

In most cases, when the infantile form clears, which is usually at about two years of age, recurrences do not occur. When the eruption does reappear, it is usually observed at pubescence, adolescence, or early adult life. Occasionally, atopic dermatitis develops with no history of an antecedent eruption in infancy. Beyond infancy, the lesions of atopic dermatitis are usually chronic in appearance with scaling, papules with crusted summits, hypertrophy and lichenification. Weeping is not a usual feature of the pattern, but when present it is observed more frequently among children rather than adolescents or adults. In long standing cases the skin becomes leathery, fissured and striated. A grayish discoloration of the involved areas is frequently observed. Scratch marks capped with crusted blood are present at all stages.

Obstruction of the sweat gland pores is a feature of all forms of dermatitis, including atopic dermatitis. Since obstruction of the sweat glands is limited to areas of dermatitic involvement, the problem is only serious when the atopic dermatitis is widespread. With poral obstruction the sweat is dissipated throughout the skin with involvement of the corium and the epithelium, which results in an inflammatory response that induces severe itching. When the sweat spreads through the epidermis, it may produce tiny vesicles similar to those observed in infantile atopic dermatitis.

Any situation that induces increased sweating, such as increased heat, excessive clothing, exposure to the sun, exercise or emotional disturbances, can precipitate very sudden severe itching of the involved regions.

If the eruption is limited to a few localized lesions, poral obstruction presents no great problem, but with widespread skin involvement itching may be not only intense but intolerable.

In the management of such cases it is important to avoid situations that induce sweating until the lesions have healed. Drugs which suppress sweating may be effective for very short periods. Their use for long periods is not recommended, as the generalized anhidrosis induced can be hazardous to the patient.

The course of atopic dermatitis beyond infancy is also subject to periods of remission, which like its onset may be related to pubescence, adolescence and early adult life.

Even in persistent cases, the condition rarely continues beyond early adult life. In most cases there is complete restoration of the skin to normal. *Very* rarely do residuals of a few small patches persist. Scarring secondary to severe infection is *not* the *usual* sequel.

Symptoms of respiratory allergy occur in over 50 per cent of individuals with a history of eczema. Respiratory symptoms may develop while the patient is still experiencing his dermatitis. In some cases the respiratory involvement appears shortly following the dermatitis, but in the majority of cases, respiratory symptoms develop following an interval of several years, which usually coincides with pubescence, adolescence and early adult life.

Etiology of Atopic Dermatitis: The literature records a wide difference of opinion regarding (1) the etiology of "eczema" and (2) the acceptance of "atopy," or the immediate type of hypersensitivity, as the etiology of both eczema and atopic dermatitis. The failure to recognize that eczema is a descriptive term with many etiologies and also the attempt to consider all eczemas as atopic in nature, contribute to a considerable degree to the wide differences in opinion.

The clinicians who consider the etiology of all eczemas to be atopy or the immediate type of hypersensitivity with pollens, environmentals and foods as the specific allergens, support their contention with the following observations:

(1) The high incidence of atopic allergic disease in the familial history.
(2) The occurrence of allergic respiratory disease, such as rhinitis, hay fever, bronchial allergy and bronchial asthma in over 50 per cent of individuals with a history of so-called "infantile eczema."
(3) The correlation in some cases of positive skin tests with the disease. In most cases of atopic dermatitis, skin tests are not reliable (see discussion on skin tests, Chapter 17).
(4) Positive provcative testing with inhalant factors and foods has been reported in some cases.
(5) The successful control of the dermatitis in some patients through management based upon the general principles of allergy treatment.
(6) The presence of increased IgE antibody in atopic skins.

The contention that atopy or the immediate type of hypersensitivity *cannot* be the cause of eczema is supported by the following observations:

(1) A cutaneous response similar to the eruption of atopic dermatitis has been observed in agammaglobulinemic patients in whom there are no humoral antibodies, a *sine qua non* for the atopic or immediate type of hypersensitivity.
(2) The histopathology does not correlate with the classical tissue reactions associated with the immediate type of hypersensitivity.
(3) The inability to relate skin test reactions with the dermatitis.
(4) The frequent failures following management based upon principles of atopic allergy.

If the thesis that eczema has multiple etiologies is accepted, then resolving the problem of the etiology of eczema would depend upon determining the factors capable of inducing the tissue response.

(1) In patients in whom the skin response does not correlate with the classical tissue reaction observed with atopy, it is conceivable that the atopic reaction induces only itching through release of lysozymes from mast cells. No other tissue reaction is necessary, the scratching and rubbing provoke acute response in infants and the chronic response in the older individual. This contention is supported by the absence of cutaneous lesions when the skin is covered to protect it against scratching.
(2) It is possible that some cases diagnosed as infantile eczema or atopic dermatitis may be due to delayed hypersensitivity.
  (a) Bacteria or bacterial components could serve as antigens to induce the delayed type of hypersensitivity. Such reactions could explain the absence of the classical involvement of the antecubital and popliteal regions which occurs in some cases.
  (b) Contactants of various types including clothing, dusts, various environmental factors, including the oleoresins of pollens and

plants, could induce contact dermatitis which is a manifestation of delayed hypersensitivity. Low grade irritants induce chronic changes rather than acute inflammation.

The distribution of the lesions may be helpful in identifying this type of response.

(c) Delayed hypersensitivity could explain the cutaneous reactions observed in some agammaglobulinemic patients.

(d) Theoretically, an auto-allergic mechanism may be involved in some patients, in which case the delayed type of hypersensitivity would be involved.

If eczema is caused by mechanisms other than atopy, it is conceivable that individuals whose dermatitis is caused by atopy provide the over 50 per cent eczematous patients who experience atopic respiratory disease later in life, while the "infantile eczemas" of nonatopic etiology fail to develop atopic manifestations in subsequent years.

Complications of Infantile Eczema and Atopic Dermatitis

1. ADENOPATHY: The nodes draining the affected areas are usually involved. With a generalized skin eruption practically all of the superficial nodes of the body become enlarged, ranging from tiny shot to pea or even lima bean in size. Enlargement of the nodes is most pronounced in infantile eczema when the cervical, axillary and inguinal nodes may show a considerable increase in size. Although quite enlarged, the nodes rarely manifest either tenderness or suppuration. It is possible that lymph node enlargement is an immune response.

II. INFECTION: Both bacterial and viral infection complicate allergic dermatitis.

1. Bacterial infection: Either streptococci or staphylococci or both are frequent invaders in allergic dermatitis and infantile eczema. The infection is usually low grade and smoldering. Impetigo is the commonest complicating infection, especially in infantile eczema. Low grade infection intensifies the pruritus which results in an aggravation of the skin condition due to either scratching or rubbing. Low grade infection should always be considered to be present in most cases of eczema and atopic dermatitis.

Upper respiratory bacterial infections will usually aggravate atopic dermatitis both in the infant and in older individuals. When there is sudden aggravation of the eczematous state, upper respiratory bacterial infection must be considered as a possible exciting agent. Specific therapy directed against the infection may often be followed by a dramatic response.

2. Viral infection: At the peak of most viral infections such as measles, chickenpox, mumps, poliomyelitis, influenza and pertussis (although not a viral infection it has the same influence), an improvement in the cutaneous manifestations and at times complete clearing of the skin may be observed. With convalescence from the infection, the skin rash recurs and frequently with a greater intensity than existed before the onset of the intercurrent viral infection. The reason for this influence upon the course of the disease by viral infection is not known.

Individuals with atopic dermatitis and particularly infants with eczema are very susceptible to infection with herpes virus and vaccinia virus (Kaposi's varicelliform infection). The eruption with these viruses appears suddenly in the form of umbilicated varicelliform lesions which usually are confined to the affected parts of the skin. The lesions become crusted and pustular; appear in waves as seen in both chickenpox and smallpox. The patients become acutely ill with high fever and extreme prostration. When complicated with viremia and encephalitis, death may occur.

A history of exposure to either a herpetic lesion or a recent vaccination for smallpox is important in making the diagnosis. On the basis of the lesions a differential between the types of virus cannot be made. When identification of the virus is possible, it may serve as a guide in treatment. Specific transfer factor has been successful in the management of the vaccinial form. Treatment should be directed aginst the secondary invaders, and when possible against the primary infection. The usual procedures for toxemia and acute infection should be instituted.

Because of the seriousness of viral complications patients with eczema should practice strict avoidance of individuals with either herpes or a recent vaccination for smallpox. Smallpox vaccination should *not* be performed in patients with infantile eczema and atopic dermititis. Siblings should not be vaccinated when an eczematous infant resides in the household.

3. The development of cataract is occasionally observed in patients with eczema. The *type* of eczema, i.e. the cause, has not been identified, nor is the interrelationship explained.

Diagnosis: The diagnosis of eczema can be made very readily from the cutaneous lesions, but determining the etiology is more difficult.

A. Infantile Eczema

A familial history of atopy is presumptive but not conclusive support for a diagnosis of *atopic* infantile eczema. Since the eruption usually presents no distinguishing features, a diagnosis of atopy must often await the full evolution of the disease.

Atopic infantile eczema must be differentiated from (1) contact dermatitis, (2) seborrheic dermatitis, (3) Letterer-Siwe syndrome (Histiocytosis X), (4) Wiskott-Aldrich syndrome, and (5) acrodermatitis chronica enteropathica.

(1) Contact Dermatitis

Contact dermatitis is the most common imitator of infantile atopic eczema. With the following distribution of the rash, contact dermatitis must be excluded:

(a) Isolated involvement of the cheeks, especially if only one cheek is involved or if one cheek shows a more intense reaction than the other.

(b) In the absence of either antecubital or popliteal involvement.

(c) Involvement of the extensor surfaces of the arms and legs.

(d) Involvement of the anterior chest, the abdomen, knees, anterior tibial regions, and the dorsum of the feet. This pattern is more common among creeping infants.

(2) Seborrheic Dermatitis of Infancy

(a) Onset may be early infancy before six weeks of age.

(b) Initial involvement is usually limited to the scalp, cradle cap.

(c) Extension of the rash to the eyebrows, postauricular areas, neck, intertriginous involvement. Usually spares the flexural areas. When the axillae and diaper area are involved, secondary infection with monilia is common.

(d) Lesions are yellowish, sharply demarcated and frequently with central clearing of involved skin areas. Scales are yellowish, oily and flaky ("potato chip" scale). Circumscribed, isolated or multiple lesions of seborrheic dermatitis occur less frequently in infancy. When present, they must be differentiated from contact dermatitis and fungus infection.

(e) Itching is either mild or absent. The *absence of itching* should exclude atopy.

Leiner's disease is a severe form of seborrheic dermatitis with secondary gastrointestinal complications and failure to thrive.

(3) Letterer-Siwe Syndrome (Histiocytosis X)

This is uncommon and begins later in infancy. There may be a mild to severe dermatitis involving the scalp and trunk. The lesions are more papular and on close inspection, petechiae are present. Systemic involvement is evidenced by hepatosplenomegaly, lymphadenopathy, lytic bone lesions, and pulmonary infiltrations. A biopsy of the lesions reveals numerous large histiocytes. The histiocyte may show giant cell formation and a vacuolated eosinophilic cytoplasm.

(4) Wiskott-Aldrich Syndrome

This is a sex-linked recessive disorder characterized by an atopic dermatitis-like picture, thrombocytopenia, recurrent infections, absent isohemagglutinins, low IgM values and impaired delayed hypersensitivity. The dermatitis is usually mild; petechiae often are present in the skin lesions. The first manifestations are usually seen later in the first year of life. (See Chapter 19)

(5) Acrodermatitis chronica enteropathica

This is often a fatal disease. The etiology is unknown but may involve a basic defect in fatty acid metabolism. It is characterized by severe diarrhea, failure to thrive, hair loss, areas of vesiculo-pustulo-bullous dermatitis about the mucocutaneous junction, the mouth, nose and anus, and the distal extremities, including the digits.

B. Atopic Dermatitis or Atopic Eczema

The rash of atopic eczema which is present beyond the period of infancy presents no distinguishing features to permit differentiating it from eczema of other etiologies. Skin test reactions do not necessarily correlate with a diagnosis of atopic dermatitis nor is there any correlation between intradermal test results and the severity of the dermatitis.

Serum IgE levels are usually higher in cases of atopic dermatitis, and in addition there is a strong correlation between serum IgE levels and the severity of the atopic dermatitis.

A family history of atopic disease is presumptive support for a diagnosis of atopy, while a history of atopic eczema in infancy strongly favors a diagnosis of atopy.

Atopic eczema must be differentiated from (1) contact dermatitis, (2) seborrheic dermatitis, (3) neurodermatitis (*Lichen simplex chronicus*), and (4) nummular dermatitis.

(1) Contact Dermatitis (see discussion below)

(2) Seborrheic Dermatitis of the Older Individual.

Seborrheic dermatitis can be differentiated by the distinguishing characteristics of (a) the distribution, and (b) the lesions.

(a) *Distribution*: The scalp is usually the initial site of involvement. When the condition is mild with a fine, flaky, slightly oily desquamation, it is labelled "dandruff."

Involvement may extend to the eyebrows, postauricular regions, the external auditory canal, the presternal, interscapular and intercervical regions.

Less frequently there is involvement of the axillae, the inframammary region, the umbilicus and the ano-genital regions.

(b) *The Lesions:* The lesions are usually multiple, discrete, circumscribed oval or nummular patches covered with fine, yellowish, slightly oily scales. Erythema may be present but occurs more commonly when the distribution of the lesions is more diffuse and widespread.

The intertriginous areas of involvement may become macerated, leading to oozing and crusting which may resemble the lesions of acute atopic eczema.

Itching may be present with seborrheic dermatitis, but it is usually mild. In the absence of itching a diagnosis of atopic dermatitis can be excluded.

(3) Neurodermatitis (*Lichen simplex chronicus*)

The lesions of neurodermatitis are usually single, but may be multiple, discrete, circumscribed areas of hyperkeratosis and lichenification. Erythema and vesiculation are not common.

As in atopic eczema, pruritus is the dominant feature of neurodermatitis, with the result that hyperkeratosis and lichenification induced by scratching is similar in both conditions.

The lesions of neurodermatitis occur most commonly in areas of the body accessible to scratching, such as the scalp, the side of the neck, the occipito-nuchal regions, the ankles, thighs and dorsum of the hands. This distribution is suggestive of neurodermatitis but does not necessarily differentiate it from atopic eczema.

An antecedent history of psoriasis, contact dermatitis or seborrheic dermatitis, upon which the lesions can be superimposed, is highly suggestive of neurodermatitis.

Very often the lesions cannot be differentiated from isolated patches of atopic eczema.

(4) Nummular Dermatitis

Nummular dermatitis is a descriptive term based upon the morphology of the lesions which are coin-shaped.

The etiology is unknown. Since the lesions usually appear after the age of thirty years, the condition is frequently considered an adult form of atopic eczema. An autoallergic mechanism for the etiology has also been proposed.

The lesions consist of inflammatory patches, variable in size and in the degree of acute reaction. Distribution is most commonly over the extensor surfaces of the arms, the neck, the anterior surfaces of the legs and the dorsum of the hands.

Since in most cases the disease is self-limiting after a course of several weeks to several months, it usually presents no clinical problem.

Treatment

I. Topical

Soaks and compresses are helpful for most forms of dermatitis. In the acute forms with crusts, the crusts are loosened and more readily removed. In the chronic forms with dry, lichenified and crusted skin, soaks and compresses help soften the skin and soften crusts which serve as a medium for infection.

For *tub soaks,* $MgSO_4$: one handful to a tub of water, for periods of fifteen to twenty minutes repeated several times daily. Long periods of soaking cause maceration. The water should be tepid or at room temperature. The *room air* should not be too cool nor too hot to avoid excessive itching upon exposure following undressing.

Do not use boric acid for tub soaks.

Compresses with either normal saline or boric solution at room temperature are effective for localized lesions and involvement of the face. Excessively wet and dripping compresses or application for unduly long periods predispose to maceration.

II. Treatment of Infection

The response of low grade infection to tub soaks and compresses is frequently so satisfactory that the need for specific therapy with antibiotics is eliminated.

When antibiotics are administered, oral preparations are favored. For acute involvement a single course of the medication is usually sufficient, while for more chronic involvement the intermittent administration of courses of antibiotics is recommended rather than prolonged therapy with the drug. The dosage should be regulated to prevent complications, particularly diarrhea.

Most topical medications, particularly antibiotics and antihistamines should be avoided, since they offer great risk of inducing contact dermatitis which will aggravate and complicate the illness.

Topical steroid therapy is frequently helpful for small, localized patches of involvement. The combination of local compresses and topical steroids is especially helpful. *Avoid* topical steroids with preservatives such as parabens which are prone to induce contact dermatitis.

Topical steroids are *not* recommended for large areas of involvement. When the skin lesions are distributed over large areas of the body, *oral steroids* are recommended (see Chapter 15 for schedule of therapy).

Steroids are not recommended for children because of the risk of side reactions, such as retardation of bony development and growth.

III. Treatment of Itching

Anything that induces increased sweating will aggravate the itching which in turn provokes scratching which results in an aggravation of the rash.

Avoid: dressing too warmly
       irritating or scratchy clothing, such as wool, crepe, *etc.* (these intensify itching)
       overheating in both summer and winter
       excessive muscular exertion
       undue exposure to hot sun
       emotional disturbances by causing increased sweating which will aggravate itching

Protective clothing such as cotton leotards and pants can be helpful.

Reassurance as to prognosis and the restoration of the skin to normal will aid in calming the patient.

Antipruritics: There are no effective *oral* medications for the control of pruritus. Antihistamines do not influence the pruritus but may offer a measure of relief because of their sedative action. *Avoid opiates* in all forms. Barbiturates may aggravate pruritus.

Contact Dermatitis

Contact dermatitis can be classified as (I.) nonallergic or irritant, or (II.) allergic.

I. Nonallergic or irritant contact dermatitis is induced by any substance that is irritating to the skin. Since the mechanism is either mechanical or chemical, no allergic reaction is involved. Any part of the body may be affected, and the intensity of the skin reaction depends upon the strength of the irritant and the duration of the exposure. Since no allergic reaction is involved, the skin response appears immediately with no history of previous exposure. The skin lesions can range from slight erythema or intense redness, through various degrees of inflammation with vesiculation and at times bullae formation. This cutaneous pattern does not differ from that induced by an allergic reaction. When the irritants are highly caustic, necrosis with sloughing may occur.

Treatment: Both prophylactic and palliative treatment depend upon identification and removal of the offending substance. Rapid clearing of the skin usually follows elimination of the irritant.

When the irritant cannot be controlled as in some industrial situations, protective clothing should be worn.

For topical treatment simple soaks or compresses of either normal saline or $MgSO_4$ or boric acid solution will usually expedite healing of the acute inflammatory reaction.

Topical medications are not recommended, as the skin is already sick; anything applied will serve as an added irritant.

Unless infection complicates the lesion, antibiotics are not indicated. In most cases compresses will also control the infection.

II. The Allergic Response: Since allergic contact dermatitis is a manifestation of the delayed type of hypersensitivity, the skin reaction has all the immunological and histological features of this type of reactivity (see Chapter i, Delayed Hypersensitivity).

In delayed hypersensitivity the latent period between initial exposure and the development of sensitivity is usually five to ten days. However, in allergic contact dermatitis there may be great variations in the latent period, i.e. the period of no reactivity may be extended to weeks, months or even years. For this reason a history of continued exposure does not exclude any material as the antigen involved. For example, a patient may offer a history of a cosmetic in use for several years with no ill effects, but suddenly a dermatitis occurs. There is no explanation for the prolonged latent period, but in attempting to identify the offending material, this behavior must be considered.

In contact dermatitis the offending agent may serve both as the irritant and the antigen, in which situation the patient will experience dermatitis in response to (1) the irritating capacity of the material, and (2) the allergic response induced by the substance serving as a hapten.

After sensitivity has been established, minute quantities of the offending material may evoke a reaction entirely out of proportion to the small quantity involved. Highly active, simple chemicals which are prone to conjugate with skin proteins are the most common causes of allergic contact dermatitis.

Only minute quantities of the specific antigen are required for either the induction of sensitivity or eliciting a skin response after sensitivity has been established.

The "Id" Reaction: In some cases of contact dermatitis a flare-up at sites remote from the point of exposure are observed. This flare-up may be due to sequestered antigen which reacts after sensitivity has developed. (See Chapter 12 for the mechanism)

The skin pattern may be either (a) acute, or (b) chronic.

(a) The acute reaction, which is usually sharply demarcated from the surrounding skin, may range from slight erythema to extreme redness with vesiculation and bullae. The degree of the response depends upon the antigenicity of the offending material and the degree of sensitivity of the patient. When the skin lesions appear immediately following exposure, simple irritation must be considered. Since the T-cells involved in the delayed type of hypersensitivity induce capillary permeability, any edema or vesiculation or bullous formation observed eighteen to twenty-four hours after exposure may be considered as an expression of the allergic reaction.

Pruritus is a constant symptom, but at times burning and even pain may be present.

(b) The chronic form shows the usual response of epithelial structures to continued irritation, which is characterized by hypertrophy, hyperplasia and lichenification of the skin. The chronic lesions may be the response to a very weak antigen acting over an extended period, or it is possible that the weak antigen induces only pruritus, when the scratching will evoke the chronic changes in the skin. Vesiculation and weeping are rarely observed in the chronic forms.

The hairy parts of the body, such as the scalp, axillae and pubis are less susceptible to contact dermatitis. For example, the apex of the axilla is usually not involved in contact dermatitis.

Diagnosis: The diagnosis of contact dermatitis and the identification of the offending factors presents a very complex clinical problem because of the great variety of material and their universal distribution. To list every possible item would be an encyclopedic undertaking. There are, however, several guidelines based upon pattern and regional distribution which can be helpful. The guidelines are also helpful in detecting contact dermatitis when, instead of an isolated condition, it occurs intercurrently with infantile eczema, atopic dermatitis, fungal infections and nummular eczema.

In many cases a thorough history will reveal the causative agent, but when history offers no clues, the various patterns and distribution of the lesions may be successful in identifying the causative agent.

In Infants

Contact dermatitis may resemble infantile eczema. When both cheeks are involved, it is difficult to differentiate from infantile eczema, but when one cheek or one cheek more intensely than the other is affected, contact dermatitis rather than atopic infantile eczema should be considered. Involvement of various body regions may occur with or without facial involvement. When body lesions occur without the classical involvement of the antecubital and popliteal regions, diagnosis of infantile eczema should be withheld until contact dermatitis is ruled out.

When the knees, anterior surfaces of the legs, anterior abdomen or anterior chest are involved, the diagnosis is more likely to be contact dermatitis.

In the infant, the eruption can be induced by a number of materials in the environment, such as:

(a) Any individual holding the child may provide contactants through clothing (wool, dyed or synthetic fabrics, permanent press garments) or cosmetics (hair spray or other cosmetics).

(b) Bedding materials, e.g. plastic covered mattresses urine causes a breakdown of the plastic coating which serves to provide chemical contactants; blankets; permanent press bed sheets, crib paint.

(c) When the infant learns to creep, a great variety of new contactants becomes available, but the most common factors are *floor coverings,* either carpets or linoleum, vinyl or waxed floors; plastic playpen covers; playpen paint.

The creeping infant usually develops the rash on the knees, anterior surface of the legs, and the dorsum of the feet and fingers. The anterior body surface and even the cheeks may become involved as the infant interrupts its creeping by lying on the floor.

(d) Plastic toys may cause lesions about the mouth and cheeks and at times between the fingers.

Hand foods may induce a similar pattern.

Childhood, Adolescence and Adulthood

The older child may be a victim of "TV dermatitis," an eruption involving the lateral surfaces of the legs, induced by contacting floor coverings while in the cross-legged position on the floor.

Regional involvement suggests the following contactants:

Forehead—hat bands

Eyes—eye drops; usually an accompanying conjunctivitis with a drip pattern of the lower lids

Eyelids—may manifest marked edema of the loose tissue in addition to dermatitis; fingernail polish; hair dyes and tints; hair rinses and shampoos; cosmetics of various types, including perfumes, powders, creams, *etc.*

Ears—postauricular eruption from perfumes, shafts of eyeglass frames

Nose—involvement of the bridge from eyeglass frames

Face and neck—smoke from burning twigs and leaves of poison oak or poison ivy (see *Rhus* dermatitis); aerosol sprays of any type, including insecticides, deodorants, hair sprays, paint sprays (especially in industry)*; dusts and pollens (involvement usually extends to the V of the neck)

Neck—contact with scarf, coat collar, permanent press garments

Apex of the axilla—antiperspirants, deodorants, clothing (especially sleeve lining), fabric dyes, permanent press materials. The apices of the axillae are usually free of rash.

Arms—lateral surfaces may show involvement from leaning on plastic, lacquered or varnished table or desk tops; chromium trim on tables (lesions develop at point of contact); linear lesions across the forearm from the handle of ladies' purses. Complete involvement of the arm suggests contact with a sleeve lining. Inner aspect of the arm suggests rubbing against an upholstered chair with the arms draped over the sides.

Body involvement—girdles, bras, garters and suspenders; cosmetics, suntan lotions; exposure during the pollinating season may manifest involvement of the exposed parts.

Ano-genital region suggests suppositories of various types, contraceptives, douches, rectal and vaginal discharges, perfumes, soaps, bubble bath, detergents in bath water.

Feet—shoes, especially the glue and dyes; foot powder and deodorants

Patch Testing. See Chapt. 17.

---

*For lists of contactants, see references by Fregert and Hjorth, and Fisher in bibliography.

Poison Oak (*Rhus diversilobia*) and Poison Ivy (*Rhus toxicodendron*)

In addition to poison oak and poison ivy there are a number of plants such as poison sumac (*Rhus venenata*), primula, oleander, chrysanthemum, and various pollens such as ragweed, which have oleoresins capable of inducing sensitivity which results in contact dermatitis. By virtue of their wide distribution, poison oak which is indigenous to the western states and poison ivy which is found in the midwest and eastern states are the most important clinically.

The active principle in poison oak and poison ivy is urushiol, an oleoresin which consists of a mixture of four catechols. In poison oak one of the catechols has a saturated side chain of seventeen carbon atoms (heptadecylcatechol), while the remaining three catechols are mono-, di-, and tri-olefins, depending upon the number of double bonds in the side chains. The composition of the urushiol in poison ivy is identical except that the saturated side chain, has fifteen carbons (pentadecylcatechols).

The exact role of each component of urushiol in the mechanism of sensitization is not known.

Clinically it is generally recognized that the oleoresins are very active sensitizers which produce a high degree of reactivity which results in very acute cutaneous manifestations following exposure to either the bark, the leaves or the smoke from burning the plants.

Except for the intensity of the reaction, the cutaneous response with poison oak and poison ivy does not differ from that observed with other forms of contact dermatitis.

Itching is a constant complaint with all degrees of response but varies with the intensity of cutaneous involvement.

The rash may vary from a small isolated, pruritic erythematous patch with vesiculation to widespread body involvement, affecting all exposed parts. The smoke of burning leaves and twigs induces the most violent reaction with involvement of the face, neck, hands, arms, and all exposed parts. The two extreme patterns are least common, so that the usual clinical picture presents a moderate degree of involvement limited to the area of skin that made direct contact with the oleoresin. Scratching can distribute the lesions to other parts. The genitals and perianal regions are frequent sites of involvement through contamination by the fingers.

The lesions are always intensely red, with vesicles, bullae and oozing. Linear scratch marks capped with vesicles are frequently observed. These may serve as diagnostic guides.

Diagnosis: Diagnosis is usually made from a history of exposure. Occasionally, exposure may be indirect through contact with an exposed hairy animal (cats and dogs) or contact with contaminated clothes of an individual exposed to the oleoresins.

The linear scratch marks, capped with vesicles, mentioned above, suggest the diagnosis.

Treatment

I. Topical

(1) Compresses and soaks as recommended for atopic dermatitis.

(2) Topical medications of any type are not recommended. The risk of aggravating the dermatitis is very great. Sensitization to the excipients of topical medications is readily induced when applied to an already inflamed skin.

(3) Steroid therapy, preferably by mouth. Injectable steroids are less satisfactory (see discussion on steroid therapy in Chapter 15).

(4) Antibiotic therapy should be administered only in the presence of infection. Infection is not a common complication of *Rhus* dermatitis except occasionally in neglected cases and in children from uncontrolled scratching. Topical antibiotics are not recommended because of the risk of additional sensitization to either the drug or the preservative.

(5) Antihistamines are usually ineffec-

tive since in the delayed type of hypersensitivity histamine is not involved. Any benefits derived from antihistamines are due to their sedative effects. Antihistamines can induce contact sensitization.

(6) Most antipruritics are ineffective. If necessary, for a period of twenty-four to forty-eight hours, mild tranquilizers such as the hydroxyzine drugs (Atarax® or Vistaril®) may be administered.

In most cases the course of the illness is very brief. Good control of symptoms will usually be observed following the simple treatment with soaks, compresses and steroids. Even in severe reactions itching is controlled after twenty-four to thirty-six hours. Resolution of the cutaneous reaction usually requires about seven to ten days, but may require two to three weeks.

Prophylaxis: The best prophylaxis is avoiding contact with the plant or its oleoresins. For individuals whose occupation predisposes to exposure, protective clothing, e.g. gloves, shoes, masks, *etc.*, can be helpful. When protective clothing is worn, caution must be employed to avoid contact with the contaminated surfaces of the clothes.

II. Principle of Prophylactic Treatment with Extracts

(1) Experimental studies in animals have demonstrated that the oral administration of a hapten can prevent induction of contact dermatitis following exposure to the hapten (contactant).

(2) Experimental studies in animals have demonstrated that in flea-bite sensitivity, which is a haptenic mechanism, the administration of the flea hapten can:

(a) prevent the development of sensitivity,

(b) prevent the reaction following exposure after sensitivity has developed.

On the basis of similar principles extracts of the oleoresins of poison oak and poison ivy can be administered to induce non-reactivity.

There are commercial products available which have been tested for toxicity. Efficacy of these products has never been confirmed by controlled studies. The general impression gathered from clinical experience suggests that some of the available products are effective. When commercial extracts are prescribed, the procedure recommended by the manufacterer should be followed.

Such extracts should never be administered while the patient has any active eruption.

Injectable extracts for prophylaxis are not recommended.

Urticaria

Urticaria is a localized edema of the skin. The lesions vary from a single, minute wheal such as observed following an insect bite, to large coalescent patches involving extensive areas of the body. When tissues are loose, as with the eyelids and scrotum, edema replaces whealing.

The lesions are usually pale or even blanched due to distention of the skin by edema. A flare, which is more pronounced in younger individuals, surrounds the whealing lesions. The lesions appear in crops; as the new ones appear, the older lesions absorb, resulting in a pattern that waxes and wanes. Itching, which is usually pronounced, precedes the development of the wheals, and as the lesions reach full development, itching is diminished or completely absent.

Pathology: Increased capillary permeability of the small vessels of the upper corium of the skin, induced by the release of histamine from mast cells, causes edema of the corium which extends to the epidermis where it is manifested as whealing. The waxing and waning observed clinically is attributed to the depletion and recovery of histamine in the mast cells.

Etiology: Since urticaria is a manifestation of increased permeability of small vessels, any mechanism that induces this small vessel alteration can serve as a cause.

Histamine, released from mast cells, is the commonest mediator of increased small vessel permeability. Since the release of histamine is a cardinal feature of the immediate or atopic type of hypersensitivity induced by foods, pollens, environmental factors, drugs and chemicals (see Chapter 1), this type of allergic response is the commonest cause of urticaria.

Histamine can be released from mast cells by *nonallergic* factors such as trauma, temperature change (either hot or cold), infection, parasitism, and some chemicals.

Cholinergic urticaria which is induced by a nonallergic mechanism involves the release of acetylcholine by an impulse initiated by heat, emotions or exercise, originating in the higher centers and traveling via cholinergic fibers of the autonomic nervous system to the skin. In this type of urticaria the lesions usually occur in clusters of small wheals, unlike the large confluent patches of involvement seen in other forms of urticaria.

Emotional disturbances are frequently mentioned as a cause of urticaria. It is frequently stated that sudden onset of urticaria in an *adult* with no previous history of allergic disease is often on an emotional basis. Although such patients may respond to treatment with the hydroxyzine drugs (Atarax and Vistaril) there is no conclusive evidence that emotions are the cause (see Chapter 11, Psychological Factors in Allergic Disease). A diagnosis of emotional urticaria is frequently offered when the specific etiologic factor has not been identified.

Chronic Urticaria: When persistent urticaria cannot be related to any food or drug sensitivity, the various chemicals which serve as food additives—colorings, flavorings, gums, stabilizers, and preservatives—should be considered as a possible cause (see Chapter 9, Management With the Elimination Diet).

Treatment of Urticaria:
(1) Identification of the cause and its elimination is the only specific measure for definitive treatment.

Aspirin, tartrazine (FD&C yellow #5) and indomethacin are frequent causes of urticaria. If the elimination of aspirin fails to control the urticaria in an aspirin-sensitive patient, the elimination of all foods containing natural salicylates, by means of the salicylate-free diet (see Chapter 9, Management with the Elimination Diet) is often met with great success. The salicylate-free diet can also be a valuable prophylactic measure in salicylate sensitive patients.

(2) Symptomatic Treatment

(a) Antihistamines are usually effective, since in most cases histamine is involved. For extensive, acute involvement, oral steroids can be administered. Steroid therapy is not recommended for long-standing chronic urticaria.

(b) The hydroxyzine drugs (Atarax and Vistaril) are very often effective in chronic urticaria.

Dermographism

Dermographism is a condition characterized by a marked whealing reaction which may appear in response to a very light physical stimulus such as simple stroking of the skin. The whealing can be induced by various physical agents including

(1) scratching
(2) pressure upon the skin
(3) temperature changes, as hot to cold or cold to hot
(4) exposure to sunlight
(5) excessive muscular exertion where the overlying skin manifests whealing

Although dermographism is frequently attributed to either vasomotor instability or physical allergy, its occurrence in some patients suggests that the condition may be latent urticaria, i.e. urticaria without wheals. The basic conditions that predispose to whealing may be present, but the urticaria does not appear unless provoked by an exciting factor, such as the various physical agents indicated above.

This concept is supported by the following observations:

(1) Individuals with a history of past penicillin disease may manifest dermographism. Following dietary control to eliminate all sources of penicillin, such as dairy products contaminated with penicillin, the dermographia will clear. The patient has a normal response to stroking.

(2) Individuals with a history of aspirin sensitivity may manifest dermographia. Following management with a salicylate-free diet, the dermographia may clear, with a completely normally reacting skin.

(3) Individuals with a history of intolerance to one or more of the various food chemicals may manifest dermographia. With dietary control to eliminate the offending food chemical, the dermographia may disappear.

These observations suggest that in some individuals factors responsible for a skin reaction may induce a degree of reactivity which is not sufficient to produce overt cutaneous manifestations unless provoked by an exciting agent. In addition to penicillin, salicylates and food additives, it is conceivable that many other factors can operate to produce this state of latent skin reactivity.

In all patients with dermographia, this latent state should be considered as a possible cause.

Angio-edema

Angio-edema is characterized by marked swelling of tissues secondary to the diffusion of edema fluids secondary to increased permeability of the larger vessels situated in the stratum corneum of the skin, or the deeper mucosal layers.

The swelling varies in degree, but very often affects the upper and lower lips, the tongue, hands, or various body parts. With marked swelling about the pharynx, airway obstruction can lead to death.

The mechanism may be either allergic or nonallergic.

Allergic involvement is usually induced by foods, drugs and chemicals. Drugs and chemicals may also induce a nonallergic response by involvement of tissue receptors which necessitates no allergic mechanism.

When angio-edema is associated with joint involvement, either arthralgia or swelling, a serum type of reaction, should be considered. This type of response is often induced by drugs, particularly penicillin.

Management: Identification and elimination of the cause is essential for absolute control. Marked swelling of the tongue and edema in the region of the pharynx can be life threatening due to interference with breathing.

Epinephrine-HCl 1-1000 in doses of 0.4 to 0.5 cc should be administered immediately and repeated at frequent intervals. This will usually arrest the progress of the edema and permit sufficient time for steroids to become effective.

Steroids should be administered in massive doses (see steroid therapy in Chapter 15). If the patient is unable to take oral steroids, parenteral steroids should be administered. It usually requires several hours for the initial response to steroids.

Hereditary Angio-edema (Quincke's Disease)

Hereditary angio-edema is a familial disease, with its usual onset at puberty or adolescence, characterized by swelling of various body parts, resulting from the congenital deficiency of an inhibitor of the serum permeability factor. A deficiency of the inhibitor C^1 esterase, whose function is related to vascular permeability, has been reported in several families with a history of the disease.

The swelling may involve any body region, e.g. the skin, muscle, mucosal linings, and various organs.

Pruritus is usually absent, but pain may

accompany extreme distention of the tissues. The disease often develops insidiously, with no awareness by the patient that swelling is present. The patient may awaken insentient of the swelling which may involve the hands or the lips or distort the face. Involvement about the pharynx can cause respiratory obstruction leading to death. Intestinal swelling can cause obstruction. Fortunately, the condition is rare, as the prognosis is poor. There is no known treatment.

REFERENCES

1. Allen, Arthur, C.: *The Skin,* 2nd ed. New York, Gruen & Stratton, 1967.
2. Arthur, R. P. and Shelley, W. B.: The nature of itching in dermatitic skin. *Ann Intern Med, 49:* 900, 1958.
3. Austen, K. F. and Sheffer, A. L.: Detection of hereditary angioneurotic edema by demonstration of a reduction in second component of human complement. *N Engl J Med, 272:* 649, 1965.
4. Baer, R. L.: *Atopic Dermatitis.* New York, NYU Pr, 1955.
5. Baer, R. L.: *Allergic Dermatoses due to Physical Agents.* Philadelphia, NYU Pr, Lippincott, 1956.
6. Baer, R. L. and Witten, V. H.: *Year Book of Dermatology, 1956 To Present.* Chicago, Year Book Publishers, Inc.
7. Baer, R. L. and Witten, V. H.: Allergic eczematous contact dermatitis, Part II, test procedures. *Year Book of Dermatology and Syphilology,* 1957–1958 series. Chicago, Year Book Publishers, Inc.
8. Baer, R. L. and Fellner, M. J.: Pathogenesis of sensitization in allergic contact dermatitis in man. In *XIII Congressus Internationalis Dermatologiae.* New York, Springer, 1968.
9. Brunsting, L. A., Reed, W. B. and Baier, H. L.: Occurrence of cataracts and keratoconus with atopic dermatitis. *Arch Dermatol, 72:* 237, 1955.
10. Chase, M. W.: Inhibition of experimental drug allergy by prior feeding of the sensitizing agent. *Proc Soc Exp Biol Med, 61:* 257, 1946.
11. Coperman, P. W. and Wallace, H. S.: Eczema vaccinatum. *Br Med J, 2:* 906, 1964.
12. De Weck, A. L. and Frey, J. R.: *Immunotolerance to Simple Chemicals.* Basel, Karger, 1956.
13. Donaldson, V. H.: Mechanisms of activation of C'1 esterase in hereditary angioneurotic edema plasma *in vitro*: The role of Hageman factor, a clot promoting agent. *J Exp Med, 127:* 411, 1968.
14. Ebken, R. K., Baushard, F. A. and Levine, M. I.: Dermagraphism. Its definition, demonstration and prevalence. *J Allergy, 41:* 388, 1968.
15. Eisen, H. N., Orris, L. and Belman, S.: Elicitation of delayed allergic skin reactions with haptens. *J Exp Med, 95:* 473, 1952.
16. Epstein, E.: Allergy to dermatologic agents. *JAMA, 198:* 517, 1966.
17. Fisher, A. A.: *Contact Dermatitis.* Philadelphia, Lea & Lebiger, 1967.
18. Fregert, S. and Hjorth, N.: The principal irritants and sensitizers. Appendix I in Rook, Arthur, Wilkinson, D. S. and Ebling, F. J. G. (Eds.): *Textbook of Dermatology.* Philadelphia, F. A. Davis, 1968, vol. 2.
19. Hill, Lewis W.: Nomenclature, classification and pathogenesis of "eczema" in infancy. *AMA Arch Derm Syph, 66:* 212, 1952.
20. Hjorth, N. and Fregert, S.: Contact dermatitis, Chapter 14. In Rook, Arthur, Wilkinson, D. S. and Ebling, F. J. G. (Eds.): *Textbook of Dermatology.* Philadelphia, F. A. Davis, 1958.
21. Holti, G.: Management of pruritus and urticaria. *Br J Med, 1:* 155, 1967.
22. Kirschbaum, B. A., Beerman, H. and Stahl, E. B.: Drug eruptions: A review of some of the recent literature. *Am J Med Sci, 240:* 512, 1960.
23. Landsteiner, K. and Di Somma, A. A.: Studies on the sensitization of animals with simple chemical compounds. VIII Sensitization to picric acid, subsidiary agents and mode of sensitization. *J Exp Med, 72:* 361, 1940.
24. Lever, Walter F.: *Histopathology of the Skin,* 4th ed. Philadelphia, Lippincott, 1967.
25. Lowenthal, L. J. A.: *The Eczemas.* London, Livingstone, 1954.
26. Montagna, W.: *The Structure and Function of Skin.* New York, Acad Pr, 1956.
27. Montagna, W.: *The Structure and Function of the Skin,* 2nd ed. New York, Acad Pr, 1962.
28. Montgomery, H.: *Dermatopathology.* New York, Harper, 1966, 2 vols.
29. Ogawa, Makio, Berger, Peter A., Ross, McIntyre, Clendenning, William E., and Ishizaka, Kimischige.: IgE in atopic dermatitis. *Arch Dermatol, 103:* 575, 1971.
30. Pillsbury, Donald M., Shelley, Walter B. and Kligman, Albert M.: *A Manual of Cutaneous Allergy.* Philadelphia, Saunders, 1968.
31. Rook, Arthur: *Progress in the Biological Science in Relation to Dermatology.* New York Cambridge U Pr, 1960.

32. Rook, Arthur J. and Walton, G. S. (Eds.): *Comparative Physiology and Pathology of the Skin.* Philadelphia, F. A. Davis, 1965.
33. Rook, Arthur J., Wilkinson, D. S. and Elbing, F. J. G.: *Textbook of Dermatology,* vols. I and II. Philadelphia, F. A. Davis, 1968.
34. Rosen, F. S., Charache, P., Pensky, J. and Donaldson, V.: Hereditary angioneurotic edema: Two genetic variants. *Science, 148:* 957, 1965.
35. Rostenburg, A., Jr. and Solomon, L. M.: Infantile eczema and systemic disease. *Arch Dermatol, 98:* 41, 1968.
36. Rothman, S.: *Physiology and Biochemistry of the Skin.* Chicago, of Chicago Pr, 1954.
37. Rovensky, J. and Saxl, O.: Differences in the dynamics of sweat secretion in atopic children. *J Invest Dermatol, 43:* 171, 1964.
38. Schorr, W. F.: Paraben allergy: A cause of intractible dermatitis. *JAMA, 204:* 889, 1968.
39. Sedlis, E.: Conference on infantile eczema. *J Pediats, 60:* 236, 1965.
40. Sulzberger, M. B. and Herrman, R.: *Clinical Significance of Disturbances in the Delivery of Sweat.* Springfield, Thomas, 1954.
41. Sutton, R. L., Jr.: *Diseases of the Skin,* 11th ed. St. Louis, Mosby, 1956.
42. Walker, R. B. and Warin, R. P.: The incidence of eczema in early childhood. *Br J Dermatol, 68:* 182, 1956.
43. Walker, R. B., Smith, J. D. and Maibach, H.: I. Genetic factors in human allergic contact dermatitis. *Int Arch Allerg Appl Immunol, 32:* 453, 1967.
44. Waldbott, G. L.: *Contact Dermatitis.* Springfield, Thomas, 1953.
45. Wheatley, V. R.: Secretions of the skin in eczema. *J Pediatr, 66:* 200, 1965.
46. Winkelman, R. K.: Non-allergic factors in atopic dermatitis. *J Allergy, 37:* 29, 1966.
47. Zelickson, A. S.: *Ultrastructure of Normal and Abnormal Skin.* Philadelphia, Lea & Febiger, 1967.

Chapter 7

HEADACHES

A. ALLERGIC HEADACHES

THE REPORT OF EYERMAN in 1931 on a study of sixty-four cases of headache introduced the term "allergic headache." Forty-four of Eyerman's cases had a definite relation to the ingestion and avoidance of certain foods. On the basis of this observation, plus a claim of positive skin test reactions for the suspected foods, Eyerman concluded that the headaches were related to an allergic mechanism and more specifically food allergy. Following Eyerman's report, the term "allergic headache" has gained wide acceptance, although the evidence to support an allergic mechanism is lacking, and the attempt to correlate skin testing with offending foods has not been successful.

The association of headaches with the ingestion of a particular food is a common complaint, but even in cases where a cause and effect relationship can be demonstrated, either by inadvertent ingestion or by well-controlled blind studies, the evidence to support allergy as a primary cause of headache is lacking. Experimentally, brain lesions have been induced by hypersensitivity tissue reactions, but none of the lesions observed can be associated with the reaginic form of allergy. It is possible, as with other adverse food reactions, there are as yet unexplained nonimmunologic mechansims which operate to produce headaches.

Headaches secondary to allergic involvement of the nose and sinuses are not infrequent. In these cases, edema of the nasal and sinus mucosa with blocking of the sinus ostiae leads to a sense of pressure and even pain over the frontal and maxillary sinus areas. With stoppage of the nose by polypoid masses, the sense of pressure and the discomfort may be extreme. At times, involvement of the sphenoid sinuses will produce occipital headaches. The presence of complicating infection can usually be demonstrated by purulent secretion and x-rays.

Management: In the management of headaches consideration must always be given to systemic diseases, intracranial lesions, and migraine.

The treatment of headaches secondary to allergic involvement of the nose and sinuses is the same as outlined for these diseases. (See Chapter 2, Allergic Diseases of the Upper Respiratory Tract.)

When foods are incriminated, they should be eliminated from the diet. In some cases various elimination diets may be required to control the headaches. (See Chapter 9, Management with the Elimination Diet.)

B. MIGRAINE

Migraine, a disease with a familial tendency, is characterized by a constellation of functional disorders of which headache with nausea are the cardinal complaints. Paguiez, Vallery-Radot and Nast (1919) were the first to implicate an allergic mechanism for migraine. In 1927 Vaughn reported on "allergic migraine," following which the association of migraine with an allergic etiology became popular in this country. Substantiating evidence for a causal relationship of migraine to allergy is still lacking. The frequent occurrence in the migraine syndrome of complaints which simulate allergic patterns may explain the tendency to attribute this condition to an allergic etiology.

Headache, which is the most common complaint that brings the patient to the physician, is only one aspect of the clinical pattern of migraine; a condition which shows great variations in symptomatology, not only from individual to individual but within the experience of a single patient. Recognition of the variety of complaints presented by the migrainous patient is essential for its differentiation from allergic disease. Because of the complexity of the clinical pattern of migraine, several interviews may be required to develop an adequate history which permits recognition of the disease.

The figures for the incidence of migraine range from 6 per cent to 20 per cent, depending upon which observations are the source of reference. This would indicate that the frequency of the disease is actually not known.

The Aura or Prodromal Symptoms

Aural symptoms may precede the fully developed clinical pattern, or they may occur as abortive symptoms without the occurrence of headache or any other symptoms of the migraine syndrome. The aural symptoms may occur singly, but more frequently are experienced as a combination of the manifestations as classified by Sacks.

1. Sensory Hallucinations: Scotomata are the best known of the visual hallucinations which may take the form of a dance of brilliant stars, sparks, flashes or simple geometric forms across the visual field.

Tactile hallucinations may be positive (paresthesia) or negative (anesthesia) and involve the tongue and mouth, the hand or hands, and less commonly, the feet. Occasionally, tactile hallucinations may start on the trunk or the thigh. These hallucinations may coexist with, precede, or follow scotomata. These are less frequent than the visual manifestations.

Auditory hallucinations in the form of hissing, growling or rumbling noises occur occasionally.

Hallucinations of smell emphasize intensely odors which are familiar, *yet* not identified.

2. Alterations in the sensory threshold may occur which are characterized by an extreme intensification of either visual, tactile, or aural sensations.

3. Alterations of consciousness and postural tone may occur which are characterized by a hyperalert, tense and vigilant phase which is succeeded by a wavering of conscious level and tonus. In mild cases only a dullness and listlessness may be present, while in extreme cases there may be a complete loss of consciousness with an almost cataleptic loss of muscular tone.

4. Changes in mood occur in rare cases.

5. Various complex cerebral symptoms, manifest as difficulties in perception, speech and language disorders, may occur.

The Migraine Headache

Distribution: The migraine headache is usually unilateral at its onset but tends to become diffuse in distribution later in the attack. One side or the other may be involved, and at times the side of involvement alternates during the same attack or with succeeding episodes. About one third of the patients experience bilateral or diffuse (holocrania) involvement from the outset.

These variations in distribution differ from the headaches which are secondary to allergic nasal or sinus involvement that present a constant pattern of involvement over the affected sinuses with occasional radiation from the primary site of the allergic reaction. Headaches following the ingestion of food usually have a more diffuse involvement, but again fail to manifest the variations characteristic of migrainous headaches.

The *quality* of the migraine headache is also variable. In less than 50 per cent of cases throbbing occurs at the onset, which soon becomes a steady aching as the illness progresses. Continued throbbing throughout the attack is uncommon. Throbbing is synchronized with arterial pulsations and may be accompanied by visible pulsations of the extracranial arteries. Throbbing may occur with allergic sinus involvement or with the complication of infection but in either case the synchronization with arterial pulsations usually is lacking.

The migraine headache is aggravated by active or passive head movements or by coughing, sneezing or vomiting. Rest or splinting the head in one position relieves the pain. Counterpressure on the affected areas also offers a measure of relief. Nonmigrainous headaches are also affected by various movements of the head and body but usually not to the degree observed with migrainous headaches. With "sinus headaches" the jolting transmitted by walking (especially placing the heel onto a firm surface) may induce severe localized pain over the involved sinus.

Duration: The duration of migrainous headaches is also very variable. In some cases (migrainous neuralgia) the pain may last only a matter of minutes. These are difficult to differentiate from the *very* transitory acute pain which may be experienced following jolting with sinus involvement. In most cases of migrainous headache the duration is between eight and twenty-four hours, but rarely less than three hours. Occasionally, the attacks may last for several days and on occasion for a week. The pattern of longer duration is more difficult to differentiate from nonmigrainous headache, the duration of which is rarely limited to hours.

Intensity: The intensity of the migrainous headache also shows great variability, ranging from extreme discomfort which incapacitates, to slight pain induced by jolting and coughing. The briefer pattern can also be observed with "sinus headaches."

Nausea

Nausea is a cardinal feature of the migrainous headache and is invariable some time during the course of the illness, regardless of the intensity of the headache. This one feature should serve as a diagnostic differential for the migrainous headache.

Increased salivation and reflux of bitter stomach contents may precede or be associated with nausea. When it precedes the nausea, it may serve as the harbinger of an impending attack.

As nausea becomes established, the patient usually experiences various patterns made up of hiccup, belching, retching and then vomiting. Following vomiting, the entire attack may terminate, which misleads the patient into attributing his illness to food sensitivity. In most cases, however, vomiting does not terminate the attack but actually aggravates it. Vomiting plus profuse sweating and diarrhea may lead to dehydration.

In addition to headache which is usually the primary complaint of migraine, there are associated a variety of physiological disturbances which are referred to as migraine equivalents.

Facial Appearance

The common appearance of the patient is one of pallor, at times even ashen with a thin, drawn, haggard expression. The eyes appear small, sunken and ringed. Pallor is also a characteristic of the allergic individual (see Chapter 13, The Allergic Patient) but never to the extreme degree of the nauseated migrainous patient.

In a small percentage of cases (less than 10%) the face may be dusky and flushed.

Facial, lingual, labial and peri-orbital edema at the inception of an attack of migraine may resemble angio-edema and lead to an erroneous diagnosis of allergy.

Ocular Symptoms

Lacrimation, bulbar injection, itching, burning, photophobia and at times edema may suggest an allergic involvement. However, the migrainous patient in addition usually experiences blurring of vision due to an involvement of the vascular bed. At times, due to exudative thickening of the cornea, the retinal vessels cannot be visualized. Another differential is the increased salivation which frequently accompanies the ocular findings.

Nasal Symptoms

Nasal stuffiness is not an uncommon accompaniment of the migrainous headache. Upon examination of the nose the mucosa appears engorged and purple rather than the bluish pallor of the classical allergic nose (see discussion of allergic rhinitis). This difference would suggest that in migraine the involvement is in the erectile tissue rather than in the superficial capillaries which are the site of allergic involvement.

The nasal blocking together with profuse watery discharge is suggestive of an allergic rhinitis which in most cases can be differentiated by the appearance of the turbinates and nasal mucosa.

Abdominal Symptoms

Abdominal symptoms which occur in about 10 per cent of migrainous patients are observed more commonly among younger individuals. Pain in the upper abdomen may resemble peptic ulcer, cholecystitis or pancreatitis, while lower right quadrant pain may simulate acute appendicitis.

In the early states of the migrainous attack, peristaltic action may be absent which leads to constipation. Later in the attack, peristalsis becomes active, leading to colicky pain and diarrhea.

Fluid Retention

Wolff's studies confirm the observation that in over 30 per cent of patients, fluid retention leads to weight gain which the patients notice as tightness of the clothes, rings, belts, shoes, *etc.*

Dizziness, vertigo, tachycardia followed by bradycardia and hypotension with postural faintness are also observed in some cases of migraine.

The migrainous headache is only one symptom of a complex aggregate of various physiological disturbances. The diagnosis and management are dependent upon the recognition of the broad spectrum of this disease. It is beyond the scope of this book to catalog all the symptoms and variations that may constitute a migrainous syndrome. The studies of Sacks have been drawn upon freely, to which source the interested reader is referred.

ETIOLOGY OF MIGRAINE

A general appraisal of the situation regarding the etiology of migraine is well stated by Sacks:

> The search for a single causative factor, Factor X, is likely to be successful if the event being studied has a fixed form and fixed determinant. But the essence of migraine . . . lies in the variety of forms it may take and the variety of circumstances in which it may occur. Therefore, though one type of migraine may be associated with Factor X and another with Factor Y, it seems impossible on *prima facie* grounds, that all attacks of migraine could have the same etiology.

Theories of the Migraine Mechanism

1. Allergy

In 1933 Balyeat claimed an allergic etiology for migraine on the basis of a statistical correlation between migraine and the incidence of allergy among a group of migrainous patients and their families. Since Balyeat's report, the allergic etiology for migraine has gained wide acceptance.

Without the demonstration of a cause and effect relationship, migraine is commonly attributed to adverse food reactions. On the other hand, many food reactions are arbitrarily considered to be allergic in nature. As a result, migraine is commonly associated with food allergy. The importance of a non-immunologic mechanism in food sensitivity has been discussed (see Chapter 8, Adverse Reactions to Foods and Food Chemicals). Such a causal association risks subjecting the patient to unnecessary allergy skin tests, long periods of injection therapy, and a highly restricted dietary program which may be not only a great inconvenience to the patient but even injurious to his nutritional state.

2. Vasomotor Theory

This concept is based upon sympathetic hyperactivity which produces vasoconstriction of cranial blood vessels followed by vasodilatation secondary to sympathetic exhaustion. Wolff has demonstrated that the intensity of the migraine headache is closely proportional to the dilatation of extracranial arteries. In the later stages of migraine headache, dilatation of the affected arteries was followed by a sequence of local changes with exudate of a polypeptide rich fluid provocative of local pain and finally a sterile inflammatory reaction.

Sacks states that the ischemic hypothesis is attractive in view of its simplicity, but is altogether too simple to account for a migraine.

3. Chemical Theory

(a) *Histamine*: In 1956 Horton described as "histamine headaches" (Horton's headaches, cluster headaches, migrainous neuralgia) a condition which he attributed to a vascular mechanism induced by endogenous histamine. Clinically, the headaches were characterized by severe, pounding, unilateral pain of short duration (10 to 60 minutes) associated with unilateral lacrimation, nasal stuffiness, rhinorrhea, conjunctival congestion and unilateral facial flushing (on the side of the headache). The symptoms occur in frequently recurring episodes (cluster headaches) for a period of a few days to a week to be followed by a free interval of months or even years. Horton claimed that injection of histamine in predisposed individuals could evoke the headaches. He also reported that gastric acidity was increased during the attack of headache and that histamine "desensitization" could avert attacks. Other investigators refute Horton's claims on the basis that the headaches induced by histamine lack the unique characteristics of migrainous neuralgia and that elevated blood histamine has not been demonstrated in headaches or any other form of migraine.

(b) *Acetylcholine*: Kunkle (1959) attributed the migrainous reactions to an increased level of acetylcholine in the spinal fluid observed in some patients with migrainous neuralgia. Confirmatory studies on acetylcholine levels in spinal fluid of migrainous patients have not been reported.

(c) *Serotonin*: The likelihood that serotonin may play a role in the mechanism of migraine was indicated initially by the studies of Sicuteri who demonstrated the therapeutic effects in migraine of lysergic acid butanolamide (methylsergide), a potent serotonin inhibitor. Lance *et al.* who studied total plasma serotonin (TPS) before, during and after migraine attacks, observed an abrupt fall of TPS at the onset of headaches in the majority of cases. Based on the observation that the intracarotid injection of serotonin causes tonic contraction of extracranial arteries, Lance postulated that an abrupt fall in levels of circulating serotonin may lead to painful distention of extracranial vessels by a rebound phenomenon. Confirmation of the studies of Lance are necessary before an evaluation of the role of serotonin can be made.

4. Electrical Theories

Over the past thirty years there have been a number of electroencephalographic (EEG) studies on migraine patients that have reported many kinds of abnormalities, such as generalized slow wave dysrhythmias, convulsive patterns, focal abnormalities, *etc.*, but there is no agreement as to the incidence of these findings or their significance. It is generally recognized that migraine generates electrical disturbances in the brain, but the nature of these disturbances is still speculative, which explains the inability to formulate specific conclusions from EEG data.

Treatment of Migraine

The greater percentage of migraine headaches is not severe in nature and can be treated with mild analgesic drugs such as aspirin. Caution must always be exercised to determine that the patient is not an aspirin sensitive individual. If nausea and vomiting prevent oral medication, the rectal administration of ergotamine is recommended. If symptoms are very mild, the patient may be ambulatory.

With more severe involvement the patient usually seeks relief in a quiet, darkened room to protect against photophobia and aggravation of the headache by external stimuli.

Rest is very important and not infrequently sleep will be followed by complete relief from symptoms. In such cases mild sedation with either barbituates or tranquilizers can be helpful. When barbituates are prescribed, only small doses, gr ¼ to gr ½ should be administered. Precaution should be exercised to avoid addiction.

Caffeine in the form of strong tea and coffee has been a therapeutic measure for migraine over the ages. Alkaloidal caffeine may be administered by mouth.

Tincture belladona in small doses can be helpful in some cases, particularly when other drugs are not effective. The patient should be observed carefully for toxic side effects.

Amphetamine, codeine and morphine are not recommended because of the risk of addiction which can be more serious than the illness.

Approximately 80 per cent of all cases with moderately severe symptoms will respond favorably to ergotamine tartrate. To be effective, the drug must be administered as soon as possible after the onset of symptoms and preferably during the aural or prodromal period. Ergotamine tartrate is usually effective within the hour following administration. If control of symptoms has not been experienced after one hour, *continued* administration of the drug is not advised; nothing will be gained from continued administration of the drug except the risk of toxic side effects.

The time required for effectiveness of the various preparations of ergotamine tartrate are as follows:

oral tablets	30 minutes on an empty stomach
sublingual tablets rectal suppositories	15 minutes
aerosol parenteral injection	5 to 10 minutes

The choice of preparation is usually governed by the speed of onset of symptoms. For patients with patterns that develop slowly, and in the absence of nausea and vomiting, *oral* tablets are effective. In the presence of nausea and vomiting, rectal suppositories are helpful. In patients who manifest a rapid development of symptoms aerosol or parenteral injections are the treatment of choice.

Dosage: For oral preparations, administer 4 to 8 mg within the first hour; for parenteral preparations, administer 1 to 2 mg within the first hour. DO NOT ADMINISTER AFTER THE FIRST HOUR.

Contraindications To the Use of Ergotamine

(1) Pregnancy
(2) Disturbance of the peripheral circulation, such as Raynaud's disease or Berger's disease
(3) Coronary disease

Side Effects of Ergotamine

(1) Majority of patients have no side effects.
(2) Nausea and vomiting
(3) Faintness, drowsiness

Diuretics: Diuretics of various types have been recommended for the treatment of migraine, especially when fluid retention is evidenced. The studies of Wolff would seem to indicate that the action of diuretics has no influence upon the headaches.

Antihistamines: Except for the analgesic action of antihistamines, this class of drugs is ineffective in the treatment of migraine. Failure to respond to the antihistamines with a good response to ergotamine is presumptive evidence in favor of a diagnosis of migraine.

Steroids: Steroids have been effective in cases when ergotamine has either failed or is contraindicated. Steroids are worth a trial in some cases. The response to steroids should not be misinterpreted that the condition is allergic.

Local Measures: Ice packs on the forehead and pressure over the affected arteries may offer some relief.

For Nausea and Vomiting: Suppositories of sedative preparations such as meprobamate are effective.

The following simple mixture can be very helpful to allay nausea and counteract dehydration:

orange juice (clear, strained through gauze)	2 oz
water	2 oz
lemon juice (strained)	2 teaspoons
Karo® syrup (light)	2 teaspoons

Pack the mixture in ice. Start with a single teaspoonful, permitting an interval of several minutes before administering a second teaspoonful. Gradually and very slowly decrease the interval and increase the dosage until the patient is able to take the mixture freely. The mixture must be ice cold.

For the extreme attack, hospitalization may be required to permit the correction of dehydration and the control of symptoms.

When a strong psychosomatic component is evident, psychotherapy is recommended.

Prophylactic Drugs for Migraine

The drugs available for prophylaxis include belladonna, ergometrine, steroids and methysergide.

Belladonna compounds such as Bellergal® (ergotamine, bellafoline and phenobarbital) are frequently effective.

Steroids have been found useful in some cases, especially when ergotamine has been unsuccessful or is contraindicated.

Methysergide (lysergic acid butanolamide) (Sansert), the most powerful of the prophylactic drugs, is effective in about 30 per cent of cases. Because of the side effects, which in some cases can be very serious and insidious in development, the drug should be administered with great caution and never unless the patient is under frequent observation and careful physical examination to detect early evidence of side reactions.

Dosage: Methysergide is available in 2 mg tablets. The dosage should never exceed 8 mg in twenty-four hours. The drug should be administered gradually, attaining maximum dosage (8 mg per day) after about seven days. Full effectiveness of the drug is usually not observed before seven days and at times even ten days. The patient should be informed of this pattern to avoid the temptation to unnecessarily increase the dosage of the drug which could increase the likelihood of adverse reaction.

Side Effects:

(1) Nausea, drowiness or abnormal wakefulness
(2) Disorders of high cerebral function, such as depression, catatonia
(3) Vasomotor disturbances, such as elevated blood pressure, disturbed circulation of the extremities, numbness, tingling of toes, coldness, etc.

(4) Fibrotic induration of the pleural, pericardial and retroperitoneal spaces.

Ergotamine Preparations Available

Cafergot® { ergotamine 1 mg / caffeine 100 mg }

Cafergot P-B® { pentobarbital / bellafoline / caffeine / ergotamine }

Migral® { ergotamine / caffeine / cyclizine (antiemetic) }

Cafergot suppositories

Cafergot P-B suppositories

Medihaler-Ergotamine®

Bellergal { ergotamine / bellafoline / pentobarbital }

REFERENCES

1. Alexander, F. and French, T. M.: *Studies in Psychosomatic Medicine: An Approach to the Cause and Treatment of Vegetative Disorders.* New York, Ronald, 1948.
2. Balyeat, R. M. and Brittain, F. L.: Allergic migraine. *Am J Med Sci, 180:* 212, 1930.
3. Balyeat, R. M.: *Migraine: Diagnosis and Treatment.* Philadelphia, Lippincott, 1933.
4. Dow, D. J. and Whitly, C. W. M.: Electroencephalographic changes in migraine. *Lancet, 2:* 52, 1947.
5. Eyerman, Charles H.: Allergic headache. *J Allergy, 2:* 106, 1931.
6. Freud, Sigmund: *A General Introduction of Psychoanalysis.* Reprinted by Washington Square Press, New York, 1952.
7. Horton, B. T.: Histaminic cephalgia: Differential diagnosis and treatment. *Proc Mayo Clinic, 31:* 325, 1956.
8. Kimball, R. W., Friedman, A. P. and Vallejo, E.: Effect of serotonin in migraine patients. *Neurology, 10:* 107, 1960.
9. Kunkle, E. C.: Acetylcholine in the mechanism of headache of the migraine type. *Arch Neurol Psychiatry, 81:* 135, 1959.
10. Lance, J. W. and Anthony, M.: Some clinical aspects of migraine. *Arch Neurol, 15:* 356, 1966.
11. Lance, J. W., Anthony, M. and Hinterberger, H.: The control of cranial arteries by humoral mechanisms and its relation to the migraine syndrome. *Headache, 7:* 93, 1967.
12. Luria, A. P.: *Higher Cortical Functions in Man,* trans. by Basil Haigh. New York, Basic Books, 1966.
13. Paquiez, P., Vallery-Radot, P. and Nast, A.: Therapeutique preventive de certaines migraines. *La Presse Medical, 27:* 172, 1919.
14. Sacks, Oliver W.: *Migraine.* Berkeley, U of Cal Pr, 1970.
15. Selye, H.: The general adaptation syndrome and diseases of adaptation. *J Clin Endocrinol Metab, 6:* 117, 1946.
16. Sicuteri, F.: Prophylactic and therapeutic properties of methyl lysergic acid butanolamide in migraine. *Int Arch Allergy Appl Immunol, 15:* 300, 1959.
17. Symonds, C.: Migrainous variations. *Trans Med Soc, Lond, 67:* 237, 1952.
18. Tourraine, G. A. and Draper, G.: The migrainous patient: A constitutional study. *J Nerv Ment Dis, 80:* 1, 1934.
19. Vaughn, W. T.: Allergic migraine. *JAMA, 91:* 1628, 1928.
20. Wolff, H. G.: *Headache and Other Head Pain.* New York, Oxford Pr, 1963.

Chapter 8

ADVERSE REACTIONS TO FOODS AND FOOD CHEMICALS

I. ADVERSE FOOD REACTIONS

ADVERSE FOOD REACTIONS are commonly recognized by both professionals and laymen, but the failure to appreciate that nonimmunologic as well as immunologic mechanisms operate to produce unfavorable food responses explains the great variety of symptoms and diseases which are arbitrarily attributed to allergic mechanisms, often without supporting evidence. This is well illustrated by the list compiled from various textbooks by Sherman.

It is important to realize that even diseases such as urticaria, angio-edema, nasal polyps and bronchial asthma, which have been traditionally cited as classical examples of the allergic response, may at times be caused by nonimmunologic mechanisms.

Nonimmunologic mechanisms which cause adverse food reactions include:

(1) Enzymatic deficiencies as occur in disaccharide intolerance; observed in milk sensitivity and in gluten intolerance in coeliac disease.

(2) Chemical irritation which induces symptoms, such as pyrosis, flatulence, cramping, and other intestinal disturbances as observed with cabbage, broccoli, onions, garlic, radishes, spices and herbs.

(3) Toxic reactions induced by tainted foods, such as fish and shellfish. Fish and shellfish which are improperly preserved may develop a high histamine content which can induce characteristic reactions.

(4) Contamination of foods by bacteria and bacterial products can produce untoward food reactions.

(5) Chemicals in foods which occur either naturally or as additives may be responsible for adverse food reactions (see Food Chemicals).

Symptomatology

Food reactions occur as either immediate or delayed, depending upon the time of on-

Table 8-I: SOME DISEASES AND SYMPTOMS ATTRIBUTED TO FOOD ALLERGY BY VARIOUS TEXTBOOKS[1]

Migraine[2]	Meniere's disease[2]
Coated tongue[2]	Belching[2]
Transient palsy[2]	Transient blindness[2]
Erythromelalgia[2]	Recurrent neuritis[2]
Renal colic[2]	Hypertension[2]
Irritable bladder[2]	Enuresis[2]
Intermittent hydrarthrosis[2]	Favism[3]
Recurrent pyuria[3]	Hematuria[3]
Fetal hiccough[3]	Urethral meatitis[3]
Hyperkinesis[3]	Fatigue[3]
Sluggishness[3]	Hyperesthesia[3]
Photophobia[3]	Torpor[3]
Depression[3]	Insomnia[3]
Irrational behavior[3]	Paranoid ideas[3]
Feeling of unreality[3]	Nervous tics[3]
Inability to concentrate[3]	Foul breath[3]
Constipation[3]	Recurrent diarrhea[3]
Anorexia[3]	Abdominal pain[3]
Acneiform eruption[4]	Recurrent corneal ulcer[4]
Recurrent herpes labialis[4]	Cheilitis[4]
Canker sores[4]	Pruritis ani[4]
Blurred vision[4]	Scintillating scotoma[4]
Dysmenorrhea[4]	Leukorrhea[4]
Fever[4]	Cardiac arrhythmia[2]
Dizziness[5]	Physical tiredness[5]
Nervousness[2]	Neuralgia[5]
Heartburn[5]	Indigestion[5]

[1] From Sherman, W.B.: *Hypersensitivity, Mechanisms and Management.* Philadelphia, Saunders, p. 158.
[2] Vaughan, W.T. and Black, J.H. (Eds.): *Practice of Allergy*, 3rd ed. Mosby, St. Louis, 1954.
[3] Speer, F.: *The Allergic Child.* Harper & Row, New York. 1963.
[4] Rowe, A.H.: *Food Allergy.* Lea & Febiger, Philadelphia, 1931.
[5] Coca, A.F.: *Nonfamilial Nonreagenic Food Allergy.* 3rd ed. Thomas, Springfield, 1953.

set of the symptoms following the ingestion of the food.

The *immediate* (under one hour) food reactions frequently occur instantaneously upon contact of the food with the lips or the mouth, causing itching, burning or swelling. More often small quantities of food are swallowed, to be followed very soon by vomiting, cramps, and at times diarrhea. The generalized reaction induced is usually characterized by flushing, itching, urticaria, angioedema but less frequently nasal symptoms and bronchial asthma. Very occasionally, extreme reactions are observed characterized by hypotension and syncope suggestive of anaphylaxis.

The *delayed* reactions usually occur one hour or more following ingestion of the food. In some cases symptoms may occur as late as forty-eight hours following ingestion, which further complicates identification of the food. The delayed adverse food reactions may involve any organ or tissue of the body, producing symptoms referable to the particular system. As with the immediate form, generalized reactions may occur which are characterized by pruritus, urticaria, angioedema, rhinitis and asthma.

The variability in the onset of symptoms is related to several factors, such as concomitant exposure to other allergens, particularly the inhalants when the individual is allergic; the time required for the digestive breakdown of the food; the quantity of a given food ingested; the variety of the foods eaten at the time the offender is ingested; and the presence of infection, particularly in children.

Identification of Foods Involved in Reactions

The immediate reactions to foods usually present no diagnostic problem. In most cases the patient or the parent, when children are involved, can identify the offender associated with the reaction and exclude it from the diet even before consulting the physician.

The identification of the foods involved in delayed reactions is a more complex problem because of the lack of reliable guidelines.

History is usually very helpful in determining that the patient is an allergic individual which is the first prerequisite in diagnosis. Since food sensitivity rarely occurs as an isolated event, the patient will usually manifest sensitivity to inhalant factors and particularly to items in the environment. Positive skin tests are usually quite reliable for confirming the sensitivity to environmental factors. When environmental factors are incriminated, food allergy cannot be determined reliably unless strict environmental control is exercised. With failure to control the environment, an adverse reaction may be falsely attributed to a food, when actually it is induced by a feather pillow, a pet animal or an item of furniture. If following strict environmental control the patient with suspected food sensitivity fails to respond, it is reasonable to try elimination of the suspected food.

When patients with seasonal symptoms supported by positive skin test reactions to pollens fail to respond to injection therapy, the possibility of food sensitivity should be considered.

Fortunately, foods do not play a very important role in respiratory allergic disease and particularly when sensitivity to inhalant factors can be supported by positive skin tests. The extreme position is held by those allergists who contend that foods are rarely if ever involved in allergic rhinitis or bronchial asthma. This position, however, is the extreme, for there are unquestionably, though they are not common, individuals whose symptoms cannot be controlled until offending foods are excluded from the diet.

Skin Tests in Food Sensitivity

It is generally recognized that skin testing for foods is quite unreliable. A positive skin test will frequently fail to correlate with the patient's tolerance for the food, while a known intolerance very often cannot be confirmed by a positive skin test reaction.

The Positive Skin Test with Food Allergens

The immediate symptoms of adverse food reactions usually parallel very closely the positive skin test responses for the offending food. This is particularly true for highly antigenic food substances, such as egg white, buckwheat, nuts, shellfish and fish. When symptoms occur immediately following contact or ingestion of the food, the patient is aware of the offending food, so that confirmation by skin testing is not only unnecessary but is contraindicated. With a positive history of food sensitivity, particularly of the immediate type, skin testing can be hazardous because of the risk of precipitating violent constitutional reactions. This is especially true for the highly antigenic foods mentioned above. When an adverse response to food is elicited in the history, the food should be excluded from the diet and no confirmatory skin test should be performed.

Challenge by ingestion of samples of known food offenders must also be conducted with great caution to avoid violent reactions.

The False Positive Food Skin Test Reaction

Since isolated allergic food reactions without involvement of other systems occur very rarely, it is unusual to observe positive skin test reactions to foods without reactions to inhalant factors. In other words, if the patient fails to react to inhalant factors on skin testing, the likelihood of obtaining reliable positive skin test reactions for food is very remote. As a corollary to this observation it can be stated that isolated gastrointestinal symptoms attributed to food allergy without supporting evidence of allergic disease elsewhere in the body is very rare. These patients usually have positive reactions to inhalant allergens (see Chapter 5, Gastrointestinal Allergy).

False positive skin tests are observed very commonly with food extracts, which add to the unreliability of the testing procedure for food sensitivity. A positive skin test reaction for a food with no adverse reactions following ingestion of the food item is a common experience in clinical allergy.

The false positive skin test for foods is well illustrated by two situations observed clinically.

(1) Bakers who experience asthma upon exposure to an atmosphere contaminated with grain dust can usually tolerate the ingested grains even when manifesting strongly positive skin test reactions to the grains.

(2) Patients with seasonal symptoms induced by pollens may react strongly to both grass pollen extracts and extracts of the grains. However, following ingestion of the grains to which the skin test reactions are *strongly* positive, the patient experiences no adverse response.

The difference in the patient's tolerance for the ingested allergen as compared with the intolerance for the inhaled allergen, in the presence of skin reactions to both, suggests that the immunologic response in each situation is not identical. This hypothesis is supported by recent observations which demonstrate that antigens applied topically to the respiratory mucosa manifest a different immunologic response as compared with the parenteral injection of the same antigen.

On the basis of this observation, in patients with symptoms induced by pollen sensitivity, the grains should *not* be excluded from the diet because of positive skin test reactions to the grains. Such positive skin test reactions for the grains may actually be *false positive* tests.

Very *rarely*, a patient with symptoms induced by pollens with positive skin test reactions to both pollens and the grains will experience a more favorable response to injection therapy following the elimination of the grains from the diet. This situation is not encountered very commonly, so that the elimination of the grains is not recommended as a routine procedure. A similar experience is observed with foods other than the grains. During the pollinating season a patient may have an intolerance for a particular food which can be ingested with impunity out of the pollinating season. This may occur with or without positive skin test reactions for the food, but it is not a common observation.

The Negative Skin Test Reaction

The negative skin test reaction with a positive history of food intolerance may be due to (1) an alteration in the chemistry of the ingested food as a result of the digestive process. In these situations the clinical response to the foods is usually of the delayed type. During the process of digestion the food proteins are degraded to polypeptides and proteoses which serve as antigens to induce allergic reactions. The only evidence to support this hypothesis is the study of Cooke who successfully demonstrated a positive reaction to a milk proteose in a milk sensitive patient with a negative skin test reaction to milk. This observation has not been confirmed by other investigators.

Another reason for the negative skin test reaction may be due to nonimmunologic mechanisms. Food chemicals either natural or as additives can induce adverse reactions which simulate allergic clinical patterns (see discussion on Food Chemicals). These reactions may be either immediate or delayed In these cases skin tests for the foods are negative.

A history of respiratory symptoms, urticaria or angio-edema with complete failure to demonstrate any positive reactions on skin testing to either inhalants or foods suggests either a response to a digestive product of food or a reaction to a food chemical occurring either naturally or as an additive (see discussion on Food Chemicals). In either situation the mechanism may be nonimmunologic, and the skin test reaction is always negative.

It is often stated that a dislike for a particular food indicates an intolerance for the food, particularly in children. This is not a reliable index, since many patients can ingest reasonably large quantities of food for which they have a dislike without untoward reactions. Food dislikes cannot be correlated with skin test reactivity.

Antibodies to Foods

The involvement of the immediate type of allergy in food sensitivity was demonstrated by Walzer as early as 1927. He injected intradermally into a nonsensitive individual the serum of a sensitive individual. When the recipient ingested the food to which the donor was sensitive, an urticarial wheal developed at the site of the transfer. This experiment also demonstrated that adults absorbed antigenically active food proteins.

Precipitating antibodies for foods, especially for milk, have been demonstrated in the sera of both allergic and nonallergic individuals. The significance of these antibodies is not known.

Schloss (1924) demonstrated that undigested food proteins are absorbed from the intestinal tracts of children and evoke precipitating type of antibodies. These antibodies caused no apparent disease and disappeared with increasing age. The gut of children seems to be more permeable to food proteins. This observation is frequently mentioned as an explanation for the higher incidence of food allergy among children.

MILK: Since milk is the chief item of food in infancy and very early childhood, it is frequently involved in adverse reactions. The higher incidence of sensitivity in infancy and early childhood as compared with later life is attributed to the increased permeability of the gut at the earlier age which permits passage of undigested proteins into the serum.

The casein of milk is species specific, while

milk whey is nonspecific. For this reason when milk casein is at fault, attempts are frequently made to substitute the milk of other species, such as goat, sheep, mare, *etc.*, but without the success one would anticipate theoretically.

Breast milk has not been observed to be allergenic; however, foods eaten by the mother and especially egg may be excreted in the milk to produce symptoms in allergic infants.

Contamination of milk with extraneous substances can also be a factor in cow's milk intolerance. Constituents of the cow's fodder, such as the grasses and pollens ingested while grazing, may be excreted in the milk to cause symptoms unrelated to milk proteins. Boiling the milk at times will destroy the extraneous proteins, but at best, heated milks, such as evaporated, condensed and various forms of powdered milk have proved to be unsatisfactory substitutes when milk sensitivity is a problem.

In penicillin-sensitive individuals the contamination of milk with penicillin must be considered. The drug is used for both prophylaxis and treatment of the udders of the cattle which results in various concentrations of penicillin in the milk. In penicillin-sensitive individuals who may experience chronic urticaria or recurrent angio-edema, it is usually necessary to eliminate from the diet all sources of milk, including cheese and particularly the natural cheeses.

An allergic individual may offer a history of milk intolerance in early life which apparently subsides at about two or three years of age. However, when such individuals experience allergic complaints in later childhood or adult life, it is important to consider milk sensitivity as a contributory factor in their management.

In nonallergic individuals with milk intolerance, a nonimmunologic mechanism or disaccharidase deficiency must be considered. Such patients have only gastrointestinal symptoms. The skin involvement and the respiratory symptoms of the allergic individual are lacking.

Individuals who experience allergic milk sensitivity in early infancy and childhood usually develop other manifestations of allergy in later life, while the nonimmunologic individuals are entirely symptom-free throughout life upon elimination of milk from the diet.

Skin tests with the various milk fractions are quite unreliable.

When milk sensitivity has been established, *total* exclusion of milk from the diet is essential for control of the patient's symptoms (see milk-free diet in Chapter 9). Elimination of milk while permitting food derived from milk, such as cheeese or foods prepared with milk, *usually* results in unsatisfactory control of the patient's symptoms.

EGGS: Egg white is a highly antigenic substance. Egg yolk is less active; however, since most commercially available yolk extracts are not absolutely free of egg white, false reactions to tests with egg yolk are observed quite frequently.

In most cases the patient who has a marked sensitivity to egg is aware of his condition. In such cases skin testing with egg extracts is not only unnecessary but actually contraindicated because of the risk of violent generalized reactions. The egg-sensitive patient can develop the violent symptoms of anaphylactic shock immediately following a prick test with egg white extract.

With lesser degrees of sensitivity it may be necessary to test the patient. If the patient offers a history of ingesting either egg or foods prepared wih egg, testing can be undertaken with a reasonable degree of safety. The patient should always be screened by the prick test technique before undertaking intradermal testing.

When egg sensitivity is established, management requires an egg-free diet (see egg-free diet in Chapter 9). If the patient is exquisitely sensitive to egg white it may be necessary to prepare his food in utensils which have not been exposed to egg. It is not possible to prepare immunologically clean utensils by routine domestic procedures.

Eggs from other fowls cannot be substituted for chicken eggs.

MEATS: Meats are rarely involved in sensitivity reactions; however, occasionally an individual sensitive to cow's milk will not tolerate beef and veal, while egg-sensitive individuals may not tolerate chicken or chicken feathers. Egg-sensitive individuals usually tolerate capon and rooster.

Papain, derived from papaya, used as a tenderizer, can be a frequent cause of reactions to meat. Individuals sensitive to papaya may exhibit an intolerance to beef, ham and luncheon meats treated with the papain tenderizers. Many housewives use meat tenderizers to improve less costly cuts of meat. Occasionally, tenderizers are administered to cattle before slaughter which results in concentrations of papain in the meat which can cause reactions of variable degrees.

CHOCOLATE: Chocolate is not a strong antigen. Although reactions to chocolate are observed, this food does not deserve the reputation it has as a common cause of reactions.

Chocolate rarely occurs in pure form as a food. The various additives employed in

Table 8-II: FOOD AND NON-FOOD SOURCES OF CORN*

Adhesives	Excipients or diluents in	Jello®	Rice, coated
envelopes, stamps,	capsules, lozenges,	Ketchup	Root beer
stickers, tapes	ointments, suppositories	Kixs®	Salt
Ale	tablets, vitamins	Kremel®	salt cellars in restaurants
Aspirin & other tablets	Fish, prepared & processed	Laxatives†	A & P 4 Seasons Salt®
Bacon	Flour, bleached†	Leavening agents	Salad dressings†
Baking mixes	Foods, fried	baking powders, yeasts	Sandwich spreads
Baking powders	French dressing	Lemonade	Sauces for:
Batters for frying	Fritos®	Linit®	sundaes, meats, fish,
Beets, Harvard	Frostings	Life Savers®	vegetables
Beers	Fruits	Liquors	Sausages, cooked or
Bleached wheat flours†	canned, frozen	Margarines & shortenings†	table-ready
Bourbon & other whiskies	Fruit juices	Meats, processed & cold cuts†	Sherbets
Breads and pastries	Fruit pies	bacon, bologna	Similac®
Breath sprays & drops†	Frying fats	cooked with gravies	Soft drinks
Cakes	Gelatin capsules	ham, cured or tenderized	Spaghetti†
Candy	Gelatin dessert	lunch ham, meat pies	String beans
candy bars	Glucose products	sausages, cooked	canned, frozen
commercial candies	Graham crackers	wieners (frankfurters)	Sobee®
box candies, all grades	Grape juice	Metrecal® cookies & wafers	Soups
Carbonated beverages	Gravies	Milk, in paper cartons	creamed, thickened,
Catsups	Grits	Monosodium glutamate	vegetable
Cereals, many processed	Gums, chewing	Mull-Soy®	Soy bean milks
Cheeses	Gummed papers:	Nabisco®	Sugar, powdered
Cheerios®	envelopes, labels, stamps,	Nescafe®	Syrups, commercially prepared
Chili, all forms	stickers, tapes	Noodles†	Cartose,® glucose, Karo,®
Chop suey	Gin	Pablum®	Puretose,® Sweetose®
Chow mein	Ginger ale	Paper containers	Tablets†
Coffee, instant	Hams	boxes, cups, plates (only	Talcums
Colas	cured, tenderized	when foods have a moist	Teas, instant
Cookies	Harvard beets	phase in contact with	Tooth paste
Confectioner's sugar	Holiday type stickers	these cartons)	Craig-Martin & Bost
Corn flakes	Ices	Pastries	Tortillas
Corn Soya®	Ice cream†	cakes, cupcakes	Vanillin
Corn Toasties®	Inhalants	Peanut butters	Vegetables
Cough syrups	bath powders	Peas, canned	canned, creamed, frozen
Crackels®	body powders	Pickles	Vinegar, distilled
Cream O Soy®	cooking fumes of	Pies, creamed	Vitamins
Cream pies	fresh corn	Plastic food wrappers	Waffles
Cream puffs	hair sprays†	(inner surfaces may be	Whiskies
Cups, paper	popcorn	coated with corn starch)	Scotch† & bourbon
Dates, confection	starch	Pork & beans†	American brandies, both
Deep fat frying mixtures	starch, while ironing	Powdered sugar	apple and grape
Dentifrices	starched clothing	Preserves	Wines, American†
Dextrose	talcums	Puddings	dessert
Egg nog	Jams	blanc mange, custards	fortified
Envelopes, gummed	Jellies	Royal® puddings	sparkling
		Ravioli	Zest®

* Courtesy Hollister-Stier Laboratories.
† Some brands are corn free.

preparing chocolate as a food may be responsible for the reactions so frequently attributed to this food.

For example, egg white is a common item used for glazing chocolate, which in egg-sensitive individuals could be the cause of reactions rather than the chocolate.

In the preparation of chocolate drinks and chocolate milk, in order to keep the chocolate in suspension, surface active agents are used in combination with hydrophilic macromolecular stabilizers or thickeners. Any of the additives may cause adverse reactions which are erroneously attributed to chocolate.

CORN: In addition to its use as a food in its natural form, derivatives of corn, such as corn starch and corn syrup have numerous applications not only in the preparation of foods but also its use for non-food purposes. Because of the wide distribution of corn in food products, it is one of the most common food offenders.

While the bulk of the starch produced in this country is from corn, starches are also milled from sorghum, potato, wheat and tapioca. The major source of commercial starch is corn which explains its extensive distribution and also accounts for its importance as a cause of unfavorable reactions. In spite of its very widespread and varied usage, the role of corn as a cause of symptoms frequently passes unrecognized and particularly when the complaints are vague, such as fatigue, listlessness and tiredness.

Isolated positive skin test reactions for corn are not rare. When corn is recognized as an offender, all contacts and all foods containing corn should be eliminated.

II. FOOD CHEMICALS

In addition to the natural composition of foodstuffs, chemicals may be incorporated either directly or indirectly during the growing, storage or processing of foods. These chemicals are termed "food additives."

Additives are classified as (1) intentional or (2) nonintentional.

(1) Intentional or direct additives include those chemicals which in accordance with governmental regulations are purposely added for specific functions.

(2) Nonintentional additives include all materials which would not usually become part of food if man could completely control food production, such as pesticides and chemicals absorbed from packages.

Table 8-III lists the classification of intentional food additives compiled by the Food Protection Committee of the National Research Council. Thirteen classes are listed which include over 2,700 individual items. In addition, there are many secret formulas used as additives in food and beverage processing which are under the jurisdiction of various governmental agencies and are not available for publication. For example, the chemicals used as additives in processing wines and other alcoholic beverages fall under the jurisdiction of the Internal Revenue Service. Information regarding these chemicals is usually not available to the public. In most cases, the Food and Drug Administration has no knowledge of the chemicals added to alcoholic beverages.

With the wide distribution of the food additives, a higher incidence of reactions would be anticipated than that indicated by

Table 8-III: CLASSIFICATION OF INTENTIONAL ADDITIVES

1. Preservatives	33
2. Antioxidants	28
3. Sequestrants	45
Chelating agents	
Metal scavengers	
Emulsifiers	
Stabilizing agents	
4. Surface active agents	111
5. Stabilizers, thickeners	39
6. Bleaching and maturing agents	24
7. Buffers, acids, alkalines	60
8. Food colors	34
9. Non-nutritive and special dietary sweeteners	4
10. Nutritive supplement	117
11. Flavorings—synthetic	1610
12. Flavorings—natural	502
13. Miscellaneous	157
Yeast foods	
Texturizers	
Firming agents	
Binders	
Anti-caking agents	
Enzymes	
Total Number of Additives	2764

the comparatively limited number of reports in the literature. This discrepancy can perhaps be attributed to the lack of awareness of both the professionals and the laity of the almost universal distribution of these chemicals and their potential for inducing unfavorable reactions. In the concentrations permitted by regulations, it is generally believed that adverse reactions to food additives occur infrequently.

In a great measure, much of the lack of awareness of the problem can be attributed to improper labelling of the various products. The label frequently fails to disclose the ingredients in a product or, when they are indicated, the disclosure is usually imprecise and incomplete, such as when the chemicals are listed as artificial coloring or artificial flavoring without specifying precisely which color or flavor is contained in the product. Very often when disclosure does appear on the label, the type is so small that it escapes the notice of the consumer.

It is possible that with greater awareness of the problem, a higher incidence of reactions will be recognized. In addition, improved techniques and procedures for the identification of chemical patterns of adverse reactions to food chemicals will increase the frequency of diagnosis.

Many food chemicals in use prior to 1958 with no record of adverse experiences were routinely approved for use in food processing and are now labelled "generally regarded as safe" (GRAS). The present status of GRAS substances is indicated by the following excerpt from the 1971 FDA Annual Report.*

In his Consumer Message of October 1969, President Nixon charged FDA to review the safety of the approximately 600 items on the list of substances "generally recognized as safe" (GRAS) published by FDA in 1959–1961. To meet the intent that all substances for addition to food have a modern toxicological evaluation, FDA is including in this major project other substances previously sanctioned or identified as GRAS in unpublished correspondence.

---

*FDA Papers. FDA Annual Report 1971, December 1971–January 1972, p. 15.

By contract to FDA the Food Protection Committee of the National Academy of Sciences–National Research Council developed and tested a questionnaire designed to obtain current production information from suppliers, manufacturers, and users of substances on the GRAS list.

Within FDA, a GRAS Review Branch was established to expedite activities connected with the review.

The first and basic regulation of many contemplated in the project was published June 28. This order established the criteria by which FDA will measure the eligibility of a specific substance to be classed as GRAS. Under the order, all substances requiring any limitations for safety must be approved by specific food additive regulations.

Taking its first action under the new criteria, FDA removed saccharin from the GRAS list and issued a provisional regulation restricting its use.

During the fiscal year, 110 new food additive petitions were received and fifty-one orders published involving food additive regulations, exclusive of veterinary products.

As of June 30, 1971, approximately 2,752 food additives were covered by formal regulations. In addition, 561 substances for direct use in food packaging, and forty-six compounds for providing trace mineral in animal food were listed as "generally recognized as safe."

Preservatives

Except for the reactions attributed to the tetracyclines which are used for the preservation of fish, shellfish and some meats, there are no reports of adverse reactions attributed to preservatives.

Stabilizers and Thickeners

The stabilizers and thickeners are chiefly gums of various types. In addition to the natural gums, there are semisynthetic products which are modified natural gums, such as carboxymethyl cellulose, methyl cellulose, modifications of starch, alginate, locust bean and agar gum.

The completely synthetic gums, such as vinyl and acrylic polymers, are not used as food additives.

All the gums have a very wide distribution in food processing.

Since 1658 the most commonly used gum was agar, imported from Japan. With the advent of World War II the agar supply was no longer available, so substitutes for agar were developed. These were principally Car-

Table 8-IV: CLASSIFICATION OF GUMS

Tree Exudates and Extracts
  Arabic
  Tragacanth
  Karaya
  Larch
  Ghatti

Seed or Root
  Locust bean
  Guar
  Psyllum seed
  Pumice seed

Seaweed Extracts
  Agar

Algae
  Carrageen
  Furcellaran
  Algin

Others
  Pectin
  Gelatin and other proteins
  Starch

Table 8-V: MAJOR USES OF GUMS IN FOOD PRODUCTS

Agar
  bakery, confectionery, meat and fish products, dairy products, laxatives

Algin
  ice cream, ice milk, water ice, sherbets
  cheese
  water dessert gels and milk puddings
  fruit drinks and other beverages
  beer
  salad dressings
  film-forming coating for meat, fish, etc.

Carrageenan*
  chocolate milk
  milk puddings, pie fillings
  water dessert gels
  ice cream, ice pops
  dietetic foods
  salad dressings
  beer
  soups, sauces, soft drinks
  syrups, toppings
  infant foods

Furcellaran*
  milk pudding
  flan or blanc mange
  jams, jelies, dietetic products
  bakers jellies
  meat and fish preservation

Gum Arabic
  citrus oil emulsions
  flavor emulsions
  spray dry flavors
  confectionery
  jellies
  glazes
  chewing gum
  beer
  icings, glazes, toppings

Ghatti gum
  substitute for gum arabic

Karaya
  salad dressings
  ice pops, sherbets
  cheese spreads
  Philadelphia® cream cheese
  meat products, as a binder
  meringues, toppings, and whipped cream products

Larch gum†
  essential oils, flavor base puddings, non-nutritive sweeteners

Tragacanth
  salad dressings
  confectionery
  ice cream
  bakery products

Guar Gum
  ice cream
  soft cheeses
  baked products
  sausage
  beverages
  salad dressings
  relishes

Locust bean
  ice cream
  bakery goods
  sauces, salad dressings
  pie fillings
  soft cheeses
  sausages

* Since World War II these gums have enjoyed a wide distribution in commercially prepared foods.
† Use is limited because it is an expensive gum.

rageenan* and Furcellaran. Currently, the most widely used gum is Carrageenan, derived from a species of red algae found off the Irish coast near the town of Carrageenan. Furcellaran, quite similar to Carrageenan is a derivative of red algae found off the coast of Denmark.

The gums are complex, long chain carbohydrates which are not subject to breakdown either by digestion or by the action of most bacteria. For this reason, the gums are usually eliminated from the body with no change in structure. Because of their chemical characteristics they are actually inert substances and, as such, are not antigenic, which means allergic reactions should not be anticipated from the gums. In addition, because of the chemical nature of gums, extracts of them cannot be prepared. However, in spite of this, for years allergists have tested with extracts of gums, such as karaya and tragacanth and have reported positive skin reactions which they have correlated with various allergic symptoms. It is very likely that these

---
* Chondrus extract (Carrageenan) (Irish moss) derived from seaweed has been removed from the approved GRAS list, Federal Register, August 2, 1972.

reactions are not a response to the gums, but rather a reaction to contaminants present in the gums. The testing materials are probably extracts of the contaminating substance rather than an extract of the gum. It is possible that the contaminants of the various gums which may be proteins could cause allergic reactions, which would explain the clinical reactions attributed to gums.

Synthetic Food Colors and Flavors

Since the clinical problems involving food colors and flavors are quite similar, the two groups can be considered together.

Of the thirty-four chemicals listed under the heading of food colors, the Food, Drug and Cosmetic (FD&C) colors are the most important. Eleven coal tar drugs are listed in this group of which the seven in Table 8–VI are used most commonly.

FD&C Red #2 is the most widely used of all food colors. Russian workers have reported that FD&C #2 had adverse effects on reproduction and was carcinogenic in rats. In the FDA laboratories rats were fed FD&C Red #2, several of its metabolites and an impurity commonly present in the color, at various levels from 2 to 200 mg/kg/day. Preliminary results confirm the Russian observation of an effect on reproduction at high levels, but the study has not been underway long enough to evaluate the possibility of carcinogenicity. Similar studies are being made of FD&C Red #40, the new color listed as a replacement for FD&C Red #2.

The group of synthetic flavors includes 1,610 chemicals, while the natural flavors include 502 items for a total of 2,112 chemicals which represents roughly 80 per cent of all the food additives listed by the Committee on Food Processing of the National Research Council and the National Academy of Sciences.

Because of the extremely wide distribution of these chemicals in the supply of foods, beverages, and pharmaceuticals, practically everyone has daily contact with one or more of the colors and flavors. A list of the foods containing these chemicals would be encyclopedic. It is important to recognize that very few processed foods are free. Frequently, the consumer is surprised to learn that a common, everyday food product contains either a synthetic color, a synthetic flavor, or both. For example, it is not generally recognized that many dry breakfast foods contain artificial colors and flavors, particularly the products designed for catering to children.

The distribution of colors in carbonated beverages is indicated in Table 8-VII. The flavors are usually disclosed on the label.

The use of these chemicals in drugs is readily apparent from the wide variety of colors employed for coating tablets and coloring capsules, while both colors and flavors are incorporated into tablets and liquid preparations of medicinals.

The most commonly incriminated color is tartrazine (FD&C yellow #5) which finds a

Table 8-VI: FD&C COLORS

Blue #1 (Brilliant Blue)	Bottled soft drinks
Green #3	Mint-flavored jelly
Red #2	Breakfast cereal
	Imitation jellies
	Bottled soft drinks
Red #3 (Erythrosine)	Canned fruit cocktail
	Fruit salad
	Cherry pie mix
Yellow #5 (Tartrazine)	Imitation strawberry jelly
	Bottled soft drinks
	Drugs
Yellow #6	Bottled soft drinks
Red #40	Replacement for Red #2

Table 8-VII: COLOR AND CONCENTRATION IN CARBONATED BEVERAGES

Flavor	Color	Parts	Concentration
Orange	FD&C Yellow No. 6	98	54 ppm
	FD&C Red No. 2	2	
Cherry	FD&C Red No. 2	100	50 ppm
Raspberry	FD&C Red No. 2	99	45 ppm
	FD&C Blue No. 1	1	
Grape	FD&C Red No. 2	94.5	55 ppm
	FD&C Blue No. 1	4.5	
	FD&C Yellow No. 5	1.0	
Strawberry	FD&C Red No. 2	80	50 ppm
	FD&C Yellow No. 6	20	
Lime	FD&C Yellow No. 5	95	20 ppm
	FD&C Blue No. 1	5	
Lemon	FD&C Yellow No. 5	100	20 ppm
Cola	Caramel color	100	400 ppm
Root Beer	Caramel color	100	400 ppm

very wide application in foods, beverages and medicinals. The adverse responses to tartrazine seem to be similar to those induced by aspirin and indomethacin (see discussion on aspirin sensitivity, Chapter 10). Samter, in a rigidly controlled double blind study, induced reactions in three aspirin-sensitive patients by the administration of 25 mg of tartrazine in aqueous solution. A case of non-thrombocytopenic vascular purpura attributed to tartrazine has been reported by Criep. Sensitivity to tartrazine was substantiated by a double blind study using capsules containing either the dye or a placebo. The author has observed a severe shock-like reaction resembling anaphylaxis in an adult male following the ingestion of Tang®, an orange drink colored with tartrazine.

There are several published reports of reactions to tartrazine (FD&C yellow #5) contained in medications. In 1959 Lockey reported that tartrazine (FD&C yellow #5), the coloring in decadron, paracortol, and deronil, was the cause of urticaria in three adults. In 1967 Chafee and Settipane reported a case of severe, intractable asthma attributed to tartrazine (FD&C yellow #5) which was included in the patient's medication and in a yellow-coated vitamin tablet. Urticaria and angio-edema have been attributed to the tartrazine (FD&C yellow #5) used in the manufacture of Provera® and Provest.®

Intractable pruritus was observed in an adult female treated with Esidrix® (Ciba), a yellow-coated tablet containing 50 mg of hydrochlorothiazide. The pruritus cleared when the patient was treated with the same drug and equal dosage by a tablet without the yellow coloring, tartrazine (FD&C yellow #5).

Rhinorrhea and asthma have been observed following the ingestion of Norinyl,® a contraceptive tablet colored with tartrazine (FD&C yellow #5).

The conditions attributed to the colors and flavors are listed in Table 8-VIII.

For discussion of emotional patterns in-

Table 8-VIII: ALLERGIC CONDITIONS INDUCED BY FLAVORS (SYNTHETIC, NATURAL) AND COLORS

1. Respiratory
   Allergic rhinitis
   Nasal polyps
   Cough
   Laryngeal edema
   Asthma
2. Skin
   Pruritis
   Dermatographia
   Localized skin lesions
   Urticaria
   Angio-edema
3. Gastrointestinal
   Macroglossia
   Flatulence & pyrosis
   Constipation
   Buccal chancres
4. Neurological Symptoms
   Headaches
   Behavioral disturbances
5. Skeletal System
   Arthralgia with edema

duced by food additives, see Chapter 11, Psychological Factors in Allergic Disease.

Diagnosis

Both the colors and the flavors may produce identical patterns with no distinguishing features to differentiate one group from the other. There are actually no specific criteria for incriminating either class of chemicals. The diagnosis must in great measure depend upon (1) an awareness that colors and flavors are a common cause of adverse reactions, and (2) a high degree of suspicion which follows the exclusion of all other possible factors. A careful history and a diet diary for a period of seven to ten days are also very helpful in making the diagnosis when reactions occur to one or more of the chemicals.

There are no skin tests for the chemicals. Since the food chemicals are low molecular weight compounds, their involvement in an immunologic reaction would mean they are serving as haptens. Since haptens cannot be demonstrated by skin testing, this procedure is not helpful in the diagnosis.

It is likely that, as in the case of tartrazine, the reaction to most food chemicals is induced by nonimmunologic mechanisms, in which case skin testing is of no value.

If an immunologic mechanism were operating, it would be reasonable to expect that some of the patients reacting to tartrazine would manifest evidence of an Arthus type reaction, such as a morbilliform eruption or a vasculitis as observed with drugs that serve as haptens. Or perhaps hematologic findings induced by a cytotoxic mechanism should occur in some patients. None of these immunologic responses has been either observed or reported in patients sensitive to tartrazine. This lends additional support to the nonimmunologic behavior of the chemical.

In the absence of test procedures and specific identifying criteria for the involvement of food chemicals, the following patterns will frequently serve as helpful guidelines for the management of patients with suspected reactions to food additives:

(1) Aspirin sensitivity
(2) Nasal polyps
(3) The failure to react on skin testing
(4) Reactions on skin testing but failure to respond to routine management

1. Aspirin Sensitivity

In aspirin sensitive patients tartrazine (FD&C yellow #5), which is a chemically unrelated compound, can induce reactions similar to those caused by aspirin. It is conceivable that among the thousands of food chemicals encountered in the food supply,

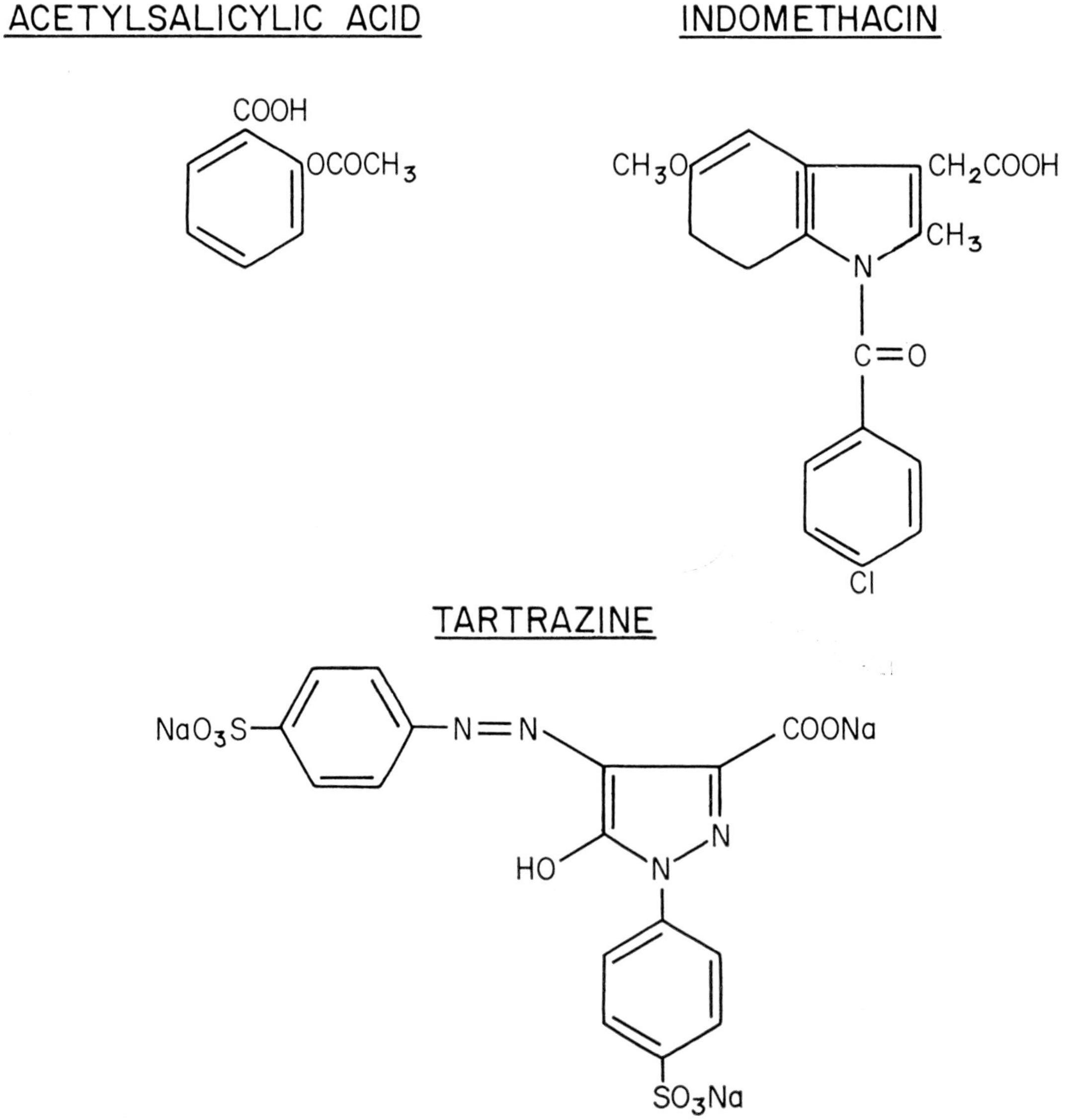

Figure 8-1

there may be additional compounds as yet unidentified which can induce identical adverse responses. On the basis of this premise it can be helpful to use a history of aspirin sensitivity as a guide for arriving at a presumptive diagnosis of sensitivity to food chemicals.

Identifying the Aspirin Sensitive Patient: The patient with a history of urticaria, angioedema or asthma following the ingestion of aspirin presents no diagnostic problem. However, the individual whose history is less obvious for aspirin sensitivity, such as the patient with only minor disturbances following the ingestion of aspirin, requires a more careful interview to disclose the intolerance. The symptoms may be only those of mild pruritus, pyrosis or slight gastric distress following the ingestion of aspirin. Very often because of the mild nature of the symptoms the patient may not consider them important, or may not attribute the symptoms to aspirin intolerance. Very often the patient reports that buffered aspirin is tolerated but not plain aspirin, while not infrequently proprietary aspirin compounds are not considered to be aspirin. All these factors must be considered in developing the patient's history. The slightest adverse response may serve as a clue to aspirin intolerance and serve as an excellent guide in the management of the patient.

When either a definite or a presumptive history of aspirin sensitivity is made, the patient should be managed by

(a) the elimination of all aspirin and aspirin containing compounds

(b) the elimination of all food flavors with a salicylate radical, (oil of wintergreen, methyl salicylate). Methyl salicylate is a commonly used flavoring for both foods and medicinals. At times methyl salicylate may be labelled as mint flavoring.

(c) The elimination of all foods containing a natural salicylate radical (see Chapter 9). Both Samter and Farr report that following the elimination of aspirin in patients sensitive to this drug, the symptoms may persist. In such cases a good response has been observed following the elimination of all foods containing a natural salicylate radical.

(d) The elimination of all foods containing synthetic coloring and flavorings. Except for tartrazine and FD&C Red #2 there are no observations to support adverse reaction to any specific food color or food flavor. However, the possibility exists that one or more of the many food additives may behave as tartrazine, FD&C Red #2 and aspirin to produce adverse reactions. A diet designed to eliminate all synthetic food colors and flavors will exclude approximately 80 per cent of all the additives encountered in the food, beverage and drug supply. Such a program can be very rewarding when the causative agent is obscure in chronic urticaria, recurrent angio-edema or persistent asthma.

2. Nasal Polyps

The association of nasal polyps with the ingestion of aspirin is generally recognized. The mechanism involved in the production of polyps by aspirin is not understood. It is possible the foods containing natural salicylates as well as some food additives may be factors in the etiology of nasal polyps. On the basis of this possibility, the following procedure is recommended for patients with nasal polyps.

The patient with nasal polyps who offers a history of known sensitivity to inhalant factors and manifests positive skin test reactions for the inhalant factors can be initially managed by routine environmental control and immunotherapy. If following a trial period of routine management (about 5 to 6 months) no response is observed, the patient should be placed on a diet which eliminates all foods containing natural salicylates as well as all synthetic colors and synthetic flavors.

3. Patients Who Fail To React To Routine Allergy Skin Tests

A patient with any of the symptoms listed in Table 8-VIII—with no known etiology—

who fails to react to allergy skin tests, may be sensitive to chemicals which are (a) serving as haptens to induce immunologic reactions or (b) causing nonimmunologic responses. In either instance the skin test will be negative. In this group of patients the possibility that food additives may be the causative factor should be considered. Management is with the appropriate elimination diet.

4. Patients Who React To Routine Allergy Skin Tests

Not infrequently a patient who reacts positively to allergy skin tests will have a good response to routine management through environmental control and immunotherapy. However, following a period of good control of the symptoms, the patient may experience a recurrence of the initial symptoms or may develop a new clinical pattern suggestive of allergic disease. It must be recognized that "suggestive of allergic disease" does not mean that the underlying mechanism is immunologic. The identical pattern may be induced by a nonimmunologic reaction. If following a careful review of the patient's routine, a causative factor cannot be identified, a trial with a diet eliminating all synthetic food flavors and colors, and also all foods containing natural salicylates, may be successful in controlling the patient's symptoms.

The Non-Nutritive Sweeteners

Sorbitol and mannitol, polyhydric alcohols, find wide use in food processing. As a sweetener, they occur as major components in most "sugar-free" confections, chewing gum and dietetic foods. Although adverse reactions have not been reported, such adverse responses would be difficult to evaluate since these compounds are usually associated with artificial colors and flavors which are common offenders.

Saccharin has been used as a sugar substitute since the turn of the century, but adverse reactions were not reported until 1951. Since that date several reports of adverse reactions, e.g. pruritus, urticaria and photosensitivity have been documented. The clinical patterns were recently reviewed Gordon.*

Recent studies suggest that saccharin may be carcinogenic for some individuals.

The first action taken under the new criteria established by the FDA for licensing food additives removed saccharin from the GRAS list and issued a regulation placing this chemical on restricted use.

REFERENCES

1. Aas, K. and Jebsen, J. W.: Studies of hypersensitivity to fish: Partial purification and crystallization of a major component of cod. *Int Arch Allergy Appl Immunol, 32:* 1, 1967.
2. Anderson, A. F. and Schloss, O. M.: Allergy to cow's milk in infants with nutritional diseases. *Am J Dis Child, 26:* 451, 1923.
3. Bayliss, T. M., Pantin, J. S. and Pantin, J. C.: Serum precipitins to milk, gluten and rice in tropical sprue. *Bull Hopkins Hosp, 120:* 310, 1967.
4. Beckwith, A. C. and Heiner, D. C.: An immunologic study of wheat, gluten proteins and derivatives. *Arch Biochem Biophys, 117:* 219, 1966.
5. Bleumink, E. and Young, E.: Identification of the atopic allergens in cow's milk. *Int Arch Allergy Appl Immunol, 34:* 521, 1968.
6. Brunner, M. and Walzer, M.: Absorption of undigested proteins in human beings: The absorption of unaltered fish proteins in adults. *Arch Intern Med, 42:* 173, 1928.
7. Chafee, F. H. and Settipane, G. A.: Asthma caused by FD&C approved dyes. *J Allergy, 40:*65, 1967.
8. Crawford, L. W. et al.: Immunologic studies on the legume family of foods. *Ann Allergy, 23:* 303, 1965.
9. Feingold, B. F.: Recognition of food additives as a cause of symptoms of allergy. *Ann Allergy, 26:* 309, 1968.
10. Francis, C.: The prognosis of operation for removal of nasal polypi in cases of asthma. *Practitioner, 123:* 272, 1929.
11. Goldman, A. S., Anderson, D. W., Jr., Sellers, W. A., Saperstein, S., Kniker, W. T., Halpern, S. R. et al.: Milk allergy I. Oral challenge with milk and isolated milk proteins in allergic children. *Pediatrics, 32:* 425, **1963.**

---

* Gordon, H. Untoward Reactions to Saccharin, *Cutis,* Yorke Medical Journal, New York, 1972.

12. Gryboski, J. D.: Gastrointestinal milk allergy in infants. *Pediatrics, 40:* 354, 1967.
13. Hanson, L. A. and Mansson, I.: Immune electrophoretic studies of bovine milk and milk prodducts. *Acta Paediatr, 50:* 484, 1961.
14. Heiner, D. C., Wilson, J. F. and Lahey, M. E.: Sensitivity to cow's milk. *JAMA, 189:* 563, 1964.
15. Heiner, D. C., Lahey, M. E., Peck, G. A. and Wilson, J. F.: Precipitins to wheat in steatorrhea. *Am J Dis Child, 102:* 446, 1961.
16. Horton, G. E. and Wruble, L. D.: Lactose intolerance syndrome mimicking milk allergy and/or functional bowel disorders. *Ann Allergy, 24:* 698, 1966.
17. Huesley, J., Asquith, P. and Cooke, W. T.: Immune response to gluten in adult coeliac disease. *Br Med J, 2:* 159, 1969.
18. Katz, J., Herskovic, T., Spiro, H. M. and Gryboski, J. D.: Coproantibodies to milk in an infant with milk sensitivity. *Gastroenterology, 52:* 1098, 1967.
19. Katz, J., Spiro, H. M. and Herskovic, T.: Milk precipitating substances in the stool in gastrointestinal milk sensitivity. *N Eng J Med, 278:* 1191, 1968.
20. Lockey, S. D.: Allergic reactions due to FD&C yellow #5, tartrazine, an analine dye used as a coloring and identifying agent in various steroids. *Ann Allergy, 17:* 719, 1959.
21. Samter, Max: The acetyl in aspirin. *Ann Intern Med, 71:* 208, 1969.
22. Samter, Max and Beers, R. F., Jr.: Intolerance to aspirin: Clinical studies and consideration of its pathogenesis. *Ann Intern Med, 68:* 975, 1968.
23. Saperstein, S., Anderson, D. W., Jr., Goldman, M. S. and Knilsen, W. T.: Milk allergy III. Immunological studies with sera from allergic and normal children. *Pediatrics, 32:* 580, 1963.
24. Schloss, O. M.: A case of allergy to common foods. *Am J Dis Child, 111:* 341, 1912.
25. Schloss, O. M.: The intestinal absorption of antigenic proteins. *Harvey Lect, 20:* 18, 1924–25.
26. Solomon, Joan: Thursday's child: A review of minimal brain dysfunction (MBD). *NY Acad Sci, 12* (no. 5): 6, 1972.
27. Van Meter, T. E., Jr. *et al.:* A controlled study of the effects on manifestations of chronic asthma in a rigid elimination diet based on Rowe's cereal free diet. *J Allergy, 41:* 195, 1968.
28. Walzer, M.: Studies in absorption of undigested proteins in human beings: I. A simple direct method of studying the absorption of undigested proteins. *J Immunol, 14:* 143, 1927.

Chapter 9

MANAGEMENT WITH THE ELIMINATION DIET

by
ALICE D. FRIEDMAN, M.D.*

IN THE CHAPTER ON Adverse Reactions to Foods and Food Chemicals it was pointed out that the attitude regarding the significance of foods in clinical allergy ranges from those clinicians who believe that foods are of no importance, particularly in respiratory allergic disease, to those who contend that foods are the chief etiologic agents in allergic disease. The role of food as a cause of symptoms undoubtedly occupies a position between the two extremes. The majority of individuals with complaints due to an allergic mechanism have no intolerance for any foods, while in a small percentage of allergic individuals, the symptoms cannot be controlled without dietary exclusions. When foods are eliminated from the diet for the control of symptoms, the dietary restrictions should be applied judiciously in order to avoid unnecessary inconvenience to the patient and also to prevent additional harm to the patient's health through nutritional disturbances which can result from extreme and prolonged dietary exclusions.

The preceding chapters have considered the significance of both positive and negative skin tests for foods as well as the following indications which may serve as guidelines for prescribing an elimination diet:

(1) A history of food intolerance
(2) Failure to control symptoms with immunotherapy and environmental control
(3) A recrudescence of symptoms not attributed to a reaction to injection therapy or an infraction of environmental control
(4) A history of nasal polyposis
(5) A history of recurrent serous otitis
(6) A history of aspirin intolerance

Procedure for Diet Elimination

When the patient experiences an immediate reaction to a food or foods, the management usually presents no problem, since in most cases the patient eliminates the offending food, even before consulting the physician.

When delayed reactions to foods are suspected, the problem is more complex. For such cases the guidelines indicated above can be helpful.

Initially, it is imperative to establish either by history, skin tests or both whether the patient is an allergic individual.

An intolerance to milk in early infancy, which may be either immunologic or non-immunologic, can be of great significance in the dietary management of the patient. In early infancy the symptoms of the adverse reaction to milk may be "spitting up," vomiting, colic, diarrhea, skin eruption or nasal snuffles. These symptoms may subside following the period of infancy so that complaints that develop in later childhood or in adult life may not be associated with the intolerance in infancy. A family history of milk

---
* Department of Allergy, Kaiser Foundation Hospital—Permanente Medical Group, San Francisco.

intolerance, particularly with a disaccharidase deficiency, helps to exclude allergy. The elimination of milk from the diet under these circumstances may be followed by a dramatic control of symptoms. Milk sensitivity is observed quite frequently in children offering a history of recurrent serous otitis.

Since egg, particularly egg white, is a very strong antigen, the reaction following the ingestion of egg by sensitive individuals is usually quite pronounced and in most cases evident to the patient. In some cases the patient may fail to relate the symptoms to the ingestion of egg because of the late onset of symptoms and at times because of the mildness of the reaction. This is observed more frequently following the ingestion of food products containing egg rather than egg itself. The correlation between egg sensitivity and skin reactivity is quite reliable so that in most doubtful cases egg sensitivity can be confirmed by skin testing. Skin testing for egg should never be attempted with a positive history for egg sensitivity. *If in doubt, do not test for egg.* When egg is proved to be a known reactor, all egg and egg products must be eliminated from the diet (see egg-free diet). Since egg is a very antigenic material, the ingestion of infinitesimal quantities—even a single drop—can in some cases precipitate violent reactions.

A history of penicillin sensitivity can be of great importance in a patient who takes milk and eats natural cheeses. Milk is commonly contaminated with penicillin which is used for the treatment of the udders of milk cows. Natural cheeses contain molds which may cross react with penicillin. In penicillin-sensitive patients both milk and natural cheese may cause symptoms. Occasionally, oranges and orange juices may be contaminated with penicillin. Elimination of these food items in penicillin sensitive patients may be followed by excellent control of symptoms (see milk-free diet).

A history of nasal polyposis, either with or without positive skin tests, is an absolute indication for management with a salicylate-free diet (see diets below).

The same rule applies to any patient who offers a history of sensitivity to aspirin (see Chapter 10, Adverse Reactions to Drugs) either with or without positive tests for any allergen.

When food intolerance is suspected in a patient who fails to react on skin testing, the following must be considered:

The sensitivity may be induced by food fragments developed during the digestive processes. The fragments, which may be peptides, proteoses or even smaller components of foods, can act either as a hapten to produce immunologic reactions or merely as chemicals to induce a nonimmunologic response. In either situation, in the absence of specific information derived from the history, the choice of a dietary program must be determined empirically.

The Role of Inhalant Factors in Dietary Management

When the skin tests are positive for inhalant factors, no foods can be incriminated unless the environmental factors, pollens and at times even molds have been excluded as a cause of the symptoms. This is achieved by strict environmental control (see Chapter 17) and injection therapy for a reasonable period (arbitrarily, no less than 6 months). Not infrequently, patients will attribute to foods the symptoms that are actually caused by inhalant factors. Seasonal symptoms caused by pollens, and at times molds, are frequently erroneously attributed to foods. On the other hand, it is possible for a seasonally occurring food to be responsible for seasonal symptoms.

When environmental control has been observed strictly and injection therapy has not proved successful in the control of symptoms, consideration may be given to a possible food factor which justifies the use of an elimination diet. In the absence of guidelines in the history, the choice of diet is determined empirically. In these situations the diet diary discussed below can be helpful in arriving at a choice of diets.

The identical analysis of the problem applies to patients who have been managed successfully with environmental control and injection therapy who suddenly experience a recrudescence of symptoms or develop new complaints.

The Diet Diary

A carefully recorded diet diary which can be of great value in the management of patients with a food intolerance will not only serve as a diagnostic aid but may be helpful in identifying any infraction when a program is ordered. The diary can explain either the patient's failure to respond or a recrudescence of symptoms that may occur following a period of good control.

The patient must be impressed with the importance of recording each item of food, beverage or medication ingested. The record should include not only items taken with meals but everything ingested between meals. Even a minute quantity such as a single bite or at times a teaspoonful of a deleterious product may be the cause of symptoms. It is important to stress that proprietary preparations such as aspirin, aspirin compounds, antacids, laxatives, vitamins and also contraceptive tablets are considered as medications that should be listed in the diary. It is important that the constituents of all home prepared foods be listed as well as ingredients of all packaged foods. This latter information is particularly important when considering the possibility of a food color or flavor as a causative agent.

If the patient's condition permits, it is often helpful to establish a profile of the patient's dietary habits by keeping a diary for about seven to ten days without any alteration in the customary eating and drinking habits. The various symptoms experienced by the patient should also be recorded chronologically. By correlating symptoms with the information in the diary, the physician is frequently able to determine the elimination diet suitable for the particular case.

The Procedure

Two weeks after starting an elimination diet the patient should be interviewed and the diary carefully reviewed for any likely infractions. In most cases if the elimination diet is successful, an improvement will be experienced within ten to fourteen days. Occasionally, a patient will require up to twenty-one days to manifest an improvement. The reason for the delay in showing a favorable response is not known.

After four weeks the patient should again be interviewed and the diet carefully reviewed whether the patient does or does not report a good response. A favorable response in the face of dietary infractions would indicate that factors other than the suspected food had been operating to produce the symptoms. If the response to dietary management is reported as unfavorable, it is important to not only review the diet for possible infractions but also the patient's environment for any possible changes either at home, at work or places visited by the patient. If the review fails to detect a cause for the failure, it is likely that the diet will not be effective. The program should be abandoned and a different dietary regimen tried.

If the dietary program outlined for the patient is effective, it is advisable to continue the routine for at least two months before attempting additions to the diet. New foods should be added individually, starting at first with very small quantities once a day then gradually increasing the quantities for fourteen days following which the food may be taken freely. If symptoms recur at any time during the period of challenge, the new food should be discontinued. Following a second symptom-free period, another challenge can be attempted. If the second attempt is not successful the food should be permanently excluded from the diet. When the tolerance for one food has been determined, the program may be repeated with other foods, each time individually until a well balanced and varied diet is provided for the patient.

It is important to impress upon the patient the importance of a continuing diary even after the symptoms are controlled so that in the event of a recurrence of symptoms an inadvertent infraction can be detected. With correction of the error, the patient can again enjoy a symptom-free period.

The Salicylate-Free Diet

It has been observed that aspirin-sensitive patients will not infrequently fail to respond following the elimination of aspirin until the foods containing natural salicylates are also excluded from the diet. Accordingly, the salicylate-free diet was initially designed as an adjunct in the management of patients sensitive to aspirin. It was also noted that flavors containing a salicylate radical also cause reactions similar to those induced by aspirin. Further, it has been learned that compounds chemically unrelated to aspirin, such as tartrazine (FD&C yellow #5) can induce similar reactions. Since the specific nature of the coloring added to food products is frequently not indicated on the package, it became necessary to eliminate all food products containing artificial coloring in order to avoid the ingestion of tartrazine. As a result, the diet excludes all foods that contain artificial color. On the premise that many synthetic compounds, though chemically unrelated to aspirin may induce similar adverse reactions, the diet was extended to eliminate all artificial flavors as well as colors. As the patient's symptoms come under control, an occasional food color or food flavor may be very carefully added, but never a food containing tartrazine and never a food containing a synthetic compound whose specific composition is not disclosed. When in doubt, it is usually safer to exclude the product.

When the diet is initially presented to the patient, a common first reaction is that the diet is highly restrictive and permits very little choice of foods. Each category of the diet should be reviewed to assure the patient that a broad choice of foods is still permitted.

On the permitted list are included fruits:

> pears
> grapefruit
> lemon
> lime
> banana
> pineapple
> melons of any variety

Bakery Goods

If prepared at home with basic ingredients which exclude all color and flavor additives, a broad assortment can be prepared.

All mixes, which contain a great variety of additives of all sorts, should be excluded from the diet.

Most cereals are permitted. Caution must be exercised to exclude the dry cereals prepared with artificial color and flavors. The ingredients on the package must be checked carefully.

All meats except processed meats, such as luncheon meats, sausages and bologna, are permitted.

All poultry is permitted.

Salad dressings can be prepared with oil and distilled vinegar or oil with lemon juice.

All vegetables are permitted.

SALICYLATE-FREE DIET

The following foods should be eliminated:

I. FOODS

Almonds	Nectarines
Apples	Oranges
Apricots	Peaches
Blackberries	Plums or prunes
Cherries	Raspberries
Currants	Strawberries
Gooseberries	Cucumbers and pickles
Grapes or Raisins	Tomatoes

II. FLAVORINGS (Omit artificially flavored foods and drinks)

Ice cream
Oleomargarine
Gin and all distilled beverages (except vodka)
Cake mixes
Bakery goods (except plain bread)
Jello®
Candies
Gum
Cloves
Oil of wintergreen
Toothpaste and toothpowder
Mint flavors
Lozenges
Mouthwash
Jam or jelly
Lunch meats (salami, bologna, *etc.*)
Frankfurters (Hot Dogs)

III. BEVERAGES

Cider and cider vinegars
Wine and wine vinegars
Kool Aid® and similar beverages
Soda pop (all soft drinks)
Diet drinks and supplements
Gin and all distilled drinks (except vodka)
All tea
Beer

IV. DRUGS AND MISCELLANEOUS

1. All medicines containing aspirin, such as Bufferin,® Anacin,® Excedrin,® Alka-Seltzer,® Empirin,® Darvon compound,® *etc.*
2. Perfumes
3. Toothpaste and toothpowder (A mixture of salt and soda can be used as a substitute or Neutragena® soap unscented)

Note: Check all labels of prepared foods or drugs for artificial flavoring and coloring.

Milk- and Egg-free Diets

Occasionally, an individual is encountered in whom both egg and milk are suspected as reactors. For such patients a combination of the milk-free and egg-free diets will usually work no greater hardship than either diet separately. For diagnostic purposes a combination of the two diets will expedite the search and shorten the period of trial.

MILK-FREE DIET

Milk (fresh, dry, evaporated)
Cheese, cheese crackers, cheese snacks
Cottage cheese
Milk chocolate and other chocolate drinks
Yogurt
Butter
Ice cream and sherbet
Puddings
Custards
Creamed soups and sauces
Cakes, cookies and pastries made with milk

Milk may be found in the following:

Bread
Margarine
Hot dogs, luncheon meats, bologna
Pastries and bakery goods
Pancakes, muffins, sweet rolls, *etc.*
White sauces and gravies
Foods dipped in butter or margarine for frying
Some salad dressings

EGG-FREE DIET

Eggs occur in the following:

Egg dishes in any form
Baked goods: Breads, rolls, muffins may contain egg or be brushed with egg for glazing.
    waffles and griddle cakes
    doughnuts
    cakes, cookies
    pie fillings
    pastries
Baking powder: some brands contain egg
Beverages: at times coffee is cleaned with either egg or egg shell
    Egg may be used in root beer for foaming.
    egg nog and other egg drinks

Candies: Egg is frequently used for glazing, especially jelly beans, chocolate candies.
Desserts: custards, blanc mange, puddings of various types
Meats: Egg is used as a binding agent in many prepared meats, such as sausages, meat loaf, croquettes, lunch meats.
Salad dressings: Many are prepared with egg—French dressing usually contains no egg.
Sauces: especially hollandaise and tartar
Soups: especially with egg noodles

MOLD-FREE DIET

Avoid the following foods:

All cheeses including cottage cheese, sour cream, sour milk and buttermilk.
Beer and wine
Cider and homemade root beer
Pickled and smoked meats and fish including sausages, hot dogs, corned beef, pastrami, and pickled tongue
Vinegar and vinegar-containing foods, such as mayonnaise, salad dressings, catsup, chili and shrimp sauces, pickles, pickled vegetables, relishes, green olives, and sauerkraut
Soured breads (e.g. pumpernickel), fresh rolls, coffee cakes, and other foods made with large amounts of yeast
All dried and candied fruits including raisins, apricots, dates, prunes and figs
Melons, especially cantaloupe
Mushrooms
Soy sauce
Canned tomatoes, unless homemade
Poultry
Fish

CORN-FREE DIET

In addition to fresh, canned or frozen corn, and corn meal, avoid corn oil, corn starch, and corn syrup. These may occur in the following:

Bakery products (other than bread)
Baking mixes
  cake or cookie
  biscuit
  pie
  doughnut
  pancake
Baking powders
Batters for frying
Carbonated beverages
Candy
Chop suey and other Chinese food
Canned fruits
Cereals, hot or cold, containing corn
Corn meal, mush and grits
Corn chips
Alcoholic beverages
  Gin
  beer
  bourbon whisky
Meats
  Any canned with gravy
  Bacon, except Swift's® and DuBuque®
  Ham
  Sausages, cooked
  Bologna
  Hot dogs
Ices, ice cream, ice milk
Jelly and jam
Jello,® gelatin, puddings
Instant tea or coffee
Salad dressing
Margarine
Syrups, Karo,® etc.
Powdered sugar
Gummed envelopes, stamps, stickers, tape
Frozen lemonade
Distilled vinegar
Lambase formula
All soy milks except Mull-Soy® and Neo-mull-Soy®
Powdered soyagen (not liquid)

The Elimination Diets of Rowe

The late Doctor Albert Rowe, Sr., a pioneer advocate of elimination diets, designed a series of diets which bear his name.

The initial Rowe diets excluded wheat,

milk, egg, fish, chocolate, the cabbage group of vegetables, orange, apple, banana, melons, berries, nuts, spices, tea and coffee. Following the original diets reported in 1926, a number of diets have been formulated:

Cereal-free elimination diet
Fruit-free cereal-free elimination diet
Cereal-free elimination diet for infants
Minimal fruit-free elimination diet

Doctor Rowe stressed the importance of glutens as an offending agent in grains and emphasized the necessity for carefully selecting the suppliers of basic food products in order to assure their freedom from undesired components and contaminants which can make for failure in management with elimination diets.

Although the incidence may not be high, there are unquestionably a limited number of patients whose symptoms are controlled by management with one of the various Rowe diets. It is possible that in some of these patients the mechanism is nonimmunologic. However, whatever the mechanism may be, if control of symptoms can be effected, management with the diets is justified. If careful management with environmental control, injection therapy, and simple dietary management has not been successful in control of the patient's symptoms, a trial with a Rowe diet is justified. When carefully administered to protect the general nutrition and health of the patient, the Rowe dietary management entails no risks. In some few cases the reward may be gratifying.

For the physician interested in the Rowe dietary management, Doctor Rowe's text* is recommended.

WHEAT-FREE DIET‡

Wheat and wheat products include white flour, bread flour, cake flour, pastry flour, self-rising flour, whole wheat flour, wheat flour, all purpose flour, cracked wheat flour, graham flour, enriched flour, entire wheat flour, and phosphated durum flour. They also include wheat, wheat germ, bran, farina and semolina as well as malt, bread crumbs and cracker meal.

In order to remain on a wheat-free diet, it is essential not to buy any packaged foods which are not labelled with all their ingredients and when eating away from home, it is essential to always take substitute foods which are known to be free of wheat.

Forbidden Foods

1. Breads, white bread, rolls, biscuits, muffins, whole wheat bread, graham bread, gluten bread, sweet rolls, doughnuts, johnny cake, pancakes, waffles, pretzels, crackers, zwieback, and popovers. Wheat is also in prepared mixes for waffles, biscuits, doughnuts, breads, rolls, pancakes and muffins. It may also be in breads which are listed as being rye bread, corn bread, soybean bread, potato bread, rice bread or rolls or muffins and, therefore, it is not safe to eat any of these unless they are clearly labelled as being free from wheat. For example, wheat-free rye bread is readily available, but ordinary rye bread does contain some wheat, and only reading the label will give confirmation of this. Breaded foods also contain wheat products.

2. Desserts: Doughnuts, dumplings, commercial sherbets, ice creams, ice cream cones, pastry, cakes, cookies, pies, puddings, and custards frequently contain wheat products as do prepared mixes for cakes, ice creams, puddings, cookies and pie crusts. Again it is essential to purchase only those which have the ingredients listed on the label.

3. Cereals: Many cereals contain wheat, and it is essential that the label be read carefully in every case.

4. Salad Dressings: Many salad dressings are thickened with wheat flour.

5. Soups: Many creamed soups contain

---

* *Food Allergy—Its Manifestations and Control and the Elimination Diets—A Compendium*, Springfield, Thomas, 1972.

‡ From Collins-Williams, C: *Pediatric Allergy and Clinical Immunology (As Applied To Atopic Disease)*. Toronto, University of Toronto, 1970.

wheat flour as do vegetable and meat soups, chowders, and bisques.

6. Sweets: Many commercial candies contain wheat products and should not be eaten unless they are clearly labelled with their ingredients.

7. Beverages: Some coffee substitutes and similar beverages contain wheat products as do malted drinks, beer and ale.

8. Sauces and gravies: Many sauces and gravies are thickened with wheat flour. It is not safe to consume these in restaurants, and if they are purchased, they should be accepted only if they are clearly labelled with their ingredients.

9. Meats, poultry, fish, seafood and game: Many fish or meat patties contain wheat products. Wheat products are frequently used for stuffing poultry and game. Swiss steak, chili con carne and croquettes frequently contain wheat.

10. Many vegetables: Vegetables must not be served with sauce thickened with wheat flour.

11. Miscellaneous: Most dumplings, spaghetti, macaroni, mostaccioli, ravioli, soup rings, soup alphabets, vermicelli, and dumplings as well as malt products contain wheat.

WHEAT-EGG-MILK FREE DIET*

Wheat and Wheat Products Include:

Wheat flour, bread flour, cake flour, pastry flour, self-rising flour, whole wheat flour, all purpose flour, cracked wheat flour, graham flour, enriched flour, entire wheat flour, and phosphated durum flour. They also include wheat, wheat germ, bran, farina and semolina as well as malt, bread crumbs and cracker meal.

Egg and Egg Products Include:

Egg dishes such as dishes with baked, creamed, devilled, scalloped, fried, scrambled, hard or soft cooked eggs, egg drinks such as egg nog, egg sauces, egg meringue and egg omelettes.

Milk and Milk Products Include:

Fresh whole milk, skimmed milk, cultured milk, buttermilk, cream, condensed milk, evaporated milk, dried milk, milk solids, casein, lactalbumin, butter, margarine (unless specifically stated on the label to be free of milk solids), curds, whey, malted milk and cheese.

It is very difficult to stay on a wheat-egg-milk free diet unless all food is prepared in the home. Use packaged foods which are labelled with their ingredients and clearly not containing any of the three forbidden foods or their products. When eating away from home, the best approach is to eat only foods such as vegetables and meats without gravies or sauces with fresh fruits as dessert. In order to avoid these three foods, the following must be avoided:

1. Breads: All breads, muffins, biscuits, crackers and rolls except those made at home without the three foods in them or commercial ones which are clearly labelled with all their ingredients. This refers also to breaded foods.

2. Egg dishes: All foods known to include egg including those with egg sauces, egg drinks, meringues, souffles and egg omelettes.

3. Fats and salad dressings: All butters and margarines, all salad dressings except true French dressings unless homemade without the above products.

4. Baking powders: These can be used only if they are clearly labelled as being free of egg or albumen.

5. Sauces and gravies: Tartar and hollandaise, cream and hard sauces, sauces or gravies thickened with wheat flour. These are preferably homemade.

6. Sweets: Most hard candies are free of these products, but no candies should be consumed unless the ingredients are on the label.

---

* From Collins-Williams. C: *Pediatric Allergy and Clinical Immunology (As Applied To Atopic Disease).* Toronto, University of Toronto, 1970.

7. Meats, poultry, fish, seafood and game: One must avoid all foods stuffed with bread or cracker stuffings, meat loaves, croquettes, Swiss steak, dealer prepared or commercially prepared meats, chili con carne. A patient sensitive to milk may be sensitive to beef, so beef should also be avoided. A patient sensitive to egg may also be sensitive to chickens, and these should be avoided, although capon is acceptable.

8. Vegetables: Creamed and scalloped vegetables may contain one or more of these products.

9. Beverages: Coffee substitutes may contain wheat products. One must also avoid coffee cleared with egg white or egg shell; chocolate or cocoa unless made with water from milk-free and egg-free chocolate and cocoa preparations; root beer, malted drinks, beer and ale.

10. Desserts: Cakes, dumplings, fritters, macaroons, meringues, sherbets, pastries, doughnuts, mousses, ice cream cones, ice cream, Bavarian cream, custard, blanc mange, prepared mixes, frostings and puddings or cookies unless homemade without the three forbidden foods. Pies must be avoided unless they are made without the use of any of these products.

11. Cereal: All cereals have to be checked for their labelled ingredients because they frequently contain wheat and/or milk.

12. Soups: Creamed soups contain milk products, also avoid mock turtle soups, bouillons, broths, consommes, thickened soups or soups containing noodles, soup rings or alphabets. Canned and dehydrated soups frequently contain wheat, egg or milk products so that usually only homemade soup is suitable unless a commercial product which is clearly labelled is obtainable.

13. Miscellaneous: Creamed and scalloped foods, fritters, timbales, rarebits, foods cooked in batter, French toast, malt products, dumplings, macaroni, ravioli, mostaccioli, spaghetti, vermicelli, alphabets in soups, and soup rings must all be avoided.

REFERENCES

1. Bowes and Church: *Food Values of Portions Commonly Used,* 11th ed. Philadelphia, Lippincott, 1970.
2. Dixon, Martin, Smith and Wood: *Salicylates.* Boston, Little, 1963, p. 170.
3. Furia, Thomas E. (Ed.): *Handbook of Food Additives.* Cleveland, Chemical Rubber Co., 1968.
4. *Handbuch der Pflanzenanalyse.* Wien, G. Klein, 1932, vol. I, pp. 538–540.
5. Moore-Robinson, M. and Warin, R. P.: Effect of salicylates in urticaria. Br Med J, 4:262, 1967.
6. Rowe, Albert H.: *Elimination Diets and the Patient's Allergies,* 2nd ed. Philadelphia, Lea & Febiger, 1944.
7. Rowe, Albert H.: *Bronchial Asthma—Its Diagnosis and Control.* Springfield, Thomas, 1963.
8. Samter, M. and Beers, Ray J.: Intolerance to aspirin. Ann Intern Med, 68:975, 1968.
9. Shelley, W. B.: Birch pollen and aspirin psoriasis. JAMA 189:985, 1964.
10. Smith, M. and Smith, P.: *The Salicylates.* London, Interscience, 1966, p. 233.
11. Williams, S.: *Nutrition and Diet Therapy.* St. Louis, Mosby, 1969, p. 652.

Allergy Cookbooks

1. Conrad, Marion L.: *Allergy Cooking.* New York, Pyramid, 1968.
2. Emerling, C. G. and Jonckers, E. D.: *The Allergy Cookbook.* New York, Doubleday, 1969.
3. Little, Billie: *Recipes for Allergies.* Grosset & Dunlop, 1971, (Paperback No. 1868).

Chapter 10

ADVERSE REACTIONS TO DRUGS

IN 1958 AT THE SYMPOSIUM ON Sensitivity Reactions to Drugs organized by the Council for International Organization of Medical Sciences, the chairman, Professor M. L. Rosenheim stated, "It is not surprising that the introduction of so many potent and toxic chemicals into clinical use has been accompanied by dangerous, unwanted effects and today, as never before, the clinician must not only know the drugs he uses and their pharmacological activities, but must always be on the lookout for ill effects induced by his therapeutic efforts."

Today, over a decade since that statement was made, the complexity of the problem is greater, due to the ever increasing number of drugs in clinical use and also by the recognition that identical clinical patterns may be caused by nonmedicinal chemicals, such as food additives, cosmetics and industrial chemicals.

Drug reactions are among the most frequently encountered clinical problems, yet the exact incidence is difficult to determine. Among the many factors that contribute to the complexity of the clinical problems and prevent exact evaluation of the reactions are:

(1) Drug reactions may simulate the disease process which is being treated, such as contact dermatitis complicated by dermatitis induced by the medicament.

(2) The interaction with other drugs in programs of multiple therapy and the interaction with nonmedical chemicals, such as food additives.

(3) Nonmedicinal chemicals, such as food additives and industrial chemicals, may be primary factors in the production of clinical patterns which may be confused with drug reactions.

Precise classification of drug reactions presents many difficulties because: (1) the conditions predisposing to the drug reactions show great variation, and (2) the various patterns frequently overlap the different suggested categories.

Classifications of Unwanted Drug Reactions*

1. Overdosage

The toxic effect is in direct relation to the total amount of the drug in the body.

(a) Absolute: resulting from an excess amount administered or as a result of accumulation in the body.

(b) Relative: the dose of the drug is minimal or even decreased, but overdosage results from an abnormality in the patient, such as:

(1.) renal disease which prevents breakdown and excretion of the drug
(2.) sensitization to effects of digitalis in presence of a low serum potassium
(3.) deficiency of an enzyme system

2. Intolerance

The exaggeration of pharmacological effects due to lowering the threshold of the patient, as for example, cinchonism with very small doses of quinine. Intolerance may result from extremes of biological variation either in absorption, metabolism, excretion or in susceptibility to the drug.

---
* Recommended by the Council for International Organization of Medical Sciences, 1958.

3. Side Effects

This term applies to the undesirable but unavoidable pharmacological effects of a drug that accompany the desired therapeutic effect.

(a) The hypnotic effect of certain antihistamines

(b) The histamine releasing action of some drugs, such as atropine, codeine, morphine, amphetamines and like salts. The histamine releasing drugs may cause prickling, itching, urticaria, vasodilatation, fall in blood pressure, headache and bradypnea. Bradypnea develops into expiratory dyspnea only in asthmatic patients. In most cases an increase in expiratory effort is felt with a definite feeling of retrosternal oppression. Bronchial or tracheal rales occur.

(c) Blood dyscrasias including megaloblastic anemia induced by:

    (1.) Mephenytoin (Mesantoin®)
    (2.) hydantoins diphenylhydantoin (Dilantin®) diphenylhydantoin sodium (Dilantin sodium®)
    (3.) barbiturates
    (4.) phenothiazines (Phenergan,® chlorpromazine)

(d) Jaundice with phenothiazines

4. Secondary Effects

These effects are not related to the pharmacological action of the drug but are caused by conditions produced by the drug, such as:

(a) Moniliasis or evidence of vitamin deficiency in patients given oral antibiotics

(b) Interference with an enzyme system

5. Idiosyncracy

True idiosyncracy implies an inherent qualitatively abnormal action to a drug, as for example, the hemolytic anemia due to an enzyme deficiency observed in American Negroes given primaquine.

6. Allergic Reactions

In this class the manifestations are caused by immunologic reactions.

The Immunology of Drug Allergy

Drugs are low molecular weight chemicals which serve as haptens. In order to become immunogenic, i.e. able to induce sensitivity, they must combine with a protein carrier.

The factors which influence the conjugation of a drug or chemical with a protein carrier are:

(1) The genetic predisposition to hypersensitivity. The ability to become sensitive varies from individual to individual. The ability to become sensitive to a particular drug also varies with individuals.

(2) Combining site: A suitable *combining site* must be present in both the drug and its protein carrier. The union with the carrier must be irreversible (covalent binding). A weak union between the hapten and its carrier is not conducive to immunogenicity.

(3) Metabolic breakdown: A drug or chemical may not have a suitable combining site that is naturally available. Through metabolic breakdown a suitable combining site may become available which permits the metabolites to unite with a protein carrier to become immunogenic. Any condition that modifies the metabolism of the drug will influence its capacity to sensitize, including:

(a) Renal deficiency
(b) Gastrointestinal disorders
(c) The disease for which the drug is administered.

There are additional factors which influence the development of sensitivity in allergy, such as:

(1) Dosage of the drug. A large dose, or small repeated doses predispose to sensitization.

(2) The route of administration can influence the incidence of hypersensitivity as well as the type of the allergic response. Oil sol-

uble chemicals induce contact dermatitis more readily. Depot preparations of drugs are more likely to induce sensitivity, which is usually more persistent in its manifestations.

(3) The interaction with other drugs administered simultaneously can be a determining factor in the induction of sensitization.

(4) Cross reactivity between drugs is an important factor. The previous administration of one drug may sensitize so that the initial dose of a cross reacting drug will cause symptoms.

(5) Sensitivity may be due to a contaminant or an excipient rather than the basic chemicals.

The Mechanism of Allergic Drug Reactions

Following the union of a hapten with its carrier, changes in the configuration of the molecule are induced. The alterations in molecular structure can uncover a buried chemical grouping which can serve as an antigenic determinant or it may cause the masking of a potential antigenic determinant (see Figures 1-2 and 1-3). As a result of the rearrangement of the protein molecule (carrier) and the drug molecule (hapten) a variety of new antigenic determinants capable of evoking different types of antibodies becomes available. The antigen formed by the conjugation of the drug with a carrier can evoke three types of antibodies:

(1) antibodies to the altered protein carrier
(2) antibodies to the altered drug (hapten)
(3) antibodies to the conjugated product.

None of these antibodies is able to recognize (specificity) either the undenatured carrier or the undenatured hapten. This failure of recognition of the undenatured molecule makes identification of the offending drug impossible with present day techniques.

The various antibodies produced in drug allergy are capable of initiating immunologic responses which can induce any of the four types of allergic tissue reaction, the immediate or anaphylactic, the intermediate or Arthus, the delayed and the cytolytic and cytotoxic.

It is conceivable that a single conjugated antigen may bear different antigenic determinants capable of evoking different types of antibodies. It is possible that a single antigen can induce more than one type of allergic reaction.

This broad spectrum of immunologic response results in many clinical patterns. In other words, drug sensitivity can produce every possible clinical pattern of allergic disease.

Clinical Manifestations

Skin Manifestations

Pruritus may occur as an isolated manifestation but more frequently it precedes the development of other manifestations of the drug reactions.

The pruritus is usually generalized but at times may be localized about the anus, in the axillae, about the nipples and the intercrural regions. Penicillin and the barbiturates are common causes of pruritus, but almost any drug capable of inducing an allergic reaction may cause pruritus. Peri-anal and genital pruritus occur frequently with the barbiturates.

Urticaria and Angio-Edema: Urticaria is the most common manifestation of drug reactions followed very closely by angio-edema. The whealing lesion of urticaria may involve any part of the body but occurs more frequently over pressure points where clothes fit tightly, or over muscle groups that have been exercised. The lesions may appear in clusters of small wheals or as large, pale confluent patches. Itching is usually intense.

Angio-edema represents the involvement by edema of loose tissue structures seen most commonly about the eyes, the lips, the scrotum and the vulva.

Any drug may cause urticaria and less frequently angio-edema, but penicillin and aspirin are the most common causes.

Swelling of the small joints of the hands and feet occurs frequently with penicillin. In most cases the urticaria and angio-edema induced by penicillin will clear within a few days after stopping the drug, but following the injection of depot penicillin, the lesions may persist for weeks or even months until all the penicillin at the site of the injection has been absorbed and eliminated. In some patients a penicillin reaction may be protracted by the ingestion of penicillin contaminants in foods, such as milk, cheese or other milk derivatives. In patients who are sensitive to antibiotics, penicillin or tetracycline, the antibiotics used for the preservation of fish and poultry may serve to keep the clinical pattern active. Although cross reactivity between penicillin and tetracycline is not a common observation, such cross reactivity has been reported.

The urticaria and angio-edema induced by an aspirin reaction may occur as an isolated observation, but more frequently it is accompanied by other complaints such as nasal polyps or asthma. (See discussion in this chapter of Aspirin Sensitivity)

Maculo-Papular Eruptions: The isolated maculo-papular lesions may occur over any part of the body but are observed most frequently over pressure areas as on the buttocks. Initially, the lesion is a pruritic, slightly reddened macule which soon becomes indurated to form a papule. With chronicity the lesion increases in size, becomes lichenified, scale covered and may show signs of localized hemorrhage. The isolated lesion is observed rather frequently following the prolonged administration of small doses of barbiturates as occur in compounded preparations.

Fixed Drug Reaction: In this reaction the eruption occurs at the identical site with each administration of the drug. The lesions which may be single or multiple are characterized by pruritic, red, edematous papular or even bullous lesions, which upon healing leave a residual pigmentation. Involvement of buccal and genital mucus membranes may accompany the cutaneous lesions.

The drugs most commonly implicated are phenolphthalein, barbiturates and sulfonamides. The mechanism involved in the fixed drug reaction is not known.

Generalized Involvement

In addition to urticaria, the body may manifest a generalized involvement characterized by:

(1) Diffuse erythema as observed with phenolphthalein.

(2) A morbilliform pattern as observed with barbiturates and sulfonamides.

(3) A maculo-papular eruption as observed most commonly with penicillin, streptomycin, the barbiturates and the sulfonamides.

When accompanied by fever, the generalized eruptions may resemble the exanthemata.

Purpuric Lesions: Purpuric lesions may be primary or secondary. The primary

Table 10-I: AGENTS CAPABLE OF CAUSING FIXED ERUPTIONS*

Acetanilid	Digitalis	Penicillin
Aconite	Disulfiram	Pentaerythritol
Acriflavin	Emetine	tetranitrate
Aminopyrine	hydrochloride	Phenacetin
Amphetamine	Eosin	Phenolphthalein
Anthralin	Ephedrine	Phenothiazines
Antihistaminic	Ergot	Potassium chlorate
drugs	Formaldehyde	Quinacrine
Antimony	solution	hydrochloride
compounds	Hydantoins	Quinine
Antipyrine	Hydralazine	Rauwolfia alkaloids
Arsenicals	Iodine	Reserpine
Barbiturates	Ipecac	Saccharin
Belladonna	Karaya gum	Salicylates
alkaloids	Legumes	Streptomycin
Chloral hydrate	Meprobamate	Sulfonamides
Chloroquine	Mercurials	Tartar emetic
phosphate	Methenamine	Tetracyclines
Cinchophen	Morphine	Tetriodofluorescein
Codeine	Opium	Thiram
Copaiba	Oxyphenisatin	Vermouth
Diethylstilbestrol	acetate	Wormseed

* Reproduced from Derbes, V. J.: The fixed eruption. *JAMA, 190*: 765–766, 1964.

hemolysis at drug concentrations that are well within therapeutic levels.

Renal insufficiency may result in high drug concentrations which can lead to hemolytic anemia.

Anaphylaxis

Life threatening constitutional reactions to drugs are not rare. These are associated with a rapid onset with all the signs and symptoms characteristic of anaphylactic shock (see discussion of anaphylaxis in Chapter 1) induced by protein antigens.

In some mild forms constitutional reactions may be limited to malaise and vertigo, while in some cases a generalized urticaria or marked angio-edema are the only presenting complaints.

It is not always possible to determine whether the reaction induced is on an immunologic basis. Nonimmunologic reactions can produce identical patterns.

Penicillin is the most common cause of anaphylactic drug reactions, but other drugs to consider include streptomycin, bromsulphalein, radiopaque iodides, sodium dehydrocholate, organic mercurials, and other heavy metals, liver extract, vitamin B_{12}, iron dextran, anesthetic agents, local and parenteral.

Aspirin causes constitutional reactions and even death, but an immunologic basis for the reaction has not been demonstrated.

Serum Sickness Syndrome

All the manifestations of serum sickness can be induced by low molecular chemicals used as drugs. The mechanism involved is apparently identical with that observed with protein antigens, except that drug induced serum type reactions, because of the multiplicity of antibody types produced, are frequently complicated by manifestations of delayed hypersensitivity and hematological involvement of the cytotoxic type of reactivity (see Chapter 1).

Following an incubation period of five to fourteen days, the initial signs are usually those of immediate hypersensitivity, such as pruritus, urticaria, angio-edema and asthma. In some cases the initial cutaneous lesions are petechiae secondary to vascular damage caused by the Arthus type reaction. At times, as observed with sulfonamides and barbiturates, delayed hypersensitivity may be operating as evidenced by a maculopapular eruption or erythema-multiforme type of lesions. When cytotoxic reactions occur, the skin lesions may be purpuric.

Fever, lymphadenopathy, arthralgia and evidence of organic involvement such as proteinuria are manifestations of the Arthus reaction component.

Vasculitis

Vasculitis, which is an important part of the pathology induced by serum sickness type of reaction, plays an important role in the symptomatology of drug reactions. The intensity of the reaction and the degree of vessel involvement which determine the symptoms are governed by the dosage of the drug, its antigenicity and the susceptibility of the patient. The pathology is that typical for the Arthus type reaction; involvement of small vessels and capillaries by inflammation of vessel walls, rupture, leading to hemorrhage and tissue necrosis. In severe reactions the involvement of vessels may be diffuse with pathology in many organs including the skin, mucus membranes, kidneys, heart, lungs, gastrointestinal tract and muscles.

In some cases, such as with depot penicillin, the development of the vascular lesions may be insidious, gradual and smoldering with no symptoms until considerable organ and tissue damage have developed.

In many cases the vascular damage may be very mild with no obvious symptoms. In the mild cases, after the drug has been stopped, there is usually rapid restoration.

The drugs most commonly involved in vasculitis are penicillin, the sulfonamides, thiouracil and the phenothiazines.

Exfoliative Dermatitis

Exfoliative dermatitis, the most violent of the cutaneous drug reactions, is characterized by widespread persistent erythema and edema with continuous exfoliation. The widespread skin involvement predisposes to heat loss, protein loss through exfoliation and exudation which, added to the increased circulatory burden from continuous vasodilatation may prove fatal, especially in elderly and debilitated patients.

The onset may be sudden with chills and fever, or develop as an extension of a pre-existing eruption when the drug is not discontinued. The most important drugs involved in exfoliative dermatitis include the heavy metals, barbiturates and the sulfonamides. Penicillin rarely causes exfoliative dermatitis.

Aspirin Sensitivity

The considerable consumption of aspirin, which in America is estimated to be thirteen million pounds annually, accounts for the position of this medicament as one of the most frequent causes of adverse drug reactions. The free use of aspirin in prescription drugs and the large traffic in over-the-counter preparations containing aspirin, undoubtedly account for a number of unrecognized reactions to the drug, which makes it difficult to accurately determine the incidence of aspirin sensitivity.

The following features of aspirin sensitivity are emphasized by those who have studied the problem.

1. Intolerance to aspirin is reasonably common.
2. Evidence for an immunologic mechanism, i.e. allergic, is inconclusive. Atopy was observed in less than 3 per cent of the aspirin-sensitive group as compared with the 20 per cent in a random population.
3. The clinical triad of nasal polyposis, bronchial asthma, and exquisite aspirin sensitivity is a definite disease entity.
4. Onset of symptoms occurs during the second and third decade of life with intermittent, profuse, watery rhinorrhea followed by perennial nasal blockage with no intermission. As symptoms become more persistent, their response to vasoconstrictors decreases.
5. Nasal and paranasal polyps develop in approximately 50 per cent of patients. Polyps tend to be bilateral, respond poorly to therapy, recur following surgery. Polypectomy commonly precipitates bronchial asthma.
6. In the early stages of the disease the bronchial asthma is readily reversible with bronchodilators and is controlled with very small doses of corticosteroids. (*Note:* We have observed control of asthma in aspirin-sensitive patients on a daily dose of 1 mg of triamcinolone.)
7. Nasal polyposis and bronchial asthma continue whether or not aspirin is ingested. In Samter's series no patient ceased to form polyps once the presence of polyps had been established.
8. Severity of the reactions is not related to the frequency with which patients had taken aspirin.
9. If the taking of aspirin is interrupted for long periods, subsequent administration of aspirin may cause more severe reactions.
10. Aspirin-sensitive patients suffer from

Table 10-III: REACTIONS TO ASPIRIN

Cutaneous
  Angio-edema
  Purpura
Gastrointestinal
  "Dyspepsia"
  Occult bleeding
  Massive GI hemorrhage
  Activation of peptic ulcers
Hematological
  Anemia, secondary to occult GI bleeding
  Leucopenia
  Thrombocytopenia
  Agranulocytosis, with bone marrow depression
  Pancytopenia
  Prolonged bleeding time
Liver
  Fatty cleavages
Kidneys
  Nephropathies with prolonged administration
  Syncope and fatal reactions
Respiratory
  Rhinorrhea
  Sinusitis
  Nasal polyps
  Asthma

either respiratory symptoms or urticaria or both.

11. Associated sensitivities in 182 aspirin-sensitive patients:

> Foods, alcohol, tartrazine (FD&C #5 yellow)
> Inhalant allergens
> Perfumes and odors
> Drugs
>> penicillin, morphine, morphine derivatives, codeine, antipyrine and aminopyrine, caine compounds, sulfonamides, isoniazid.

12. Intolerance to aspirin is not intolerance to salicylates.

The mechanism involved in aspirin sensitivity is not known. Samter attributes the adverse reactions to aspirin to an unusual responsiveness of the bradykinin receptors of the nasal and bronchial mucus membranes.

The studies by Farr on aspirin sensitivity indicate that in sensitive individuals the ingestion of aspirin results in acetylation of albumin, neuroreceptors, neuroreceptor synthesizers, glomerular basement membranes, bradykinin receptors and perhaps other body structures that lead to nonimmunologic responses.

Studies by British investigators on the pharmacology of aspirin and aspirin-like* drugs attribute their clinical effects to the inhibition of the synthesis of prostaglandins which are a group of biologically active substances that occur in many tissues of the body. Aspirin and aspirin-like drugs block the production of prostaglandins in several systems, presumably by interfering with an enzyme or enzymes involved in the synthesis of prostaglandins from arachidonic acid.

The interpretation of the behavior of aspirin in adverse reactions must await a better understanding in many areas, such as the possible immunologic factors, the behavior of the neuroreceptors and chemoreceptors and the role of known and unknown mediators.

In the absence of more precise information, the diagnosis and management of these reactions must depend upon (1) an awareness of the diverse patterns induced by the adverse reactions, and (2) the history of the patient.

The prime prerequisite in diagnosis is the awareness that aspirin can produce a wide variety of untoward reactions, particularly pruritus, rhinitis, urticaria, angio-edema and asthma. Gastrointestinal bleeding of various degrees is also a common complication. With any of these diseases as presenting complaint, in the absence of a demonstrable etiologic agent, the possibility of aspirin sensitivity should be considered. A history of the ingestion of aspirin for long periods preceding the onset of symptoms is strong suppporting evidence for aspirin sensitivity rather than excluding such a diagnosis. This feature of the patient's history supports Farr's contention that "the explosive symptom-complex of full blown aspirin intolerance is an end-stage of slowly accumulative acetylating effect, which proceeds over the years and is hastened by repeated and often indiscriminate use of small doses of aspirin." Elimination of the drug is not always followed by immediate improvement of the symptoms.

When the symptoms fail to clear following the discontinuance of aspirin, a good response may be observed upon elimination from the diet of food chemicals including:

(1) The foods containing natural salicylates (see salicylate-free diet, Chapter 9).

(2) All coloring and flavorings, both natural and synthetic (see food additives, Chapter 8).

Allergic Reaction to Antibiotics

Antibiotics have been one of the great contributions of the twentieth century in the field of antimicrobial therapy. Many com-

---

* An aspirin-like drug is any compound that combines antipyretic, anti-inflammatory and analgesic effects. The compounds are not chemically related except that all are organic acids. Included as aspirin-like drugs are: salicylates and congeners, phenacetin and congeners, antipyrines and congeners, and indomethacin.

plex clinical problems have been resolved by the antibiotics, but they have also created many new ones. The hopes of developing a perfect antibiotic, free of deleterious side effects has spurred considerable research in both natural and synthetic antibiotic chemicals. Since the effectiveness of all antibiotics is dependent upon their action as a protoplasmic poison, it is questionable whether such an ideal product will ever be developed.

The antibiotics presently in clinical use vary greatly in structure, mechanism of action, antimicrobial spectrum and inherent toxicity. However, with the recognition of the factors that predispose to unwanted drug reactions of any type, the various antibiotics can be prescribed effectively and with a reasonable degree of safety.

It is beyond the scope of this book to consider the toxicology of the various antibiotics. Even a detailed consideration of the allergic reactions of each of the many available antibiotics is beyond a simple text.

To assist the reader in obtaining information when unusual situations arise, several references with more detailed information are indicated in the bibliography.

PENICILLIN

Penicillin is a generic term applied to the group of antibiotics comprising all drugs derived either from 6-aminopenicillanic acid or from 7-aminocephalosporanic acid. (Fig. 10-1)

Since biochemists have learned to synthesize the penicillin nucleus, thousands of compounds have been produced, resulting in four families of penicillins,* as follows:

---

* For detailed information on the pharmacology and the variety of products available the reader is referred to Goodman, Louis and Gilman, Alfred (Eds.): *Pharmacological Basis of Therapeutics*, 4th ed. New York, MacMillan, 1970 and *AMA Drug Evaluations*, 1st ed. 1971.

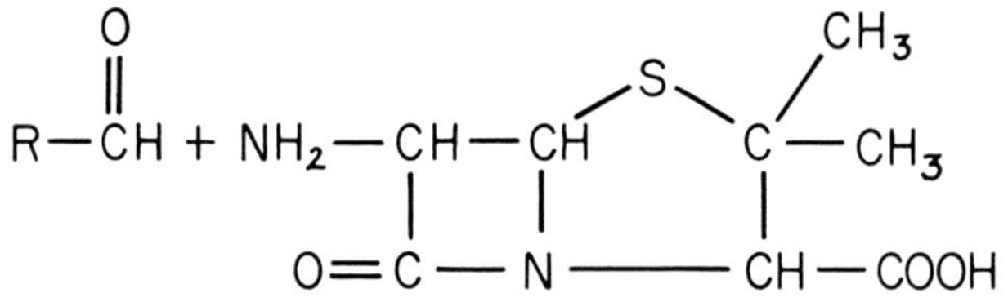

R + 6-AMINOPENICILLANIC ACID

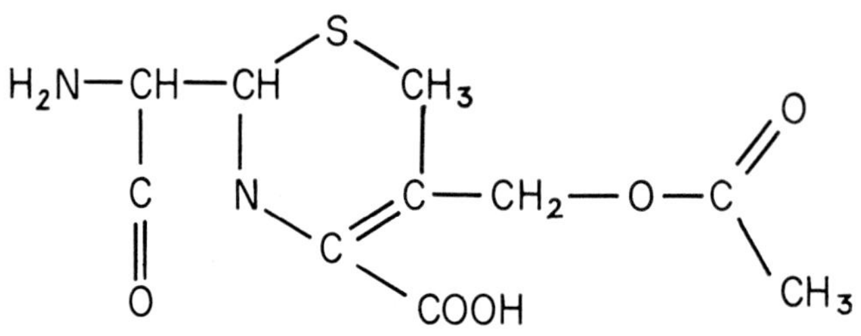

7-AMINOCEPHALOSPORANIC ACID

Figure 10-1

(1) The benzyl group which includes penicillin G and ampicillin. Allergic reactions to this group are discussed below.

(2) The phenoxyl group which includes potassium penicillin V, Compocillin-VK,® Pen-Vee K® and V-Cillin.®

This group of congeners of penicillin G has the same antibacterial spectrum as benzyl penicillin (pencillin G), but since these drugs are more stable in acidic media, they can be administered orally and are well absorbed from the gastrointestinal tract.

Reactions occur with oral preparations but less frequently than with parenteral products.

(3) The isoxazolyl group includes cloxacillin sodium monohydrate (Tegopen®) and discloxacillin sodium monohydrate (Dynapen,® Pathocil,® Veracillin®).

This group has shown remarkably few untoward reactions within the therapeutic range (20 to 80 mg per kg per day). These penicillins seem devoid of direct toxicity, except for mild gastrointestinal disturbances. The main reactions to this group have been allergic in nature, which are similar to those observed with other forms of penicillin.

(4) The methicillin group includes methicillin (dimocillin RT, Staphcillin®) and nafcillin (Unipen®).

Methicillin is administered parenterally but usually in much larger doses (50 to 200 mg per kg per day) than other forms of penicillin. For this reason, it is more toxic for patients than benzyl penicillin. Allergic reactions of almost every type are quite common following the administration of methicillin.

Nafcillin is available for either oral or parenteral use. The usual allergic responses are observed with this drug. Bone marrow toxicity with nafcillin may be a problem.

THE CEPHALOSPORINS: The cephalosporins are derivatives of cephalosporium A which has as its nucleus aminocephalosporanic acid. Side chain manipulation has produced cephalothin (Keflin®) and cephalordine. These drugs have a low acute and subacute toxicity, but the allergic reactions are similar to those observed with derivatives of 6-aminopenicillanic acid.

All penicillins should be regarded as immunologically cross reactive. Anaphylactic reactions have been reported in patients known to be penicillin sensitive following the administration of cephalosporin derivatives. These drugs should not be used in penicillin-sensitive patients. There is no safe substitute for penicillin.

Immunological Considerations in Penicillin Reactions

Like all other drugs, penicillin is a low molecular weight chemical which behaves as a hapten. Since penicillin is a hapten, it must combine with a protein carrier to achieve immunogenicity. In its pure form penicillin is not antigenic because it is lacking in available chemical groupings which can serve as combining sites for union with a protein carrier. Following entrance of penicillin into the body, and also at room temperature with an altered pH, the penicillin molecule is rearranged to form an isomer, benzyl penicillanic acid, which offers two combining sites for irreversible union with a protein carrier and accordingly can become immunogenic. The studies of Bernard Levine have demonstrated that in addition to benzyl penicillanic acid, a variety of haptenic groups are formed. Some of the groups have been identified but others have not been identified. Any or all of the haptenic groups formed are associated with penicillin sensitivity.

Antibodies to Penicillin

The union of the various haptenic groups on the penicillin molecule with the body proteins make available, on the conjugated antigen, a variety of antigenic determinants which can evoke a heterogeneous population of antibodies. Any type of allergic response can be induced. The function of the antibody will determine the type of allergic reaction produced. If the antibody response is homogeneous, only a single type of allergic reaction will occur, as, for example, the immediate type of reactivity which will cause urticaria, angio-edema and asthma. If the antibody response is heterogeneous, a mixture of allergic reactions will result as observed in the serum disease type of reaction. In some cases the newly formed antigen will sensitize T cells, resulting in the delayed type of hypersensitivity.

Identification of the specific function of the antibodies involved in penicillin hypersensitivity is complicated by the inability to demonstrate

(1) the protein carrier involved,
(2) the structural alterations induced in both the carrier and the hapten following their conjugation.

The isolated hapten is ineffective in demonstrating or identifying the antibody. In the absence of adequate information concerning the structure of the antigen involved in penicillin sensitivity, the correlation of antibodies with function and with chemical reactions has not been successful. For example, the demonstration of skin sensitizing antibodies does not necessarily indicate susceptibility to adverse clinical responsiveness. For identical reasons, attempts to design reliable clinical and laboratory test procedures to predict penicillin sensitivity have failed.

PENICILLIN CONTAMINANTS: Clinical reactions may be induced by contaminants derived from (1) the culture media used when preparing penicillin by microbiological techniques, and (2) from the penicillanic mold used for the extraction of penicillin.

Preparations available from reliable pharmaceutical manufacturers usually present no such problems.

Clinical Patterns of Penicillin Hypersensitivity

(1) The immediate type of hypersensitivity due to IgE antibodies leads to the liberation of histamine and SRS-A. The onset of symptoms may range from seconds to twenty minutes. Symptoms of this type include:

anaphylactic shock
urticaria
angio-edema
rhinitis
asthma

(2) The serum sickness type of reaction involves both IgE and precipitating form of IgG, resulting in both immediate type symptoms and intermediate or Arthus type symptoms. In previously sensitized patients, the onset may be immediate to forty-eight hours. In cases of initial sensitization symptoms usually appear after five to ten days.

The immediate symptoms are pruritus, urticaria, angio-edema, rhinitis and asthma. These symptoms are usually followed by polyadenopathy, arthralgia and petechiae. When vasculitis develops, organ involvement such as nephritis is evident. Symptoms may be accompanied by fever which is not a constant complaint.

(3) The delayed type of hypersensitivity is manifested after twenty-four hours in previously sensitized patients but after five to eight days in patients experiencing an initial exposure. The usual symptoms are those of contact dermatitis and a maculopapular eruption. Some patients may have a cutaneous reaction resembling erythema multiforme.

(4) In cytolytic or cytotoxic reactions the penicillin serves as a hapten to conjugate with cellular proteins. The event is usually delayed for a few days, but in some cases symptoms may become evident within several minutes to several hours. Symptoms are those induced by damage to blood elements, as purpura secondary to thrombocytopenia, anemia due to red cell damage, and general debilitating symptoms secondary to agranulocytosis.

Although most patients present a clinical pattern related to one of the four types of allergic response, it is not unusual to observe a mixture of reactions representing various combinations of the different types of allergic reactions.

Since penicillin can induce any type of allergic reaction, it can serve as a prototype for studying the adverse reactions of other low molecular chemicals used as drugs.

Diagnosis of Penicillin Sensitivity

Tests

Screening tests to determine a patient's sensitivity include:

(1) Skin tests with a variety of penicillin derivatives are not only unreliable but carry the additional hazards of:
  (a) inducing an anaphylactic reaction, and
  (b) sensitizing the patient
(2) The basophil degranulation test
(3) Various immunologic and electrophoretic techniques.

There is lack of agreement regarding the clinical usefulness of any of the screening tests in predicting hypersensitivity to penicillin. A positive test should exclude therapy with penicillin, but a positive test does not always correlate with adverse clinical responses.

A careful and thorough history is the only reliable diagnostic procedure, but even with careful questioning and exclusion of previous outward clinical responses, there is no absolute guarantee that a severe or even fatal reaction may not take place.

If the patient's history fails to disclose treatment with penicillin but the possibility of a penicillin reaction is suspected because of unexplained pruritus, urticaria, angioedema, asthma or involvement of the small joints of the hands and feet, other possible sources of subtle exposure to penicillin must be investigated. These are listed below.

(1) Large quantities of penicillin are used by dairy farmers in the treatment of bovine mastitis, resulting in a significant concentration of penicillin in milk. Ingestion of penicillin-containing milk and milk products, such as cheese, ice cream, *etc.* has produced allergic reactions in sensitive individuals. It is possible that penicillin ingested with such contaminated foods can induce sensitivity in individuals.

(2) Penicillin is used as a bacteriostatic in biological products such as polio vaccine.

(3) Drugs manufactured and packaged under conditions that do not completely control penicillin contamination can be an inadvertent source of penicillin.

(4) Contamination of syringes occurs very easily. It is almost impossible to destroy the antigenic properties of penicillin by either boiling or steam sterilization. Disposable syringes are recommended for the administration of penicillin.

(5) Contact in environments of employment, such as nurses, dental personnel and pharmaceutical personnel.

(6) Inhalation of penicillin-contaminated air in pharmaceutical laboratories, hospitals, *etc.*

Desensitization Procedure for Specific Situations

The administration of penicillin to a patient with a history of sensitivity to the drug is occasionally indicated as a life saving procedure. For these patients the desensitization procedure outlined in Table 10-IV is recommended.

Depot Penicillin

The repository forms of penicillin, such as procaine penicillin or penicillin in oil provide a reservoir for a continuous and sustained release of antigen. This can lead to:

(1) A higher incidence of reactivity
(2) A higher degree of sensitivity, and
(3) A persistence of the reaction for long periods.

Following the administration of depot penicillins, particularly those in oil, symptoms may persist for weeks or even months.

In cases with the serum sickness type of reaction following depot penicillin therapy,

Table 10-IV: METHOD FOR CAUTIOUS ADMINISTRATION OF INCREASING DOSES OF PENICILLIN*

A. *Preparation of solutions, using aqueous crystalline penicillin G*
  Dilute 20,000,000-unit vial to 20 ml = 1,000,000 units/ml (Solution 1)
  Dilute 1 ml of Solution 1 to 10 ml = 100,000 units/ml (Solution 2)
  Dilute 1 ml of Solution 2 to 10 ml = 10,000 units/ml (Solution 3)
  Dilute 1 ml of Solution 3 to 10 ml = 1,000 units/ml (Solution 4)
  Dilute 1 ml of Solution 4 to 10 ml = 100 units/ml (Solution 5)

B. *Application*
  1. Administer scratch test (15 minutes) with 1 drop of Solution 3 on forearm†
  2. Administer intradermal test (15 minutes) with 0.02 ml of Solution 5.
  3. Proceed with penicillin administration as outlined in C. Record blood pressure, pulse, and respiration at frequent (5 minute) intervals and have antianaphylactic equipment‡ always at hand.
  4. Immediately begin continuous therapy with intravenous penicillin G.

C. *Details of penicillin administration for Step B-3*
Penicillin Solution

Solution Number	Concentration (units/ml)	Injected each 15 minutes (ml)	Injected Subcutaneously (units)
5	100	0.05	5
		0.1	10
		0.2	20
		0.4	40
		0.8	80
4	1,000	0.15	150
		0.3	300
		0.6	600
		1.0	1,000
3	10,000	0.2	2,000
		0.4	4,000
		0.8	8,000
2	100,000	0.15	15,000
		0.3	30,000
		0.6	60,000
		1.0	100,000
1	1,000,000	0.2	200,000
		0.4	400,000
		0.8	800,000

* Reproduced with permission from Green, G. R., Peters, G. A. and Geraci, J. E.: Treatment of bacterial endocarditis in patients with penicillin hypersensitivity. *Ann Intern Med*, 67: 239, 1967.
† Preliminary skin tests with penicilloyl-polylysine (Cilligen,® (Sigma Chemical Co., St. Louis) may be helpful, but this agent is available only on an investigational basis at present.
‡ Syringes, hypodermic needles, alcohol, sponges, and drugs for injections: epinephrine (aqueous, 1:1,000) and ephedrine; intramuscular chlorpheniramine (Chlor-Trimeton®); metaraminol or phenylephrine; levarterenol (Levophed®); sodium bicarbonate; aminophylline; corticosteroids.
Equipment for intravenous infusion and tracheostomy, including tourniquet, venous cutdown equipment, and 5 per cent glucose: sphygmomanometer and stethoscope; oxygen tank, with mask or intranasal tube, or bag and valve equipment; endotracheal tube.

the persistent supply of antigen can lead to serious disseminated vasculitis.

The incidence of penicillin reactions has been reported highest with penicillin in oil (2.5%) followed by procaine penicillin (0.7%).

Ampicillin

With ampicillin sensitivity, cutaneous involvement is the most frequent manifestation.

The rash usually occurs after the drug has been administered for at least ten days. During the course of administration of the drug, the eruption does not appear, but usually develops about four to five days following withdrawal of the drug.

The eruption is maculo-papular in character which, when occurring after discontinuance of therapy, may be misdiagnosed as measles. The maculo-papular nature of the rash suggests the involvement with the delayed type of hypersensitivity.

Anaphylactic shock induced by oral ampicillin has been reported.

The Tetracylines

Chlortetracycline (Aureomycin®)
Tetracycline
Oxytetracycline (Terramycin®)
Dimethylchlortetracycline (Declomycin®)

Extensive clinical experience with tetracyclines has shown them to have a low but significant level of toxicity.

Hypersensitivity reactions to the tetracyclines are quite uncommon during the clinical use of these drugs. Anaphylactic reactions following either oral or systemic administration of tetracyclines have been reported in less than twenty cases (until 1966), some of which were fatal. The highest incidence has been associated with orally administered dimethylchlortetracycline.

Cutaneous allergic reactions with the tetracyclines are exceptionally rare.

Most adverse effects are related to toxic actions rather than hypersensitivity. The most common unfavorable reaction is gastrointestinal irritation characterized by anorexia, nausea, vomiting, flatulence, pyrosis, epigastric distress and diarrhea. These symtoms are dose related, occurring in patients receiving 2.0 grams or more of one of the tetracyclines.

The main danger with the tetracyclines is the overgrowth of resistant micro-organisms following suppression of normal bacterial flora in the gastrointestinal, respiratory and genito-urinary tracts. This manifestation is a biological disturbance and not an allergic reaction.

This disturbance of the enteric bacterial balance by the tetracyclines is held responsible for stomatitis, glossitis, black hairy tongue, vesiculo-papular lesions of the oropharynx, sore throat, dysphagia, hoarseness, and inflammatory lesions of the vulva, vagina and peri-anal regions (candidiasis).

The Macrolides*

The macrolide antibiotics comprise:
erythromycin (Ilosone,® Ilotycin,® Erythrocin®)
oleandomycin (Matromycin®)
triacetyloleandomycin (Cyclamycin,® Tao®).

All the macrolide antibiotics have a relatively low order of toxicity except for triacetyloleandomycin.

Hypersensitivity reactions occur but are extremely rare. Maculo-papular eruptions, urticaria and angio-edema have been reported.

Streptomycin

The allergic reactions observed with streptomycin are similar to the patterns induced by the penicillins.

Blood dyscrasias, which are a frequently encountered untoward reaction to streptomycin, are probably on an allergic basis, although a toxic dose-related etiology cannot be ruled out.

---

* The macrolide antibiotics are so named because they contain a many-membered lactone ring to which are attached one or more deoxy sugars. (Goodman and Gilman, *The Pharmacological Basis of Therapeutics* p. 1275).

Labyrinthine damage, a very common complication of therapy with streptomycin, is a toxic reaction.

The Sulfonamides

With the development of the antibiotic drugs the indications for prescribing the sulfonamides have been reduced appreciably. In addition, the increased resistance of organisms to this class of drugs has limited their clinical usefulness.

Allergic reactions to the sulfonamides are common. The great capacity of the drug to serve as a hapten predisposes to a broad spectrum of responses including:

Pruritus: Skin eruptions of various morphology, such as scarlatinal, morbilliform, urticarial, erysipeloid, pemphigoid, erythema nodosum, purpuric, petechial and, in extreme cases, exfoliative dermatitis.

Vasculitis with organ damage is not uncommon.

A *serum disease type reaction* with polyadenopathy, urticaria and polyarthralgia is not rare with the sulfonamides.

In addition to the various allergic manifestations, dose-related toxic complications are not unusual.

Diagnosis of Drug Sensitivity

The various tests* designed to predict and diagnose drug hypersensitivity have not

---

* Skin tests include scratch, prick and intradermal; serological tests include hemagglutination, immunodiffusion and immunoelectrophoresis; histamine release; lymphocyte transformations; provocative tests.

All the tests listed are based upon immunologic reactions between antigens with their specific antibodies. Drugs are haptens which must conjugate with a protein carrier to become antigenic. The process of conjugation induces alterations in the steric structure of both the protein carrier and the hapten. As a result the antibodies induced by these altered structures are not recognized by the natural protein or the natural chemical which serves as a hapten. Therefore, the natural or unconjugated chemical or drug cannot induce a demonstrable Ag-Ab interaction. Actually, the hapten can prevent a reaction. Since the altered protein or the conjugated protein and chemical cannot be identified. the attempts to design tests demonstrating chemical sensitivity to drugs has not been successful.

proved to be dependable. Fortunately, clincal management does not rely upon a differentiation between toxicity and hypersensitivity. The absence of tests to differentiate the two mechanisms does not affect diagnosis and treatment of drug reactions. In the absence of reliable test procedures, the diagnosis of adverse drug reactions must depend upon:

(1) A high index for suspicion of drug toxicity and drug hypersensitivity, and
(2) A careful history.

If in the course of a patient's illness the progress is not in accordance with the expectations for the disease which has been diagnosed, the case must be carefully scrutinized to make sure that the medications used for treatment are not causing reactions which can contribute to the clinical pattern. It is important to emphasize that no drug is exempt. Under the proper circumstances, any medication can induce an adverse reaction. The recognition of this fact and the familiarity with the wide variety of clinical patterns produced by adverse drug reactions will aid the practicing physician in the diagnosis of adverse drug responses and also resolve many puzzling clinical problems.

There is no clinical pattern which is diagnostic for a given drug. There are some drugs that develop one pattern more frequently than another, as, for example, erythema by phenophthalein, a morbilliform eruption by the sulfonamides and the barbiturates, urticaria and asthma by aspirin. There is, however, nothing absolute about the relationship of any drug to any pattern; considerable diversification and crossing over occurs. For example, aspirin commonly causes urticaria and asthma, but the same pattern can be caused by penicillin or less frequently it can be induced by tartrazine (FD&C yellow #5), a food dye. A great variety of drugs can cause hematological diseases.

The diagnosis of drug sensitivity is usually made on the basis of history. To obtain an accurate history is not always simple; it requires all the ingenuity of the physician and complete, intelligent cooperation on the part of the patient. It is important to uncover all medications and at times all food factors taken by the patient prior to the appearance of symptoms.

A history of using aspirin over a long period, either months or even years may offer the patient a false sense of security, since the experience of receiving the drug over long periods does not exempt it from acting adversely. Farr has pointed out that in aspirin sensitivity the patient may not infrequently offer a history of aspirin ingestion for many years with no apparent adverse response.

In some cases the initial experience with a drug may serve as a sensitizing dose, as the first dose of penicillin which may be followed by an adverse reaction following subsequent administration of the drug.

In hospitalized patients this usually offers no problem, except in situations when the patient may surreptitiously self medicate. Very often it is not the patient's intent to deceive but rather one of innocence. He may not consider taking a customary vitamin tablet, a daily laxative or an occasional proprietary aspirin compound as an irregular procedure.

In the ambulatory case, one of the chief problems is the memory of the patient. It is imperative to impress upon the patient the importance of obtaining accurate historical data. One must explain what is included as drugs. The patient may not consider a daily cathartic taken routinely for years as medication. A proprietary antacid taken regularly for "dyspepsia" is usually not classed as a drug by the patient. At times the patient who is accustomed to relying upon a sedative tablet at bedtime is reluctant to reveal the information because of the fear of restriction. It is necessary to review every habit and every routine procedure of the patient. In many cases this can be accomplished more effectively with a daily diary including every activity and every item eaten or used by the patient.

Treatment of Drug Reactions

Prophylaxis

(1) The best prophylaxis is to avoid every unnecessary contact with the drug. It is important to avoid unnecessary administration of any drug which always carries the risk of sensitizing an individual so that subsequent treatment of future ailments may be greatly hampered.

(2) Before administering any medication, the patient should always be questioned concerning known adverse reactions to drugs. This is particularly true of medications with a comparatively high incidence of reactions, such as penicillin, aspirin, barbiturates, phenothiazines, *etc.*

(3) Testing the patient for drug sensitivity is not only unreliable but not without hazards. Skin testing to determine sensitivity or provocative testing by the administration of small doses of the drug are *not recommended*. In case of doubt it is always safer to resort to a different class of medication or to omit the doubtful medication completely.

(4) With a confirmed diagnosis of a drug reaction and identification of the medication at fault, the only procedure is to *immediately stop* the administration of the drug.

In the case of multiple drug therapy, if the causative item cannot be specifically pinpointed, the safest procedure is the discontinuance of all medications. Many patients have recovered from complex syndromes following the cessation of drug therapy.

In most cases, with early diagnosis, recovery is usually prompt following withdrawal of the drug. Upon recovery it is not wise to attempt diagnostic challenges either by skin tests or provocative challenge. The risk of precipitating violent reactions is usually very great.

(5) Pruritus, urticaria and mild angio-edema are treated with antihistamines. Caution must be exercised so that a reaction is not induced by the antihistaminic drug. This is best controlled by avoiding excessive dosage, monitoring the hemogram and carefully observing the patient's response. In the event that symptoms persist or become aggravated following antihistamine therapy, suspicions should be raised and the drug discontinued.

Corticosteroid therapy should be initiated for control of symptoms.

For more severe reactions which include severe angio-edema, asthma and serum sickness type of response, corticosteroids are the drug of choice (see discussion of therapy with corticosteroids in Chapter 15).

For hematological reactions, corticosteroids are recommended to arrest progress of the disease until the offending agent can be eliminated.

REFERENCES

1. AMA Council on Drugs: *AMA Drug Evaluations*, 1st ed. Chicago, 1971.
2. Baer, R. L. and Harber, L. C.: Photosensitivity induced by drugs. *JAMA, 192:* 989, 1965.
3. Boyd, E. M.: Expectorants and respiratory tract fluid. *Pharmacol Rev, 6:* 21, 1954.
4. Chafee, F. C. and Settipane, G. A.: Asthma caused by FD&C approved dyes. *J Allergy, 40:* 65, 1967.
5. Council on New Drugs and Development in Therapeutics: Penicillin and other antibiotics in milk. *JAMA, 171:* 49, 1959.
6. Cutting, Windsor C.: *Handbook of Pharmacology*, 4th ed. New York, Meredith, 1969.
7. Drill, V. A. (Ed.): *Pharmacology*. New York, McGraw-Hill, 1952.
8. Farr, Richard S.: The need to re-evaluate acetylsalicylic acid (aspirin). *J Allergy, 45:* 321, 1970.
9. Giraldo, B., Blumenthal M. N. and Spink, W. W.: Aspirin intolerance and asthma. A clinical and immunological study. *Ann Intern Med, 63:* 109, 1965.
10. Goth, A.: *Medical Pharmacology*, 4th ed. St. Louis, Mosby, 1968.
11. Green, G. R., Peters, G. A. and Geraci, J. E.: Treatment of bacterial endocarditis in patients with penicillin hypersensitivity. *Ann Intern Med, 67:* 235, 1967.
12. Grossman, M. I., Matsumoto, K. K. and Lichter, R. J.: Fecal blood loss produced by oral and intravenous administration of various salicylates. *Gastroenterology, 40:* 383, 1961.
13. Hammond, A. L.: Aspirin: New perceptions. *Science, 174:* 48, 1971.

14. Hjorth, N.: Drug reactions. In Rose, B. *et al.* (Eds.): *Allergology*. Amsterdam Excerpta Med Foundation, 1968, pp. 360–365.
15. Idsoe, O. *et al.*: Nature and extent of penicillin side reactions with particular reference to fatalities from anaphylactic shock. *Bull WHO, 38:* 159, 1968.
16. Krantz, J. C., Jr., Carr, C. J. and LaDu, B. N., Jr.: *The Pharmacologic Principles of Medical Practice,* 7th ed. Baltimore, Williams & Wilkins, 1969.
17. Levine, B. B. and Price, V.: Studies on the immunological mechanism of penicillin allergy. II. Antigenic specificities of allergic wheal and flare skin response in patients with histories of penicillin allergy. *Immunology, 7:* 542, 1964.
18. Levine, B. B., Redmond, A. P., Fellner, M. J., Voss, H. E. and Levytska, V.: Penicillin allergy and the heterogeneous immune responses of man to benzylpenicillin. *J Clin Invest, 45:* 1895, 1966.
19. Levine, B. B.: Immunochemical mechanism of drug allergy. *Ann Rev Med, 17:* 23, 1966.
20. Meyler, L. and Herxheimer, A. (Eds.): *Side Effects of Drugs,* Baltimore, Williams & Wilkins, 1965–1967, Vol. VI, Excerpta Med Found, Amsterdam.
21. Moser, R. H. (Ed.): *Diseases of Medical Progress: A Study of Iatrogenic Disease.* 3rd ed. Springfield, Thomas, 1969.
22. Mull, M. M.: The tetracyclines. *Am J Dis Child, 112:* 483, 1966.
23. Queng, J. T., Dukes, C. D. and McGovern, J. P.: Antigenicity of the tetracyclines. *J Allergy, 36:* 505, 1965.
24. Reidenberg, M. M. and Lowenthal, D. T.: Adverse non-drug reactions. *N Engl J Med, 279:* 678, 1968.
25. Rook, A. and Rowell, N. R.: Drug reactions. In Rook, A., Wilkinson, D. S. and Ebling, F. J. G.: *Textbook of Dermatology,* Philadelphia, F. A. Davis, 1968.
26. Rosenheim, M. L. and Moulton, R.: *Sensitivity Reactions to Drugs.* A symposium organized by the Council for International Organizations of Medical Sciences, established under the joint auspices of UNESCO and WHO. Oxford, Blackwell, 1958.
27. Samter, M. and Berryman, G. H.: Drug allergy. *Ann Rev Pharmacol, 4:* 265, 1964.
28. Siegel, B. B.: Hidden contacts with penicillin. *Bull WHO, 21:* 703, 1959.
29. Spector, W. G.: Substances which affect capillary permeability. *Pharmacol Rev, 10:* 475, 1958.
30. Van Meter, T. E., Jr.: Adverse effects of inhalation of excessive amounts of nebulized isoproterenol in status asthmaticus. *J Allergy, 43:* 101, 1969.
31. Wintrobe, M. M. *et al.:* The problem of adverse drug reactions. *JAMA, 196:* 404, 1966.
32. Zolov, D., Redmond, A. P. and Levine, B. B.: Immunological studies of desensitization in penicillin allergy. *J Allergy, 39:* 107, 1967.

Chapter 11

PSYCHOLOGICAL FACTORS IN ALLERGIC DISEASE*

THAT PSYCHOLOGICAL EVENTS are primary factors as a cause of allergic disease is an opinion held by many professionals and particularly by laymen. The association between psychological disturbances and allergic disease is a common observation, but there is no conclusive evidence to support a primary psychogenic origin for allergic disease. On the other hand, secondary contributory psychogenic factors which precipitate or aggravate the allergic attack seem well established.

There are three main deficiencies which have detracted from most studies on the relationship between allergic disease and psychological behavior.

First, any chronic illness may induce a personality difference.

In attempting to differentiate personality characteristics of asthmatic and normal individuals, Neuhaus indicated that the differences may not be specific for asthma but rather a reaction to the experience of chronic illness. He found that asthmatic children, children with another chronic illness, and the siblings of those patients, responded similarly to psychological tests and differed from a matched group of normal children.

Second, a large portion of all allergic subjects studied have been patients referred for or already undergoing psychiatric treatment. As a result, only a very select segment of the allergic population has been studied, and very little is known about allergic persons as a general group. This means that when differences were found between "psychiatric" allergic patients and groups of individuals not in psychiatric treatment, the researchers may have inadvertently contrasted neurotic and non-neurotic persons while their intention was to compare allergic and nonallergic groups.

That allergic patients in psychiatric therapy cannot be compared to other asthmatic individuals or to the general asthmatic population has been demonstrated by the findings of Leigh and Marley who reported that asthmatic patients in psychiatric therapy admitted to more neurotic symptoms than other asthmatic subjects or the general population.

A *third* major weakness in most studies in the field of psychological factors in allergic disease is the absence or weakness of criteria for designating a person as allergic. In some studies the diagnosis of allergy depends upon the mere self-description that one is "allergic." Many investigators simply lump together all persons with clinical symptoms suggestive of allergic disease and label them as *allergic subjects* with no attempt to confirm the diagnosis through history, physical findings or skin testing, either direct or passive transfer (PK) techniques.

Nonimmunologic mechanisms may induce clinical patterns resembling allergic disease as, for example, the urticaria, angio-edema and asthma induced by aspirin or tartrazine (FD&C yellow #5).

In many studies, histories taken previously for other purposes provided the data for per-

---

* Supported in part by NIH Grant AI 06188-01.

sonality ratings. In such histories pertinent information is frequently absent or inaccurate.

SPECIFIC HYPOTHESES CONCERNING THE RELATIONSHIP OF PSYCHOLOGICAL BEHAVIOR AND ALLERGIC DISEASE

I. The Psychoanalytic View of Alexander and French

A number of authors of psychoanalytic persuasion have hypothesized a psychological cause in allergic respiratory disease. The most influential reports have been those published by Alexander and French and their colleagues. These investigators propose a specific psychogenesis for asthma arising from an excessive dependence of the infant on the mother. Asthmatic attacks are precipitated when the individual is threatened with separation from the mother. The asthmatic attack itself is held to be symbolic of suppressed crying. Difficulty in crying and the increased capacity to cry following improvement are reported as common findings in asthmatics by these observers. They further hypothesize that a combination of sensitivity to allergens and conflict activation produced symptoms and that treatment of either factor could bring relief.

A complex body of theory, case reports and research grew out of Alexander and French's basic formulations. While case histories are an excellent source of ideas, their fruitfulness, however, depends upon casting these ideas into testable hypotheses. All too often the criteria for classifying the patient as allergic is omitted, and the history of the illness is not described. Similar deficiencies occur on the psychological side, when the basis for a conclusion that a subject suffers, for example, from conflicts over hostility or dependency is not specified. The conclusions of Alexander and French are further complicated by the fact that the patients studied had two conditions: neuroses for which they were being psychoanalyzed and allergic asthma. In view of this, there is no evidence to prove that the psychologic conflicts were the primary cause of the asthma. It is very possible that identical conflicts may be observed in any patient with a similar neurosis but without asthma.

Despite the considerable time lapse since the original Alexander and French publication, a definitive statement about the general usefulness or applicability of their views cannot be made. In surveying the literature one gets the impression that investigators have often used their observations or data to confirm or illustrate analytic formulations rather than to test their validity.

II. Allergy as Response to Stress

The general view of Selye and of Wolff and colleagues. based on studies of patients with a variety of bodily diseases, is that under stress many physiological changes occur. If these protective physiological aberrations, used originally as emergency measures, become habitual ways of coping with continuous daily stresses, then permanent tissue damage may result, with concomitant clinical patterns of asthma, rhinitis, hay fever, hypertension, and so forth. Different kinds of stresses can combine with each other to produce symptoms, when any one of them might be below the response threshold. Thus, the exposure of pollen-sensitive and pollen-insensitive subjects to a ragweed-pollen room was well tolerated when the mucus membranes were functioning well, but very poorly tolerated when there was previous hyperfunction due to already clinically manifest allergy or infection. Further, when pollen-sensitive subjects were exposed to a high pollen concentration in a setting of conflict and anxiety, hay fever symptoms were exacerbated. When sensitive subjects who were reacting only mildly to pollen discussed repugnant material, their hay fever symptoms became more extreme.

This group of studies was reported before the observations of Connell, who demonstrated the triggering effect of previous exposure to a dose of allergen which may lower the threshold for a response to subsequent exposure. The observations of Connell will undoubtedly influence the interpretation of responses to cumulative effects of stress factors.

III. Asthma and Psychosis

There is a widely shared conviction, or myth, that asthma seldom occurs among psychotic patients, that psychosomatic illness in general and asthma in particular cannot coexist with a functional psychosis. In the psychosis-prone individual, it is expected that periods of psychosomatic illness will alternate with periods of psychosis; for the population as a whole, significantly fewer psychotics will have psychosomatic disturbances. Research evidence is quite contradictory, with some workers confirming the hypothesized relationship and others refuting it. The contradictory findings appear to result from methodological weaknesses. This area is particularly handicapped by the following practices: relying on self-reports of psychotic individuals to establish the diagnosis of allergy, assuming that psychotic subjects can adequately describe their current condition, and relying upon completeness of medical charts gathered for other purposes to provide information essential for a diagnosis of allergy. Further, these studies have all used statistics gathered in 1928 for incidence of allergic disorders in the general population. It is unlikely that these figures accurately reflect the picture in the current population.

Some studies have indicated that, when patients are skin tested and relatives interviewed about symptoms, allergy incidence among hospitalized psychotic patients is equal to the rate in the general population. Such methods are more objective, but still insufficient for a diagnosis of allergic disease in the absence of careful history and physical examination.

Substantial differences in use of the term *psychotic* from one study to another certainly contribute to conflicting results. Work by Sabbath and Luce indicates that severity of personality disorganization in psychosis may be an important differentiating variable; for example, the more severe the psychosis, the less likely is concomitant asthma. Therefore, description of psychotic patients with respect to extent of personality disturbance becomes an important part of sample definition.

A few experimental studies have provided interesting leads. Funkenstein reported that in two small samples asthma and psychosis alternated, and there were concomitant shifts in autonomic functioning in response to Mecholyl® injections. When the patient was actively psychotic, Mecholyl led to transient systolic blood pressure change and minor wheezing; when temporarily not psychotic, blood pressure reactions to Mecholyl were marked, and asthma attacks occurred. To test the hypothesis that psychosis involves diminished ability to manifest an allergic reaction. Freedman, Redlich and Igersheimer skin tested chronic hospitalized schizophrenic patients and control subjects with allergens, histamines, and cantharides. The patients did not show a lesser reaction to allergens as compared to control subjects, but they did have smaller wheal responses to histamines.

Thus, at this time, speculation about an alternating relationship between asthma and psychosis has been neither confirmed nor denied. It may be myth or it may be that certain clinical observations hold under certain clinical conditions and not others. Not all the parameters of the issue have been adequately tested.

IV. Psychosomatic Specificity

A number of hypotheses, advanced originally by psychoanalytic writers, Alexander and French, Dunbar, and Weiss, propose a specific constellation of psychological conflicts for each psychosomatic disease syndrome.

The assumption is that a particular psychosomatic illness develops from the physiological accompaniments to particular psychological stresses or conflicts, such as dependency conflict in asthma, or hostility conflict in hypertension. Most writers believe that these relationships pertain only to types of psychological conflict and not to superficial traits of personality. Groen, however, favors a dual hypothesis relating psychosomatic specificity with personality traits and areas of conflict.

Since hypotheses differ considerably from one study to the next, it is difficult to arrive at substantive conclusions from the body of work as a whole. Many studies have used poorly defined psychological terms and have separated groups of patients on a *post hoc* basis. Although any study proceeding on this basis requires cross validation, it has almost never been performed. Two projects, however, by Ring and Graham and colleagues, deserve special notice because of their careful execution and their success in identifying psychological differences accompanying different illnesses. For example, raters made physical diagnoses on the basis of psychological characteristics and frequently were correct.

V. Emotional Precipitation of Allergy Symptoms

Some workers have reasoned that, if emotional factors are important in producing asthma or hay fever, it should be possible to demonstrate a specific role for such stresses in the precipitation of individual attacks. Very little formal research has been done to test this hypothesis, although there have been casual reports for centuries of such emotional precipitation. Recently, Dekker and Groen were able to produce asthma attacks in the laboratory with a few patients by duplicating emotional precipitating factors that the patients described as important. Similarly, Wolf *et al,* found that emotional arousal in an experimental setting could exacerbate hay fever symptoms.

Most workers have relied on patients reports, but Knapp and Nemetz have done so in a particularly thorough and intensive fashion. They studied intensively the circumstances around several hundred asthmatic attacks in nine chronic asthmatic patients being seen in psychoanalytic psychotherapy. For these cases it was possible to classify moods accompanying and preceding attacks of asthma as well as environmental changes occurring around the attacks. Excitement and arousal were frequent prodromal features, and depression was often experienced during the attack. In a study of one case, Bursten found a relationship between similar psychological qualities, sputum-eosinophil count and asthma attacks.

Both the method of experimental manipulation and the use of patient reports have serious difficulties; the solution is probably a gradual accumulation of material derived from work performed by both methods. The experimental method requires the isolation of specific kinds of stresses, assignment of relative degrees of importance to each, and then duplication of them under controlled conditions. For example, various emotional stresses may cause an acceleration of the respiratory rate, which in an asthmatic individual with an increment of edema, bronchiolar spasm or both may result in obvious wheezing. In this situation the emotional stress should not be interpreted as a primary cause of the wheezing. Walking, running or any activity that accelerates the respiratory rate may induce wheezing in the asthmatic individual. (See Chapter 4, Allergic Diseases of the Lower Respiratory Tract.)

On the other hand, use of patients' reports relies heavily on their awareness of emotional factors, the rapport between patient and interviewer, the effect of the interviewer's theoretical biases on what a patient reports, and the time lag between symptoms and interviewing. A neglected but possibly very fruitful approach would be the close observation of patients in an institutional setting, with an attempt to delineate *in vitro* the important precipitants, be they allergy, infection, weather, or social encounters and their psychological meanings.

VI. Allergic Persons as a Psychologically Heterogeneous Population

Clinicians sometimes observe that allergic factors appear to be the major cause of symptoms in some of their patients, while emotional factors seem relatively more important precipitants for certain other patients. They also note that some of their patients, while suffering from symptoms suggestive of allergy, present negative immunological findings. A recent hypothesis makes use of these observations and suggests that allergic patients can be classified roughly into groups on the basis of greater or lesser skin reactivity to allergens and that there may be important psychological differences associated with these groupings.

It has been observed that individuals who reacted strongly on skin testing manifested fewer psychological disturbances than those who failed to react. In evaluating this aspect of the problem, the patterns, simulating allergic disease, induced by nonimmunological factors must be considered. For example, the author has observed behavioral disturbances in both children and adults which have been attributed to food additives.

In children, the behavioral disturbances included hyperactivity, lack of concentration, distractibility, impulsivity and learning difficulties. These children were poorly adjusted at home and disruptive at school. The primary complaint in each case was either pruritus or urticaria which was attributed to the ingestion of synthetic flavorings and colorings as encountered in various types of soft drinks, particularly Kool-Aid® and Funny Face®; artificially colored and flavored breakfast foods and chewable vitamins. Following management with a diet excluding all synthetic flavors and colors (see salicylate-free diet, Chapter 9), not only were the pruritus and urticaria controlled, but in addition the parents observed a striking and at times dramatic change in the child's behavioral pattern. The parents reported that the child became docile, was better adjusted to its home environment and showed a definite improvement in achievement at school. Several of the children under observation experienced a return of symptoms with a reversal of the behavioral pattern following the inadvertent ingestion of the additives.

The following case history illustrates the observations in adult patients:

Case History: An adult white female, forty years of age, reported to the Allergy Department with the complaint of peri-orbital edema and urticaria which, following a thorough investigation, was attributed to food additives. The patient was managed with a salicylate-free diet, which resulted in complete control of the angioedema and urticaria, and in addition, a striking change in her behavioral pattern. The patient who had been under psychiatric care for over two years because of her hostility to all individuals including her husband, and because of her inability to hold any employment, experienced a striking change in her personality pattern when she observed the salicylate-free diet. All the complaints for which she sought psychiatric care cleared completely on the salicylate-free diet but returned when the diet was not observed.

Following the experience with this patient, other adults were noted with personality problems which cleared following treatment of their allergic or pseudo-allergic complaints by elimination of the food additives.

It is important to note that although the primary complaints of the patients observed simulated allergic disease, it is possible that the clinical response is induced by a nonimmunologic mechanism as occurs with tartrazine (FD&C yellow #5) and with the salicylates. The emotional and behavioral disturbances observed in this group of patients were coincidental findings, noted upon developing the history, while the psychological improvement followed treatment directed to the chief complaint. It is conceivable that similar emotional and behavioral disturbances are induced by food additives, but are unrecognized because somatic complaints to serve as a clue are lacking. The clinical patterns observed in this group of patients bear a striking similarity to many reports for individuals diagnosed as having minimal brain dysfunction (MBD). This raises a question, "Is it possible that some cases of so-called MBD may be manifestations of neuro-physiologic disturbances induced by certain chemicals such as the food additives?"

This is an area which deserves further investigation, and one in which the practicing clinician, although not trained specifically in either psychology or psychiatry, can undertake successfully. Following a careful history, the procedure of the elimination diet is quite simple (see sections on elimination diets, Chapter 9). The favorable responses at times are quite dramatic and usually do not require the expert to recognize that a favorable response has been achieved. It is also quite simple to confirm the results by the administration of the suspected offender as a blind control. The reactions induced are usually mild and do not involve the risk observed with atopy and anaphylaxis.

VII. The Relevance of Animal Conditioning Studies to Asthma

A number of studies, largely with animals, have suggested that symptoms with varying degrees of clinical similarity to asthma may be produced by means of conditioning procedures. Some of these observations have emerged as by-products of the experimental setting or of the conditioning of other responses. These are to be differentiated from studies in "experimental asthma" *per se*. The term "experimental asthma" as used in the literature has generally referred to laboratory induction of sensitivity to an allergen such as egg white or pollen. When this response is established, some authors have reported that the response can be conditioned to a previously neutral stimulus such as a tone, a bell, or the experimental chamber itself. One such study was reported by Ottenberg *et al*. Noelpp and Noelpp-Eschenhagen have reported similar findings with laboratory animals.

A study by Dekker, Pelser, and Groen, one of the few successful studies with human subjects, is illustrative. An allergen known to be effective with each of two subjects was paired with a neutral solvent. After repeated pairings, inhalation of pure oxygen was sufficient to cause respiratory changes, as measured by clinical signs and respiratory distress. After additional trials the mouthpiece alone was sufficient to bring on symptoms.

A more typical finding is that there are respiratory accompaniments to classical Pavlovian conditioning: respiratory enhancement can be an unconditioned response to noxious stimuli. Changes in breathing pattern appear to be but one physiological accompaniment of the conditioning situation, a part of a generalized stress response, and resemble asthma less closely than does experimental asthma. That these changes in breathing pattern have little explanatory value for the development of asthma was demonstrated in a study by Schiavi, Stein, and Sethi. A group of animals given electric shock developed a breathing pattern of shortened inspiration and lengthened expiration, but there was no evidence of bronchiolar obstruction as measured by body plethysmograph. Tracheotomies demonstrated that the respiratory pattern was due to the animals' screeching. Animals sensitized to egg white (experimental asthma), on the other hand, did show bronchiolar obstruction.

Although work with conditioned experimental asthma suggests that conditioning could be an important process in the establishment and maintenance of asthma, the studies with humans have not yet been successfully repeated. Indeed, both Knapp and Dekker, who have continued careful studies of conditioning in humans, fail to replicate previous positive results. Again methodological considerations appear to be paramount. When clinical indices of an asthmatic attack have been used, the observed changes in breathing pattern were considered to be indicative of asthma; however, when more precise measurements were taken, as with Stein's use of the whole body plethysmograph, results were less conclusive. Here again, the influence of accelerated respiration from any cause must be considered as a positive factor in causing wheezing in an asthmatic individual who has persistent narrowing of the terminal air pathways. (See Chapter 4, Allergic Diseases of the Lower Respiratory Tract.)

Psychological Treatment of Allergic Individuals

The major portion of studies on psychological aspects of allergic disease has been based upon data derived from allergic persons referred for treatment to psychologists or psychiatrists. Almost every psychological treatment technique used with neurotic patients has been applied to the allergic patient: individual psychotherapy, psychoanalysis, group therapy, tranquilizing drugs, and environmental manipulation. Accounts of success have usually been subjective statements such as, "This treatment seems to work." With the exception of a few practitioners of group therapy who have taken initial steps toward controlled studies, there have been no attempts to test the relative merits of various therapeutic techniques.

There are enough anecdotal accounts of successful psychological treatment with allergic patients to conclude that at least sometimes it is of benefit in controlling allergic symptoms, but these represent isolated clinical reports of success. Treatment failures are seldom published. A germane question is, what kind of allergic patient benefits from which psychological treatment? Further, are successfully treated patients actually allergic individuals, or have they been labelled allergic because of current suggestive symptoms without careful allergy history or immunological investigation (skin test or passive transfer)?

An additional caution applies in evaluating psychological treatment research. The results from studies where psychotherapy was given to selected neurotic, allergic patients cannot be compared with those where psychotherapy was assigned randomly to allergic patients. The former represents highly select group and limits the extent to which results can be generalized regarding the role of psychological factors.

REFERENCES

1. Block, J., Jennings, P. H., Harvey, E. and Simpson, E.: Interaction between allergic potential and psychopathology in childhood asthma. *Psychosom Med, 26:* 307, 1964.
2. Bursten, B.: Psychological state and sputum eosinophia. *Psychosom Med, 24:* 529, 1962.
3. Collier, R. O. and Stunkard, C. L.: An analysis of variance of multiple measurements on subjects classified in unequal groups of one dimension. *J Exp Educ, 25:* 255, 1957.
4. Dekker, E., Barendregt, J. T. and De Vries, K.: Allergy and neurosis in asthma. *J Psychosom Res, 5:* 83, 1961.
5. Dekker, E. and Groen, J.: Reproducible psychogenic attacks of asthma. *J Psychosom Res, 1:* 58, 1956.
6. Dekker, E., Pelser, H. E. and Groen, J.: Conditioning as a cause of asthma attacks. *J Psychosom Res, 2:* 97, 1957.
7. Dunbar, F.: *Emotions and Bodily Changes, A Survey of Literature on Psychosomatic Interrelationships, 1910–1953,* 4th ed. New York, Columbia U Pr, 1954.
8. Feingold, B. F., Gorman, F. J., Singer, M. T. and Schlesinger, K.: Psychological studies of allergic women. *Psychosom Med, 24:* 195, 1962.
9. Feingold, B. F., Singer, M. T., Freeman, E. H. and Deskins, A.: Psychological variables in allergic disease: A critical appraisal of methodology. *J Allergy, 38:* 143, 1966.
10. Freedman, D. X., Redlich, F. C. and Igersheimer, W. W.: Psychosis and allergy: Experimental approach. *Am J Psychiatry, 112:* 873, 1956.
11. Freeman, E. H., Gorman, F. J., Singer, M. T., Affelder, M. T. and Feingold, B. F.: Personality variables and allergic skin reactivity. *Psychosom Med, 29,* 1967.
12. Freeman, E. H., Feingold, B. F., Schlesinger, K. and Gorman, F. J.: Psychological variables in allergic disorders: A review. *Psychosom Med, 26:* 543, 1964.
13. French, T. M. and Alexander, F.: Psychogenic factors in bronchial asthma. *Psychosom Med Monographs 4,* Washington, D.C., 1941, National Research Council.
14. Funkenstein, D. H.: Psychophysiological relationship

of asthma and urticaria to mental illness. *Psychosom Med, 12:* 377, 1950.
15. Funkenstein, D. H.: Variations in response to standard amounts of chemical agents during alterations in feeling states in relation to occurrence of asthma. *Res Publ Assoc Res Nerv Ment Dis, 29,* 1950.
16. Graham, D. T., Lundy, R. M., Benjamin, L. S., Kabler, J. D., Lewis, W. C., Kunish, N. O. and Graham, F. K.: Specific attitudes in initial interviews with patients having different "psychosomatic" diseases. *Psychosom Med, 24:* 257, 1962.
17. Greenfield, N. S.: Allergy and the need for recognition. *J Consult Clin Psychol, 22:* 230, 1958.
18. Groen, J.: Emotional factors in the etiology of internal diseases. *Mt Sinai J Med NY, 18:* 71, 1951–1952.
19. Groen, J. J. and Pelser, H. E.: Experiences with, and results of, group psychotherapy in patients with bronchial asthma. *J Psychosom Res, 4:* 191, 1960.
20. Herxheimer, H.: Induced asthmas in humans. *Int Arch Allergy Appl Immunol, 3:* 192, 1953.
21. Holmes, T. H., Trenting, T. and Wolff, H. G.: Life situations, emotions and nasal disease, evidence on summative effects inhibited in patients with "hay fever." *Psychosom Med, 13:* 71, 1951.
22. Knapp, P. H.: Acute bronchial asthma. II. Psychoanalytic observations on fantasy, emotional arousal, and partial discharge. *Psychosom Med, 22:* 88, 1960.
23. Knapp, P. H. and Nemetz, S. J.: Sources of tension in bronchial asthma. A study of forty patients: Notes on mood, self-image, and the role of the voice. *Psychosom Med, 19:* 466, 1957.
24. Knapp, P. H. and Nemetz, S. J.: Acute bronchial asthma. I. Concomitant depression and excitement, and varied antecedent patterns in 406 attacks. *Psychosom Med, 22:* 42, 1960.
25. Leigh, D.: Asthma and the psychiatrist: A critical review. *Int Arch Allergy Appl Immunol, 4:* 227, 1953.
26. Leigh, D. and Marley, E.: A psychiatric assessment of adult asthmatics: A statistical study. *J Psychosom Res, 1:* 128, 1956.
27. Liddell, H.: The influence of experimental neuroses on respiratory function. In Abramson, H. A. (Ed.): *Treatment of Asthma.* Baltimore, Williams & Wilkins, 1951.
28. Little, S. W. and Cohen, L. D.: Goal-setting behavior of asthmatic children and of their mothers for them. *J Personality, 19:* 376, 1951.
29. Loewenstein, J.: Psychotherapy of asthma. *Med Klin, 22:* 994, 1926.
30. Margolis, M.: The mother-child relationship in bronchial asthma. *J Abnorm Psychol, 63:* 360, 1961.
31. McDermott, N. T. and Cobb, S.: Psychiatric survey of fifty cases of bronchial asthma. *Psychosom Med, 1:* 203, 1939.
32. Miller, H. and Baruch, D. W.: Psychosomatic studies of children with allergic manifestations. I. Maternal rejection: A study of 63 cases. *Psychosom Med, 10:* 275, 1948.
33. Mohr, F.: *Psychophysische Behandlungsmethoden.* Leipzig, Hirzel, 1925.
34. Moos, E.: Zur Behandlung des Asthma bronchiale. *Munch Med Wochenschr, 75:* 1841, 1928.
35. Neuhaus, E. C.: A personality study of asthmatic and cardiac children. *Psychosom Med, 20:* 181, 1958.
36. Noelpp, B. and Noelpp-Eschenhagen: I. Das Experimentelle Asthma Bronchiale des Meerschweinhens. II. Mitterlung die Ralle Ludingter Reflexes in de Pathogenese des Asthma Bronchialle. *Int Arch Allergy Appl Immunol, 2:* 321, 1951.
37. Noelpp, B. and Noelpp-Eschenhagen: I. Des Experimentelle Asthma Bronchiale des Meerschweinhens. III. Mitterlung. Studien zur Beduntung Bedingter Reflexe. Bahnung-Slureitschaft und Hastfahigkeit inter "Stress." *Int Arch Allergy Appl Immunol, 3:* 108, 1952.
38. Ottenberg, P., Stein, M., Lewis, J. and Hamilton, C.: Learned asthma in the guinea pig. *Psychosom Med, 20:* 395, 1958.
39. Purcell, K.: Distinctions between subgroups of asthmatic children: Children's perceptions of events associated with asthma. *Pediatrics, 31:* 486, 1963.
40. Purcell, K.: Some observations on psychosomatic studies of asthma. *Pediatr Dig, 6:* 59, 1965.
41. Purcell, K., Bernstein, L. and Bukantz, S. C.: A preliminary comparison of rapidly remitting and persistently "steroid-dependent" asthmatic children. *Psychosom Med, 23:* 305, 1960.
42. Purcell, K., Turnbull, J. W. and Bernstein, L.: Distinctions between subgroups of asthmatic children: Psychological tests and behavior rating comparisons. *J Psychosom Res, 6:* 283, 1962.
43. Ratner, B.: Experimental asthma. In Abramson, H. A. (Ed.): *Somatic and Psychiatric Treatment of Asthma.* Baltimore, Williams & Wilkens, 1951, pp. 62–92.
44. Ratner, B., Jackson, H. C. and Gruehl, H. L.: Respiratory anaphylaxis: Sensitization, shock, bronchial asthma and death induced in the guinea pig by the nasal inhalation of dry horse dander. *Am J Dis Child, 34:* 23, 1927.
45. Ring, F. O.: Testing the validity of personality profiles in psychosomatic illnesses. *Am J Psychiatry, 113:* 1075, 1957.

46. Rogerson, C. H.: Psychological factors in asthma-prurigo. *Q J Med, 30:* 367, 1937.
47. Sabbath, J. C. and Luce, R. A.: Psychosis and bronchial asthma. *Psychiatr Q, 26:* 562, 1952.
48. Schiavi, R. C., Stein, M. and Sethi, B. B.: Respiratory variables in response to a pain-fear stimulus and in experimental asthma. *Psychosom Med, 23:* 485, 1961.
49. Sclare, A. B. and Crockett, J. A.: Group psychotherapy in bronchial asthma. *J Psychosom Res, 2:* 157, 1957.
50. Selye, H.: *The Physiology and Pathology of Exposure to Stress.* Montreal, Acta, 1950.
51. Solomon, Joan: Thursday's child: A review of minimal brain dysfunction (MBD). *The Sciences,* N Y Acad of Sci, *12* (mo. 5): 6, 1972.
52. Tuft, H. S.: The development and management of intractable asthma of childhood. *Am J Dis Child, 93:* 251, 1957.
53. Weiss, E.: Psychosomatic aspects of certain allergic disorders. *Int Arch Allergy Appl Immunol, 1:* 4, 1950.
54. Wittkower, E. and Petow, H.: Beiträge zur Klinik des Asthma bronchiale und verwandter Zustände. Zur Psychogenese des Asthma bronchiale. *Z Klin Med, 119:* 293, 1932.
55. Wolf, S.: Causes and mechanisms in rhinitis. *Laryngoscope, 6:* 601, 1952.
56. Wolf, S., Holmes, T. H., Treuting, T., Goodell, Helen and Wolff, H. G.: An experimental approach to psychosomatic phenomena in rhinitis and asthma. *J Allergy, 21:*1, 1950.
57. Wolff, H. G.: Life stress and bodily disease—a formulation. *Res Publ Assoc Res Nerv Ment Dis, 29:* 1059, 1950.
58. Zeller, M. and Eolin, J. V.: Allergy in the insane. *J Allergy, 14:* 564, 1942.
59. Ziskind, Eugene: Psychosomatic aspects of asthma. An eclectic therapeutic orientation for the nonpsychiatrist physician. *Ann Allergy, 24,* 1966.

Chapter 12

INSECT ALLERGY

CLINICALLY, the allergic response to insects can be classified as: (1) allergic response to biting insects, (2) allergic response to stinging insects, and (3) allergic response to insect parts as inhalant factors.

ALLERGIC RESPONSE TO BITING INSECTS

Fleas, Mosquitoes, Bedbugs, Body Lice, Sand Flies, and Triatoma (Kissing Bug, Blunt-Nosed Beetle)

Flea Bites*

The antigen in flea bite hypersensitivity is a low molecular hapten, less than 1,000, which conjugates with skin collagen to form a complete antigen which induces the delayed type of hypersensitivity (DH).

There are five stages in the reactivity to flea bites:

Stage I. Induction—no observable skin reaction
Stage II. Delayed reactivity
Stage III. Immediate followed by delayed reactivity
Stage IV. Immediate reactivity only (no delayed)
Stage V. No response

I. THE INDUCTION STAGE: Following the initial bite or bites, nonsensitive individuals require five to eight days for sensitivity to develop. During this latent or induction period no skin lesions are observed.

II. THE STAGE OF DELAYED REACTIVITY: Following the development of sensitivity, reaction to the bite appears after twenty-four to forty-eight hours. The initial lesion is a very pruritic, slightly indurated papule induced by the monocytic infiltration characteristic of delayed hypersensitivity (DH). Occasionally a tiny vesicle may cap the lesion, which is an expression of increased permeability that can accompany DH. Scratching induced by the pruritus may cause excoriations of the papule, leading to a punctate hemorrhage which upon drying forms small crusts. The papule may persist for days and at times weeks. As the papule heals, it leaves no apparent residual in the skin, except that in some dark-skinned individuals pigmented areas may persist at the bite site for long periods, at times even for months.

Papular Urticaria: During the induction or latent period an individual may experience a number of insect bites, but since skin manifestations do not appear until sensitivity is fully developed, such patients will manifest no lesions. When sensitivity is fully developed, about the fifth to eighth day following the initial exposure, all the bite sites may flare up, producing a shower of pruritic papular lesions which are usually diagnosed as "papular urticaria." The condition is observed more frequently in children.

III. THE STAGE OF IMMEDIATE AND DELAYED REACTIVITY: If following the development of DH the individual continues to be bitten for several days, instead of a papule, the initial lesion that develops is a wheal that appears within twenty minutes after the

---

* The studies on fleas were supported in part by NIH grants AI E-1389 and AI E-3966.

bite and persists for about one hour, to be supplanted after twenty-four hours by the papule of DH. The papule has the identical characteristics, both microscopically and macroscopically of the lesion of stage II. These papules may persist for days and at times for weeks. In stage III, an individual subjected to repeated bites on successive days may simultaneously manifest both wheals and papules.

IV. STAGE OF IMMEDIATE REACTIVITY: If the individual experiences flea bites for an additional sixty to ninety days, he responds with only the whealing reaction. No papules occur. In most cases the whealing lesion is very transitory, lasting for about one hour. The size of the wheal may show an individual variation. In some cases the immediate response may be vesicular or even bullous, with extreme pruritus and persisting for days.

V. STAGE OF NONREACTIVITY: In the experimental animal, following continued exposure for a period of ninety days or more, no skin reaction occurs. Even the histological pattern is normal at this stage. In areas where fleas are indigenous, following exposure to flea bites for long periods of time (many months), individuals fail to manifest a skin response. This explains the initial, sometimes violent response experienced by newcomers in an area indigenous to fleas, followed by complete nonreactivity with continued residence in the area. Nonsensitivity does not develop in all individuals since some individuals experience a persistence of the cutaneous response for indefinite periods.

Cross Reactivity: Cross reactivity among species of fleas has been demonstrated for both humans and animals, so that an individual sensitized to one species will react to all other species. The degree of reactivity which may vary with different species is greatest with *Pulex irritans,* the human flea, which is a very avid feeder that induces multiple lesions that are larger than those observed with most common varieties such as the cat flea *(Ctenocephalides felis felis),* the rat flea *(Xenopsylla cheopsis),* and the dog flea *(Ctenocephalides canis).*

Treatment

Prophylaxis: The only effective prevention is extermination of the insects and elimination of their ova and pupae. In the immediate home environment, control must be directed against infested pets, such as cats and dogs that serve as natural hosts for the propagation of the insects. The flea prefers its natural host so that cat fleas prefer cats, dog fleas, dogs, and human fleas, humans. Although fleas will attack animals other than their natural host, they are less prone to do so when the natural host is available. Since control is not effective unless all ova and pupae in and about the premises are destroyed, the services of professional exterminators may be required.

In areas where fleas are endemic, it is often difficult to avoid exposure. When *Pulex irritans* is the offender in the area, the local public health agencies will usually control the infested premises.

Palliative Treatment: Oral medications which include antipruritics, antihistamines, and steroids are ineffective for the control of pruritus. Thiamine chloride has been recommended as a repellant, but the effectiveness of such therapy has never been confirmed.

Topical Treatment: The treatment of a small number of lesions with the various anesthetic lotions, creams and ointments is often helpful in controlling the intense itching. In the use of topical agents care must always be exercised against the development of contact dermatitis, especially following repeated applications of products containing the anesthetic "caines" and the mercurial and paraben preservatives.

For widespread involvement as may be encountered in papular urticaria, tub soaks at room temperature may be effective.

Infection: Secondary infection of the lesions introduced by scratching occurs more commonly in children. Infection in most cases is not severe and often can be controlled by simple compresses. For widespread secondary infection, antibiotic therapy is recommended.

Hyposensitization: Since flea bite sensitivity is induced by a hapten present in flea salivary secretion, none of the products presently available are effective for inducing nonreactivity, since they do not provide the *free* hapten which theoretically can induce nonreactivity. Experimentally, the administration of the flea hapten derived from flea salivary secretions has been demonstrated to induce nonreactivity. Were a similar product available for human use, it is possible it would be effective.

A controlled study on humans, using whole body flea extracts administered over variable periods up to two years, followed by challenge with live fleas, demonstrated that such therapy fails to eliminate the reactivity to bites. While in some cases an increase in the degree of reactivity was induced. The studies reporting a good response following the administration of whole body flea extracts did not use live fleas for challenge, but based their conclusions upon subjective reports by the patients. It is possible that the favorable experiences of the patients in these studies were associated with the commonly observed seasonal decrease in the incidence of fleas.

Mosquitoes, Bed Bugs, Body Lice and Sand Flies

The allergic reaction to flea bites which has been studied extensively both clinically and experimentally in animals, can serve as the prototype for the allergic response to the *bites* of most insects. The identical sequence of reactivity observed with flea bites has been reported for the mosquito, bed bug, body louse and sand fly.

Controlled experiments in humans have demonstrated the sequence of response for both mosquitoes and bed bugs, but the reactions reported for lice and sand flies are based upon clinical observations. It is commonly recognized that an individual living in an area endemic for a specific insect will fail to react to bites after prolonged repeated exposure. Such failure to react following repeated bites has been reported for the body louse, sand fly, bed bugs, mosquitoes and fleas.

The Mosquito: Immunologic studies on the mosquito bite have succeeded in locating the specific antigen in the salivary secretion of the mosquito. Although the antigen has been neither isolated nor characterized, its behavior is haptenic in nature.

The lesions observed with mosquito bites are identical with those induced by flea bites, except that mosquitoes are more likely to attack the exposed areas of the body including the face and neck, which are rarely attacked by fleas.

The time required for nonreactivity to mosquito bites to develop is not known, but Mellanby has reported that individuals exposed repeatedly to thousands of bites lost their sensitivity.

Treatment

The palliative measures for mosquito bites are identical with those for flea bites.

Hyposensitization: Reports on the injection of whole body mosquito extracts into mosquito bite-sensitive humans indicate a decrease in the delayed reactivity but no change in the immediate reactivity. The most notable feature of the reports on desensitization with mosquito extracts is the conflict in the claims. Differences in opinion with regard to clinical hyposensitization may stem from the fact that in most cases conclusions were based on subjective reports of patients rather than on controlled experiments in which the treated individuals were challenged by an insect bite.

Bed Bugs: The sequence of reactivity to bed bugs has been reported both by Kemper and by Usinger who made the observations by feeding the insects upon themselves. These investigators noted that the sequence of reactivity was identical to that of other biting insects, such as the flea and the mosquito. They also observed that following repeated exposure to the bites of bed bugs at intervals of two days for a period of eleven months, the bites failed to elicit reactivity. Since bed bugs are secretive insects, the lesions, which are both papules and wheals, are usually confined to covered areas of the body. A residual pigmentation and at times ecchymosis (macula cerulea) are common.

Hyposensitization for bed bugs has never been reported.

Lice and Sand Flies: No immunologic studies have been reported for either lice or sand flies. As has been indicated above, following *repeated* long term exposure, nonreactivity is observed.

Triatoma:
  cone-nosed beetle
  blood sucker
  big bed bug
  Mexican bed bug
  Texas bed bug
  assassin bug
  cannibal bug (Europe)

Triatoma have been described throughout the world, but fifteen species of the insect

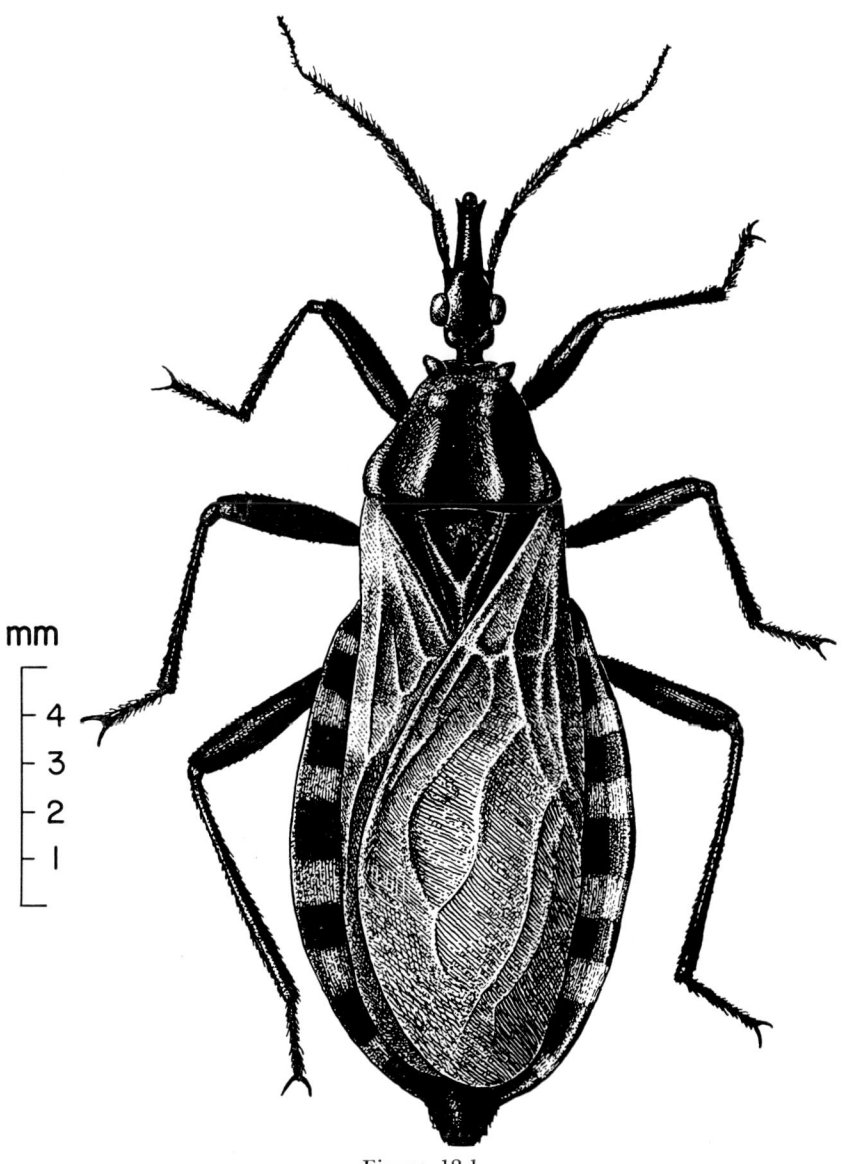

Figure 12-1
TRIATOMA

are endemic throughout the southern half of the United States with particular concentration in Texas and California from which states most of the clinical reports have emanated.

The insect is dark brown to black in color with orange markings about the periphery of the posterior two thirds of the body. Although the insects are winged, they are not strong fliers. Triatoma are blood sucking insects which accept as their host any warm blooded mammal, including man. For this reason they are usually found in proximity to stables, barns, animal houses and residences, or the nests of various wild animals, such as rats, armadillo, opossum, *etc.* They are secretive creatures for whom cracks and crevices, pieces of bark or the nests of animals serve as their lairs from which they crawl out at night to attack their prey. In bedrooms, they crawl out late at night from cracks and crevices, in walls, the floor, in brick work, or in furniture and attack the exposed parts of the body, usually an arm, a leg, or the face and eyes. Or they gain access beneath the bed coverings to attack undressed parts of the body. The entrance of the proboscis through the skin is usually painless and imperceptible, so that the host is rarely aware of the bite.

The Bite Reaction: Wood, a Los Angeles entymologist who permitted the insects to feed upon himself, observed that following the *initial* exposure, about four days elapsed before itching was experienced at the point of contact which was marked by a reddened discoloration of a slightly elevated area about 3 mm in diameter. Itching persisted for about thirty minutes, but the point of penetration was visible for about six days.

The evolution of the bite reaction is very ably described by Shields and Walsh.

Following the initial bite, there is a period of induction or sensitization of four to eight days following which a pruritic papule develops which persists for about six to eight days. With subsequent bites the latent period is shortened to about forty-eight hours, but with successive bites the lesions become larger and persist for longer periods, frequently up to ten days.

As is observed with most biting insects, with continued exposure reactivity is lost.

Shields and Walsh, in their excellent report on "kissing bug" bites, classify the bite reaction as follows:

(1) Papular lesions with central puncture. The lesions are usually larger than those observed with other species of biting insects. When the lesions are grouped, secondary to multiple probings, they have been misdiagnosed as atypical Herpes zoster. Biopsy at this stage revealed a lymphocytic infiltration which is the histological pattern observed with the stage of delayed reactivity of flea bites.

(2) Grouped small vesicles, with moderate swelling and slight redness but no visible central puncture may occupy an area 2 to 3 cm in diameter. These may be the product of a single bite.

(3) Giant urticarial lesions, characterized by firm wheals 10 to 16 cm in diameter.

(4) Hemorrhagic nodular to bullous lesions on the hands and feet which are the most characteristic for the Triatoma bite reaction. When such lesions are present, Triatoma bites should be suspected, especially when they are on one extremity. The bullae may occur as isolated lesions or be accompanied by papular lesions nearby, or on other parts of the body. The same investigators state that the bullous lesions have been erroneously attributed to "spider bites" but except for the black widow, spiders seldom bite and when they do, the lesions are not bullous.

Lymphangitis and lymphadenitis may accompany the urticarial and bullous lesions but are not a manifestation of secondary infection.

Various degrees of *constitutional* allergic reactions have been reported by several observers. These range from a localized urticarial reaction to diffuse edema of an extremity. Swelling of the hands and feet and face and eyes may develop remote from the

Entomologically authentic pictures of
STINGING INSECTS

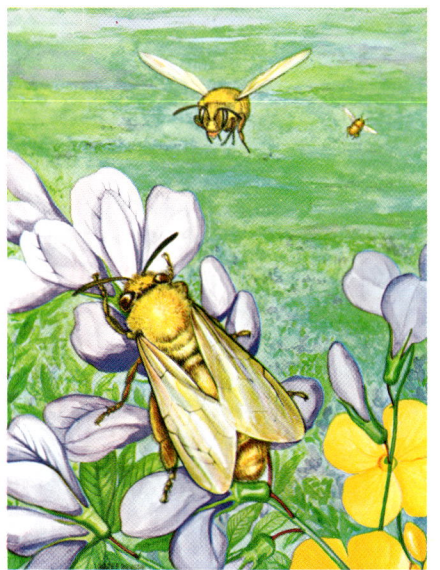

Apis mellifera
(Honey Bee)

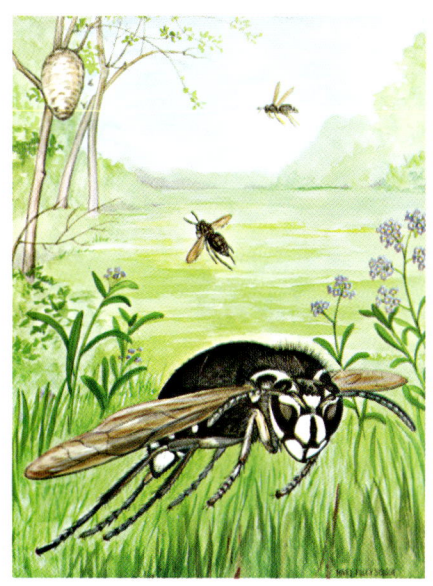

Dolicho vespula maculata
(Black Hornet or White-Faced Hornet)

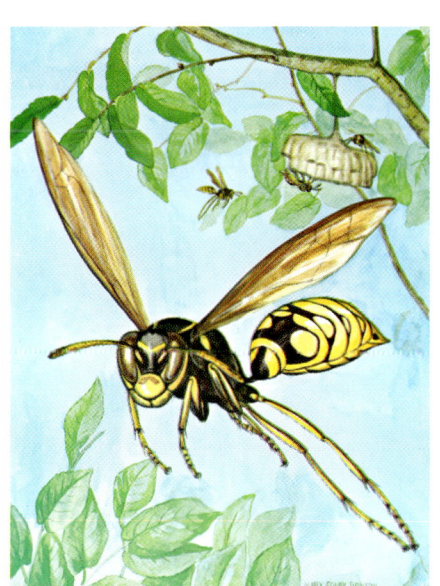

Polistes annularis
(Wasp)

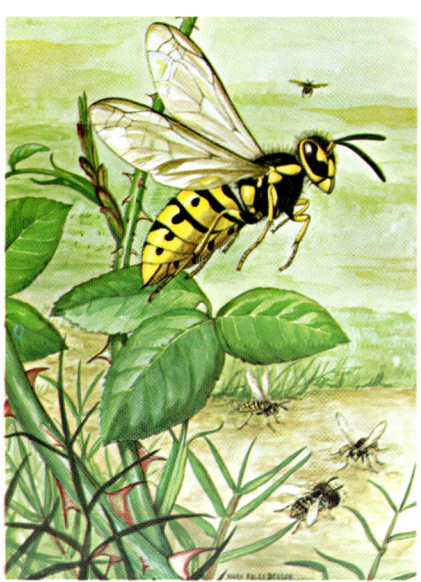

Vespula pennsylvanica
(Yellow Jacket)

Four Allergically Important Members of the Order

HYMENOPTERA

The four insects which constitute the allergically important members of the Hymenoptera are the Honey Bee and three of the social vespids or Paper Wasps.

Apis mellifera, the Honey Bee, is pictured at the upper left.

The insect pictured at the upper right is **Vespula (Dolichovespula) maculata,** variously called the "Black," "White-faced," or "Bald-faced Hornet."

The **Polistes** species pictured at the lower left is a showy yellow and black wasp. However, throughout the eastern half of the U.S. the more common species appears to the untrained eye to be a uniform reddish brown.

On the lower right is the Western Yellowjacket, **Vespula pennsylvanica.** The Eastern species, *Vespula maculifrons,* is so similar that it is doubtful if the layman could detect the difference. Yellowjackets are ground-nesting as distinct from the other Paper Wasps.

The three Paper Wasps are pictured with their distinguishing nests. Since wasp colonies are annual, the size of the nest increases as the season progresses, unlike the perennial hive of the Honey Bee which starts with a swarm rather than a single queen.

Severe general allergic reactions have been reported from the sting of all three Paper Wasps. With the Honey Bee both the sting and airborne body fragments have caused severe allergic reaction.

bite. Laryngeal edema, asthma, generalized weakness and loss of consciousness have also been reported.

Diagnosis: An absolute diagnosis can be made only by detecting and identifying the insect.

A presumptive diagnosis can be made when a unilateral or a localized cluster of lesions is observed, and particularly hemorrhagic bullae.

With such efflorescences, in areas where Triatoma are indigenous, a search should be made to detect the insect. Every available crack and crevice should be investigated. Spraying the suspected areas with aerosol insecticides may be effective in routing the insects from their lairs.

In view of the wide distribution of the insects, particularly in Texas and in southern California, one would expect a higher incidence of bite reactions than are reported in the literature. Failure to diagnose Triatoma bite reactions may be attributed to:

(1) The lack of awareness that the insect is indigenous in the area.

(2) The failure to recognize that the bite reaction occurs from two to seven days following the bite.

(3) The absence of any residual evidence, such as fecal deposits, that the insect has been present. Defecation usually occurs thirty minutes or longer following engorgement with blood.

(4) The symptomless bite, the secretive and nocturnal habits of the insect make detection difficult.

Treatment

For the papular lesions, cool boric compresses may be effective.

For urticarial lesions, antihistamines can be effective.

For constitutional reactions, epinephrine by hypodermic is very effective in controlling symptoms.

Susceptible individuals living in an area where the insects are indigenous should be taught emergency procedures as recommended for Hymenoptera stings. The emergency kits provided for Hymenoptera stings are satisfactory.

The transmission of the trypanosome responsible for Chagas' disease has no relation to the allergic response. Transmission is by fecal deposits, inoculated through scratching.

HYMENOPTERA STINGS

Because of the hazard to life, the stings of hymenoptera which include honey bees, yellow jackets, hornets and wasps, create very serious clinical problems. United States vital statistics report a yearly average of approximately twenty-nine deaths from hymenoptera stings. The figures available are no doubt quite conservative as there is no accurate method for determining the true incidence of fatalities to hymenoptera stings, since the cause of sudden death may be wrongly diagnosed, as for example, coronary disease.

Hymenoptera Venoms

The various constituents in hymenoptera venoms are listed in Table 12-I and 12-II.

Table 12-I: PHARMACOLOGICALLY AND BIOCHEMICALLY ACTIVE CONSTITUENTS OF HYMENOPTERA VENOMS*

	Bee	Wasp	Hornet
Biogenic Amines			
Histamine	X	X	X
Serotonin	O	X	X
Dopamine	X	X	O
Noradrenalin	X	X	O
Acetylcholine	O	O	X
Protein Polypeptide Toxins (Non-enzymatic)			
Melittin	X	O	O
Apamin	X	O	O
MCD peptide	X	O	O
Minimine	X	O	O
Kinins	O	wasp kinin	hornet kinin
Enzymes			
Phospholipase A	X	X	X
Phospholipase B	?	X	X
Hyaluronidase	X	X	—

* Derived from Haberman, E.: Bee and wasp venoms. *Science, 177:* 314, 1972.
An extensive survey has been reported by E. Haberman: *Ergeb Physiol, 60:* 220, 1968.

Table 12-II: SYNOPSIS OF SOME BIOCHEMICAL AND PHARMACOLOGICAL PROPERTIES OF BEE VENOM COMPONENTS*

	Histamine	Melittin	Apamin	MCD Peptide	Hyaluronidase	Phospholipase A
Content % (approx, dry venom)	0.1–1	50	2	2	1–3	12
Molecular weight	111	2,840	2,038	2,593	>20,000	14,500
Surface activity	0	++	?	?	0	0
General toxicity (mg/kg, mouse intravenously)	192–445	4	4	>40	0	7.5
Increase of capillary permeability	++	++	+	++	Indirectly	+
Pain production	++	++	?	?	0	?
Cellular damage	0	++	?	+	0	+
Neurotoxicity	0	+	++	+	0	0
"Direct" hemolysis	0	++	0	0	0	0
Indirect hemolysis	0	0	0	0	0	++
Circulatory effects	++	++	0	+	0	+
Neuromuscular effects	0	++	0	?	0	0
Smooth muscular effects	++	++	0	0	0	+
Ganglionic blockade	0	++	0	?	0	0
Histamine release	0	++	0	++	0	+
Thromboplastin inactivation	0	+	?	?	0	++
Spreading	0	0	0	0	++	0
Antigenicity	0	?	?	?	++	++

++ strong
+ significant
? not yet tested
0 not demonstrable

* Derived from Haberman, E.: Bee and wasp venoms. *Science*, 177: 314, 1972.

Histamine: The most predominant of the low molecular agents in bee venom with a concentration of 0.5 to 1.5 per cent. The histamine content of venom is perhaps only sufficient to cause a local reaction characterized by flaring and edema due to local dilatation of capillaries and arterioles, with ensuing increased permeability resulting in fluid escape that causes swelling at the site of the sting.

It is likely that the more severe pharmacological actions of histamine are induced by endogenous histamines released from organs and tissues involved in the allergic reaction induced by the venom. These include contraction of smooth muscle, especially of the bronchioles, the uterus and gall bladder; the stimulation of glands of external secretion and especially the gastric glands; increased capillary premeability leading to edema and generalized dilatation of vessels with a drop in blood pressure, even leading to shock.

Serotonin: (5-hydroxytryptamine) Serotonin is a common "sting agent" of plants and animals, so it is not surprising to find that it is a constituent of hymenoptera venom. Although the pharmacological actions of serotonin are chiefly contraction of smooth muscle and increased capilliary permeability, it is doubtful that the drug plays a very important role in the stings in man. Perhaps in invertebrates where the dosage may be more significant, it is of greater importance.

Dopamine and *noradrenalin*: recently identified as constituents of the bee and yellow jacket reservoirs *in vivo* but not of the secreted dried venom.

Acetylcholine: Hornet venom contains considerable amounts (about 5% dry weight). This is the most concentrated biological source of this amine. Acetylcholine produces vasodilatation, especially of the smaller blood vessels, with a resulting fall in blood pressure. It stimulates salivary, lacrimal and sweat glands. Acetylcholine produces pain. The combination of acetylcholine with histamine produces much more pain than would be expected from the simple addition of the individual components.

Melittin: the major component of beevenom (50% by weight). It causes local pain and inflammation. It is a powerful hemolysin and liberates histamine and serotonin from mast cells and thrombocytes. Melittin raises capillary permeability and blocks synaptic transmission. It causes smooth muscle contraction and may affect oxidative phosphorylation. Thus, melittin appears to have broad pharmacological activity. The LD 50 per kg of melittin revealed that it is a dialyzing basic peptide having a molecular weight of approximately 3,000, but apparently existing in solution as the tetramer.

Higginbotham and Karnella have reported that local tissue mast cells were found to rapidly secrete their heparin-containing granules in a dose-related response to subcutaneous injection of relatively small amounts of bee venom. The shed granules formed complexes with cationic protein *in vivo* and these complexes were subsequently ingested by adjacent mononuclear cells. Addition of heparin to bee venom *in vitro* resulted in the formation of complexes with reduction in both cytolytic and lethal activities of the venom. It is suggested that mast cell granules may, during transfer from mast cells to phagocytic cells, sequester noxious cationic proteins of bee venom and that dermal mast cells may thus be strategically situated and uniquely adapted to serve as a local means of resistance to bee sting.

Apamin: the smallest necrotoxic peptide known. Its mode of action as a neurotoxin is not known. Apamin raises vascular permeability of the rat cutis and affects the central nervous system in mice, rats and rabbits. The LD of apamin is approximately 4 mg/kg in mice and 2 mg/kg in rats. Death is preceded by extreme hyperexcitation and convulsions. Gel filtration studies revealed that apamin is of relatively low molecular weight—lower than melittin. Like melittin, apamin is strongly basic.

Mast Cell Degranulating (MCD) Peptide: MCD is only 1 to 2 per cent of bee venom. Depending upon the test system used, it is ten to one hundred times more active than melittin against rat mast cells. Both MCD and melittin contribute to the mastocytolysis of bee venom. MCD peptide is in the 48/80 class of substances.

Minimine: a small peptide with an undetermined function.

Kinins: Jacques and Schachter in a very comprehensive study of wasp venom, reported that they detected a slow-reacting substance which they labelled as kinin. This substance was a slower but powerful mediator that induced contraction of smooth muscle, lowering of arterial blood pressure, marked vasodilatation and increased permeability of vessels. Only the venom of *V. polistes* has been sufficiently purified for study. Suitable experiments with hornet kinin are still lacking.

Hyaluronidase: an enzyme which is known as a spreading factor, achieves its action by depolymerizing hyaluronic acid which results in lowering the viscosity of the normal connective tissue gel and in so doing destroys the normal tissue barriers. Without possessing local or systemic toxicity of its own, the enzyme opens the way for the other venomous constituents.

Phospholipase A: widely present in many animal venoms, so it is not surprising that this enzyme is a component in the venom of bees, wasps and hornets. Phospholipase A is capable of producing a series of pharmacological effects: contraction of smooth muscles, lowering of blood pressure with successive tachyphylaxis, increase of capillary permeability and destruction of mast cells. The most prominent actions are the modification of structure-bound enzymes or enzyme chains.

The hemolytic effect of the enzyme is based on the conversion of lecithin to lipolecithin, a powerful hemolytic substance. Whereas phospholipase A removes the unsaturated fatty acids, phospholipase B hydrolyzes both saturated and unsaturated acids from lecithin.

The complex nature of the venom creates very involved problems regarding both toxicity and allergenicity. It is not always possible to distinguish between a toxic response to the venom and an allergic reaction. The insect injects approximately 0.3 to 0.6 mg of venom with each sting, which is less than the LD_{50} for a mouse, and a dose that one would expect to be below the threshold of toxicity for a human. But recent studies on venoms by Elliot of the University of Buffalo indicate that even small amounts of venom may cause generalized reactions and even fatalities. This investigator postulates that in individuals who respond with violent reactions to small doses of venom, one of the following conditions may exist:

(1) A synergistic action of the various components of venom following injection.
(2) The activation of an enzyme system.
(3) The inhibition of enzymatic activity.
(4) An enzyme deficiency.

Size and extent of the reaction are not reliable differential indices to determine either toxicity or allergenicity. A small localized lesion, extensive involvement of an extremity or generalized and even fatal reactions may be either toxic or allergic in nature.

It is possible that the inability to differentiate between toxic and immunologic responses may explain the failure of many studies to correlate the immunologic findings with the clinical patterns observed.

The complexity of the venom creates a very intricate immunologic pattern indicated by the great number of antigens and antibodies observed by various investigators. Langlois, Shulman and Arbesman by the immunoelectrophoretic technique have detected nine antigens for bees, twelve to thirteen for wasps, and nine to ten for yellow jackets.

Although none of the antigens has been characterized nor the antibodies identified, the immunologic studies on hymenoptera extracts offer several clinical guidelines.

1. THE DISTRIBUTION OF ANTIGEN IN THE INSECT: Antigens are present in both the body of the insect and the venom. Shulman *et al.* who studied the sera from sting sensitive patients and beekeepers, reported that skin sensitizing antibodies were more frequent in

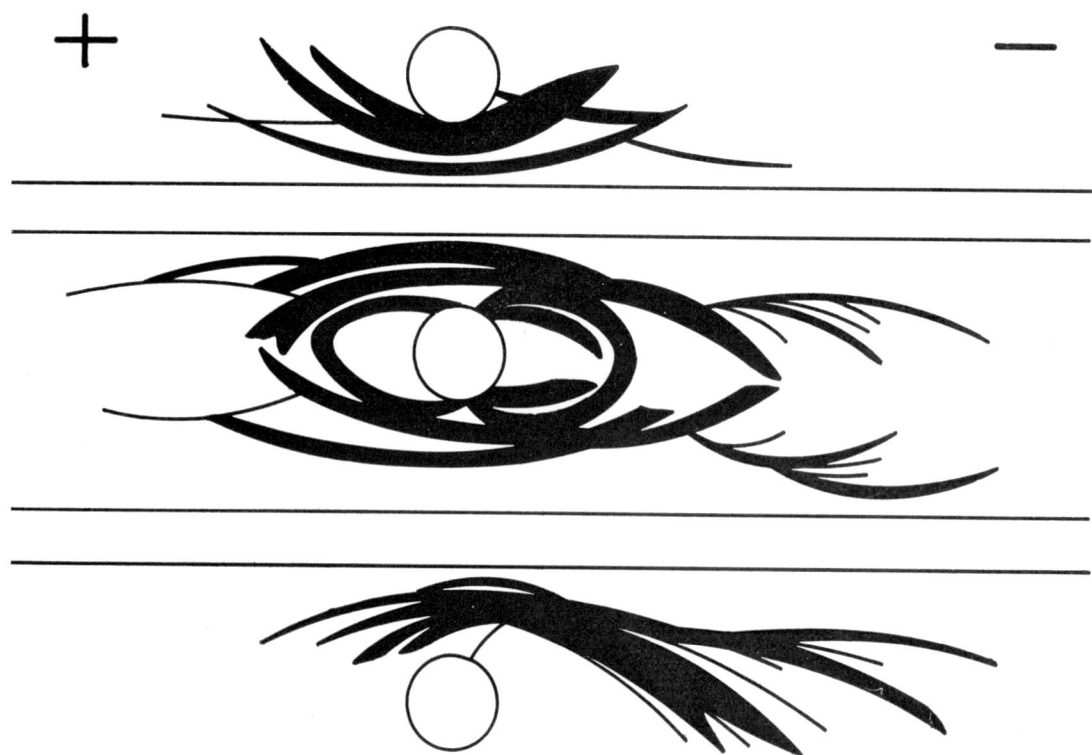

Figure 12-2. Immunoelectrophoretic pattern of bee venom illustrates the multiplicity of antibodies. (From Langlois, Shulman and Arbesman: The allergic response to stinging insects. III. The specificity of venom sac antigens. *J Allergy, 36*:109, 1965.)

sera of sting sensitive patients, while the beekeepers more frequently had antibodies against bee bodies.

2. THE PRESENCE OF SPECIFIC ANTIGEN IN THE VENOMS: It has been demonstrated that the insect venoms contain a specific antigen which is not found in the body of the insect. In addition, venom also has an antigen specific for the insect's body. The importance of this observation will be considered under hyposensitization.

3. THE PRESENCE OR ABSENCE OF CROSS REACTIVITY AMONG THE SPECIES: There have been many studies devoted to determining whether an individual sensitive to the sting of one insect may also be sensitive to other hymenopterous stings; and also to demonstrating whether or not the antigens and allergens derived from one species show immunological cross reactivity with those derived from heterologous species. Apart from the academic interest, the establishment of cross reactivity among hymenopterous insects is of great practical value. Often the identity of the stinging insect is obscure, but if cross reactivity indeed exists, hyposensitization should be achieved with preparations of any hymenopterous species. In addition, the scarcity of many species, particularly the wild insects, would not pose a problem if substitutes could be made with more readily available species.

Cross reactivity between wasp and yellow-jacket venoms has been demonstrated, while the honey bee venom does not react with either wasp or yellow-jacket.

4. THE VALUE OF SKIN TESTS IN STING SENSITIVE PATIENTS: There are several reports in the literature that indicate there is *no* correlation between skin testing and clinical hypersensitivity to hympenoptera stings. An individual with a strong reaction on skin

testing may offer a history of little or no response to stings, while individuals who fail to react on testing may experience violent constitutional responses. Some fatal cases have offered a history of no response on skin testing.

Passive transfer tests do not correlate with clinical reactions.

Skin testing is of no value for determining sensitivity to a specific insect.

Skin tests with specific extracts used for treatment can be reliably titrated for *tolerance* for the extract.

Clinical Patterns

The response of an individual to a hymenoptera sting may vary from a punctate lesion with a small surrounding area of pallor at the sting site to a generalized reaction with all the signs and symptoms of anaphylaxis which in some cases can lead to death within fifteen minutes.

Local Reaction: Immediately following the sting, intense burning pain is experienced at the site of the sting to be followed after several minutes by swelling and intense itching. The swelling may be localized to a few centimeters immediately surrounding the sting or the edema may involve an entire extremity or other segment of the body. With honey bee stings the stinger is usually *in situ* at the site of the sting. Edema usually subsides within twenty-four hours but in some cases it may persist for several days.

The local lesions may be soft and easily pitted upon pressure, or in some cases the localized edema may cause stretching of the skin, feel tense to the touch and resist pitting on pressure. Erythema of the involved area may be present, while with secondary infection, which is more common with yellow jacket and wasp stings, streaks of acute lymphangitis with some lymphadenopathy may develop.

When areas of loose tissue such as about the eyes and neck are involved, even a mild reaction may induce extensive involvement. Involvement of the soft tissues of the neck, by impinging upon the major airways may be a hazard to life.

Constitutional Reactions: Constitutional involvement may be mild and marked by a slight urticaria either near the site of the sting or at a remote area. Urticaria and edema which occur in proximity to the initial lesion but are not continuous with the primary lesion are indicative of a constitutional response.

The symptoms of more severe reactions are those of varying degrees of anaphylaxis which include:

massive edema and urticaria
generalized hot flush
severe dyspnea, cough and wheezing
tachycardia, hypotension
diarrhea
polyuria
collapse
loss of consciousness
death

Delayed Reactions: In some cases the reactions may be delayed for twenty-four hours or even longer following the sting. It is important to note that of fifty fatal cases reported by Barnard, 38 per cent had their onset of symptoms more than one hour following the sting, while 14 per cent of the fatalities developed symptoms more than twenty-four hours following the sting. The absence of an immediate reaction following the sting does not rule out the potential seriousness.

In some cases, the delayed response is characterized by serum sickness type of response with fever, arthralgia, urticaria and lymphadenopathy. With these symptoms an allergic mechanism is unquestioned. But the role of toxicity and hypersensitivity in each situation is not always clear. In view of the behavior of venoms as reported by Elliot and the lack of precise information concerning the immune response involved, it is not always possible to differentiate a toxic reaction from an allergic response.

Diagnosis and Identification

Unless the offending animal is seen, an absolute diagnosis of hymenoptera sting cannot be made. Stings may be induced by other arthropods such as scorpions, spiders, fire ants which also cause burning pain with itching, swelling and at times even urticaria at the site of the sting. The urticaria in these cases is considered to be a chemical response rather than an immunological reaction. It is likely that the response to stings of all animals other than hymenoptera is toxic which may explain the absence of reports of hypersensitivity reactions to the stings of animals that are not hymenoptera.

The problem of identification is complicated by the thousands of species of hymenoptera capable of inflicting stings. To attempt to classify them is not only impractical but almost impossible because of the difficulty in drawing distinction between the various divisions, and also because of the many exceptions that arise when classification is attempted. In allergy, only the social insects that nest in or about areas inhabited by humans are important. From a clinical standpoint it is probably correct to recognize two superfamilies, (1) bees, and (2) wasps.

(1) Bees
  (a) Honey bees—Apis: nest in artificial hives or natural hives in tree hollows, under floor boards, *etc.*
  (b) Bumble bees—Bombus: nest underground.
(2) Wasps
  (a) Polistes wasps: nest in tree branches or under eaves.
  (b) Hornet (Dolichovespula): football-shaped nests under eaves or on branches.
  (c) Yellow jacket (Vespula): nests underground.

Clinically, such a classification is practical since:

(1) Bees leave the venom sac *in situ* following the sting.
(2) Wasps do not lose the venom sac and induce multiple stings.
(3) Bee venom does not react with wasp.
(4) Various wasp venoms cross react.

Skin testing is not recommended as a diagnostic procedure for either determining hymenoptera sensitivity or for identification of the species. A negative skin test does not rule out the offending insect, while a positive skin response does not confirm the identity of the insect at fault. In addition, diagnostic skin test procedures carry the risk of inducing sensitivity to the insect.

Treatment

Emergency Treatment: With a history of a previous sting, epinephrine-HCl 1-1000 in doses of 0.4 cc by hypodermic should be administered as soon as possible following the sting. Since a previous mild reaction is no index to the severity of subsequent reactions, it is advisable to administer epinephrine to all patients with a history of previous sting. For epinephrine to be effective, it must be administered immediately, without waiting for the development of symptoms. Once the reaction is established, reversal is very difficult. If signs and symptoms develop following the initial dose, repeat the epinephrine within fifteen to twenty minutes.

Honey bees leave their stingers and venom sacs attached at the site of the sting. The stinger should be removed promptly and carefully, avoiding squeezing the venom sac. This can be accomplished by scraping motions with a knife blade, fingernail or tweezer. *Do not grasp* the venom sac between the fingers, as compression will inject additional venom.

Tourniquet: If a tourniquet is available, it can be helpful in slowing absorption of venom into the body, when the sting occurs on an extremity. Apply the tourniquet above the sting (between the sting and the body). Caution should be exercised so as not to apply the tourniquet too tightly. The pulse at the wrist or foot should be detectable while the tourniquet is in place. The tourniquet should be loosened every three to five minutes and discontinued entirely as symptoms are brought under control.

Cold compresses to the sting will also prevent rapid dissemination of toxin and in addition, offer some relief from the immediate burning and pain.

Antihistamines may be administered either orally or parenterally. Because of the slow onset of action of antihistamines, they should not be used as a substitute for epinephrine. Antihistamines can be helpful in controlling edema, especially when it occurs about the neck and becomes a threat to breathing.

Steroids are recommended for patients with severe edema or for those with signs of a constitutional response. (See steroid therapy in Chapter 15.)

Hyposensitization

There are no reliable criteria to indicate the effectiveness of hyposensitization. Neither the specific antigen nor the antibodies involved in the reaction can be identified. In spite of the lack of specific data concerning efficacy, hyposensitization for hymenoptera sensitivity is a generally accepted practice which is supported by favorable reports in the literature and particularly by the surveys of the Insect Allergy Committee of the American Academy of Allergy. These reports seem to indicate that hyposensitization with whole body extracts of hymenoptera is an effective procedure for either reducing the severity of reactions or preventing constitutional reactions.

Commercial extracts derived from either a single insect or a mixture of insects are available. It is important to obtain the extracts from a reputable firm.

The administration of extracts derived from a single insect is recommended. The only advantage of extracts from multiple insects is the decrease in the number of injections administered. The *advantages* of the single insect extract far outweigh *this* single factor.

(1) When the specific offender is identified, there is no indication for including other species in the hyposensitization program. Actually, such a procedure is contraindicated because of the risk of inducing sensitivity to other species.

(2) With a history of multiple sensitivity, extracts for each insect are preferable in order to regulate the dosage required for each specific insect. The patient may not react identically to each species, and by the same token his tolerance may vary from species to species. Extracts prepared from a single insect permit a more accurate tailoring of dosage to the specific needs of the patient.

(3) When the history of specificity is vague and the decision to hyposensitize is made, treatment with extracts from individual insects is again preferable to permit evaluation of tolerance to each individual insect. Hyposensitization is always recommended for patients who offer a history of a constitutional reaction no matter how mild.

It has been reported by Brown and Benton that patients who experience the serum sickness type of response will frequently *not tolerate* extracts at even very high dilutions.

Hyposensitization should be discontinued in any patient who manifests an adverse response, either severe local or constitutional signs and symptoms, following a reduction in dosage.

Procedure

Since extracts from hymenoptera are among the most potent antigens available, they should be respected and administered judiciously. It is always advisable to determine the patient's reactivity to the *extract* to be administered, by serial titration. This is performed as follows:

Provide the following dilutions of extract:

1 - 1,000,000,000 wgt/ml
1 - 100,000,000
1 - 10,000,000

1 - 1,000,000
1 - 100,000
1 - 10,000
1 - 1,000
1 - 100
1 - 10

Initial screening should be performed by a prick test technique (see Chapter 17 for skin testing) using 1-10 or 1-100 dilution. With a negative prick test, intradermal testing may be started with 1-1,000,000,000 dilution. For intradermal testing inject the smallest volume that will produce a small wheal. Never exceed 0.025 cc per single test. The test should be applied to either the arm or the forearm.

If after twenty minutes the test is negative, i.e. no flare and no wheal, the next dilution may be tested.

Proceed in this manner until a level of reactivity is reached. It will rarely be necessary to go beyond dilutions of 1-1,000,000 or 1-100,000. If patients fail to react, one must suspect (a) a weak or impotent antigen, or (b) the antigen is not suited to the patient's requirements. It is not advisable to complete more than three dilution tests a a single visit to avoid too rapid absorption of materials. An interval of twenty-four to forty-eight hours can be allowed between groups of tests. Do not extend the interval between tests beyond five days. The complete serial dilutions should be completed within three to four days.

When the reactivity of the patient is determined, the first dilution administered should be one or even two dilutions higher than the first level of reactivity. For example, if the serial test shows a patient reactive at the level of 1-1,000,000, start the treatment injection at 1-10,000,000 or even at 1-100,000,000. Injections should be administered at intervals of three to five days for dilution up to 1-100 and then at intervals of seven days. There are *no indices* to determine when to extend the *interval* between injections when the *undiluted* extract is being administered. Many programs advocate prolonging the interval between injections when full concentration is reached. Such a program has hazards. With *very* active extracts it is advisable not to exceed an interval of seven days. If treatment is interrupted, creating longer than seven day intervals, it is advisable to drop back to a higher dilution. If treatment has been interrupted for several months, it is advisable to repeat the serial dilution tests to determine the level of the patient's reactiviy.

There are no guidelines to determine when densensitization has been accomplished. An arbitrary period of two to three years for uninterrupted treatment is the program recommended by the Insect Allergy Committee of the American Academy of Allergy.

Some clinics administer extracts prepared from the avulsed venom sacs of the insects. This technique permits relating dosage to venom sacs, so that the physician is able to determine when the patient is receiving the equivalent of a whole venom sac. When the patient can tolerate the equivalent of two or even three venom sacs, it is reasonable to believe that he should tolerate a natural sting. As has been indicated, the antibodies detected in sera of sting sensitive patients are directed against the venom, while that of beekeepers is more frequently directed against the body of the insect. Since venom sac extract contains body antigens as well as higher concentration of venom antigens, it is the product of choice. Unfortunately, venom sacs extracts are not yet available commercially.

If during the course of treatment the patient experiences a sting with no reaction, it is usually safe to discontinue therapy. Such favorable responses to stings are rarely experienced before the patient has received injections for one year.

When a program of hyposensitization is instituted, the patient should be advised that protection cannot be expected for at least two years and in some cases, three years. For this reason he should exercise precaution

(1) to avoid hymenoptera stings, and (2) to provide himself with an emergency kit.

(1) To decrease the likelihood of stings:
avoid the use of perfume and colognes
avoid walking barefoot through grass and especially clover
avoid bright colored garments
if in proximity to insects, use an aerosol spray as a deterrent.

(2) The Emergency Kit
Several types of emergency kits are available commercially.

These contain adrenalin in a sterile syringe and an antihistamine. Such kits are useful, but the patient can provide himself equally well with a bottle of 1-1,000 adrenalin and a few sterile disposable syringes with needles attached. A tourniquet and antihistamine tablet may also be included if a kit is improvised.

Immediately following the sting the patient should receive at least 0.4 cc of epinephrine, and apply the tourniquet if possible. The application of cold compresses is helpful. The antihistamine drug should be taken following the injection of epinephrine.

Upon completion of emergency first aid procedures, professional assistance should be sought from the nearest clinic, hospital or physician.

URTICATING (STINGING) HAIRS AND SPINES

The present state of knowledge regarding the urticating hairs and spines of lepidopterous larvae (caterpillars of butterflies and moths) is not decisive regarding their true venomous nature, but the observations reported permit a classification of responses based upon allergic and nonallergic responses.

(1) Hairs and spines of some species contain proteinaceous substances which can serve as antigens to induce hypersensitivity reactions. These reactions manifest all the signs and symptoms of the allergic response including both local erythema, edema (whealing) and systemic responses.

(2) Local reactions characterized by erythema, vesiculation, urticaria, swelling and burning pain at the site of contact, may be secondary to (a) mechanical action of the hairs and spines as observed with the fibers of glass wool, and (b) chemical irritation of constituents in the hairs and spines. These chemicals are not true venoms, and may actually be a structural constituent of the hair or spine.

The type of response varies with the species, and in the case of allergic reactions, with sensitivity of the individual. This can explain the great variety of responses reported for urticating hairs and spines.

ARTHROPODS AS INHALANTS

There are numerous clinical reports that indicate that arthropods and arthropod parts frequently play an important role in respiratory allergy. With the presence of millions of arthropods per acre of surface soil, the presence of substances derived from them in soil dust is not surprising. The identification and characterization of these various soil constituents contributed by arthropods is a very formidable and complex problem which can be appreciated from the fact that the class Insecta, only one of five of the phylum Arthropoda, constitutes between 65,000 to 1,500,000 insect species (according to Saborsky, 1952).

As early as 1913 Wilson incriminated the May fly (Ephemera) as a cause of asthma. Following Parlato's studies (1929, 1930, 1932) on caddis fly (order Trichoptera) the role of insects and insect parts as etiologic agents in respiratory allergy found wider recognition. An increased number of reports soon appeared in the literature which, in addition to the May fly and caddis fly, implicated a wide variety of arthropods.

Arthropod Species Which May Serve As A Source of Antigenic Material

I. Class Insecta
Coleoptera—beetles, weevils

Lepidoptera—moths, butterflies
Hymenoptera—honey bees, hornets, wasps, yellow jackets
Diptera—flies, mosquitoes
Orthoptera—grasshoppers, locusts, cockroaches
Hemiptera—box elder bugs, squash bugs
Ephenoptera—May flies
Trichoptera—caddis flies
Neuroptera—lacewings
Homoptera—aphids, leafhoppers, cicadas, scales
Thysanura—silverfish
II. Class Arachnida
Aranea—spiders
Acarina—mites and ticks
III. Class Crustacea
Isopoda—sowbugs
Branchiopoda—Daphnia, fairy shrimp
IV. Class Myriopoda
Chilopoda—centipedes
Diplopoda—millipedes
V. Class Crustacea
Copepoda—plankton, shrimp

In most instances the reports were concerned with a single species as the etiologic agent of either allergic rhinitis, hay fever of asthma. The diagnosis was usually aided by skin tests, ophthalmic tests and by passive transfer tests with patiest's sera, using extracts of the insect as antigens. Reactions to these tests indicated that an allergen was present in these extracts. In most instances the extracts for both testing and treatment of patients were prepared from the whole body of the insect. In several cases, insect parts or even excreta were used for the preparation of extracts. The seasonal increase in the number of insects, at times even in swarms (as exemplified by the caddis fly and the May fly) served as additional support for the clinical reports of seasonal hay fever and asthma attributed to arthropods. This was particularly significant when other seasonal factors, such as pollens could not be incriminated as the etiologic agents.

There are a number of studies reporting cross reactivity among various species, and at times even between taxonomically unrelated arthropods. No doubt cross reactivity, such as is observed with pollen allergens, may be present, but the role of contamination as a contributing factor must be considered in almost every study. In his own studies, Pruzansky raises the possibility of common bacterial associates as a source of common antigens. There are additional considerations regarding the possibility of the presence of contaminants in the insect extracts used for study and at times for treatment. The method for obtaining the arthropod material can be a very important determining factor. Most studies were conducted with wild insects. It is conceivable that many elements in the environment could serve to contaminate the extract, either through coating the individual animal or by their ingestion of materials from the environment.

In the case of a biting insect such as the bed bug, which has been reported as a source of inhalant allergen (Steinberg, 1929), the blood meal could be a contaminating factor. In the case of inhalant allergy caused by the mushroom fly *(Aphiochaeta agarica)* reported by Keen (1938), it would be important to consider manure as a source of contamination. The house fly, which Jamieson (1938) reported as a cause of allergy could certainly carry many contaminants. The Indian meal moth *(Plodia interpunctella)* which was implicated by Wittich (1940) as a cause of allergy may have been contaminated with mill dust in which it lives, and in the reports by the same investigator in allergic reactions to the Mexican bean weevil *(Zabrotes subfasciates)* bean dust as a possible contaminant must be considered. Almost every report suggests some possible environmental contaminant which could serve to explain the wide range of cross reactivity to arthropod extracts demonstrated by skin testing and other immunologic techniques.

Arthropod parts, serving as inhalant antigens to produce skin reactivity, may serve to complicate the diagnostic problem when skin testing with hymenoptera extracts. The anitbodies attributed to the various allergens derived from arthropods have been demonstrated *in vitro* and belong to the nonreaginic type of humoral antibodies. Inhalant allergy is induced by IgE class of humoral antibodies, which until recently were not demonstrated by *in vitro* procedures. The identification of IgE as a separate class of antibody will permit the development of more refined immunologic techniques, which may serve to resolve many of the concepts regarding arthropods in inhalant allergic disease, which at the present time are still mainly speculative, based upon circumstantial evidence.

Silk

The antigenicity of silk has been well demmonstrated by the studies of Cebra (1961). In view of the widespread distribution of silk throughout the arthropod world, and because of its varied application in daily life, silk is a substance that deserves serious consideration as an inhalant factor in allergic disease.

Mites

Mites are arachnids, which are receiving considerable attention as a possible inhalant factor in allergic disease because of their high incidence and distribution in house dust. There is no question about the presence of mites almost universally in house dust, but the role of these animals in inhalant allergy is subject to the same problems confronted in resolving the role of any arthropod in inhalant allergic disease. The development of pure cultures of mites is confronted with many problems. A pure mite culture will provide a controlled source of antigenic material which can serve to demonstrate specific antibodies related to clinical patterns. This will permit the evaluation of treatment with antigens derived from mites. Until such information is available, it is reasonable to believe that the various dust extracts available will contain components derived from mites, which may have therapeutic benefits when routinely administered as house dust extracts.

THE IMPORTED FIRE-ANT
(Solenopsis Saevissima Richteri)

The name "fire-ant" is derived from the painful sting induced by this insect.

The fire-ant *(Solenopsis Saevissima Richteri)* made its entrance into the United States from South America, at the port of Mobile, Alabama, where they were first noticed in 1918. However, because of their similarity to the domestic species of ant, the spread of the fire-ant throughout the southern states was overlooked until about 1930. Due to the inability of insecticides and control measures to contain these insects within the already infested areas, they are spreading toward California and are becoming an important economic and health problem.

A species of fire-ant or red ant *(Solenopsis geminata)* has been reported from Hawaii. This ant can induce a painful sting which can lead to anaphylaxis.

The fire ants are found in pasture lands but are particularly concentrated in row lands, e.g. cotton, corn and sorghum. At times, homes may become infested, where they feed upon meats, butter, cheese and nuts. Occasionally, the ants gnaw holes into clothing.

The ants produce grass-covered mounds which can vary in size from an average of about eighteen to thirty-six inches in diameter and height.

Five types of adult ants have been reported, which range in length from one-eighth to one-fourth inch. The commonest species is dark brown, almost black, with a honey-colored band across the mid-dorsum of the abdomen of the larger workers and the females. At times the color may be reddish-tan. In New Orleans, where they are more nearly red, the insects are called "red ants."

MacConnell *et al.* have reported the actions of the fire-ant toxin to be:

(1) A potent necrotoxin
(2) A pronounced hemolytic agent
(3) Phytotoxic
(4) Insecticidal
(5) Antibiotic

In order to study the evolution of the sting reaction and its histopathology, Caro, Derbes and Jung enlisted volunteers who permitted themselves to be stung by the ants. The following discussion draws freely upon the details reported by these investigators.

The Sting Reaction

Initially, the ant fixes itself to its assailant by pinching a small amount of skin with its mandibles and raises it slightly which produces a definite sensation of pain, even before the insertion of the stinger. The pain is reported as less severe than that following the sting of the bee or wasp. The ant then arches its back and proceeds to jab its stinger, often repeatedly, into the elevated peduncle of skin. This clustering of stings is helpful in diagnosis.

At the sting site, there is an almost immediate appearance of a 25 to 30 mm flare. Within a minute of the appearance of the flare, a wheal develops which can range from two to ten millimeters in diameter. The wheal persists for about one hour, to be supplanted within sixty to ninety minutes by small prominences, which after four hours are recognized as small superficial vesicles containing a thin, clear fluid. The fluid either escapes by rupture of the vesicles or dries to form crusts. Following an additional eight to ten hours, a cloudy vesicular fluid is noted which soon becomes purulent. After twenty-four hours, the sting sites are slightly umbilicated pustules, surrounded by either a narrow red halo or a large, extremely edematous painful area. In one subject under observation the area of involvement was eleven by seven centimeters. The lesion in this patient was edematous, firm and painful, while the pustules themselves were pruritic. Similar large uncomfortable areas of involvement are frequently seen clinically. The pustule remains for three to ten days, then ruptures with crust formation. Cultures of the pustules are sterile. Pigmented macules may persist for days, particularly on the lower extremities, while scar formation is common. Fibrotic nodules about two to three millimeters in diameter may be noted, especially in older persons. At the sites of the ant stings, and particularly over the lower extremities, patches of persistent eczematoid dermatitis may develop. These may be secondary to the irritation of scratching.

Features of the histopathology of the reaction to the fire-ant sting are the early appearance of intracellular edema in the epidermis, the early necrosis in the upper corium, the constant development of pustules at the site of the sting and the great degree and depth of necrosis beneath the pustule. The histopathologic changes are not the type generally seen following other insect stings or bites. The consistent formation of pustules is a differentiating feature, while the presence of tissue necrosis leads to scar formation. The sting of the mud dauber wasp may on occasion be followed by secondary infection with pustule formation. However, this is not a constant sequel as observed with the sting of the fire-ant.

Signs and Symptoms

The signs and symptoms of fire-ant stings are both local and systemic.

The local changes include the immediate punctum induced by the sting, usually in clusters; the flare and wheal followed by the pustule. All these lesions are both painful and pruritic.

It is likely that the flare and wheal are induced by an allergic response which would imply previous exposure for sensitization. This is supported by the progressive increase in size of the flare and wheal response following repeated exposure. The pustules which are an expression of the necrotoxic action of the venom are usually constant in size.

Mild fever of twenty-four to forty-eight hours duration, accompanied by severe apprehension, nausea and throbbing in the temples may usher in the systemic reaction. Systemic reactions include generalized prurutus, large plaques of urticarial wheals and angio-edema of varying degree, involving the eyelids, the tongue, face, neck and throat. Swelling of the eyes may interfere with vision, while the swollen tongue may protrude and interfere with deglutition. Salivation may be an accompaniment.

Angio-edema may be extensive over the face, causing distortion of the features, while swelling of the pharynx can interfere with breathing and even threaten life.

Although precordial anginal pain may be present, the pulse is not necessarily accelerated. Bronchial asthma has been reported as well as extreme shock with hypotension and cyanosis.

Treatment

Because of the necrotizing nature of the local sting reaction, topical therapy is not successful.

The systemic reactions which are similar to the reactions observed with other stings of hymenoptera, calls for identical therapeutic measures. These include the immediate hypodermic administration of epinephrine-HCl 1-1000; antihistamines, either orally or parenterally; corticosteroids and when shock develops, the necessary supportive procedures (see above the treatment of reactions to hymenoptera stings).

Extracts† of fire-ants for immunotherapy are available. The only reported experience with these extracts is that of Triplett who treated eighteen patients from 1962 to 1971. The sample of patients included eight children under four years of age, four older children, three adolescents, and three adults. Injections were administered either weekly or biweekly for periods up to two years or more. The results of this observer are listed in Table 12-IV.

Since the necrotic lesions are a nonimmunologic response, they should not be influenced by injection therapy.

Table 12-IV: FIRE-ANT SENSITIVITY: RESULTS OF TREATMENT‡

Status of Treatment	No. of Patients	No. Re-stung	No. with Reactions
Completed two years	6	5	0
Presently on treatment	9	3	0
Discontinued before completion	3	0 (one unknown)	0

‡ Reproduced with permission from Triplett, R. Faser: *Imported Fire-Ant Sensitivity: Successful Treatment with Immunotherapy.* 1970. To be published.

Table 12-III: GENERALIZED SYMPTOMS FOLLOWING FIRE-ANT STINGS IN EIGHTEEN SENSITIVE PATIENTS*

Symptom	Number	Percentage
Generalized urticaria	15	84
Generalized angio-edema	14	78
Respiratory symptoms	9	50
wheezing	5	31
coughing	2	11
"couldn't talk"	2	11
difficulty in breathing	1	5
choking	2	11
hoarseness	1	5
tightness in chest	1	5
Gastrointestinal symptoms (nausea and vomiting)	2	11
Shock symptoms	3	16
fall in blood pressure	1	5
cyanosis and collapse	1	5
unconsciousness	1	5

* Reproduced with permission from Triplett, R. Faser: *Imported Fire-Ant Sensitivity: Successful Treatment with Immunotherapy.* 1970. To be published.

REFERENCES

Biting Insects

1. Allen, A. C.: Persistent "insect bites" (dermal eosinophilic granulomas) simulating lymphoblastomas, histocytoses, and squamous cell carcinomas. *Am J Pathol, 24:* 367, 1948.
2. Allen, J. R.: *Some Properties of Oral Secretion of Mosquitoes.* Doctoral thesis, Queen's University, Kingston, Ontario, 1964.
3. Allen, J. R. and West, A. S.: Recent advances in studies on reactions to mosquito bites. In Corradetti, A.: *Proceedings of the International Congress of Parasitoly, 1st, Rome, 1964.* Pergammon Pr, 1964, vol. 2, pp. 1091–1092.
4. Arean, V. M. and Fox, I.: Dermal alterations in

† Available from Hollister-Stier Laboratories.

severe reactions to bites of the sandfly *Culicoides furens*. *Am J Clin Pathol, 25:* 1359, 1955.
5. Benjamini, E.: The immunochemistry of flea bite hypersensitivity. In Corradetti, A.: *Proceedings of the International Congress of Parasitology, 1st, Rome, 1964.* Pergamon Pr, 1964, vol. 2, p. 1090.
6. Benjamini, E., Feingold, B. F. and Kartman, L.: Allergy to flea bites. III. The experimental induction of flea bite sensitivity in guinea pigs by exposure to flea bites and by antigen prepared from whole extracts of *Ctenocephalides felis felis*. *Exp Parasitol, 10:* 214, 1960a.
7. Benjamini, E., Feingold, B. F. and Kartman, L.: Antigenic property of the oral secretion of fleas. *Nature, 188:* 959, 1960b.
8. Benjamini, E., Feingold, B. F. and Kartman, L.: Skin reactivity in guinea pigs sensitized to flea bites. The sequence of reactions. *Proc Soc Exp Biol Med, 108:* 700, 1961.
9. Benjamini, E., Feingold, B. F., Young, J. D., Kartman, L. and Shimizu, M.: Allergy to flea bites. IV. In vitro collection and antigenic properties of the oral secretion of the cat flea, *Ctenocephalides felis felis* (Bouche). *Exp Parasitol 13:* 143, 1963a.
10. Benjamini, E., Feingold, B. F. and Kartman, L.: The physiological and biochemical role of the host's skin in the induction of flea bite hypersensitivity. I. Preliminary studies with guinea pig skin following exposure to bites of cat fleas. *Exp Parasitol, 14:* 75, 1963b.
11. Benson, R. L.: Diagnosis and treatment of sensitization to mosquitoes. *J Allergy, 8:* 47, 1936.
12. Boycott, A. E.: The reaction of flea bites. *J Pathol, 17:* 110, 1913.
13. Brown, A., Griffiths, T. H. D., Erwin, S. and Dyrenforth, L. Y.: Arthus phenomenon from mosquito bites. *South Med J, 31:* 590, 1938.
14. Cavanaugh, D. C. and Randall, R.: The role of multiplication of *Pasteurella pestis* in mononuclear phagocytes in the pathogenesis of flea-borne plague. *J Immunol, 83:* 348, 1959.
15. Cherney, L. S., Wheeler, C. M. and Reed, A. C.: Flea-antigen in prevention of flea bites. *Am J Trop Med Hyg, 19:* 327, 1939.
16. Cornwall, J. and Patton, W.: Some observations on the salivary secretions of the common blood sucking insect and ticks. *Indian J Med Res, 2:* 569, 1914.
17. De Meillon, B.: The relationship between ectoparasite and host. IV. Host reactions to the bites of arthropods. *The Leech,* 43–46, August 1949.
18. Dienes, L. and Mallory, T. B.: Histologic studies of hypersensitive reactions. *Am J Pathol, 8:* 689, 1932.
19. Dubin, N., Reese, J. D. and Seamans, L. A.: Attempt to produce protection against mosquitoes by active immunization. *J Immunol, 58:* 293, 1948.
20. Feingold, B. F.: Clinical and immunological aspects of hypersensitivity to flea bites. In Corradetti, A.: *Proc Intern Congr Parasitol, 1st, Rome, 1964.* Pergamon Press, 1964, vol 2, pp. 1089–1090.
21. Feingold, B. F. and Benjamini, E.: Allergy to flea bites: Clinical and experimental observations. *Ann Allergy, 19:* 1275, 1961.
22. Feingold, B. F., Benjamini, E. and Shimizu, M.: Induction of delayed and immediate types of skin reactivity in Guinea pigs by variation in dosages of antigens. *Ann Allergy, 22:* 279, 1964.
23. Feingold, B. F., Benjamini, E. and Michaeli, D.: The allergic responses to insect bites. *Ann Rev Entomol, 13:* 137, 1968.
24. Fox, I. and Berman, N. S.: A preliminary report on biting mosquitoes in Puerto Rico together with some experimental work on natural and acquired sensitivity of man to insect bites. *Biol Assoc Med Puerto Rico, 52:* 89, 1960.
25. Goldman, L.: Parasitic infections of the skin. *Pediatr Clin North Am, 3:* 625, 1956.
26. Goldman, L.: Tick bite granuloma: Failure of prevention of lesion by excision of tick bite area. *Am J Trop Med Hyg, 12:* 246, 1963.
27. Goldman, L., Johnson, P. and Ramsey, J.: The insect bite reaction. I. The mechanism. *J Invest Dermatol, 18:* 403, 1952.
28. Goldman, L., Rockwell, E. and Richfield, D. F.: Histopathological studies on cutaneous reactions to the bites of various arthropods. *Am J Trop Med Hyg, 1:* 514, 1925.
29. Gordon, R. M. and Crewe, W.: The mechanism by which mosquitoes and tsetse flies obtain their blood meal, the histology of the lesion produced, and the subsequent reactions of the mammalian host; together with some observations on the feeding of *Chrysops* and *Cimex*. *Ann Trop Med Parasitol, 42:* 334, 1948.
30. Hartman, M. M.: Flea bite reactions. Clinical and experimental observations and effect of histamine-azoprotein therapy. *Ann Allergy, 4:* 131, 1946.
31. Hase, A.: Weitere Beobachtungen uber die Lauseplage. *Zentralbl Bakteriol [Natur Wiss], 77:* 153, 1916.
32. Hatoff, A.: Densensitization to insect bites. *JAMA, 130:* 850, 1946.
33. Hecht, O.: Die Hautreaktionen auf Insektenstiche als allergische Erscheinungen. *Arch Shiffs Tropenhyg, 33:* 364, 1929.
34. Hecht, O.: Hautreaktionen auf die Stiche blutsaugender Insekten und Milben als allergische

Erscheinungen. *Zentralbl Haut- und Geschlechtskrank, 44:* 241, 1933.

35. Hecht, O.: Las reacciones da la piel contra las picaduras de insectos como fenomenos alergicos. *Rev Sanid Asist Soc, 8:* 945, 1943.
36. Heilesen, B.: Studies on mosquito bites. *Acta Allergol (Kbh), 2:* 245, 1949.
37. Hindle, E.: *Flies in Relation to Disease. Blood Sucking Flies.* New York, Cambridge U Pr, 1914.
38. Hudson, A., Bowman, L. and Orr, C. W. M.: Effect of absence of saliva on blood feeding by mosquitoes. *Science, 131:* 1730, 1960.
39. Hudson, A., McKiel, J. A., West, A. S. and Bourns, T. K. R.: Reaction to mosquito bites. *Mosquito News, 18:* 249, 1958.
40. Hudson, B. W., Feingold, B. F. and Kartman, L.: Allergy to flea bites. I. Experimental induction of flea-bite sensitivity in guinea pigs. *Exp Parasitol, 9:* 18, 1960.
41. Hudson, B. W., Feingold, B. F. and Kartman, L.: Allergy to flea bites. II. Investigations of flea bite sensitivity in humans. *Exp Parasitol, 9:* 151, 1960.
42. Kartman, L.: Insect allergy and arthropod-borne infection: A hypothesis. In Corradetti, A.: *Proc Intern Congr Parasitol, 1st, Rome, 1964.* Pergamon Press, 1964, pp. 1092–1093.
43. Kartman, L.: Insect allergy and arthropid-borne infection: A hypothesis. *Zoonoses Res, 00:* 000, 1965.
44. Kemper, H.: Beobachtungen über den Stech-und Saugakt der Bettwanze und seine Wirkung auf die menschliche Haut. *Z Desinfekt, 21:* 61, 1929.
45. Kissileff, A.: The dog flea as a causative agent in summer eczema. *J Am Vet Med Assoc, 46:* 21, 1938.
46. Kissileff, A.: Relationship of dog fleas to dermatitis. *Small Animal Clin, 2:* 132, 1962.
47. Larrivee, D. H., Benjamini, E., Feingold, B. F. and Shimizu, M.: Histologic studies of guinea pig skin: Different stages of allergic reactivity to flea bites. *Exp Parasitol, 15:* 491, 1964.
48. Lawlor, W. K.: *Immunological Studies of Antigens Extracted from Mosquitoes and Their Application in Taxonomy.* Doctoral thesis, Sch. of Hygiene and Public Health, Johns Hopkins Univ., Baltimore, Md., 1949.
49. Lester, H. M. O. and Lloyd, L.: Notes on the process of digestion in tsetse flies. *Bull Entomol Res, 19:* 39, 1928.
50. Manalang, C.: Origin of the irritating substance in mosquito bite. *Phillippine J Sci, 46:* 39, 1931.
51. McIvor, B. C. and Cherney, L. S.: Studies in insect bite desensitization. *Am J Trop Med, 21:* 493, 1941.
52. McIvor, B. C. and Cherney, L. S.: Clinical use of flea-antigen in patients hypersensitive to flea bites. *Am J Trop Med, 23:* 377, 1943.
53. McKiel, J. A.: *Reactions to Mosquito Bites. Studies of Causation and Remedial Measures.* Doctoral thesis, Queen's Univ., Kingston, Ontario, 1955.
54. McKiel, J. A.: Sensitization to mosquito bites. *Can J Zool, 37:* 341, 1959.
55. McKiel, J. A. and Clunie, J. C.: Chromatographic fractionation of the nondialyzable portion of mosquito extract and intracutaneous reactions of mosquito bite-sensitive subjects to the separated components. *Can J Zool, 38:* 479, 1960.
56. McKiel, J. A. and West, A. S.: Nature and causation of insect bite reactions. *Pediatr Clin North Am, 8:* 795, 1961.
57. McKiel, J. A. and West, A. S.: Effects of repeated exposures of hypersensitive humans and laboratory rabbits to mosquito antigens. *Can J Zool, 39:* 597, 1961.
58. Mellanby, K.: Man's reaction to mosquito bites. *Nature, 158:* 554, 1946.
59. Metcalf, R. L.: The physiology of the salivary glands of *Anopheles quadrimaculatus. J Natl Malaria Soc, 4:* 271, 1945.
60. Michaeli, D., Benjamini, E., Young, J. D. and Feingold, B. F.: Biochemical studies on hypersensitivity to flea bites. In Freeman, P.: *Int Congr Entomol, 12th.* London, 1965, p. 832.
61. Michaeli, D., Benjamini, E., de Buren, F. P., Larrivee, D. H. and Feingold, B. F.: The role of collagen in the induction of flea bite hypersensitivity. *J Immunol, 95:* 162, 1965.
62. Michaeli, D., Benjamini, E., Miner, R. C. and Feingold, B. F.: *In vitro* studies on the role of collagen in the induction of hypersensitivity to flea bites. *J Immunol, 97:* 402, 1966.
63. Moore, W. and Hirschfelder, A. D.: An investigation on the louse problem. *Res Publ Univ Minnesota, 7.* (Minneapolis, Minnesota, 1919).
64. More, E. S.: Acquired immunity from insect stings. *Nature, 55:* 533, 1897.
65. Muller, G. H.: Flea allergy dermatitis. *Small Animal Clin, 1,* June 1961.
66. Orr, C. W. M., Hudson, A. and West, A. S.: The salivary glands of *Aedes aegypti.* Histological-histochemical studies. *Can J Zool, 39:* 265, 1961.
67. Perlman, F.: Insect allergens as injectants. Severe reactions to bites and stings of arthropods. *Calif Med, 96:* 1, 1962.
68. Rockwell, E. M. and Johnson, P.: The insect bite reaction. II. Evolution of the allergic reaction. *J Invest Dermatol, 19:* 137, 1952.
69. Roxburgh, A. C.: The treatment of insect bites and stings. *Lancet, 212:* 1146, 1927.
70. Theodor, O.: A study of the reaction of *Phlebotomus*

bites with some remarks on "harara." *Trans R Soc Trop Med Hyg, 29:* 273, 1935.
71. Usinger, R. L.: Monograph of Cimicidae. *Entomol Soc Am Thomas Say Found, 7:* 585, 1966.
72. Wilson, A. B. and Clements, A. N.: The nature of the skin reaction to mosquito bites in laboratory animals. *Int Arch Allergy Appl Immunol, 26:* 294, 1965.
73. Wood, S. F.: Reactions of man to the feeding of reduviid bugs. *J Parasitol, 28:* 43, 1942.
74. Young, J. D., Benjamini, E., Feingold, B. F. and Noller, H.: Allergy to flea bites. V. Preliminary results of fractionation characterization, and assay for allergenic activity of material derived from the oral secretion of the cat flea, *Ctenocephalides felis felis. Exp Parasitol, 13:* 155, 1963.

Triatoma

1. Arnold, H. L. and Bell, D. B.: Kissing bug bites. *Hawaii Med J, 3:* 121, 1944.
2. Balzac, J.: Anaphylactic phenomena caused by Triatoma bite. An Insti Med Req. *Univ Nac Tucumán, 3:* 35, 1950.
3. Jones, J. P.: *Public health significance of Triatoma protracta uhler in Sierra Nevada foothill areas.* State of California Department of Public Health, Bureau of Vector Control, Bulletin 70, 1961.
4. Packchanian, A.: Infectivity of Texas strain of *Trypanosoma cruzi* to man. *Am J Trop Med, 23:* 309, 1943.
5. Shields, T. L. and Walsh, E. N.: "Kissing bug" bite. *Arch Dermatol, 74:* 14, 1956.
6. Usinger, R. L.: Triatominae of North and Central America and the West Indies and their public health significance. *Pub Health Bull, 288,* 1944.
7. Wood, F. D.: Natural and experimental infection of *Triatoma protracta uhler* and mammals in California and American human trypanosomiasis. *Am J Trop Med, 14:* 497, 1934.
8. Wood, S. F.: Reactions of man to the feeding of reduviid bugs. *J Parasitol, 28:* 43, 1947.

Hymenoptera

1. Arbesman, C. E., Langlois, C. and Shulman, S.: The allergic response to stinging insects. IV. Cross reactions between bee, wasp, and yellow jacket. *J Allergy, 36:* 147, 1965.
2. Barnard, J. H.: Severe hidden delayed reactions from insect stings. *N Y J Med, 66:* 1206, 1966.
3. Barnard, J. H.: Allergic and pathologic findings in fifty insect sting fatalities. *J Allergy, 40:* 107, 1967.
4. Benjamini, E. and Feingold, B. F.: Immunity to arthropods. *Immunity to Parasitic Animals, 2:* 1601, 1970.
5. Benson, R. L. and Semenov, H.: Allergy in its relation to bee sting. *J Allergy, 1:* 105, 1930.
6. Bernton, H. S. and Brown, H.: Studies on hymenoptera. I. Skin reactions of normal persons to honeybee (*Apis mellifera*) extract. *J Allergy, 36:* 315, 1965.
7. Crewe, M. and Gordon, R. M.: The histology of the lesions caused by the sting of the hive-bee (*Apis mellifica*). *Ann Trop Med Parasitol, 43:* 341, 1949.
8. Feinberg, A. R., Feinberg, S. M. and Benaim-Pinto, C.: Asthma and rhinitis from insect allergens. I. Clinical importance. *J Allergy, 27:* 437, 1956.
9. Feingold, B. F.: Allergic reactions to hymenoptera stings. *J Asthma Research, 9:* 55, 1971.
10. Foubert, E. L. and Stier, R. A.: Antigenic relationships between honeybees, wasps, yellow hornets, black hornets, and yellow-jackets. *J Allergy, 29:* 13, 1958.
11. Haberman, B.: Bee and wasp venoms: The biochemistry of their peptides and enzymes are reviewed. *Science, 177:* 314, 1972.
12. Haberman, E. and El-Karemi, M. M. A.: Antibody formation by protein components of bee venom. *Nature, 178:* 1349, 1956.
13. Higginbotham, R. D. and Karnella, S.: The significance of the mast cell response to bee venom. *J Immunol, 106:* 233, 1970.
14. Kailin, L. W.: Interim report of the committee on insect allergy. *J Allergy, 36:* 190, 1965.
15. Langlois, C., Shulman, S. and Arbesman, C. E.: The allergic response to stinging insects. III. The specificity of venom sac antigens. *J Allregy, 36:* 109, 1965.
16. Loveless, M. D.: Sudden death from insect venom allergy reported often mistaken for coronary. *Medical Tribune,* Sept. 5, 1960.
17. Loveless, M. D.: Immunization in wasp-stings allergy through venom-repositories and periodic insect stings. *J Immunol, 89:* 204, 1962.
18. Loveless, M. D.: Antibody of atopy and serum disease in man. In Elliott, H. W., Cutting, W. S. and Dreisbach, R. H. (Eds.): *Annual Review of Pharmacology.* Palo Alto, Annual Reviews Inc, 1966, vol. 6, pp. 309–326.
19. Loveless, M. H. and Fackler, W. R.: Wasp venom allergy and immunity. *Ann Allergy, 14:* 347, 1956.
20. Mohammed, A. H. and El-Karemi, M. M. A.: Immunity of bee keepers to some constituents of bee venom: Phospholipase-A antibodies. *Nature, 189:* 837, 1961.

21. Mueller, H. L.: Insect allergy. In Samter, M. (Ed.): *Immunological Diseases*. Boston, Little, 1965, pp. 682–689.
22. Perlman, F.: Insects as inhalant allergens. *J Allergy, 29:* 302, 1958.
23. Perlman, F.: Insect allergens: Their interrelationship and differences. *J Allergy, 32:* 93, 1961.
24. Perlman, F.: Insect allergens as injectants. Severe reactions to bites and stings of arthropods. *Calif Med, 96:* 1, 1962.
25. Perlman, F.: Arthropods as causes of allergy. In Harris, M. C. and Shure, N. (Eds.): *Sensitivity Chest Diseases*. Philadelphia, F. A. Davis, 1964, pp. 157–168.
26. Schwartz, H. J.: Skin sensitivity in insect allergy. *JAMA, 194:* 113, 1965.
27. Shulman, S.: Allergic responses to insects. In Smith, R. F. and Mittler, T. E. (Eds.): *Annual Review of Entomology*. Palo Alto, Annual Reviews Inc, 1967, vol. 12, pp. 323–346.
28. Waterhouse, A. T.: Bee sting anaphylaxis. *Lancet, 2:* 946, 1914.

Fire-Ants

1. Adrouny, G. A.: The fire-ant's fire. *Bull Tulane Univ Med Fac, 25:* 67, 1966.
2. Blum, M. S.: Physiological activity of fire-ant poison. Professor of Entomology, University of Georgia.
3. Brand, J. M., Blum, M. S., Fales, H. M. and MacConnell, J. G.: Fire-ant venoms: Comparative analyses of alkaloidal components. Pergamon Press, *Toxicon, 10:* 259, 1972.
4. Caro, M. R., Derbes, V. J. and Jung, R.: Skin responses to the sting of the imported fire-ant (*Solenopsis saevissima*). *Arch Derm, 75:* 475, 1957.
5. Favorite, F. G.: The imported fire-ant. *Public Health Representative, 73:* 446, 1958.
6. Green, H. B.: Biology and control of the imported fire-ant in Mississippi. *J Econ Entomol, 45:* 593, 1952.
7. Helmly, B. R.: Anaphylactic reactions to fire-ant. *Hawaii Med J, 29:* 368, 1970.
8. Jung, R. C. and Derbes, V. J.: The imported fire-ant, *Solenopsis saevissima* var *richteri*, an agent in disease. *Am J Trop Med Hyg, 6:* 372, 1957.
9. Larson, P. P. and Mervin, W.: *All About Ants*. New York, World Publishers, 1965.
10. MacConnell, J. G. and Blum, M. S.: Alkaloid from fire-ant venom: Identification and synthesis. *Science, 168:* 840, 1970.
11. MacConnell, J. G., Blum, M. S. and Fales, H. M.: The chemistry of fire-ant venom. *Tetrahedron, 26:* 1129, 1971.
12. Russell, F. and Buffkin, D.: Some chemical and pharmacological properties of the venom of the imported fire-ant (*Solenopsis saevissima richteri*). To be published, 1972.
13. Sonnet, P.: Fire-ant venom: Synthesis of a reported component of Solenamine. *Science, 156:* 1759, 1967.
14. Surveys of physicians in Alabama, Georgia and Mississippi in September 1971. Conducted by the State Health Departments in Alabama, Georgia and the Mississippi Allergy Clinic in Mississippi. To be published.
15. Triplett, R. F.: Imported fire-ant sensitivity. Successful treatment with immunotherapy. To be published.

Chapter 13

THE ALLERGIC PATIENT

A CAREFULLY DOCUMENTED clinical history is the most important procedure not only for arriving at a diagnosis of the patient's ailment but also for determining the indications for testing, the assessment of skin test results, and the management of the patient.

Heredity in Allergic Disease

It is generally recognized that the allergic constitution or the ability to react in a hypersensitive manner is hereditary. The demonstration of an allergic familial background can be helpful in establishing the allergic diathesis of the patient. However, demonstrating a familial background for allergy is not always possible since the determination depends upon anecdotal data which is not necessarily reliable. Not infrequently, a milk intolerance is attributed to allergy when actually an intestinal disaccharidase deficiency is at fault. A diagnosis of either emphysema or bronchitis is often mistakenly reported as allergic respiratory disease or even bronchial asthma. What is frequently reported as "sinus disease" may actually be undiagnosed allergic rhinitis. Urticaria which is generally attributed to allergy may be induced by nonimmunologic mechanisms. To the layman, most skin ailments are considered to be allergic.

It is generally stated that children of "nonallergic" parents have less than a 10 per cent chance of having an allergic diathesis. If one parent offers a history of allergic disease, 50 per cent of the offspring may sooner or later manifest allergic disease, while if both parents are allergic, the incidence of allergy in the children rises to 75 per cent.

These figures are not absolute, since it is not unusual to encounter very allergic patients with nothing in the family history suggestive of allergic disease, while very allergic parents will have children with no manifestations of allergic disease.

One additional point must be considered. With the high incidence of allergic disease among humans, if one searches far enough, at least one allergic individual can be identified in every family.

THE PATTERNS OF CLINICAL ALLERGY

Although by definition allergy includes all types of altered immune reactions, the majority of the problems observed in clinical allergy are induced by the atopic or reaginic (immediate) type of hypersensitivity. Clinical patterns, such as drug allergy and serum disease involving the intermediate or Arthus mechanism, contact dermatitis caused by delayed hypersensitivity, and hematological disturbances produced by immune cytotoxic reactions, constitute only a small percentage of the patients presenting themselves with allergic disease.

Since it is generally recognized that the atopic or reaginic constitution is inherited, the patient's presenting complaint at the time the history is taken is usually the culmination of a series of allergic episodes, frequently dating back to infancy. In some cases the symptoms of infancy and early childhood abate ("growing out"), so that at the time of the interview the patient may not relate the early symptoms to the current illness. Allergy is frequently an insidious, smoldering disease that gradually encroaches upon the patient's functional reserve. The tissue changes may progress very slowly, so that the patient accommodates and learns to live with his ailment. Very often the patient does not seek relief until the functional reserve has been encroached upon or until the symptoms have become severe and annoying. Even with very acute symptoms as observed with seasonal hay fever, or bronchial asthma, many patients experience a degree of persistent perennial involvement which the patient considers his normal level.

Every clinical incident should be explored for its possible contribution toward (1) establishing a diagnosis, (2) determining the indications for skin testing, and (3) as a guide for management of the patient.

Since IgE has been established as the chief antibody involved in atopic allergy, it is possible to determine a potentially atopic individual by demonstrating an increased level of serum IgE. Mean values for IgE of 0.16 mg/100 ml of serum have been demonstrated for atopic individuals as compared with 0.03 mg/ml sera, the normal level. To date, this laboratory assay has not been developed sufficiently to permit its routine clinical application.

In the absence of specific indices for identifying the allergic individual, the diagnosis must depend upon clinical observation and the history of the patient. There are a number of clinical patterns which are generally identified with atopic hypersensitivity. Development of these patterns in the patient's history can be helpful toward achieving the three objectives indicated above.

Tension Fatigue Syndrome

The "tension fatigue syndrome" is characterized by the subjective symptoms of extreme fatigue, lassitude, listlessness, and irritability with the objective findings of facial pallor without anemia and circles of discoloration beneath the eyes. The syndrome can occur either isolated or associated with specific allergic organ involvement such as the respiratory tract, gastrointestinal tract, and the skin. Deamer also includes headaches and myalgia of the legs as common complaints. Although this pattern has been emphasized by many pediatric allergists, it has not received the general recognition it deserves as an allergic syndrome. The symptoms can be observed in both children and adults, but the incidence seems higher among the younger age group and particularly the prepubescent child. When the symptoms of fatigue, listlessness, irritability and behavioral disturbances occur as an isolated syndrome, they may not suggest an allergic etiology, and as a result the diagnosis if frequently overlooked.

In most cases, the usual allergens which include pollens, environmentals and foods are at fault. Deamer emphasizes food as the important factor in most cases.

When the symptoms present themselves in a potentially allergic individual, management on the basis of allergy can lead to dramatic responses with loss of the subjective symptoms and general improvement in the behavior and appearance of the patient.

Patterns in Infancy

The most common allergic complaints in infancy are atopic dermatitis, gastrointestinal disturbances, and nasal snuffles.

A confirmed diagnosis of atopic dermatitis in infancy is absolute confirmation of allergy in the older individual (see discussion on atopic dermatitis in Chapter 6).

A history of a feeding disturbance in infancy attributed to milk, can serve as a guide in determining milk sensitivity in later life. In the older individual milk sensitivity may be manifested by respiratory symptoms such as allergic rhinitis or bronchial allergy. Skin tests for milk are not reliable. A negative skin test reaction for milk does not exclude milk sensitivity, while a positive skin test response does not necessarily indicate milk sensitivity. A combination of milk intolerance in infancy plus a positive skin test is strong support for the elimination of all milk products from the patient's diet.

With a positive history of milk intolerance in infancy and a negative skin test for milk in a patient whose response to allergy treatment has not been satisfactory, management with a milk-free diet should be considered. This interpretation of milk sensitivity is applicable to adults as well as children, but only if the patient is an allergic individual. All milk intolerance in infancy is *not* allergic.

Patterns in Childhood

Any of the following complaints occurring in childhood, either as an isolated event or in various combinations, are suggestive of allergic disease.

The Tension Fatigue Syndrome (See discussion above)

Recurrent Otitis

A history of recurrent otitis in childhood is highly suggestive of an allergic etiology. The contributing factors are (1) the anatomy of the eustachian tube in infancy and early childhood, (2) the encroachment of lymphoid tissue upon the eustachian ostiae, and (3) the obstruction of the eustachian canals induced by the edema of the allergic reaction.

Recurrent serous otitis is also attributed to an allergic mechanism (see discussion on allergy of the ears in Chapter 2).

Upper Respiratory Symptoms

Allergic rhinitis in children usually presents a rather typical pattern. Features of tension fatigue syndrome such as facial pallor without anemia and circles beneath the eyes are commonly associated. Itching of the nose leads to constant rubbing with an upward movement of the hand (allergic salute). This frequently leads to a creasing across the nose, just above the tip. Itching also leads to picking of the nose, which together with rubbing, traumatizes the mucosa just within the nares, which results in frequent epistaxis.

Rhinorrhea with a seromucoid discharge is almost always present. Postnasal mucoid discharge causes elongation of the uvula which may induce a tickling cough, while the accumulation of the mucoid discharge in the naso-pharynx may lead to a productive cough which at times is mistaken for one of bronchial origin.

Because of the small nasal air passages, the small naso-pharyngeal compartment and the liberal distribution of lymphoid tissue in the child, obstruction to breathing can be induced by even a small increment of allergic tissue reaction. Nasal obstruction leads to mouth breathing with pursing of the lips (fish mouth), facial deformity and dental malocclusion. Obstruction also predisposes to *recurrent upper respiratory infections* which are a common hallmark of the allergic child.

As the child grows older, the anatomical parts increase in size and provide a considerably greater breathing space. As a result, mild tissue reactions may not produce obstructive symptoms. It is possible for an individual who experienced recurrent upper respiratory symptoms of allergy in early childhood to experience no complaints, although a mild allergic reaction may persist. Such an allergic individual can enter adult life with few or no symptoms of upper respiratory allergic disease.

Children experience seasonal patterns (hay fever) induced by seasonal factors. In many cases the residual mild perennial tissue reaction causes only mild or no symptoms.

Recurrent Laryngitis

Laryngitis, particularly when associated with croup, is a common complaint among infants and young children. The condition is usually associated with allergic rhinitis with marked mucosal edema and profuse seromucoid discharge. The sudden onset of symptoms, usually at night, are secondary to nasal obstruction that induces mouth breathing which in turn predisposes to sudden laryngeal edema caused by cold air currents accompanying a drop in room temperature. The children have a crowing respiration and at times a degree of suprasternal retraction. The allergic children with croup usually do not appear toxic, have a normal temperature and good color in contrast to the laryngeal croup induced by infection which is usually accompanied by purulent nasal secretions, an elevation in temperature, a toxic appearance, and frequently cyanosis.

Lower Respiratory Tract Involvement

Bronchial allergy, with and without complicating infection, is the commonly observed form of allergic pulmonary disease in children. Bronchial asthma and status asthmaticus in children are not rare, but are much less frequent than bronchial allergy (see discussion on lower respiratory tract allergy in Chapter 4).

Atopic Skin Manifestations in Children

The incidence of urticaria and angio-edema is low in children and particularly in the prepubescent period. At the time of the menarche, girls will manifest a higher incidence of urticaria. In children the whealing response to insect bites is frequently mistaken for urticaria. Papular urticaria, often classified as a chronic urticaria, is not an atopic reaction but rather the delayed hypersensitivity response to flea bites (see discussion on Insect Allergy in Chapter 12).

Atopic Dermatitis (See discussion under skin allergy in Chapter 6.)

Adult Patterns

The list below indicates most of the clinical patterns encountered in the history of an allergic adult. At a given age the patient may have experienced one or a combination of ailments. As the individual develops, the clinical pattern may change. For example, the infant with atopic dermatitis may be entirely free at two years of age. The free interval *may* be present for a number of years to be followed by recurrent otitis and upper respiratory symptoms. The patient may again experience an interval free of clinical symptoms followed by persistent upper respiratory symptoms and bronchial allergy or even bronchial asthma. Each event in the patient's history should be studied for information which can be helpful in understanding subsequent complaints, and serve as a guide for designing a test program and the management of the patient.

Each of the conditions listed is discussed under the appropriate chapter.

Fatigue, lassitude, listlessness, and *irritability* of unexplained etiology in an allergic individual

   Headaches—usually associated with nasal symptoms

   Eyes—itching, burning, injection and lacrimation

   Ears—recurrent otalgia and otitis, tinnitus, intermittent and constant aerotitis

   Sinusitis—acute, recurrent and chronic

   Rhinitis—acute, recurrent and chronic
     sneezing
     itching
     epistaxis
     crusting
     polyps
     seasonal symptoms

   Laryngitis—recurrent

   Lower respiratory involvement—
     bronchitis, chronic and recurrent
     cough, dry or productive
     dyspnea on exertion with and without overt wheezing
     bronchial asthma, perennial and seasonal
     status asthmaticus

   Cutaneous involvement—
     pruritus
     urticaria
     angio-edema
     allergic dermatitis, atopic and contact
     petechiae
     purpura

The Chief Complaint (Presenting Complaint)

The "chief complaint" is the clinical pattern that brings the patient to the physician.

Since the patient was born with his allergic constitution, it is important to determine what factors have aggravated the allergic state so that the patient now seeks relief.

An acute onset of symptoms may indicate either a change in the patient's environment or a physiologic change in the individual.

I. *Environmental changes*:

(1) Seasonal aeroallergens as observed in seasonal hay fever and bronchial asthma.

(2) *Changes in residence* from one area to another or from one geographical region to another.

After moving into a new area the patient's initial exposure may serve as a sensitizing experience with no symptoms. Symptoms may not develop until the second year and at times several years later. Variations occur with the different concentrations of aeroallergens from season to season.

A change in residence may expose the patient to a variation in *air pollutants* (pollens, organic dusts). These may be either allergenic or non-allergenic (irritating dusts and fumes).

(3) Changes in the *home environment*:

The acquisition of a *pet cat* or *dog* or any other furry animal.

The acquisition of *new furniture*, particularly down upholstered.

The acquisition of new floor coverings, especially with *felt carpet pads*.

Changes in the *heating* and *ventilating system* can serve to introduce aeroallergens.

The environment of homes visited—neighbors, grandparents, *etc.*—must be considered.

(4) Changes in the occupational environment—type of occupation, location of work, or a change in routine of duties; a change in the materials handled by the patient.

(5) With children, the school environment must be considered. Are hairy animals present, as in kindergarten? The ground covering of the playground must be considered. What is the environment to and from school?

II. *Changes in the individual*

Infection: A viral infection may antedate the onset of symptoms. The symptoms may appear immediately following the infection or be delayed for several months. In the case of pollen sensitivity, symptoms may appear during the first pollinating season following the viral infection.

Bacterial infections may usher in the initial acute episode of allergic symptoms.

Physiological changes in the individual may account for a change in the patient's clinical pattern. During pregnancy a woman may experience either an aggravation or a suppression of her allergic symptoms. Some women with bronchial asthma are improved during pregnancy, while others experience an aggravation of symptoms. The reason for these differences is not known.

Variations in the level of clinical response are also noted with the establishment of puberty, with the menarche and with the climacterium in both the male and the female.

Moderate symptoms either seasonal or non-seasonal may be related to the same factors that operate in the acute patterns.

Chronic symptoms are usually the culmination of long standing smoldering allergic reactions that have encroached upon the patient's functional reserve. As has been indicated previously, in many cases the symptoms may date back to childhood and even to infancy.

Chronic symptoms are induced by the usual allergenic factors, aeroallergens, environmental factors and foods.

Bacteria and bacterial products induce the delayed type of hypersensitivity and should not be considered as primary etiologic agents in atopic or reaginic allergic disease.

Since the patient who complains of seasonal symptoms of allergic disease has an allergic constitution twelve months of the year, it is not surprising that many individuals who present themselves with seasonal symptoms such as hay fever and bronchial asthma also experience perennial allergic tissue changes which may produce a minor or even a moderate degree of symptoms such as itching of the eyes with lacrimation, recurrently stopped ears, nasal itching, sneezing, rhinorrhea, postnasal drip, cough either dry or productive, and even bronchial allergy of mild degree. The patient has learned to live with his symptoms and often fails to report his complaints unless they are elicited by the examining physician. This observation is extremely important in evaluating all patients who offer a history of seasonal symptoms.

Physical Examination

The physical examination of the allergic patient, regardless of the complaint, should be as thorough and complete as any other medical examination. It is unusual for only a single organ to be involved by the allergic reaction; the common pattern is multiple involvement.

Pallor without anemia, circles beneath the eyes, mouth breathing with facial deformity and malocclusion suggest upper respiratory involvement by the allergic process.

Allergic conjunctivitis is rarely observed without concomitant involvement of the upper respiratory tract. With conjunctivitis it is important to examine the nose and throat. Classical bluish pallor of the nasal mucosa may be observed, or if the condition is of long standing, the nasal mucosa may be reddened, crusted and even atrophic. Following topical therapy, the mucosa may appear reddened. Examination of the nose may not be remarkable, but the throat may reveal a pattern suggestive of allergic involvement, such as postnasal drip, with an elongated uvula, succulent fauces, lymphoid hyperplasia of the post-pharyngeal wall, enlarged tonsils, or tonsilar tags when the tonsils have been surgically removed.

Retraction, scarring and calcareous deposits of the membrani tympani indicate eustachian tube involvement by the allergic process. This may be accompanied by post-pharyngeal hyperplasia.

Bronchial allergy and bronchial asthma rarely occur as isolated syndromes. They are usually associated with allergic involvement of the upper respiratory tract. The diagnosis of lower respiratory allergic disease is supported by observing the pattern of allergic rhinitis and the presence of hyperplasia and edema of Waldeyer's ring. Bronchial asthma associated with polyps may be either allergic or nonallergic.

Gastrointestinal allergy is *not* a common primary complaint, but when it is the chief complaint, it rarely occurs as an isolated syndrome. The usual accompaniment is upper respiratory allergic disease. The associated upper respiratory allergic symptoms may be very mild and not reported by the patient. Unless this aspect of the pattern is pursued in both the history and the physical examination, the respiratory allergic involvement may be completely overlooked. Positive findings of allergic upper respiratory involvement support a diagnosis of gastrointestinal allergic disease. Without evidence of allergic disease in another system, it is difficult to make a diagnosis of gastrointestinal allergy.

Atopic dermatitis may occur as an isolated finding, especially under two years of age. In the older individual the classical flexural involvement with lichenification, hypertrophy, and discoloration is usually associated with allergic respiratory involvement, and particularly allergic rhinitis. When the presenting complaint is atopic dermatitis, the patient should always be examined for evidence of respiratory allergic involvement.

REFERENCES

1. Crook, W. G.: Systemic manifestations due to allergy (allergic toxemia or T.F.S.). *Pediatrics*, 27: 790, 1961.
2. Deamer, Wm. C.: Allergy in childhood. *Adv Pediatr*, 11: 147, 1960.
3. Fontana, V.: *Practical Management of the Allergic Child*. Appleton, 1969, pp. 180–181.

4. Fries, J. H.: The cocoa bean and the allergic child. *Ann Allergy, 24:* 484, 1966.
5. Gerrard, J. W.: Familial recurrent rhinorrhea and bronchitis due to cow's milk. *JAMA, 198:*605, 1966.
6. Gerrard, J. W.: Milk allergy: Clinical picture and familial incidence. *Can Med Assoc J, 97:* 780, 1967.
7. Glaser, J.: *Allergy in Childhood.* Thomas, 1956, chap. 56 (out of print).
8. Kaufman, W.: The overall picture of rheumatism and arthritis. *Ann Allergy, 10:* 49, 1952, and *Int Arch Allergy Appl Immunol, 6:* 361, 1955.
9. Marks, M. B.: Allergic shiners: Dark circles under the eyes in children. *Clin Pediatr (Phila), 5:* 655, 1965.
10. Randolph, T. G.: Allergy as a causative factor of fatigue, irritability, and behavior problems of children. *J Pediatr, 31:* 560, 1947.
11. Randolph, T. G.: Musculoskeletal allergy in children. *Int Arch Allergy Appl Immunol, 14:* 84, 1959.
12. Roth, A.: Detection of food allergy. *Postgraduate Medicine, 32:* 432, 1962.
13. Rowe, A. H.: Allergic toxemia and fatigue. *Ann Allergy, 8:* 72, 1950 and *17:* 9, 1959.
14. Speer, F.: The allergic tension-fatigue syndrome. *Pediatr Clin North Am,* Nov. 1954, pp. 1029–1036, and *Intern Arch Allergy Appl Immunol, 12:* 207, 1968, *Ann Allergy, 12:* 168, 1954.
15. Speer, F.: *The Allergic Child.* Harper & Row, 1963, pp. 329–341.
16. Tuft, L. and Mueller, H.: *Allergy in Children.* Saunders, 1970, pp. 142, 386, and 406.

Chapter 14

ALLERGY IN INFANCY

by
Donald F. German, M.D.*

ALLERGY IN INFANCY presents a number of unique problems. Although the immune system and the barriers to sensitization are not as fully developed as in the older child, the infant is capable of staging an allergic response. Lacking the homeostatic mechanisms of the older child and adult, the infant cannot deal as effectively with the allergic reaction. This chapter concerns allergy in the first year of life.

The Immune Response

The neonatal period and to some degree early infancy represent an immunological transitional zone from intrauterine to extrauterine life. In order to change from an intrauterine existence, the newborn must make a number of physiologic adjustments. Unless the infant develops active immunity during the first year of life, he is liable to serious infection.

The newborn possesses all the organs necessary for the immediate and delayed immune response: the thymus, the spleen, the lymph nodes, and the leukocytes. However, the newborn and neonate do not respond to antigenic stimuli to the same degree as the older infant (1). A number of hypotheses have been offered to explain the impeded response, such as a deficiency in antigen capture and processing by the reticuloendothelial system (2); the newborn lacks the nonspecific priming of previous antigenic exposure (2); transplacentally acquired maternal antibody may exert an inhibitory effect on the immune response (3,4); and the great number and variety of antigens the neonate is exposed to in a short span of time reduces the response to any one antigen (5). Despite this, the newborn and for that matter the fetus during the last half of pregnancy are capable of mounting some immune response.

The Fetus: The human fetus produces cells capable of immunoglobulin synthesis and of cellular immunity. Studies using labelled amino acids have shown that immunoglobulins and immunological competence are present in early fetal life. In tissue culture, spleen cells obtained from live born fetuses at twenty weeks gestation have been shown to produce IgM and IgG. Immunofluorescent staining of the fetal spleen has revealed plasma cells containing both these immunoglobulins (6).

IgM is produced by the fetus and is generally detectable at low levels in the cord blood. A small amount of IgG is produced by the fetus (7). IgG levels in cord blood exceed those of the mother. However, the vast majority of this is derived from the mother by active transplacental transmission. Transplacental transmission of other immunoglobulins has not been demonstrated. Viral infection of the fetus constitutes a potent antigenic stimulus for the intrauterine production of IgA and IgM antibodies (8). This is reflected in elevated cord blood levels of these immunoglobulins. Another potential source of stimulation is the transplacental transfer of exogenous soluble antigens, such as foods, drugs and other chemicals.

---
* Chief, Department of Allergy, Kaiser Foundation Hospital—Permanente Medical Group, San Francisco.

The Neonate and Infant: The placenta which acted as the barrier to antigenic stimulation in the fetus is lost at birth. New barriers, the skin, the respiratory tract, and the mucosa of the gastrointestinal tract assume importance. The infant is now exposed to a multiplicity of antigens and must respond to many of them in order to remain viable. Bacterial flora rapidly populate the skin, the respiratory and the gastrointestinal tracts. As the infant matures, if he fails to produce active immunity, he will succumb to serious infection.

At birth the neonate has a titer of IgG equal to or exceeding the mother (1,031 ± 200 mg per cent) (9). The infant is able to synthesize IgG by four weeks of age (10). In spite of its active synthesis by the infant the total IgG decreases over the first four months, reaching a nadir of approximately 430 mg per cent. Thereafter, it begins to rise, and at one year it reaches a level of approximately 600 mg per cent (9). The IgG provides the infant with resistance to a number of viral and Gram positive bacterial infections in the first few months of life.

The neonate has virtually no IgM at birth. This is the first immunoglobulin the infant produces after birth. IgM is particularly important in affording protection against Gram negative infections. Until this is produced in sufficient quantity, usually by the age of three months, the infant is very susceptible to Gram negative infections. IgM gradually increases from a low of 11 ± 5 mg per cent at birth to 55 mg per cent at one year of age (9).

IgA is present in one third of all term cord sera at a mean concentration of 2 ± 3 mg per cent. Levels greater than 11 mg per cent are suggestive of intrauterine infection (8). Production of IgA begins at about two to four weeks of age, reaching a level of 30 to 40 mg per cent at one year of age (9). As detailed in the chapter on immunology, it is present in two forms: as secretory immunoglobulin, with the secretory piece attached, and as serum immunoglobulin.

Although IgA is essentially undetectable in cord blood, it is present in the colostrum and to a lesser extent in the milk of most mammals. In ruminants this colostral IgA plays an important role in host defense. The newborn horse receives virtually no immunoglobulin from the mother during gestation but is capable of absorbing intact immunoglobulins concentrated in the colostrum of the mare for twenty-four to forty-eight hours after birth. After the first few feedings, immunoglobulin levels of the newborn horse approach those of the mother (11).

In the human, immunoglobulins, especially IgA are also found in colostrum and to a lesser extent, milk. Although it is possible that colostral antibodies serve some protective function, it has as yet not been demonstrated that newborn infants necessarily benefit from colostrum rich in IgA. In a recent study it was suggested that breast fed newborns in the first ten days of life were more resistant to hematogenous spread of infection by bacteria of enteric origin (12).

IgE does not normally cross the placenta (13). Only scanty amounts are produced by the fetus *in utero*. Johansson reported a mean cord level of IgE of 36.3 Nanograms per milliliter contrasted with the mean IgE serum level of 286 Nanograms per milliliter in the atopic mother. Maturation results in increasing IgE levels throughout infancy and childhood paralleling IgA development (14).

Cellular Immunity

Delayed or cellular immunity is mediated not by humoral antibody but by small lymphocytes, specifically, T cells. This response can be passively transferred by viable small lymphocytes. The transfer of maternal delayed hypersensitivity to the fetus has not been reported.

By twenty weeks gestation the fetus possesses all of the elements necessary to mount a delayed hypersensitivity response. But it is not known when the fetus can exhibit such a response. Newborn premature infants can be sensitized to topically applied 2-4-dinitrofluorobenzene (15). Newborn term infants immunized with BCG at birth develop a positive tuberculin skin test at three weeks of age (16). Homograft rejection is a form of cellular immunity also mediated by T cells; the fetal sheep, which has a gestation period of 150 days, is capable of rejecting a homograft while still *in utero* after the eighty-fifth day of gestation (17). It is possible that the human fetus also is capable of homograft rejection. From this evidence, it is apparent that the neonate and probably the fetus have intact cellular immunity.

Sensitization: With the loss of protection from external antigens by the placenta and uterus, the newborn is immediately exposed to a rich variety of exogenous antigens. During the first few weeks of life, which corresponds to the period of sensitization, the infant is usually free of allergic symptoms. When the infant is exposed to bacteria, viruses and parasites, protective immunity usually develops, while exposure to common allergens, such as ingestants and inhalants, may lead to the development of hypersensitivity.

The factors that predispose to the development of hypersensitivity in the infant include:

(1) the inherent predisposition or the atopic constitution
(2) the state of the digestive tract
(3) the food requirements of the infant
(4) allergenic factors in the environment
(5) infection

(1) The importance of heredity in determining the atopic constitution has been pointed out in Chapter 1. The factors that constitute an atopic constitution and predispose to hypersensitivity are not known, but it is generally recognized that the individual has the ability to respond to an appropriate allergen with a higher than normal titer of IgE antibody. Although all infants are exposed to allergens, only the atopic individuals become sensitized.

(2) The digestive tract of the young infant has not fully matured, which results in the inability to completely digest the large quantities of food required for its rapid growth. The average infant triples its weight in the first year. In addition, the infant's digestive tract is more permeable than that of the older individual which permits the assimilation of undigested food proteins. These undigested proteins as well as degradation products of food can serve as allergens to sensitize the infant.

(3) Added to these anatomical and physiological differences is the comparatively large quantities of food ingested by the infant to meet the rapid growth requirements. This large supply of food serves as a rich source of antigenic material. It is for this reason that in the early months of infancy, foods are the most common and most important allergenic factors.

Since cow's milk is the principal source of food in early infancy, it serves as the richest source of allergens and accordingly, milk is the most common cause of food allergy in infancy (18). By the age of one year a twenty-one pound infant conservatively has ingested sixty gallons or 480 pounds of milk. As that infant grows older, each additional food can serve as a potential allergen. Most common among the allergenic foods are eggs, wheat and beef.

Infants who are exclusively breast fed may be sensitized not to breast milk proteins, but rather to antigenic materials derived from the maternal diet, which are excreted in the breast milk. Once sensitization has been established, subsequent feedings of breast milk containing the antigenic substances will induce allergic symptoms.

(4) Allergenic factors in the environment. Although foods are the most common allergens in early infancy, environmental factors must always be considered as potentials. The presence of feathers, animal danders as provided by cats and dogs, carpet pads and upholstered furniture are all possible factors to be considered. Although the environmental factors are of lesser frequency than the

foods, they must always be considered when present and excluded as possible allergens before the incrimination of foods. In some cases both foods and environmental factors are at fault. When the symptoms of allergy first appear in later infancy, environmental factors are usually a more common cause than foods.

(5) Infection (see discussion of infection in Chapter 4) is always a factor to be considered as a provocative agent in allergy of infancy but not as a primary allergen. Infection serves to increase the permeability of the gut which permits freer passage of undigested proteins which may induce sensitivity.

CLINICAL MANIFESTATIONS OF ALLERGIC DISEASE IN INFANCY

The epithelial surfaces of the gastrointestinal tract, the respiratory tract and the skin form the first line of defense against exogenous antigenic materials, which consist of inhalants, foods, chemicals, bacteria, viruses and parasites. Because of the constant exposure, these tissues, in the atopic infant, are readily sensitized and become susceptible to allergic reactions following subsequent exposure.

Gastrointestinal Allergy in Infancy

Since food is the most common cause of allergic disease in early infancy, a natural sequel is the frequent occurrence of gastrointestinal allergic involvement during this age period. The identical five factors that favor the development of hypersensitivity in the infant also operate to induce the gastrointestinal response.

The incidence of gastrointestinal allergy in infancy is not known, but it is probably greater than the usual conservative estimate of one per cent (19). Many so-called feeding problems in infancy may actually be allergic in origin, which is implied from the close relationship between the incidence of feeding problems in infancy and the subsequent development of allergic disease in later life. Colicky infants, relieved by the elimination of cow's milk, often develop allergic symptoms at a later age. A recent prospective survey at the Kaiser Foundation Hospital in San Francisco revealed that of fifty patients who were treated surgically for pyloric stenosis, many subsequently developed major manifestations of allergy.

Symptoms: The onset of symptoms usually occurs after two weeks of age which corresponds to the period of sensitization. Symptoms may appear within minutes following the ingestion of the offending food, but more frequently, the symptoms are delayed for hours.

The most common symptoms are abdominal pain, vomiting, diarrhea and constipation.

The pain is colicky and its paroxysmal nature associated with severe crying, restlessness and flexing of the legs on the abdomen produces a pattern similar to the colic of unknown etiology so frequently observed in infancy. As with all colic it occurs in both breast fed and artificially fed infants.

Spitting and vomiting which are constant symptoms of gastrointestinal allergy in infancy may either slow the rate of weight gain or cause a very insignificant weight loss. Vomiting is usually not projectile. Because of their frequent occurrence in this disease, the symptoms of spitting and vomiting should always be considered as an expression of gastrointestinal allergic disease.

Diarrhea, which is also a frequent symptom of gastrointestinal allergy, may be characterized by frequent explosive stools which often contain mucus and at times blood. A peri-anal rash is not uncommon, secondary to irritation from the stools.

Constipation which is also common may alternate with diarrhea.

The symptoms of gastrointestinal allergy are frequently associated with those due to either upper respiratory allergic disease or atopic dermatitis and occasionally with both.

Diagnosis: Since the symptoms of gastrointestinal allergy are not specific, the diagnosis of the disease involves a high degree of suspicion, which is frequently supported by a familial history of atopy. The laboratory studies which usually show no abnormality are not particularly helpful. Blood eosinophilia may or may not be elevated. Recent studies on gastrointestinal allergy to milk reported a high titer for coproantibodies to milk (20,21), but this observation has not been confirmed (22). Skin tests are of little value in these patients.

The diagnosis is usually made by the exclusion of other possible causes and by dietary trials. Since the diet of the young infant is quite limited as to the number and variety of foods, the identification of the offending food is much simpler than with the older child.

Differential Diagnosis: Excluding infection and anatomic abnormalities, there are a number of conditions that have symptom complexes similar to gastrointestinal allergy. They will be listed in relation to their major symptoms.

(1) Diarrhea

(a) *Coeliac disease*: The etiology of this disorder is unknown. It possibly represents an inherited metabolic defect of the gastrointestinal tract. As a result, gluten is not digested and assimilated. The undigested gluten acts as a toxin and produces the clinical picture of diarrhea and progressive malnutrition. The diagnosis is made by trial elimination of gluten from the diet and subsequent challenge with a recurrence of symptoms.

(b) *Disaccharidase deficiency*: This may be primary, genetically determined, or secondary, often transient, and seen as a sequel to infectious diarrhea. It is characterized by a deficiency of intestinal enzymes necessary for the hydrolysis of the disaccharides, maltose, sucrose and lactose. The main symptoms are diarrhea, hyperperistalsis and malnutrition. The stool pH is acid because of the conversion of lactose to lactic acid within the gut lumen. The diagnosis is confirmed by oral disaccharide tolerance tests. The condition is readily corrected by removing the offending carbohydrate from the diet.

(c) *Cystic fibrosis*: Pancreatic achylia in cystic fibrosis is a common cause of severe malabsorption in the pediatric age group. The disorder is due to a deficiency in exocrine gland excretion. There is a lack of pancreatic enzyme secretion leading to poor fat absorption, resulting in diarrhea. The respiratory mucus is thick and viscid and obstructs the bronchial tree, leading to chronic respiratory infection. There is often a family history of the disorder. Sweat chlorides are elevated. Examination of the duodenal aspirate reveals a marked deficiency in pancreatic enzymes.

(d) *Immune deficiency disorders*: Diarrhea is commonly associated with many of the immune deficiency disorders. The diagnosis is made by the presence of repeated infection, a positive family history of immune deficiency disorder, and the finding of defects in the immune mechanism (see Chapter 19, Immune Deficiency States).

(2) Vomiting

Excluding neurological abnormalities, infection and improper feeding techniques, pyloric stenosis is probably the most important cause of protracted vomiting in early infancy. Vomiting due to pyloric stenosis usually starts between two to four weeks of age. The infant, despite a voracious appetite, loses weight from dehydration and lack of nutrition. The vomiting is forceful and projectile. An olive-sized pyloric tumor is often palpated. Roentgenograms, if performed, reveal an elongation of the pyloric canal.

Treatment

When food allergy is involved, the treatment consists of identification of the food factors and its elimination. In the young infant whose food supply is usually milk, the problem of identification and elimination is usually simple. If the infant fails to respond to dietary change, consideration must be given to the possibility of environmental items acting as either contributing factors or primary agents (see discussion on environmental control in Chapter 17). In some cases the symptoms cannot be controlled until the environment is fully controlled. This practice applies even in the absence of upper respiratory or dermatologic complaints.

Prognosis: In some infants a food intolerance will abate after the first or second year of life; however, in many cases the intolerance persists throughout life, but the organ of involvement changes. Respiratory symptoms (allergic rhinitis, bronchial allergy, bronchial asthma); ear symptoms (serous otitis and recurrent otalgia); skin symptoms (atopic dermatitis) may supplant the gastrointestinal pattern. It is not unusual for patients to experience a free period between infancy and the recurrence of allergic symptoms in later childhood or even in adult life. In such patients, regardless of the system or organ involved, consideration must always be given to the possibility that the identical allergens (foods and environmentals) operating in early infancy may be the cause of the symptoms in later life (see Chapter 6 for discussion of infantile eczema).

Respiratory Allergic Disease in Infancy

Like the gastrointestinal tract, the respiratory system of the infant is also a frequent site of involvement.

Allergic Rhinitis

Allergic rhinitis characterized by sniffles, nasal obstruction of various degrees and at times sneezing, is a common observation in infancy. The symptoms may occur alone or in association with gastrointestinal symptoms, in which case the latter involvement dominates the clinical pattern. The nasal mucosa is boggy and pale but rarely has the bluish pallor of the older individual. Obstruction of varying degrees together with the discharge produce the sniffles so characteristic of the allergic infant. A similar pattern occurs in congenital lues and hypothyroidism. The obstruction may be severe enough to cause mouth breathing and at times interfere with nursing. The discharge, which is either serous or seromucoid, may be profuse and at times cause excoriation of the nares. Dripping postnasally into the pharynx, the discharge may cause coughing and at times even vomiting.

The Pharynx: The pharynx participates in the allergic reaction of the infant's upper respiratory tract. The fauces are succulent and glistening, while not infrequently, the soft palate appears pale. In infancy the tonsils and adenoids are usually not prominent, so that when enlarged tonsils and lymphoid hyperplasia of the post pharyngeal wall are observed in infancy, it is usually indicative of allergic involvement.

Pharyngeal involvement in the allergic infant is never isolated but is always associated with allergic rhinitis.

The Allergic Ear in Infancy

Involvement of the upper respiratory tract in the allergic reaction induces edema that causes obstruction which predisposes to recurrent middle ear infections, a common complication of upper respiratory allergic disease in infancy.

Serous otitis is also a common observation in the allergic infant. Following the exclusion of anatomical defects, such as cleft palate, and the immune deficiency diseases, allergic involvement is frequently recognized as a cause of serous otitis (23). The mechanism that operates to produce serous otitis is not clear. Serous otitis may be secondary to the obstruction induced by edema and lymphoid hyperplasia of the upper respiratory tract in allergic disease, or it may be in response to a primary involvement by the allergic reaction of the mucosal lining of the middle ear. In either instance the onset may be abrupt or insidious. When the onset is sudden, the symptoms are usually acute, leading to fretfulness, restlessness and irritability of the infant. If insidious, the condition may be completely overlooked and persist into later childhood when the child is brought to the physician because of either impaired hearing or impaired speech development or both.

Although the common allergens may be at fault, milk is generally considered the most frequent offender.

Bronchial Allergy

The precise incidence of bronchial allergy in infancy is not known, but it is estimated that 22 per cent of childhood asthma dates its onset to infancy (24). Anatomical features of the infant's lung readily permit the development of airway obstruction by nonimmunologic as well as immunologic mechanisms, so that the resulting clinical pattern cannot always be differentiated.

Initially, growth of the lung is achieved by an increase in the number of terminal bronchioles, alveolar ducts and alveoli and later in life by an increase in size of these components. The conducting airways of the infant and young child are narrow in comparison with the older child and adult. It is not until after the third year of age and as late as the fourth year that a significant increase in the airway conduction is achieved (25).

Because of the very small caliber of the airways of the infant's lungs, any process that produces either inflammation, edema or an increased production of mucus causes obstruction of varying degree. With partial obstruction due to mucus, rhonchi of various qualities are produced, while partial narrowing due to edema and inflammation increases turbulence with resulting wheezing. Complete obstruction results in atelectasis.

The clinical patterns induced by obstruction caused by both allergic and nonallergic mechanisms may be identical, but to designate a difference Aas has applied the term "pseudoasthma" to the nonallergic form (26).

Viral respiratory infection accompanied by wheezing is observed commonly before the age of eighteen months (27). Viral respiratory infections, which are common before twenty-four months of age, may be accompanied by wheezing or a pattern of "pseudoasthma." A number of infants may experience recurrent episodes of cough and wheezing (pseudoasthma) with viral infections, but as older children have no bronchial symptoms nor any evidence of atopic disease.

Pathology: The tissue alterations with bronchial allergy in the infant are similar to those observed in the older child except that because of the short duration of the process, the basement membrane may not be thickened, and the bronchial smooth muscle may not be hypertrophied. Inspissated secretions, eosinophilic infiltrations, mucosal edema and microatelectatic areas are seen.

Symptoms and Signs: Both cough and wheezing are prominent symptoms. They may occur separately but are usually associated. In the older infant persistent nocturnal cough with wheezing on excitement or exertion are frequent patterns of the disease.

On physical examination the infant does not always appear ill, and except when complicated by infection, the temperature is usually not elevated. Dyspnea rather than wheezing is a frequent finding. Instead of wheezing, rhonchi may be heard which are reported by the parents as a "rattling in the chest." The expiratory phase is shorter, and the young infant displays less evidence of expiratory effort than in the older child. However, with more severe involvement alar flaring, the use of the accessory muscles of respiration, and intercostal retractions may be present. When hypoxic, the infant may be irritable, restless, cyanotic and pale. With marked respiratory distress and bronchial obstruction, there may be evidence of right heart failure with tachycardia, fluid retention and hepatomegaly.

Laboratory Findings: The hemogram

may reveal an eosinophilia of over five per cent. Eosinophils may be evident in the nasal and bronchial secretions. Parenthetically, it should be noted that infants under three months of age often have nasal smear eosinophilia.

In the infant with acute wheezing the roentgenogram will reveal hyperaeration of the lungs as well as various complications of asthma, such as atelectasis, mediastinal emphysema, pneumothorax and pneumonia.

Skin tests for identifying the allergens are usually of little value in early infancy.

Diagnosis: Since none of the signs and symptoms of bronchial allergy are specific for the disease, it is virtually impossible to make a diagnosis at the time of the first episode of wheezing. It is usually necessary to observe the infant for several months, and at times the diagnosis can not be made until beyond infancy.

Obtaining the history is the most important procedure in evaluating an infant with recurrent episodes of wheezing. The history should be detailed and include the date and circumstances of the onset of the first and all subsequent episodes of wheezing, provocative and ameliorative factors, complete information concerning the environment, and a detailed diet diary.

The history often reveals frequent changes in formula associated with gastrointestinal disturbances. A family history of atopy and the presence of atopic dermatitis in the infant strongly support an atopic constitution.

Differential Diagnosis: Asthma in infancy must be distinguished from a number of other anatomical, infectious and metabolic causes of wheezing. It is important in evaluating any patient to remember the time honored statement of Chevalier Jackson that "all that wheezes is not asthma."

(1) *Foreign body:* Asthma at any age must be distinguished from foreign body aspiration. To diagnose this condition it is important to have a high index of suspicion in any child wheezing for the first time. The history, noting the circumstances of the first episode of wheezing, is often helpful. Classically, there is a sudden onset of wheezing in a perfectly well infant, and subsequent to this there is persistence of the wheezing. There may be a shift of the trachea from the midline. Auscultation may reveal unilateral wheezing or absence of breath sounds. Roentgenograms, particularly inspiratory and expiratory films, may indicate the location of the foreign body or suggest its presence because of emphysema, atelectasis or mediastinal shift. The roentgenograms and fluoroscopy may reveal a lack of diaphragmatic movement on the affected side.

(2) *Vascular ring*: This may be formed by a double aortic arch, a right aortic arch with left ligamentum arteriosum, an anomalous innominate or aberrant subclavian artery. The vascular ring may cause compression of major bronchi and resultant wheezing. The diagnosis is suggested in patients with persistent wheezing not responding to ordinary therapeutic measures. Roentgenograms, particularly an esophagram, which show compression of the esophagus by the aberrant arteries are important in the evaluation of this condition.

(3) *Cystic fibrosis:* Recurrent lower respiratory infections are common in cystic fibrosis. Frequently there is a positive family history of this disorder. Gastrointestinal difficulties, such as meconium ileus in the neonate, and foul, bulky stools and fat intolerance in infancy and childhood may be seen. There is evidence of failure to thrive. The diagnosis is made by an abnormally elevated sweat chloride or an absence of pancreatic enzymes in duodenal aspirate.

(4) *Tracheoesophageal fistula*: A history of cough and wheezing during or after feedings and recurrent episodes of pneumonia suggest this diagnosis. Symptoms are present in the neonatal period, often with the first feeding. Roentgenographic studies using contrast media and proper positioning of the infant are necessary in making the diagnosis.

(5) *Bronchitis*: Bronchitis in infancy is often associated with wheezing and cough, producing a clinical picture similar to bronchial allergy. When infants who develop cough and wheezing with respiratory infection are followed into childhood, a number will develop frank evidence of bronchial allergy. In these cases there is often a family history or a personal history of other atopic manifestations. Many children will outgrow these wheezing episodes by the age of four or five years; it is these children who probably have "pseudoasthma" as detailed above.

(6) *Bronchiolitis*: This condition represents another form of "pseudoasthma" and presents a most difficult problem in differential diagnosis. Bronchiolitis, although relatively common in infancy, is rare after the third or fourth year of life because of the previously noted increase in diameter of the peripheral airways. It is usually caused by a viral infection, particularly with the respiratory syncitial virus (28). There is peribronchial inflammation. This reduces the diameter of the peripheral airways and causes partial respiratory obstruction, resulting in dyspnea, wheezing, and hyperexpansion of the chest. Fever, leukocytosis and the response to adrenalin are not differential aids in this condition.

Up to 50 per cent of these infants have repeated episodes of bronchiolitis-like symptoms. Many patients have a strong family history of allergy. In these latter two situations asthma is often a sequel to the bronchiolitis (28,29,30).

(7) *Immunological disorders*: Infants with immune deficiency diseases often have recurrent respiratory infections with wheezing. Infants with recurrent infections should be screened for immunological deficiencies. It is important to note the presence or absence of lymphoid tissue, particularly in the upper respiratory tract. Laboratory studies should include a hemogram with special attention to the number and type of lymphocytes, isohemagglutinins, monilia skin test, Schick test, quantitative immunoglobulins, chest x-ray with attention to the thymic shadow and lateral view of the skull to show lymphoid tissue in the nasopharynx (see Chapter 19, Immune Deficiency States).

(8) *Heiner's Syndrome* (31): This condition probably represents a form of extrinsic allergic bronchopneumonia in infancy. The syndrome usually begins in early infancy and is characterized by chronic respiratory disease with multiple circulating precipitins to cow's milk demonstrated by agar gel technique. These patients have recurrent episodes of coryza, cough, wheezing and pneumonia and exhibit poor weight gain, pallor, frequent vomiting and diarrhea. They may have recurrent otitis media and hemoptysis. Chest x-rays show a variable pattern from mild peribronchial infiltrate to patchy, segmental consolidation. The infiltrates often shift in pattern, location and intensity. The symptoms clear with the withdrawal of all milk products from the diet. The presence of precipitins and the evanescent pattern found on chest x-ray are suggestive of an Arthus mechanism similar to that seen in extrinsic allergic bronchopneumonia. Direct skin testing for milk is not an aid in making the diagnosis of this condition. (See Chapter 4 for discussion of extrinsic allergic bronchopneumonia.)

Management

TREATMENT OF THE ACUTE CONDITION

Hydration: Routine management should always be directed toward the assurance of an adequate fluid intake which is the most effective procedure for liquefying bronchial secretions.

Vaporizers may be helpful for the treatment of some upper respiratory conditions but is of little value in the management of lower respiratory disease. The mist particles produced by the ordinary home vaporizer are of such large size that they are actually removed from the inspired air by the time they reach the carina. A vaporizer often makes for a cold damp infant in a warm "sticky" room which is conducive to the growth of mold, which may further complicate the problem. Ideally, the relative humidity should be maintained at 35 to 50 per cent, which is best achieved by the use of an automatically controlled humidifier.

Medication: (see Chapter 15) Bronchodilators are useful for the relief of symptoms.

Ephedrine: For home use, ephedrine is probably one of the most effective and safest medications. The dosage is 3 mg/kg/24 hours, divided into four to six equal doses.

Since ephedrine frequently induces hyperactivity, it is usually combined with a sedative agent, such as Atarax®.

Syrup of Ephedrine N.F.® and Atarax consists of equal parts of Syrup Ephedrine N.F. and Syrup of Atarax. The resulting mixture delivers ephedrine 10 mg and Atarax 5 mg per 5 cc.

Epinephrine-HCl: When the infant is seen intially with wheezing, a good response is often observed following one or two subcutaneous injections of aqueous epinephrine 1-1000 given at twenty to thirty minute intervals. The dosage is 0.01 cc per kilogram body weight.

Cough Mixtures: Cough mixtures are not recommended. There is no justifiable indication for a mixture that contains an antihistamine, decongestant, an expectorant to loosen secretions and finally a cough suppressant. In such mixtures one constituent counteracts the effect of another, resulting in little if any therapeutic benefit.

Antihistamines are not only valueless but are contraindicated in the treatment of bronchial allergy and asthma. The atropine-like action of the antihistamines has a drying effect on secretions, decreasing their viscosity which leads to inspissation and further airway obstruction. Most infants with a dry persistent cough due to allergy will respond to ephedrine.

Barbiturates and sedatives in general should be avoided in all age groups with bronchial allergy and bronchial asthma because of their depressant effect on the respiratory center.

Antibiotics

The administration of antibiotics for the treatment of acute episodes of bronchial allergy is the subject of some controversy. When infection is present, there is no objection to the use of antibiotics; however, the determination of the presence or absence of infection is often difficult. Fever, leukocytosis, purulent mucus and wheezing which persist for twenty-four hours or more are certainly indicative of infection and justify the use of antibiotics.

In the infant the transition from a state of no infection to one when infection is operating can be very rapid and very subtle. In view of all these factors, if in doubt, it is usually advisable to start treatment with antibiotics as early as possible.

Appropriate cultures should be obtained, but because the infection exists at or beyond the obstruction, cultures may not reveal the offending organism.

In this age group erythromycin or ampicillin are the most effective antibiotics.

Definitive Treatment

Definitive treatment consists of the identification of offenders and their elimination.

Since foods and environmental factors are the chief offenders in bronchial allergic disease, when indicated, immediate attention must be given to correcting these factors. Skin testing is not reliable at this age period, so guidance must be obtained from a detailed history.

Pollens are rarely a factor in causing symptoms in early infancy. The first year of life serves as the period of primary exposure and sensitization, so that subsequent exposures during the second or even the third year of life may cause clinical symptoms.

For details of environmental control, see Chapter 17.

Dietary Management

The only effective method for determining allergy is by the use of an elimination diet which is both therapeutic and diagnostic. If the diet is successful, results will be noted within the first two weeks, but it may require as long as four weeks. The reason for the prolonged interval between the start of the diet and improvement is unknown. Dietary therapy in the infant is simplified by the fact that the infant has not been exposed to an appreciable variety in his diet. The most important allergens that are encountered are milk, egg and cereals, particularly wheat and corn. When an elimination diet is attempted in the infant, it is best to begin with a milk substitute. Mull-Soy® and Neo-Mull-Soy® have advantages in that they are relatively easy to use and provide all the necessary nutrients of early infancy, and unlike many other milk substitutes, they lack corn sugar. It is important to remember that soy is a potential allergen. Also some infants develop gastrointestinal difficulties, such as colic or diarrhea when on soy milk. If soy is not tolerated or if the allergic condition persists or worsens, meat base formula may be substituted. Some infants do not tolerate meat base formula because of cross reactivity between beef and milk. In such instances lamb base formula which has corn sugar as a source of carbohydrate may be tried.

In addition to the milk substitute, other foods such as green and yellow squash, yams and sweet potato and pears also may be started at the same time or ideally added at five to seven day intervals when the condition of the infant improves and stabilizes. White potato, banana and beets may be introduced at a later time. Lamb should be used if meat is added. If available, artichoke and asparagus also may be added. Ideally, to avoid additives and sweeteners such as corn syrup, all foods should be freshly prepared.

Once the baseline diet is established, oat, rice and rye cereals and other fruits and vegetables may be individually added. Challenge with suspected foods should not be attempted for a period of six months.

If the infant has immediate systemic sensitivity to any food, this should be excluded indefinitely from the diet. In this situation even exposure to the cooking food may precipitate symptoms. When there is known severe immediate systemic reaction to a food, challenge or even testing with the food is contraindicated.

Except for the foods which cause immediate systemic reactions, the infant with food allergy is often able to tolerate these foods when older. This is particularly the situation with milk. However, after a quiescent period, milk and other food allergies may be manifest by other symptoms in childhood or adult life. For example, the infant may have severe colic or diarrhea or vomiting as a result of a food allergy and as an older child may have bronchial asthma, serous otitis media or colitis.

Unless directions are meticulously followed, dietary therapy will fail.

It is important to have the cooperation of all family members when a diet trial has been instituted. A common source of failure is the well-meaning grandparent or baby sitter who feeds the infant a small amount of an omitted food, because "it won't hurt him" or her. Another common source of failure of dietary therapy is not trying the diet for a long enough period of time. The diet is often discontinued after a period of a week because of a lack of improvement. Another source of failure is the inclusion in the baseline diet of a food to which the infant is allergic.

It is useful to have the parents keep a diet diary, listing all the foods the infant ingests each day. By bringing this in the day of the physician visit, appropriate corrections, changes or additions to the diet can be made.

Prophylaxis of Allergy in Infancy

Allergic parents or parents of allergic children often ask, "How can I prevent allergy from occurring in my baby?" Jerome Glaser and Douglas Johnstone addressed themselves to this question (32). They cited earlier work, noting that breast-fed infants had only one seventh the incidence of atopic dermatitis as bottle-fed infants. Glaser also noted the frequent intolerance to egg yolk when this was introduced at three months of age; however, if egg yolk was introduced after nine months, intolerance was rare. Based on the above information in a retrospective study, they reviewed the course of a group of potentially allergic infants. These infants had at least one allergic parent or sibling. These infants were fed a soy bean formula (breast feeding was not in vogue at that time), and milk, beef, egg and wheat were excluded from the diet for the first six to nine months of life. They reported that the incidence of major respiratory allergy or eczema in this group of children was only twenty-five per cent that of a control group of siblings.

Because this was a retrospective study and the control group was open to question, Dutton and Johnstone repeated this work prospectively, studying a group of 283 potentially allergic children (33). Although their results were not as spectacular as the earlier study by Glaser and Johnstone, only 7 of 115 who were placed on the diet developed asthma as compared to 18 of 120 control patients. In this study the control group was fed evaporated milk formula, and during the first six months, oats, barley, rice, beef and lamb were added to the diet.

Although this work is controversial, the diet is safe, practical and easy to employ. According to these authors the exclusive use of soy milk and the late addition of single foods at five to seven day intervals, avoiding wheat, egg, fish, milk, beef, offers some protection against the later development of allergic disease.

In addition to dietary prophylaxis, control of the environment is also important in these infants. Pets with fur and feathers should be excluded from the environment. Household furnishings containing feathers, kapok, jute and animal hair should be avoided. The heating outlet into the child's bedroom should be filtered or completely closed.

Despite the fact the whole subject of the prophylaxis of allergy is debatable, the methods outlined above can be practiced without risk and can give the physician and parent an approach to the problem.

REFERENCES

1. Evans, D. G. and Smith, J. W.: Response of the infant to active immunization. *Br Med Bull, 19:* 225, 1963.
2. Williams, G. M. and Nossal, G. J.: Ontogeny of the immune response. I. The development of the follicular antigen trapping mechanism. *J Exp Med, 124:* 57, 1966.
3. Fink, C. W., Miller, W. E., Doward, B, and LoSpalluto, J.: The formation of macroglobulin antibodies. II. Studies in neonatal infants and older children. *J Clin Invest, 7:* 1422, 1962.
4. Reilly, C. M., Stokes, J., Buynak, E., Goldner, H. and Hilleman, M.: Living attenuated measles virus vaccine in early infancy. *N Engl J Med, 265:* 165, 1961.
5. Allansmith, M.: Development of immunity. In Falkner, Frank (Ed.): *Human Development.* Philadelphia, Saunders, 1966, p. 586.
6. van Furth, R., Schuit, H. and Hijmans, W.: The immunologic development of the human fetus. *J Exp Med, 122:* 1173, 1965.
7. Martensson, L. and Fudenberg, H. H.: Gm genes and γG globulin synthesis in the human fetus. *J Immunol, 94:* 914, 1965.
8. Stiehm, E. R., Ammann, A. J. and Cherry, J. D.: Elevated cord macroglobulins in the diagnosis of intrauterine infection. *N Engl J Med, 275:* 971, 1966.
9. Stiehm, E. R. and Fudenberg, H. H.: Serum levels of immune globulins in health and disease: Survey. *Pediatrics, 37:* 715, 1966.
10. Zak, S. J. and Good, R. A.: Immunochemical studies of human serum gamma globulins. *J Clin Invest, 38:* 579, 1959.
11. Brambell, F. W. R.: The passive immunity of the young mammal. *Cambridge Philosophical Society Biological Reviews, 33:* 488, 1958.
12. Winberg, J. and Wessner, G.: Does breast milk protect against septicemia in the newborn? *Lancet, I:* 1091, 1971.
13. Bazaral, M., Orgel, H. A. and Hamburger, R. N.: IgE levels in normal infants and mothers and inheritance hypothesis. *J Immunol, 107:* 794, 1971.
14. Johansson, S. G. O.: Serum IgND levels in healthy children and adults. *Int Arch Allergy Appl Immunol, 34:* 1, 1968.

15. Uhr, J. W., Dancis, J. and Neuman, C. G.: Delayed type hypersensitivity in premature neonatal humans. *Nature, 187:* 1130, 1960.
16. Gaisford, W.: The protection of infants against tuberculosis. *B Med J, 2:* 1164, 1965.
17. Silverstein, A. M., Thorbecke, G. J. and Kraner, K. L.: Homograft rejection in the fetal lamb, role of circulating antibody. *Science, 142:* 1172, 1963.
18. Clein, N. W.: Symposia on pediatric allergy: Cow's milk allergy in infants. In *Pediatric Clinics of North America.* Philadelphia, Saunders, 1954, pp. 949-962.
19. Bachmank, D. and Dees, S. C.: Milk allergy. I. Observations of symptoms and incidence in well babies. *Pediatrics, 20:* 393, 1957.
20. Katz, J., Spiro, H. and Herskovic, T.: Milk precipitating substance in the stool in gastrointestinal milk sensitivity. *N Engl J Med, 278:* 1191, 1968.
21. Self, T. W., Herskovic, T. Czapek, E. *et al.*: Gastrointestinal protein allergy: Immunologic considerations. *JAMA, 207:* 2393, 1969.
22. Davis, S. D., Bierman, C. W., Pierson, W. E., Maas, C. W. and Iannetta, A.: Clinical nonspecificity of milk coproantibodies in diarrhea stools. *N Engl J Med, 282:* 612, 1970.
23. McGovern, J. P., Haywood, T. J. and Fernandez, A. A.: Allergy and secretory otitis media. *JAMA, 200:* 134, 1967.
24. Bray, G. W.: The asthmatic child. *Arch Dis Child, 5:* 237, 1930.
25. Hogg, J. C., Williams, J., Richardson, J. B., Macklem, P. T. and Thurlbeck, W. M.: Age as a factor in the distribution of lower airway conductance and in the pathologic anatomy of obstructive lung disease. *N Engl J Med, 282:* 1283, 1970.
26. Aas, K.: Allergic asthma in childhood. *Arch Dis Child, 44:* 1, 1970.
27. Freeman, G. L. and Todd, R. H. *Am J Dis Child, 104:* 330, 1962.
28. Simon, G. and Jordan, W. S., Jr.: Infectious and allergic aspects of bronchiolitis. *J Pediatr, 70:* 533, 1967.
29. Wittig, H. J. and Glaser, J.: The relationship between bronchiolitis and childhood asthma. *J Allergy, 30:* 19, 1959.
30. Eisen, A. and Bacal, H.: The relationship of acute bronchiolitis to bronchial asthma—a 4 to 14 year follow-up. *Pediatrics, 31:* 859, 1963.
31. Diner, W. C., Kniker, W. T. and Heiner, D. C.: Roentgenologic manifestations in the lungs in milk allergy. *Radiology, 77:* 564, 1961.
32. Glaser, J. and Johnstone, D. E.: Prophylaxis of allergic disease in the newborn. *JAMA, 153:* 620, 1953.
33. Johnstone, D. E. and Dutton, A. M.: Dietary prophylaxis of allergic disease in children. *N Engl J Med, 274:* 715, 1966.

Chapter 15

DRUGS USED IN TREATMENT OF ALLERGIC DISEASE

ANTIHISTAMINES

THE VALUE OF THE antihistaminic drugs in the treatment of allergic diseases is dependent upon their antagonism for histamine, which is based upon the competition of these drugs with histamine in their attachment to cell receptors. Antihistamines do not prevent the release of histamine from the tissues in the allergic reaction and accordingly do not cure disease, but are merely palliative. This fundamental pharmacological behavior characterizes practically every one of the numerous antihistamines which have been synthesized mostly from ethylamine.

$$X-CH_2CH_2N\begin{array}{c}R_1\\R_2\end{array}$$
Ethylamine

$$\begin{array}{c}H\\HC-N\\\parallel\quad\diagup CH\\NH_2CH_2CH_2C-N\end{array}$$
Histamine

It is for this reason that practically every text on pharmacology supports the statement of Goodman and Gilman: "There is a needlessly large number of antihistamines and little distinction can be made between them on the basis of efficacy as histamine antagonists."

Absorption, Fate and Excretion of Antihistimines

Following oral administration, symptomatic relief is usually experienced within twenty to forty-five minutes which would indicate this is the time required for absorption from the gastrointestinal tract. Absorption from parenteral sites is quite similar.

The effects following a single dose of the drug usually disappear within three to four hours following the administration of a single dose. This would indicate that the drug is either inactivated or excreted during that period. For this reason, the drug must be repeated every three or four hours to experience a sustained clinical reponse. Some of the newer slow-release antihistamines can maintain their effectiveness for periods of ten to twelve hours.

Adverse Reactions

The incidence and severity of untoward effects and the dose required to produce them vary with each drug. It may be necessary for the physician to determine through trial which antihistamine performs best for the patient, both on the basis of effective control of the allergic symptoms and avoidance of untoward reactions.

Sedation

Sedation and drowsiness, the most common side effects, are induced in varying degree by practically every antihistamine. In most cases sedation and drowsiness are minor and will disappear with continuance of the drug for about two or three days. In some cases these side effects may interfere with the patient's normal daytime activity. Every patient receiving antihistaminics should be cautioned regarding the possibility

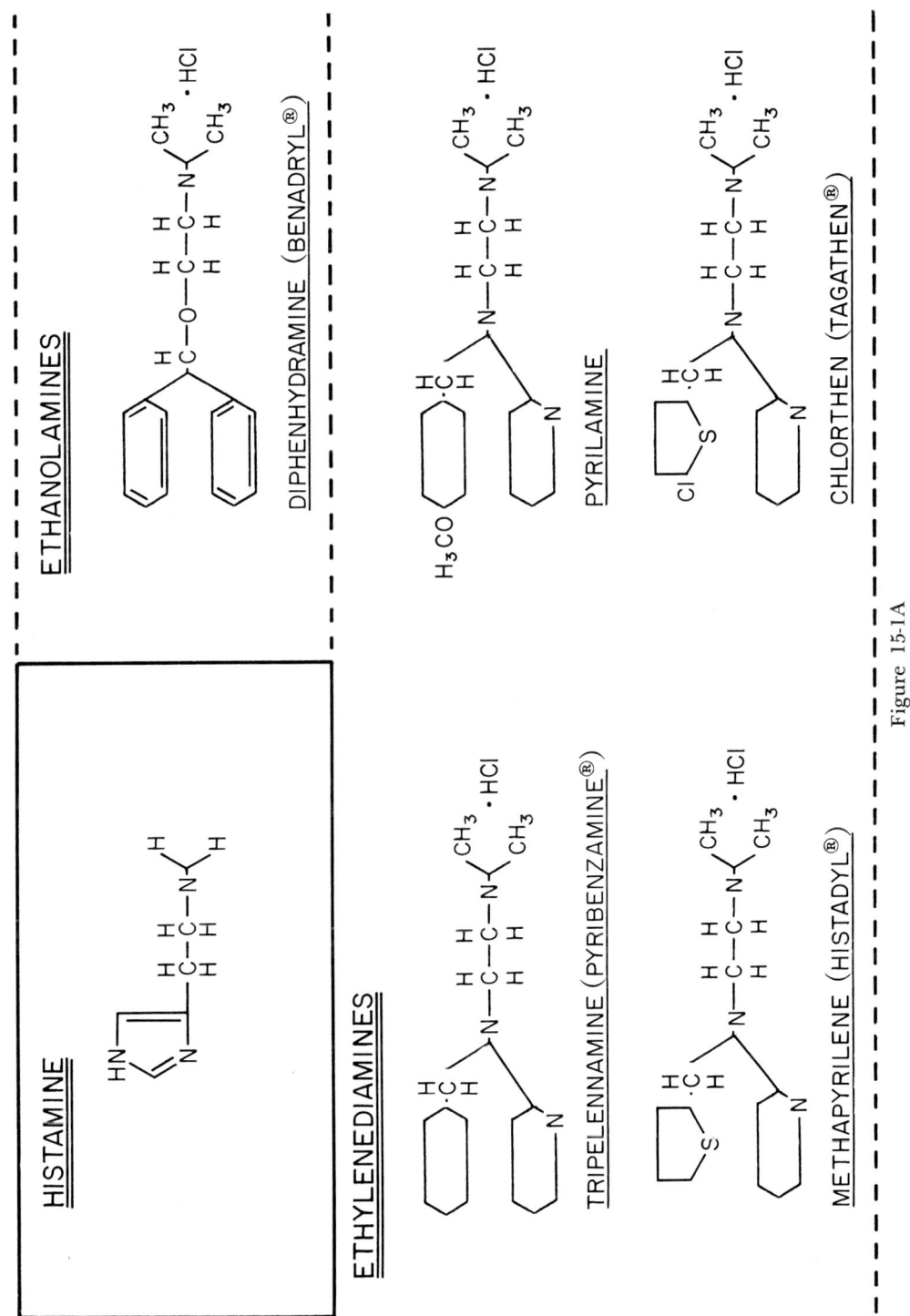

Figure 15-1A

of sedation and somnolence. The ingestion of alcoholic beverages seems to accentuate the side effects. It is particularly important to instruct individuals who are driving a car, since sudden onset of somnolence can lead to serious accidents.

When the side effects of sedation and drowsiness are severe, it may be counteracted in some cases by combining the drugs with central stimulants, such as ephedrine and methylphenidate (Ritalin®). Amphetamine is not recommended because of the

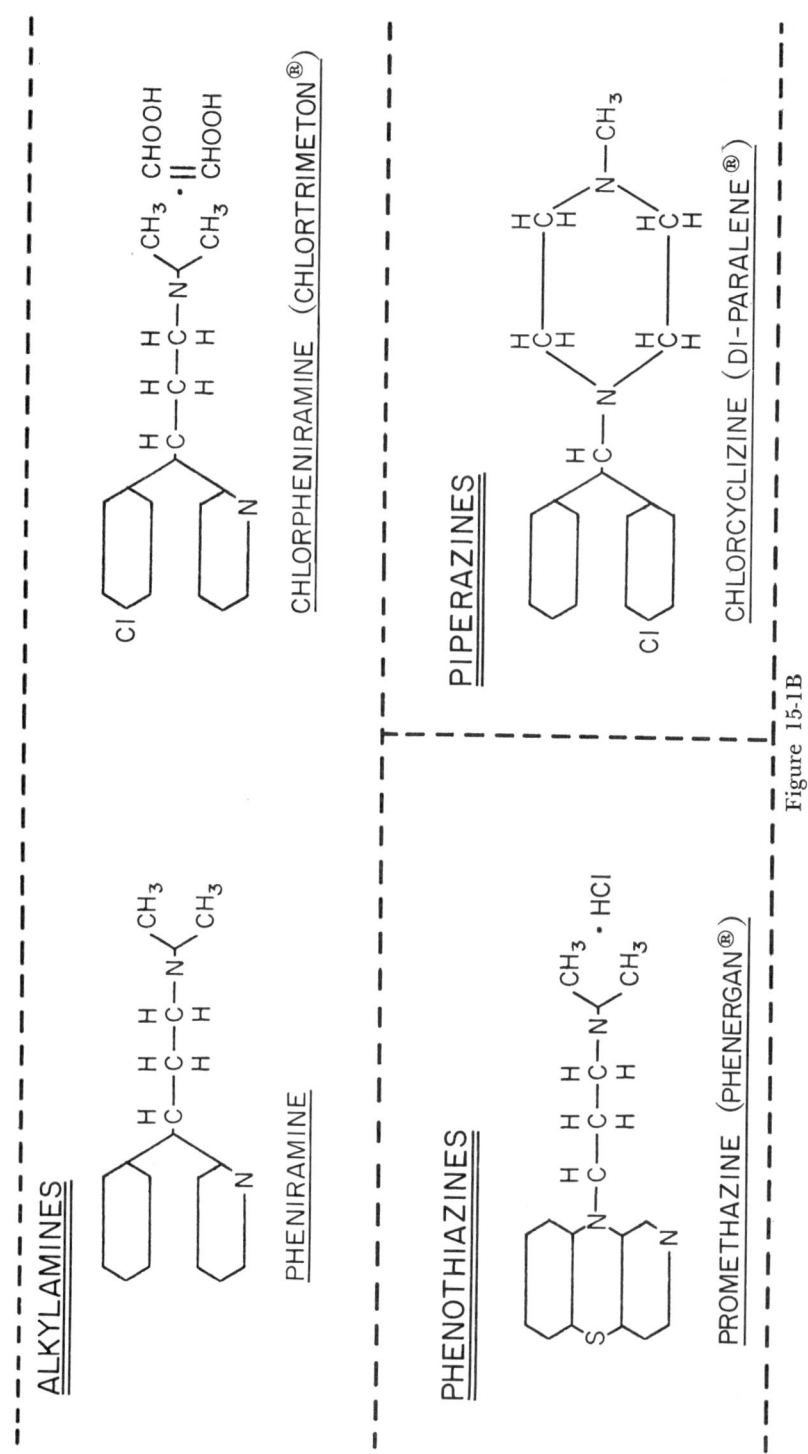

Figure 15-1B

risk of addiction. The stimulants should not be used unless substitution of other antihistamines has failed to eliminate the sedation and drowsiness.

Occasionally, the atropine-like action of the antihistamines predominates. The most common anticholinergic effect is dryness of the mouth. Symptoms of excitation, such as insomnia, tremors, nervousness, irritability, palpitation and even convulsions may occur. In cases of overdosage or accidental ingestion, death may occur. This should be guarded against in children particularly. Disorientation, vertigo, confusion and delirium have been reported occasionally. Acute labyrinthitis, hysteria and neuritis have occurred rarely.

The most commonly observed adverse response to antihistaminic drugs is depression.

The most potent sedative action is observed with:

Promethazine (Phenergan®)
Diphenhydramine (Benadryl®)
Antazoline (Antistine®)
Chlorpheniramine (Teldrin®)

Intermediate sedative action is observed with:

Tripelennamine (Pyribenzamine®)
Pheniramine (Trimeton®)

The least sedation is observed with:

Phenindamine (Thephorin®)

Blurred vision, urinary retention and tachycardia may occur with large doses of the drugs.

The depth and duration of barbiturate narcosis is increased with antihistamines.

Gastrointestinal Side Effects

Symptoms referable to the digestive tract are the second most common side effects. These include anorexia, nausea, vomiting, epigastric distress, constipation or diarrhea. The administration of the drug following meals may help eliminate these side reactions.

Blood Dyscrasias

Agranulocytosis, thrombocytopenia, pancytopenia and hemolytic anemia have on rare occasions been associated with the antihistamines. Although these reactions are rare, their possibility as a complication should be recognized, especially when patients are receiving prolonged antihistamine therapy.

Allergic Reactions to Antihistamines

Urticaria and skin eruptions may occur rarely following oral administration. Contact dermatitis following topical application is a common complication.

Antihistamines in the Common Cold

Despite the widespread indiscriminate self medication of the "common cold" with proprietary preparations, there is no evidence to support its efficacy in such cases. The observations of Fuller *et al.* (1950), have demonstrated by carefully controlled experiments that antihistamine drugs neither prevent nor cure the "common cold." The work of these investigators was based upon the course of infection in volunteers inoculated with the "cold virus."

Antihistamines may in some cases influence the serverity of the symptoms of the "common cold," but the cause remains unaffected, and the course of the illness is not shortened. The atropine-like action of the antihistamines may decrease the secretions, but this usually is not desirable physiologically. The use of antihistamines with aspirin, caffeine or acetophenetiden seems to be unwarranted.

Use of antihistaminic drugs in allergic disease is limited to those complaints caused by the action of released histamine upon the tissues, causing pruritus, erythema, and edema. This includes generalized or localized pruritus, urticaria, angio-edema, allergic rhinitis and hay fever. Antihistamines are not effective in bronchial asthma caused chiefly by the action of SRs-A which is not influenced by antihistamines. Because of the drying atropine-like action of the antihistamines, these drugs are contraindicated in all cases where there is either bronchial or pulmonary involvement. It is common practice to administer cough mixtures containing antihistamines, plus sympathomimetic drugs, such as ephedrine and cough suppressants. Such mixtures are not recommended. The antihistamine may aggravate the bronchial involvement, while suppression of the cough prevents natural elimination of bronchial secretions.

The efficacy of antihistamines as a prophy-

Table 15-I: CURRENTLY USED ANTIHISTAMINIC PREPARATIONS*

Trade Name	Generic Name	Dosage Forms
Acitidil® (Burroughs Wellcome)	Triprolidine HCl	Tablets: 2.5 mg; Syrup: 1.25 mg/5 ml.
Aliecur® (Roerig)	Clemizole HCl	Tablets: 20 and 40 mg.
Ambodryl® (Parke, Davis)	Bromodiphenhydramine HCl	Kapseals: 25 mg; Parenteral (i.v. or i.m.): 10-ml vials, 5 mg/ml; Elixir: 10 mg/4 ml.
Antistine phosphate (Ciba)	Antazoline phosphate, N.F.	Solution (nasal): 5 mg/ml.
Benadryl hydrochloride® (Parke, Davis)	Diphenhydramine HCl U.S.P.	Capsules: 25 and 50 mg; Kapseals and Emplets: 50 mg; Elixir: 10 mg/4 ml; Parenteral: 10- and 30-ml vials, 10 mg/ml.
Chlor-Trimeton maleate (Schering)	Chlorpheniramine maleate U.S.P.	Tablets: 4 mg; Repetabs: 8 and 12 mg; Parenteral; 1-ml ampul, 10 mg/ml; 2-ml ampul, 100 mg/ml; Syrup: 2 mg/4 ml.
Clistin® maleate (McNeil)	Carbinoxamine maleate N.F.	Tablets: 4 mg; R-A Tablets: 8 and 12 mg; Elixir: 4 mg/5 ml.
Decapryn® succinate (Merrell)	Doxylamine succinate U.S.P.	Tablets: 12.5 and 25 mg; Syrup: 6.25 ml/5 ml.
Diafen® (Riker)	Diphenylpyraline HCl	Tablets: 2 mg.
Diatrine® (Warner-Chilcott)	Methaphenilene HCl N.F.	Tablets: 50 mg.
Dimetane® (Robins)	Brompheniramine maleate	Tablets: 4 mg; Sustained release tablets: 8 and 12 mg; Elixir: 0.4 ml/ml; Ampul: 10 mg/ml; 200 mg/2 ml.
Diminic® (Durst)		Tablets: 25 mg pyrilamine maleate + 25 mg methapyrilene HCl.
Disomer® (White)	Dexbrompheniramine maleate	Tablets: 2 mg; Syrup: 0.4 mg/ml.
Dozar® (Tutag)	Methapyrilene HCl	Capsules: 25, 50, and 100 mg.
Forhistal maleate® (Ciba)	Dimethindene maleate	Drops (oral): 0.8 mg/ml; Syrup: 0.2 mg/ml; Tablets: 1 mg; Tablets (sustained release): 2.5 mg.
Hispril Spansule® (S.K.F.)	Diphenylpyraline HCl	Capsules (sustained release): 5 mg.
Hista-Clopane® (Lilly)		Pulvules: 25 mg Histadyl + 12.5 mg Clopane HCl; Solution: Histadyl 0.5% + Clopane HCl 0.5%
Histadyl Hydrochloride® (Lilly)	Methapyrilene HCl	Pulvules: 25 and 50 mg; Syrup: 4 mg fumarate/ml; Parenteral: 10-ml vial, 20 mg/ml; Solution 0.5%; Ointment Ophthalmic 0.5%.
Hydryllin® (Searle)		Tablets: 25 mg diphenhydramine + 100 mg aminophylline; Elixir: 12.5 mg diphenhydramine + 100 mg aminophylline/4 ml.
Neo-Antergan maleate® (Merck, Sharp & Dohme)	Pyrilamine maleate	Tablets: 50 mg.
Neohetramine® (Warner-Chilcott)	Thonzylamine HCl U.S.P.	Tablets: 25 and 50 mg.
Novahistine® (Pitman-Moore)		Tablets: 12.5 mg chlorpheniramine maleate + 5 mg phenylephrine HCl.
Perazil® (Burroughs, Wellcome)	Chlorcyclizine HCl U.S.P.	Tablets: 50 mg.
Phenergan (Wyeth)	Promethazine HCl U.S.P.	Tablets: 12.5 mg; Syrup: 6.25/5 ml.
Plimasin (Ciba)		Tablets: 25 mg tripelennamine HCl + 5 mg methylphenidyl HCl.
Polaramine® (Schering)	Dexchlorpheniramine maleate N.F.	Tablets: 2 mg; Syrup: 0.4 mg/ml; Repetabs: 4 and 6 mg.
Pyribenzamine Citrate® (Ciba)	Tripelennamine citrate U.S.P.	Elixir: 7.5 mg/ml.
Pyribenzamine HCl® (Ciba)	Tripelennamine HCl U.S.P.	Tablets: 25 and 50 mg; Lontabs Tablets: 50 mg; Solution (nasal): 0.5%; Tablets: 25 mg + 12 mg ephedrine sulf.; Parenteral (i.v. or i.m.): 1-ml ampuls, 25 mg/ml.
Pyronil® (Lilly)	Pyrrobutamine phosphate N.F.	Tablets: 15 mg.
Pyrrolazote (Upjohn)	Pyrathiazine HCl U.S.P.	Tablets: 25 and 50 mg (laminated tablets) 50 mg.
Semikon HCl® (Massengill)	Methapyrilene HCl U.S.P.	Tablets: 50 mg.
Statomin Maleate® (Bowman)	Pyrilamine maleate U.S.P.	Tablets: 25 mg.
Tacaryl® (Mead Johnson)	Methdilazine HCl	Tablets: 8 mg; Syrup: 0.8 mg/ml.
Tagathen® (Lederle)	Chlorothen citrate N.F.	Tablets: 25 mg.
Teldrin Spansule (S.K.F.)	Chlorpheniramine maleate U.S.P.	Capsules: (sustained release) 8 and 12 mg.
Temaril® (S.K.F.)	Trimeprazine tartrate	Capsule: (sustained release) 5 mg; Syrup 0.5 mg/ml; Tablets: 2.5 mg.
Theophorin® (Hoffmann-LaRoche)	Phenindamine tartrate N.F.	Tablets: 10 and 25 mg.
Trimeton (Schering)	Pheniramine maleate N.F. (prophenpyridamine maleate)	Tablets: 25 mg.

*From Krantz, John C., Jr. and Carr, C. Jelleff: Response to histamine and antihistaminic agents. In *Pharmacological Principles of Medical Practice*, 7th ed. Baltimore, Williams and Wilkins, 1969.

lactic against parenterally administered medications or blood transfusions has never been confirmed.

The choice of a particular drug is related to the incidence of side effects that it produces. Although the incidence of side effects and particularly drowsiness can be stated generally, the actual tolerance for a drug can only be determined by the patient's response. The selection of a drug is usually governed by the experience or personal preference of the physician.

SYMPATHOMIMETIC DRUGS

Drugs which emulate the action of epinephrine and norepinephrine are termed sympathomimetic drugs. There are two classes of sympathomimetic drugs: the catecholamines which are direct acting and the non-catecholamines which are indirect acting. The direct acting drugs, such as epinephrine, norepinephrine and isoproterenol produce their effect by acting upon the tissue receptor sites directly. The indirect acting drugs, such as amphetamine and ephedrine induce their effect indirectly by provoking the release of norepinephrine from stores in adrenergic nerve terminals.

Drugs which influence the same receptors as norepinephrine and epinephrine are called *adrenergic drugs*.

The effect of a sympathomimetic drug is determined by the type of receptor with which it can react to elicit a response.

In 1948 Alquist classified the receptors as alpha (α) and beta (β) on the basis of their response to six sympathomimetic amines.

Alpha receptors are associated with the excitatory response of smooth muscle. Interaction of a catecholamine with an alpha receptor in smooth muscle causes contraction.

Beta receptors cause relaxation of smooth muscle and also increase the heart rate and the strength of cardiac contractions. Stimulation of the beta receptors is very important in the management of bronchial asthma because of the relaxation of bronchiolar smooth muscle secondary to the beta receptor stimulation.

The Catecholamines

Epinephrine: Because of its action upon alpha and beta receptors epinephrine is perhaps the most valuable drug in the treatment of acute allergic conditions. In bronchial asthma stimulation of the beta receptors relieves the bronchospasm, while stimulation of the alpha receptors relieves the edema of the bronchial tree. Urticaria, angio-edema and anaphylaxis are controlled through vasoconstriction secondary to stimulation of alpha receptors.

Epinephrine is usually administered subcutaneously as epinephrine-HCl 1-1000 in doses of 0.3 to 0.4 ml for adults and lesser doses for children. The drug may be repeated at intervals of five to thirty minutes depending upon the response of the patient.

Epinephrine suspended in sodium thioglycollate (Sus-Phrine®) provides a depot for slow release over a period of several hours which eliminates the necessity for repeated hypodermic injections. With such injections it is important to make certain that the patient is showing a good response to the depot epinephrine. Unless the patient is observed carefully for a favorable response to the epinephrine, a sense of false security may be created which can permit the development of status asthmaticus.

Epinephrine fastness (the failure to respond to epinephrine) is usually secondary to dehydration and acidosis which accompany status asthmaticus. When the patient fails to respond to epinephrine, the intravenous administration of fluids (5% glucose in water), even in quantities as small as 500 cc will frequently correct the failure to respond.

Levarterenol (Norepinephrine): Norepinephrine acts primarily on the alpha receptors and as such has no value in the management of bronchial asthma.

Isoproterenol (Isuprel®): Isoproterenol has a very strong action on beta receptors and almost no action on alpha receptors. Because of this behavior, isoproterenol has a very strong bronchodilator action. However, lacking the effect of epinephrine on the alpha receptors, it is less effective in the control of bronchial asthma which also has a component of edema secondary to vasodilatation with increased vascular permeability.

It is *not* effective in anaphylaxis which has a strong component of vascular collapse.

Isoproterenol is available clinically as Isuprel as sublingual tablets (10 and 15 mg), as an aerosol (0.25%), and as solution (0.5 and 1%).

The most useful form for treatment of asthma is the sublingual tablet which in some cases offers immediate relief from acute attacks of asthma. (For discussion of Isuprel aerosol, see discussion below on aerosol sprays.)

Salbutanol is a beta-adrenergic receptor stimulant which does not produce the tachycardia that accompanies isoproterenol. The drug is still under study and not yet in general use in this country.

The Noncatecholamines

Amphetamine: Because of the very weak bronchodilator action of amphetamine, it has no application in clinical allergy.

Ephedrine: Ephedrine is effective following oral administration, but because of its slower absorption, the action of the drug is delayed as compared with both epinephrine and isoproterenol which are absorbed rapidly and act rapidly. Although ephedrine is much less effective than epinephrine, because of its prolonged action, it finds useful clinical application for the control of both bronchial allergy and bronchial asthma. The stimulation of the higher centers is quite marked in many patients, necessitating the simultaneous administration of a sedative drug to counteract these undesirable side effects.

This is the principle involved in various acute-asthmatic mixtures which combine ephedrine with phenobarbital, seconal or hydroxyzine drugs.

In some young children ephedrine is somewhat relaxing and sedating.

Methoxyphenamine Hydrochloride (1) *Orthoxine®*) : This is similar in action to ephedrine but has fewer cardiovascular effects. Orthoxine is tolerated by older males who develop spasm of the neck of the urinary bladder following ephedrine.

AEROSOL SPRAYS: Aerosol sprays incorporating epinephrine, isoproterenol and salbutanol are in common usage for self medication by the patient.

Preparations:

Vaponefrin®: 2.25 per cent racemic epinephrine-HCl

Aludrine® }
Isuprel } 1:200 concentration of isoproterenol

Salbutanol: Available in England, similar to isoproterenol with few side effects upon heart

Most sprays are propelled by a fluorinated propellant (freon) and deliver a measured dose of the medication with each inhalation from the apparatus. Some devices are available for delivering aqueous epinephrine-HCl 1-1000 in mist form.

A marked increase in the number of asthmatic deaths in England, Australia, and in this country, attributed to the rise in utilization of aerosol sprays for the treatment of asthma, has raised considerable controversy regarding the advisability of prescribing this form of therapy and permitting the over-the-counter sale of aerosol sprays.

It is generally recognized that aerosol sprays are frequently effective in relieving the symptoms of acute asthmatic attacks, but the unreliability of the procedure and the risk of abuse by the patient cancel the benefits claimed by the proponents of this method of therapy. The claim is made, and no doubt correctly, that aerosol sprays are safe with restricted use. The physician is advised to carefully inform the patient regarding the hazards from excessive use and to instruct the patient not to exceed three inhalations of the spray at each session and limit the use of the spray to three or four times in twenty-four hours. Theoretically, such instructions seem judicious; however, it is not reasonable to expect the patient who becomes panicky, anxious and apprehensive with an acute asthmatic episode to practice the self discipline required to refrain from the excessive use of the spray, which is usually in close proximity to the patient. In the absence of strict supervision by the physician, the spray becomes a crutch which can lead to unfavorable reactions or even death. The fatalities are estimated at 5 percent of the patients using this form of therapy. However, when a patient falls into the fifth percentile, the price is too high when more conservative procedures are available.

The precise cause of death is not determined, since most of the fatalities occur when the patient is alone and is found clutching the spray with the hand. Adverse reactions may be induced by either the drug or the propellant. The drug may aggravate the bronchospasm and induce cardiac arrhythmias leading to cardiac arrest.

Death induced by the freon propellant has been attributed to various causes:

(1) direct depression of the heart
(2) indirect cardiac mechanisms, e.g. fibrillation or arrest
    (a) reflex vagal and sympathetic influences
    (b) adrenal medulla influences
    (c) asphyxia
(3) local bronchopulmonary factors, e.g. bronchospasm, pulmonary edema and congestion
(4) secondary respiratory failure
(5) primary respiratory failure—reflex-respiratory muscles

The controlled administration of Isuprel sprays for respiratory function studies conducted under the supervision of trained personnel should present no problems.

The use of sprays for nonallergic chronic respiratory complaints should be determined by the judgment of the attending physician, but in every instance the patient should be informed of the hazards and carefully instructed regarding the use of the spray.

XANTHINES

The methylated xanthines, theophylline, theobromine and caffeine are the most commonly used xanthine preparations in clinical medicine. The three drugs have similar pharmacological responses, e.g. cerebral stimulation, coronary and bronchial muscle dilatation and diuresis, but the degree of each type of response varies with each drug in different tissues. Since theophylline manifests the strongest bronchodilator action of the three, it has the greatest effectiveness in the clinical management of bronchial allergy and bronchial asthma.

The broncho-dilator action of the methyl xanthines is due to the following sequence:

(1) *adenyl cyclase* is an enzyme that activates the β-receptors of bronchial musculature
(2) *phosphodiesterase* is an enzyme that inactivates *adenyl cyclase*
(3) *methyl xanthines* inactivate phosphodiesterase, which permits
(4) *uninhibited adenyl cyclase* to act upon the bronchial musculature to produce *bronchodilatation*.

Theophylline, which occurs as a white, crystalline, bitter powder of very low solubility in water (1-120) produces very low blood levels following oral administration, which decreases its clinical effectiveness. Theophylline is more frequently employed in the form of soluble derivatives or mixtures, such as aminophylline, oxtriphylline (Choledyl®), elixophyllin and theophylline olamine. Of these, aminophylline is the most popular.

1. *Aminophylline*

Aminophylline is a combination of theophylline and ethylenediamine. The ethylenediamine renders the compound soluble and effects a more dependable absorption from the gastrointestinal tract.

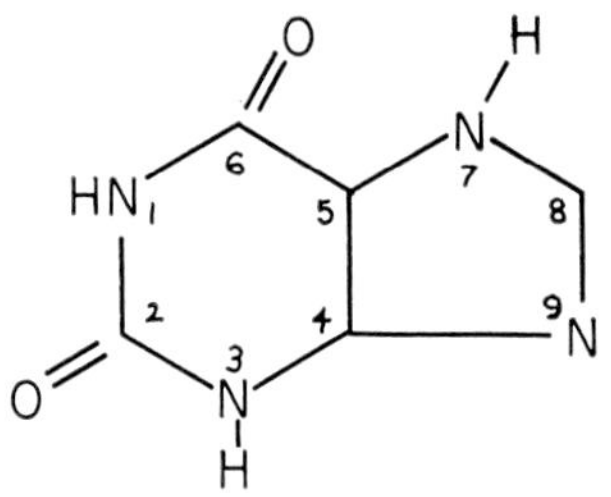

XANTHINE

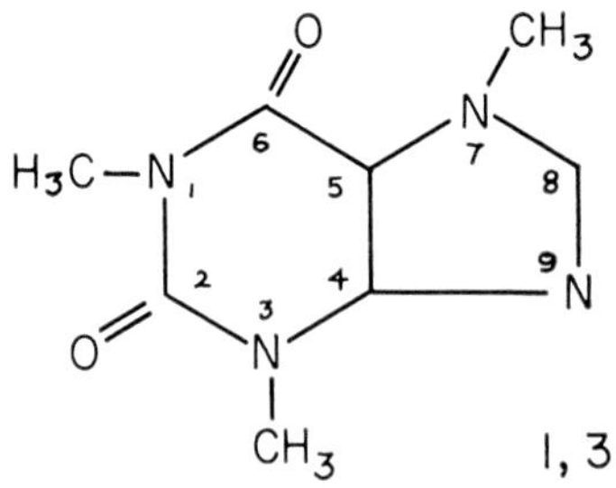

CAFFEINE
1, 3, 7 TRIMETHYL XANTHINE

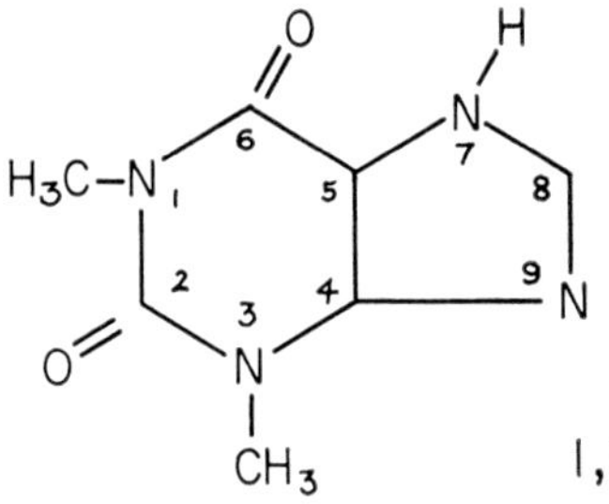

THEOPHYLLINE
1,3 DIMETHYL XANTHINE

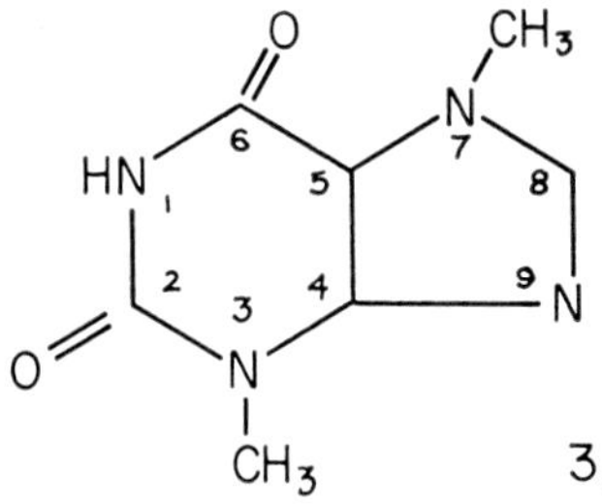

THEOBROMINE
3,7 DIMETHYL XANTHINE

Figure 15-2

(a) The oral administration of tablets (100–200 mg) is not particularly effective and in addition may cause gastric irritation.

(b) To avoid gastric irritation, suppositories (120, 250 and 500 mg) are frequently administered. Most patients who do not tolerate oral aminophylline because of gastric irritation will experience the same adverse reaction upon rectal administration. This suggests that gastric irritation may not be entirely a local response. Prolonged use of suppositories causes rectal irritation.

(c) The intravenous administration of aminophylline produces the most effective response.

The drug is often administered in 25 and 50 mg doses in volumes of 10 ml and 20 ml, respectively, for mild cases of asthma. When administered in this fashion, the drug should be introduced very slowly (10 ml in ten minutes or 20 ml in a period of twenty minutes or more). If the patient manifests any untoward response, the injection should be discontinued. Aminophylline in this form is not the treatment of choice for mild cases of bronchial asthma, since a more effective and safer procedure is the hypodermic administration of epinephrine 1-1000 followed by depot epinephrine, such as Sus-Phrine, 0.25 cc.

When dehydration is marked, the administration of an ampule of aminophylline is usually not effective, since such patients require correction of the fluid balance which will help dislodge inspissated mucus plugs, an important factor in persistent asthma.

The most effective reponse to aminophylline, and particularly in status asthmaticus, is observed following the administration of the drug as a supplement to or part of an intravenous drip. For adults 0.5 gm can be administered with a 500 cc drip of water or dextrose with water over a period of one to two hours.

For children the dose can be calculated on the basis of 4 mg/kg over a six hour period.

The aminophylline may be included in the intravenous fluid or offered as a supplement (piggy back through the intravenous tube).

When administered to either adults or children an intolerance to aminophylline should be ruled out and the history checked for possible cumulative effect from oral or rectal use of the drug just prior to the intravenous drip.

Side Effects: The commonest side reaction following oral administration of aminophylline is gastric irritation with nausea and vomiting, and epigastric distress. Similar symptoms may occur following any form of administration of the drug.

Following intravenous administration of aminophylline, particularly when administered too rapidly, serious reactions may occur with mental excitation, vomiting, hypotension and collapse.

Untoward and even fatal reactions are observed more commonly in children, especially during the first three years of life. Children do not tolerate aminophylline as well as adults, and great caution must always be exercised when the drug is administered to children. Aminophylline is not recommended for children three years of age or under. Deaths in children have been reported following the administration of a single suppository or aminophylline. Gastric hemorrhage in children following rectal aminophylline has been observed.

2. Elixophyllin

Elixophyllin which contains 80 mg of theophylline in 15 ml of 20 per cent alcohol is absorbed rapidly with little gastric irritation, which makes it a desirable preparation for oral administration.
Dose: 30 to 60 ml every four hours.

3. Oxtriphylline (NF) (Choline theophylline or Choledyl)

Oxtriphylline is a true salt of theophylline in which a choline group is substituted for a hydrogen atom. The preparation is more soluble than aminophylline and is more readily absorbed from the stomach with less gastric irritation. Available in tablets of 100 and 200 mg.

Theophylline Mixtures: The theophylline preparations indicated above have disadvantages which make long term administration unsatisfactory. Combinations of theophylline containing smaller doses of theophylline or a derivative have found widespread use. The AMA Drug Evaluations for 1971 lists sixty-four such mixtures. Only a few can be discussed in this book.

Tedral® contains: theophylline
ephedrine sulfate
phenobarbital

Preparations including other forms of barbiturates are also on the market. The small dose of phenobarbital or other forms of barbiturates is included to counteract the adverse symptoms secondary to stimulation of the higher centers by the theophylline and especially the ephedrine. Great caution must be exercised, since such preparations containing barbiturates (three or four times daily for several months) can lead to barbiturates dependence.

Marax® contains: theophylline
ephedrine
hydroxyzine HCl
(Atarax®)

The formula of Marax is similar to Tedral except for the hydroxyzine HCl which is substituted for the phenobarbital. A patient who has been on Tedral who states that Marax fails to offer equal relief should be held in suspicion for barbiturate dependence.

Mixtures with Expectorants: The inclusion of expectorants such as potassium iodide or glycerol guaiacolates is of questionable value and presents definite disadvantages.

When an expectorant is indicated in addition to the theophylline or ephedrine present in a mixture, it is advisable to administer the expectorant separately so that the required dosage can be effectively controlled. Combinations including expectorants lead to either an inadequate or an excess dose of the expectorant. Potassium iodide which is commonly included in the mixtures can lead to hyperkalemia or iodism if administered over long periods. Excessive guaiacolate may cause gastric irritation.

The use of mixtures containing antacids is not recommended. The antacids are included to counteract gastric symptoms which may be evidence of gastric irritation. The antacid can mask the toxic side effects of the theophylline which could be hazardous in some cases.

EXPECTORANTS

Drugs which augment respiratory secretions, reduce their viscosity, and facilitate the expulsion of secretions through ciliary action are termed expectorants. Adequate methods have not been developed for evaluating the effectiveness of any expectorant in influencing the volume and viscosity of bronchial secretions. The efficiency of mucolytic agents also cannot be satisfactorily evaluated. It is for this reason that, although expectorant drugs have enjoyed wide clinical acceptance, their effectiveness is based upon tradition rather than experimental evidence.

Our understanding of the physiology of the reflex mechanism involved between gastric irritation and nausea and vomiting has been advanced by the studies of Bronson and Wang (1953). It is believed that an identical reflex function influences respiratory tract secretions. The action of most of the commonly prescribed expectorants is attributed to reflex action upon the respiratory mucosa following irritation of the gastric mucosa. Drugs included in this group are potassium iodide, hydriodic acid, ammonium chloride, glyceryl guaiacolate (Robitussin®), and iodinated glycerin (Organidin®).

The volatile oils such as terpin hydrate are believed to act by direct effect upon the bronchial secretory cells.

Convincing experimental evidence to support the action of drugs in either class is lacking.

Expectorant Drugs

Water

Although water is not classified as a drug, clinical experience indicates that water is actually the best of all expectorants. Dehydration is the most important contributory factor in the bronchial obstruction of bronchial allergy and bronchial asthma. Without an adequate fluid intake the various expectorant drugs are ineffective in correcting the viscosity of the mucus and releasing inspissated plugs.

For the average adult 2,000 to 3,000 by mouth in twenty-four hours, and for children, smaller amounts are recommended. In some patients even large quantities of water by mouth are ineffective, while an early good response may be observed following the intravenous (IV) administration of fluids; even as little as 500 to 1,000 ml of 5 per cent glucose in water may be effective.

When fluids by mouth are not retained, intravenous fluids must be administered. Initially, 1,000 ml by rapid drip (forty-five to sixty minutes) followed by an additional 1,000 to 2,000 ml by slow drip. (For use of water in dermatitis see Chap. 6)

Steam Inhalation

It is well to recognize that efficient functioning of the cilia is dependent upon optimal humidity (40–50%). Dry air aggravates the symptoms caused by inspissated mucus and plugs.

It is not necessary to have the patient's room dripping with moisture to produce the desired conditions. In many environments, particularly when the humidity of the region is not low, no provision for additional moisture is necessary. However, when the vapor tension drops below 40 per cent, which is common in dry climates, additional moisture in the air can be very beneficial. In many cases this can be accomplished by placing a container with water with a large exposed surface in the patient's room. In some regions with a very dry climate a vaporizer may be helpful. When a vaporizer is used, the concentration of moisture in the room should be checked carefully. Excessive moisture, particularly over prolonged uninterrupted periods (twenty-four to forty-eight hours or more), predisposes to the growth of molds which can complicate the clinical picture.

Aerosol Inhalation Preparations

Various aerosol procedures and medications have been advocated for the management of respiratory diseases. These drugs and procedures have no application to the treatment of bronchial allergy or bronchial asthma, except when these conditions are complicated by chronic pulmonary changes as observed with bronchiectasis and chronic bronchitis. In the presence of bronchial asthma, care must always be exercised in the use of such preparations to avoid the induction of bronchospasm.

In some cases the use of nebulized water or hypertonic saline may be helpful agents for increasing respiratory fluid volume. The hypertonic solution induces its effect by osmosis.

Propylene glycol with glycerin is added to most aerosols to draw water into the bronchial secretions through its hygroscopic action.

Acetyl cysteine (Mucomyst®) is used to reduce the viscosity of abnormal bronchial secretions. It finds greater application in patients with chronic bronchitis, emphysema and bronchiectasis complicating the allergic state. The drug when used should serve as an adjunct to therapy and not as a substitute for routine measures.

Experimental studies are not conclusive as to the value of Mucomyst; however, clinical experience seems to indicate it may be of some value.

Great caution must be exercised in the use of this drug in asthmatics because of the risk of serious bronchospasm. Stomatitis and ulcerations occur occasionally, while nausea and vomiting may be induced by the increased volume of sputum.

Probable sensitization to the drug has been reported in three cases.

Dosage: 1 to 10 ml of a 10 to 20 per cent solution is nebulized through a face mask or a mouthpiece every four to six hours.

When used in an oxygen tent, bed tent, or croup tent, enough 20 per cent solution (50-300 ml) is used to provide a heavy mist.

Precautions: In administering the drug, contact with metals and rubber should be avoided because of the reaction with these materials. Polyethylene tubing is recommended.

Because severe bronchospasm may occur, close observation by the physician is mandatory. With bronchospasm the drug should be discontinued promptly and a bronchodilator administered. Close supervision is necessary, particularly in aged or severely debilitated patients to prevent drowning due to excessive secretions.

Alevaire® is a detergent mixture which increases wetting and thereby increases the liquefaction of mucus. Available evidence is not convincing that Alevaire or other detergent preparations are more effective than plain water or sodium chloride solutions.

Pancreatic dornase (Dornavac®), an enzyme, has been advocated because it reduces viscosity of secretions and particularly purulent mucus.

The effectiveness of this and other enzymes in the treatment of asthma is questionable, while the risk of sensitivity reactions is great. These medications are not recommended to allergic patients.

None of the aerosols has proved to be of greater therapeutic benefit than adequate humidification.

Potassium Iodide

Potassium iodide (KI) is perhaps the most commonly prescribed expectorant drug. Potassium iodide is administered in saturated solution.

Dosage: 10 to 15 drops *tid, pc* in water for adults
4 to 6 drops *tid, pc* for children, depending upon age and weight

Potassium iodide should be administered for short term therapy (ten to fourteen days). Prolonged administration may lead to complications. In some patients the adverse reactions may appear after the first few doses of the drug.

Adverse Reactions: Iodism is characterized by a fine papulo-pustular eruption, parotitis, fever and a profuse watery rhinorrhea which causes a burning, painful excoriation of the nares. When reactions occur, the drug should be stopped immediately.

Potassium iodide or any of the iodinated expectorants may cause thyroid enlargement and interfere with the interpretation of thyroid function.

Potassium iodide should not be administered during pregnancy, since it crosses the placental barrier and may cause thyroid enlargement of the fetus.

Sodium Iodide

Sodium iodide is often added to intravenous solutions for treatment of severe asthma or status asthmaticus. The dose is 0.5 to 1.0 gm added to 500 and 1,000 ml, respectively, of intravenous fluid.

Syrup of Hydriodic Acid (Syr. H.I.)

This is commonly prescribed for children who will not tolerate the unpleasant taste of potassium iodide. Syr. H. I. is not considered as effective as K.I.

Ammonium Chloride

Ammonium chloride is administered in doses of 0.5 to 2.0 gm, *pc*. Its effectiveness is attributed to reflex action on the respiratory mucosa through gastric irritation. Its usefulness is doubtful.

Glycrol Guaiacolate (Robitussin®)

The effectiveness of this drug is also attributed to reflex action upon bronchial mucosa generated by gastric irritation. There is inadequate evidence to support this contention.

>Dosage: 100 to 200 mg, two to four times daily by mouth Robitussin (Robins) 100 mg/5 ml

Side Reactions: Gastrointestinal upset and drowsiness occur rarely.

Syrup of Ipecac

Ipecac is a time honored drug whose expectorant quality has been recognized for many years. Recent studies seem to indicate the emetic drugs (ipecac, apomorphine) in small doses may elicit subthreshold stimulation of the chemoreceptor trigger zone in the medulla. The vomiting center is not activated, and emesis does not result, but the secretory reflex for salivation and increased respiratory tract secretions is intensified, followed by a typical expectorant action.

Dosage: (should not be confused with fluid extract of Ipecac which is much more powerful)

>Syrup of Ipecac for adults, 0.5 to 2 ml every six hours
>Not recommended for children

Expectorant Mixtures

The AMA Drug Evaluations for 1971 lists thirty-seven expectorant mixtures which have been formulated in most cases as preparations to combat the "common cold" rather than allergic respiratory diseases.

Most of the mixtures contain at least one and sometimes two antihistamines, which, because of their atropine like action, are contraindicated in allergic bronchial disease. Every mixture contains either one or two expectorants which are usually ammonium chloride or glyceryl guaiacolate. An occasional preparation contains potassium iodide or ipecac. Some mixtures, in addition to an expectorant and an antihistamine, contain codeine which apparently is included as a cough suppressant. The opiates cancel any possible effectiveness of the expectorants and in addition are contraindicated in the management of disease of the bronchial tree or lung parenchyma.

A review of the various mixtures is reminiscent of the old Galenical preparations which were designed to cover all bases and hopefully provide for the patient's complaint. None of the mixtures is an expression of good clinical practice. The clinician can treat allergic bronchial diseases more effectively by prescribing individual medications chosen for a specific purpose to cover the needs of each individual patient.

CORTICOTROPIN (ACTH) AND ADRENAL CORTICOSTEROIDS

Corticotropin (ACTH)

ACTH, the hormone derived from the anterior pituitary, stimulates the adrenal medulla to produce corticosteroids. ACTH has no direct therapeutic action. The secretion of ACTH is governed by (1) the blood level of the corticosteroids which serve as a reverse feedback mechanism to control the rate of secretion of ACTH, and (2) by the corticotropin releasing factor (CRF) which is produced in the hypothalamus and transported to the anterior pituitary by means of the hypophyseal-portal vessels. Through this relationship with the hypothalamus various stress factors, such as trauma, emotional disturbances, anesthesia and some illnesses stimulate an increased production of CRF which leads to increased release of ACTH which in turn stimulates the production of corticosteroids (see discussion below).

With the development of the synthetic glucocorticoids, ACTH is no longer the drug of choice in the treatment of allergic disease. ACTH, which must be injected either intramuscularly or intravenously, offers no advantages and perhaps many disadvantages over the oral preparations of glucocorticoids.

Although ACTH is frequently administered to re-establish adrenal responsiveness following the suppression induced by glucocorticoids, this procedure is not reliable. ACTH does not hasten re-establishment of adrenal responsiveness if administered during the withdrawal of glucocorticoids. In addition, ACTH may induce adrenal hypertrophy which can result in failure of the pituitary-adrenal system.

The administration of ACTH has the following disadvantages:

(1) Its use during withdrawal of glucocorticoids does not hasten re-establishment of adrenal responsiveness.

(2) It produces adrenal hypertrophy which can lead to failure of the pituitary-adrenal system.

(3) It stimulates the secretion of deoxycorticosterone and androgens which have no anti-inflammatory effect.

(4) Deoxycorticosterone can produce edema and hypokalemia.

(5) The androgens can produce acne, hirsutism and amenorrhea.

(6) ACTH is a protein which can induce allergic reactions following repeated injections.

The drug is administered either intramuscularly, subcutaneously or intravenously. Various preparations are available for this purpose, e.g. aqueous suspension, suspension in zinc chloride and Gelfoams® for repository administration. The dosage and method of administration for the parenteral preparations are included in the package by the pharmaceutical manufacturer.

ACTH is not the drug of choice for the treatment of allergic conditions.

Corticosteroids

Stimulation of the adrenals by ACTH leads to the production of a number of corticosteroids which have been divided into two types:

(1) *Mineralocorticoids* which are strong on sodium retention but with little or no effect on liver glycogen deposition. The prototype of this group is deoxycorticosteroid.

(2) The *glucocorticoids* which manifest a strong action on liver glycogen storage but have a weak or no effect upon sodium retention. The prototype is cortisol (hydrocortisone), which is the principal glucocorticoid excreted in man. Cortisol and cortisone are naturally occurring steroids, but cortisone was the first steroid to be synthesized.

Actions of Glucocorticoids

(1) Glucocorticoids influence the metabolism of carbohydrates, proteins, fats and

purines. They cause a marked accumulation of glycogen in the liver and can produce hyperglycemia and glycosuria. Because of these actions they tend to aggravate diabetes and may bring on an insulin resistant disturbance of carbohydrate metabolism in latent diabetics.

Glucocorticoids promote the breakdown of protein and tend to inhibit the anabolism or synthesis of proteins. These factors contribute to growth retardation in children receiving glucocorticoids. Wound healing is also impaired by these steroids.

The action on fat metabolism is not understood but is evidenced clinically by the accumulation of fat as seen with the "buffalo hump."

Glucocorticoids have a complex effect upon ketone metabolism.

The influence upon purine metabolism is evidenced by increased excretion of uric acid.

(2) They *influence electrolyte* and *water metabolism* by increasing sodium retention which leads to water retention and edema; increased potassium excretion leads to hypokalemic alkalosis especially in patients on long term therapy.

The disturbance in sodium and potassium excretion influences the distribution of electrolytes between the cellular and extracellular compartments.

(3) Glucocorticoids influence the inflammatory process. The precise mechanism of the anti-inflammatory action is not known, but it is proposed that corticosteroids halt the inflammatory process by increasing the resistance of cells to cytotoxic activity of phlogogenic substances. At the molecular level corticosteroids protect the cell by rendering it impermeable to the deleterious effects of breakdown products of injured cells.

The anti-inflammatory effects of glucocorticoids can perhaps be attributed to their capacity to suppress the cell's activity in producing the chemical agents responsible for inflammation. On the other hand, their action in the presence of infection provides an opportunity for the proliferation of bacteria because of the suppression of the chemical mediators involved in inflammation, particularly leukocytosis-promoting factor (LPF).

Steroids produce improved capillary tone and induce selective permeability which diminish the exudation of plasma into the tissues. These are important factors in allergic responses characterized by edema, such as urticaria and angio-edema.

(4) Cardiac arrhythmias may develop following the hypokalemia induced by prolonged administration of corticosteroids. In patients with marked renal impairment caution must be exercised when administering corticosteroids because of the electrolyte imbalance which can result in cardiac disturbances and even cardiac arrest.

(5) Muscle weakness especially of the upper extremities can follow prolonged administration of corticosteroids. The symptoms respond to a decrease in dosage.

(6) Gastric symptoms frequently result from the increased gastric acid and pepsin production. The protective mucus barrier is disturbed which interferes with gastric repair, leading to peptic ulcers and gastritis.

(7) Central nervous system effects: Large doses of corticosteroids may cause euphoria, nervousness, irritability, increased motor activity and insomnia. Patients suffering from convulsive disorders and psychoses must be observed very carefully when receiving corticosteroids.

(8) Ocular effects: Glaucoma and posterior subcapsular cataracts have been observed with corticosteroid therapy, usually with administration over long periods.

(9) Osteoporosis is a common adverse response to long term glucocorticoid therapy. Patients on long term therapy with steroids should be reviewed frequently with x-ray studies to rule out the development of osteoporosis which can predispose to painless vertebral compression fractures and involvement of fractures of other parts of the skeleton.

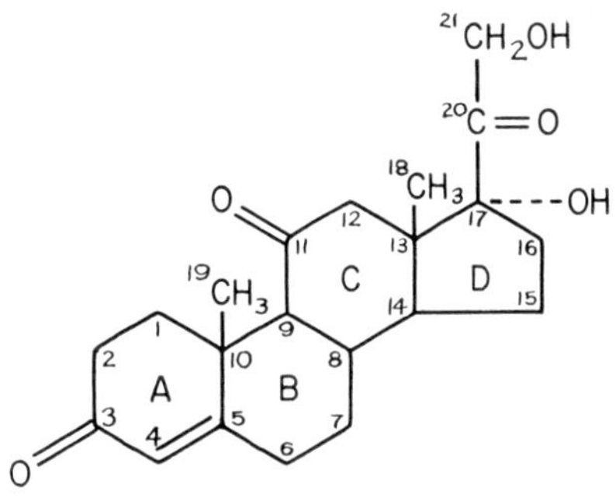

Drugs Used in Treatment of Allergic Disease

Cortisone
(Compound E)

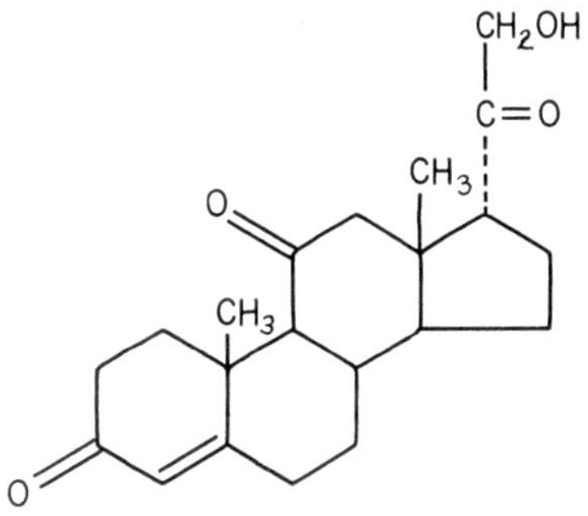

11-dehydrocorticosterone
(Compound A)

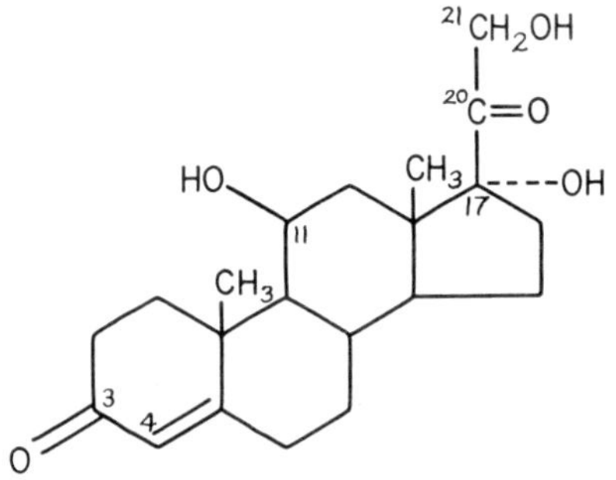

Hydrocortisone
(Compound F)

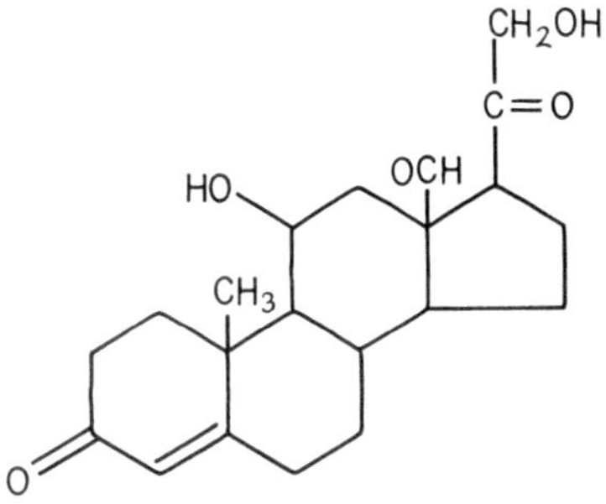

Aldosterone

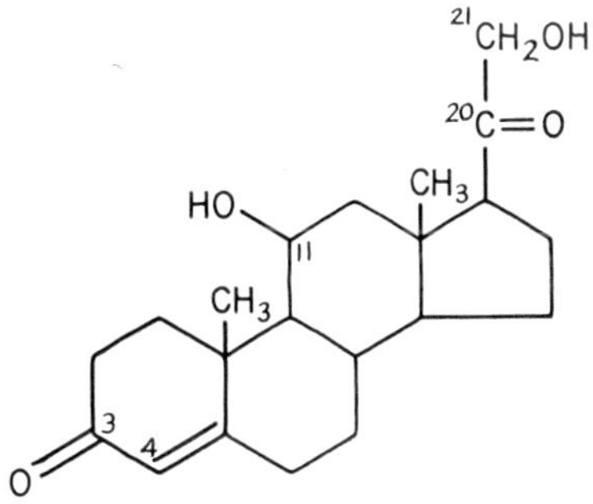

Corticosterone
(Compound B)

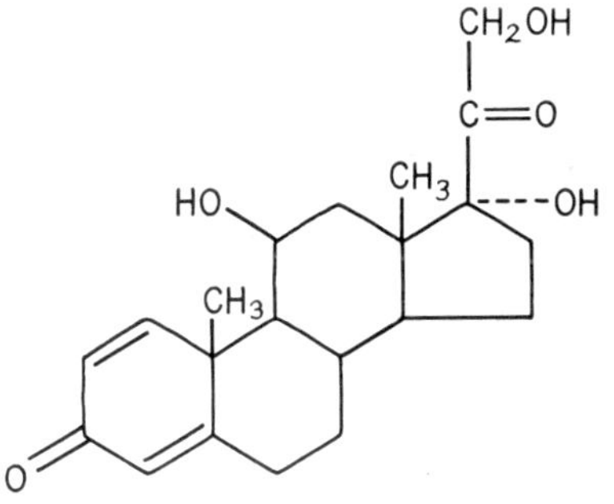

Δ^1-Hydrocortisone
(Prednisolone®)

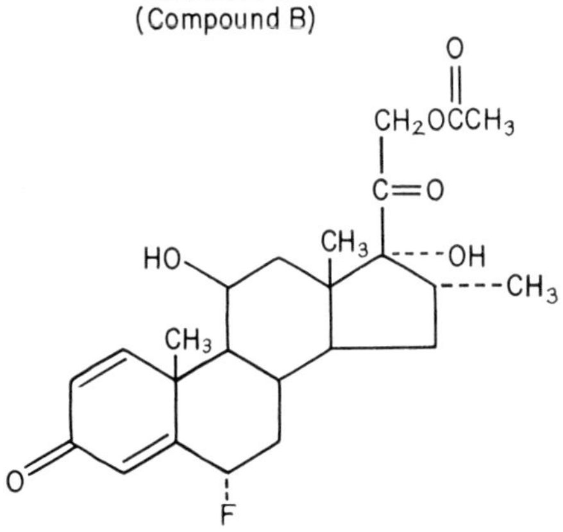

Paramethasone Acetate, Haldrone®
6α-fluoro-16α-methylprednisolone
21-acetate

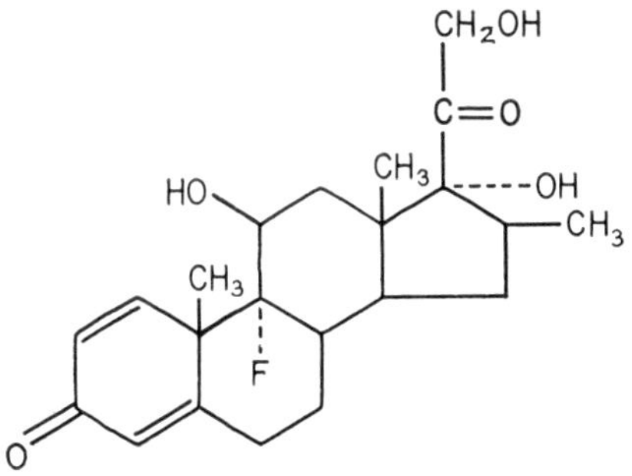

Betamethasone, Celestone®
9α-fluoro-16-β-methylprednisolone

Figure 15-3A

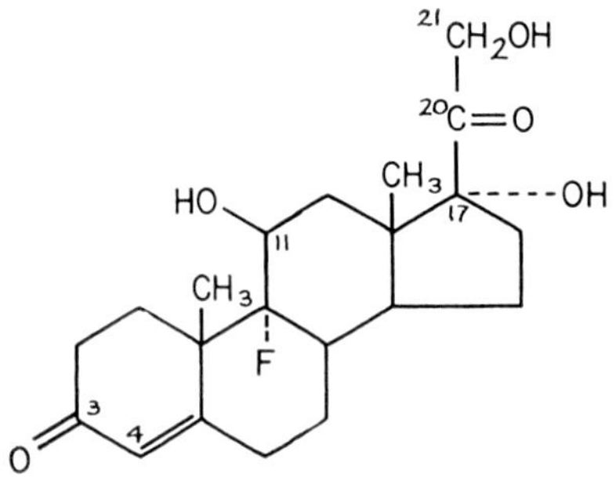

9α-Fluorohydrocortisone

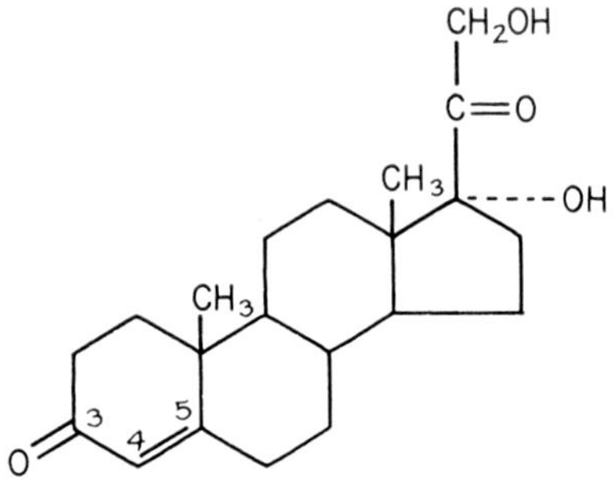

Compound S

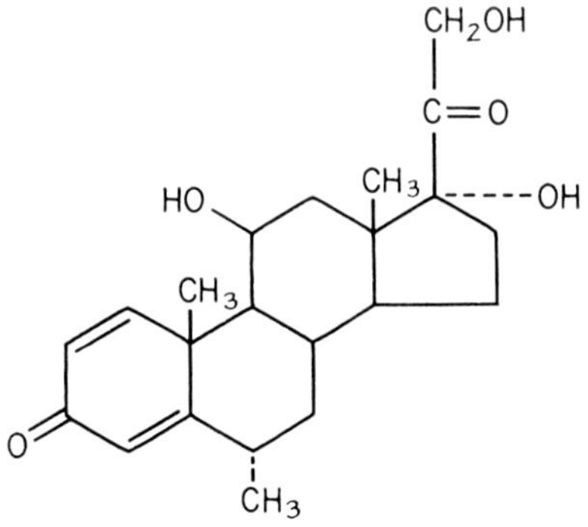

6α-Methylprednisolone
Medrol®

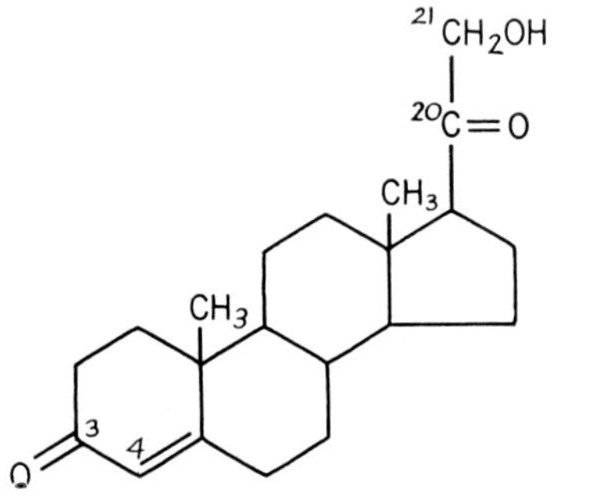

Desoxycorticosterone

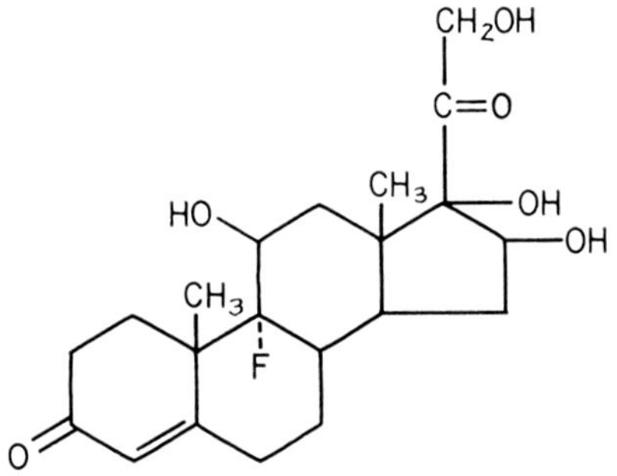

Aristocort,® Kenacort®
9α-fluoro-16α-hydroxyprednisolone

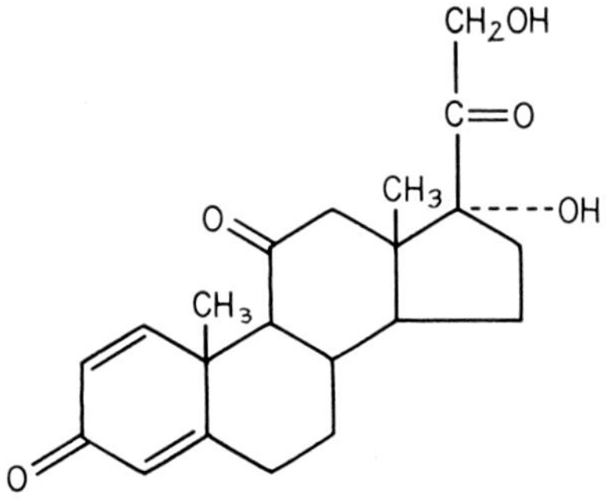

Δ¹-Cortisone
(Prednisone®)

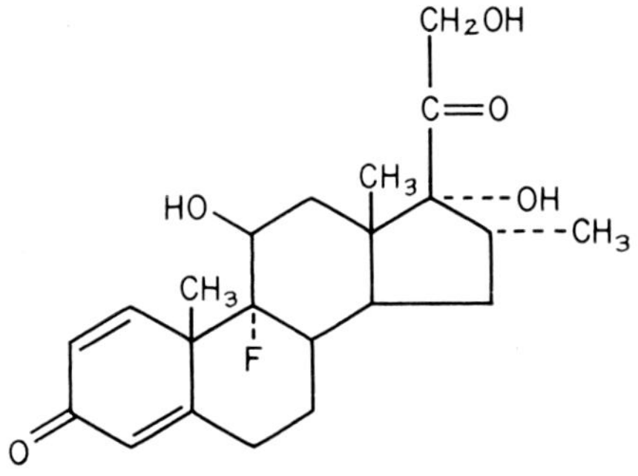

Dexamethasone
9α-fluoro-16α-methylprednisolone
Decadron,® Gammacorten,® Deronil®

Figure 15-3B

(10) Steroids cause a decrease or total absence of blood eosinophils and a decrease in lymphocytes, and an involution of lymphoid tissues.

(11) Patients receiving large doses of corticosteroids are unusually susceptible to fungal infections, e.g. candidiasis, pneumocystic pneumonia, cryptococcosis, aspergillosis and sporotrichosis.

Corticosteroids may mask the incidence and severity of bacterial and viral infections which may become servere before they are recognized.

Corticosteroids reverse a positive tuberculin reaction. When tuberculin testing is performed, it should be done before the administration of steroids.

Large doses of corticosteroids will prevent the development of the Arthus reaction.

(12) Miscellaneous side effects: Acne, hirsutism, menstrual disorders, facial rounding (moon face), weight gain from retained fluids and increased appetite, headache, hypertension, increased sweating, increased flushing, vertigo, weakness, pancreatitis, intestinal perforation, and hepatomegaly.

Indications for Steroid Therapy

In the management of allergic diseases and conditions simulating allergy, steroids are not a substitute for good environmental control, food and drug elimination when indicated, and immunotherapy. When specific management fails, steroid therapy is justified for certain situations.

Indications for Allergic Rhinitis and Nasal Polyps

Most patients with allergic rhinitis who fail to get adequate control of symptoms following definitive management will usually experience an improvement in symptoms with antihistaminic drugs and vasoconstrictors so that steroid therapy is not indicated. The risk of undesirable side effects following the prolonged administration of steroids precludes their use in the management of perennial allergic rhinitis. The exception to this rule is nasal polyposis caused by nonimmunologic mechanisms, e.g. aspirin, tartrazine, and perhaps other food chemicals. Patients of this class will very frequently experience excellent control of symptoms on very low maintenance levels of steroids following an initial high dose schedule.

An adult with nasal polyps with no reactions on skin testing and no other evidence of an allergic mechanism can be treated according to the schedule for high level dosage.

Under basal conditions the adrenal glands secrete 20 to 40 mg of corticosteroids each day, which are released into the blood stream in a diurnal pattern with the greatest amount secreted between 2:00 AM and 8:00 AM. For this reason current programs for long range steroid therapy recommend:

(1) The entire twenty-four hour dose should be administered in the morning, preferably following breakfast.

(2) The maintenance dose should be calculated to permit alternate day therapy, i.e. every forty-eight hours or at longer intervals if possible.

The program outlined will usually protect against a suppression of adrenal function unless the maintenance dose is exceedingly high.

In most cases improvement will be noted following the third to sixth day. If sufficient regression of the polyps does not occur following the sixth day, the sixth day dosage may be repeated for an additional day or two. When the polyps fail to show some improvement following the large doses of the drug, the patient's record should be carefully reviewed to determine the possibility of in-

Table 15-II: SCHEDULE OF DOSAGE FOR ADMINISTRATION OF GLUCOCORTICOIDS

Day	Prednisone	Triamcinolone or equivalent*
1	30 mg	24 mg
2	25 mg	20 mg
3	20 mg	16 mg
4	15 mg	12 mg
5	10 mg	8 mg
6	5 mg	4 mg

* See Table 15-III for list of comparative doses and actions.

advertent ingestion of salicylates or tartrazine either as a drug or in a food (see salicylate-free diet in Chapter 9).

The maintenance level must be determined by trial and error and may vary from patient to patient. Most patients will experience good control on 2.5 mg of prednisone or equivalent every forty-eight hours. Not infrequently a patient can be controlled on 1.25 mg of prednisone or 1.0 mg of triamcinolone every forty-eight hours. This program can be continued successfully without evidence of side effects for long periods (many years).

During the period of medication, even when it extends over several years, the patient should be under constant supervision to detect any signs of side effects to the drug and studied to determine if possible a causative agent that might have been overlooked. In some cases the causative agent is not identified until the patient's living habits have been reviewed repeatedly for a period of several months and the diet diary carefully examined at the time of each interview.

Indications for Hay Fever

Hay fever sufferers following a year or two of specific therapy usually show a good response requiring no medication or at most an occasional antihistamine or vasoconstrictor.

Steroid therapy for hay fever patients is indicated with:

(1) Inadequate time to institute immunotherapy
(2) Failure of immunotherapy
(3) Failure to control the symptoms with nonsteroid medications.

The program of gradually decreasing dosage outlined in Table 15-II is recommended. The steroids should be reduced to the lowest possible level for maintenance throughout the season which is usually a matter of weeks. The maintenance dose with pollinosis is usually higher than that required for treatment of nasal polyps. In some patients, supplementing steroid therapy with antihistamines and vasoconstrictors may be helpful in attaining a lower level of maintenance steroid therapy.

Steroid therapy for upper respiratory allergy in children is not recommended.

Indications for Bronchial Allergy and Bronchial Asthma

Most cases of bronchial allergy, particularly if uncomplicated by the inflammatory tissue changes of chronic bronchitis, emphysema and bronchiectasis will respond to nonsteroid anti-asthmatic drugs and mixtures. In many instances the presence of infection complicates the pattern. Supplementary therapy with antibiotics will usually permit successful management with sympathomimetic drugs and methylxanthines either separately or in combinations. When symptoms persist under such a regimen, the patient's program should be carefully reviewed for infractions of environmental or dietary control. When receiving immunotherapy, attention must be given to the possible role of overdosage of antigen, which is a common cause for aggravation of the clinical pattern.

Most children will respond to a conservative regimen using sympathomimetic drugs and antibiotics. Steroids are rarely indicated for children.

For acute asthma a short course of steroids following initial treatment with epinephrine is usually successful in controlling the patient's symptoms. If the patient fails to respond to repeated injections of epinephrine, management for status asthmaticus should be considered rather than resorting to steroids. Steroids will not correct infection nor dehydration. Steroids do not cure; they are for symptomatic relief.

If the acute asthmatic shows a good response to epinephrine, continued control with steroids and/or anti-asthmatic preparations is usually necessary until the patient's allergic state is again in homeostasis.

The chronic asthmatic presents a different problem. Chronic bronchitis, emphysema and bronchiectasis usually complicate the clinical pattern, leading to recurrent acute episodes complicated by infection and not infrequently by status asthmaticus. In such cases the patient must be treated symptomatically, constantly on the alert for complicating infection. A maintenance level of steroids can be prescribed, supplemented by nonsteroid medication which will be helpful in maintaining the patient at the lowest possible level. The patient should be examined at frequent intervals to determine the status of the cardiovascular system, the efficiency of the kidneys, the status of the electrolytes and the presence of osteoporosis.

Indications for Urticaria and Angio-edema

Many cases of mild urticaria will respond to antihistamines; however, more severe cases of acute urticaria and angio-edema should receive a graduated course of steroid therapy.

It is preferable to treat the patient initially with epinephrine to relieve the acute symptoms. Steroids are particularly indicated for angio-edema, especially when threatening vital anatomical parts such as the larynx, pharynx and the neck. The pharmacological response to steroids is slow, so that patients with angio-edema should always be treated initially with epinephrine.

If the symptoms recur during the course of reducing the dosage of the steroids, it usually indicates that the patient is not free of the offending allergen. This situation may be observed with serum disease type of reaction or in drug allergy, particularly with depot preparations.

In cases of chronic urticaria every effort must be made to identify the offending allergen. If prolonged therapy is indicated, the patient should be maintained on minimal doses of steroids administered on alternate days. Supplemental antihistamines are usually helpful in reducing the dose of steroids required.

Indications for Drug Allergy

Mild cases of drug allergy manifesting urticarial lesions can usually be treated with antihistamines. In cases of drug allergy with definite evidence of the intermediate or Arthus type of reaction with manifestations of purpura, ecchymosis, maculo-papular eruptions, renal involvement or evidence of vascular involvement, glucocorticoid therapy in large doses should be instituted as early as possible. The initial dose of steroids should be large enough to arrest the progress of the inflammatory tissue response induced by the Arthus reaction. This dose is usually greater than the initial dose indicated in Table 15-II. The steroids should be reduced as rapidly as the condition permits. The failure of the lesions to flare up is the *only* clinical guide available to regulate the dose of steroids. This procedure is important in order to prevent residual organ and tissue damage which may lead to chronic disease. *Epinephrine* is ineffective against tissue reactions induced by the Arthus mechanism.

In severe drug reactions it may be necessary to increase the initial dose of glucocorticoids to two or three times (prednisone 60 to 90 mg or triamcinolone 48 to 72 mg or equivalent) to effect this initial arrest. The drug can be reduced very rapidly depending upon the response of the patient. Regulation of the dose must be governed by the needs of the patient.

Indications for Allergic Dermatitis

Contact dermatitis including Rhus dermatitis is preferably treated with oral glucocorticoids rather than topical medication. For a very small patch of involvement, one of the newer topical steroids (Synalar®, triamcinolone, dexamethasone, *etc.*) can be prescribed. For extensive areas topical treatment is not recommended. Local applications of saline or boric compresses supplemented with oral steroid therapy is most effective. The dosage schedule as recommended above, decreasing on a daily basis, is recommended. For short term therapy an alternate day program is not indicated.

Atopic dermatitis, if acute, requires the same management with steroids as for most

Table 15-III: RELATIVE POTENCIES OF THE SYSTEMIC CORTICOSTEROIDS

Compound (or its esters)	Glucocorticoid Potency Compared to Hydrocortisone (mg for mg basis)	Mineralocorticoid Potency	Equivalent Dose (in mg)
Hydrocortisone (Cort-Dome,® Cortef,® Cortril,® HEB-Cort,® Hydrocortone,® Hydrin-2,® Cortiphate®)	1.0	++	20 mg
Cortisone (Cortone®)	0.8	++	25 mg
Prednisolone (Delta-Cortef,® Meticortelone,® Meti-Derm,® Predne-Dome,® Nisolone,® Sterane,® Hydeltrasol,® Hydeltra-T.B.A.®)	4	+	5 mg
Prednisone (Delta-Dome,® Deltasone,® Delta,® Paracort,® Meticorten®)	4	+	5 mg
Methylprednisolone (Medrol, Depo-Medrol,® Solu-Medrol®)	5	0	4 mg
Triamcinolone (Aristocort, Aristoderm,® Aristospan,® Kenacort, Kenalog®)	5	0	4 mg
Paramethasone (Haldrone, Stemex®)	10	0	2 mg
Fluprednisolone (Alphadrol®)	10	0	2 mg
Dexamethasone (Decadron, Deronil, Dexameth,® Gammacorten, Hexadrol®)	30	0	0.75 mg
Betamethasone (Celestone)	30	0	0.60 mg
*Fludrocortisone (F-Cortef,® Florinef®)	15	+++++	—

* Used only for mineralocorticoid effect and topically.

allergic conditions. For chronic involvement the maintenance dose should be as small as possible and administered on alternate days. Consideration must always be given to complicating low grade infection which will usually respond to antibiotic therapy.

Choice of Preparation

Following the synthesis of cortisone, attention was directed toward producing a product with increased anti-inflammatory effect with either reduced or no sodium retention, which is an adverse response that limits the size of the effective dose. Great success has been achieved with the synthesis of a number of glucocorticoids which differ in effective dosage, anti-inflammatory action and the degree of sodium retention. The products currently available are listed in Table 15-III.

The choice of preparation is governed by two factors:

(1) The duration of treatment

For short term therapy as required for acute allergic conditions, any one of the available synthetic products is suitable unless contraindications are present. Since prednisone and prednisolone are the least costly, they are the products of preference.

(2) Age of the patient is always a determining factor in the choice of a preparation.

Younger individuals are less likely to have cardiovascular and renal involvement. Involvement of the cardiovascular system and kidney impairment are encountered more frequently in the older age group of patients, but at any age the presence of cardiovascular or renal impairment requires the choice of a product that induces no sodium retention. Both prednisone and prednisolone cause sodium retention, but unless they are contraindicated, they should be given preference because of the great difference in cost to the patient.

For the dosage schedule outlined in Table 15-II products with moderate anti-inflammatory action are preferable. The products with very strong anti-inflammatory action are difficult to regulate at the low dosage level. For example, when prednisone, prednisolone, triamcinolone or methyl prednisolone are administered, very small doses such as 0.5, 0.075 or 1.0 mg can be conveniently controlled. With the stronger anti-inflammatory glucocorticoids it is difficult to prescribe the very minute doses required.

Injectable Products

For routine clinical use injectable preparations and particularly the depot forms are not recommended, since the dosage cannot be regulated to meet the day-to-day requirements of the patient. For prolonged therapy they are certainly not advisable, since they do not permit the interrupted program which guards against adrenal suppression.

Intravenous forms of glucocorticoids can be administered with intravenous drips, when indicated, in the management of status asthmaticus. But even with status, if the patient is able to take oral medication, it is the method of choice.

Topical Steroids

There are a number of preparations of steroids and mixtures of steroids with other drugs available for topical therapy of dermatological, ophthalmic, otic and rectal conditions.

The use of mixtures of steroids with any other drug is not recommended. Effective therapy with steroids depends upon careful regulation of the dosage which is difficult with any topical preparation and almost impossible when the steroids are incorporated into mixtures.

Dermatological Preparations

Steroid creams and ointments can be applied to small localized lesions of allergic dermatitis. Caution must be exercised to rule out a complicating infection of the lesion which can become aggravated and cause dissemination of the lesion. Dermatitis may be induced by the vehicle or by the preservative. The steroid content of the preparation does not protect against the development of such localized sensitivities.

For more extensive involvements, topical therapy with steroids is not recommended. The risk of absorption in sufficient quantities to produce side effects when used over an extended period must constantly be recognized.

If steroids are indicated when widespread dermal involvement is present, the preferred method of treatment is with oral preparations which permit accurate control of the dosage.

Topical application of *antibiotics* with or without steroids is not recommended. The risk of sensitization is very great. The steroids offer no protection against the development of such sensitivities.

When topical steroids are used, the newer fluorinated preparations are recommended, e.g. triamcinolone (Aristocort®); flurandrenolone (Cordran®); fluocinolone acetonide (Synalar®); fluorometholone (Oxylone®).

Ophthalmic Preparations

The corticosteroids are potentially toxic agents and should never be used topically to treat minor disorders of the eye that respond to decongestants, such as phenylephrine (Neo-Synephrine®); ephedrine; Visine® and Vasocon-A®.*

More severe eye conditions should be referred to the ophthalmologist for management.

Otic Preparations

Otic preparations of steroids are not recommended for the same reasons indicated for dermatologic and ophthalmic conditions.

Rectal Suppositories

Suppositories containing steroids are available for rectal conditions. These may be effective, but absorption of the steroid must be considered. Continued uncontrolled use of rectal suppositories containing steroids can lead to undesirable side effects.

SEDATIVES

The greater majority of patients with allergic complaints do not require sedatives. With control of allergy symptoms, the rest-

---

* Topical use of antihistamines is usually not recommended, but antazoline is the exception because it rarely induces sensitization. Sensitization to the phenylmercuric acetate preservative must be considered as a possibility.

lessness, anxiety and insomnia which usually accompany these ailments are also controlled. In some patients in whom emotional disturbances contribute to the clinical pattern, control of the patient's restlessness, anxiety and insomnia are very helpful in achieving control of the allergic manifestations.

Upper Respiratory Allergic Disease

Antihistamines are the usual drug of choice for the control of allergic upper respiratory complaints. The *sedative action* of antihistamines, which varies with both the choice of drug and the patient, will usually control any accompanying anxiety, restlessness or insomnia. (See discussion of antihistamines in this chapter.)

Lower Respiratory Allergic Disease

Tension, anxiety, restlessness and insomnia are observed quite commonly as accompaniments of lower respiratory tract allergic disease.

In some patients, when the tension and anxiety are pronounced, sedative medication may be necessary during the period of evaluation and until the complete program of management is instituted. In most cases successful management of the allergic condition will also control the emotional manifestations. However, when a routine program fails, a dramatic response may often be observed following the use of sedative drugs.

Barbiturates

Although barbiturates are considered the most effective sedative drugs, they are not recommended for the allergic patient because:

(1) Barbiturates are respiratory depressants, affecting both the drive to respiration and the mechanism responsible for the rhythmic character of respiratory movements. The effect upon the respiratory center varies with patients and is not always dose dependent.

(2) The risk of dependency is incurred by the prolonged use of the drug frequently necessitated by the chronic nature of allergic respiratory disease in many patients. (The reader is referred to Goodman and Gilman for a discussion of drug addiction and drug abuse.)

The most commonly administered barbiturates include:

(1) *Long-acting*
Phenobarbital

Dosage:
For adults, 30 to 100 mg daily in divided doses.
For children, 6 mg/kg of body weight in divided doses over twenty-four hours.

(2) *Intermediate duration*
Amobarbital (Amytal®)

Sedative dosage:
For adults and children over twelve years, 50 to 300 mg daily in divided doses or 100 to 300 mg at night.
For children under twelve years, 6 mg/kg body weight in divided doses.

Butabarbital sodium (Butisol sodium®)

Sedative dosage:
For adults, 50 to 120 mg daily in divided doses; 50 to 100 mg. at night.
For children, 6 mg/kg body weight in divided doses.

(3) *Short-acting*
Pentobarbital (Nembutal®)

Dosage:
Oral, for adults, 100 to 500 mg daily in divided doses; 200 mg at night.
For children, 6 mg/kg body weight daily in divided doses.

Never administer parenterally to the allergic patient.

Secobarbital (Seconal®)

Sedative dosage:
Oral, for adults, 100 to 500 mg in divided doses in twenty-four hours.

(4) Ultra short-acting
Thiopental (Pentothal®):
This should never be administered to the patient with bronchial allergy or bronchial asthma.

Non-Barbiturate Sedatives

Chloral hydrate is a relatively safe and rapidly effective sedative. To avoid the unpleasant taste, chloral hydrate can be administered in capsule form (250 mg and 500 mg) or by suppository of 500 mg.

In therapeutic doses respiration and blood pressure are affected by chloral hydrate little more than by ordinary sleep.

Chloral hydrate accelerates the inactivation of coumarin anticoagulants. Its withdrawal may sharply accentuate the anticoagulant effects of coumarin. Patients receiving anticoagulants should have the dose of chloral hydrate adjusted or another sedative substituted.

Dosage: For relief of insomnia, 1.0 to 2.0 gm.

Chloral betaine, a complex of chloral hydrate has the same pharmacological action but lacks the unpleasant taste. The drug is available as Beta-Chlor,® oral tablets of 870 mg (equivalent to 500 of chloral hydrate).

Tolerance, physical dependence and addiction may occur if chloral hydrate is given continuously. The chloral habit is similar to alcohol addiction, and sudden withdrawal may result in delirium (Goodman and Gilman).

Paraldehyde is a rapidly acting sedative with reasonable safety that does not have popular acceptance because of its very unpleasant odor. Since about 30 per cent of the drug is excreted by the lungs, the resulting unpleasant breath makes it a very unsatisfactory preparation for the ambulatory patient.

Dosage: Oral or rectal, for adults, as a sedative 10 to 30 ml.
children 0.15 ml/kg.

Can be given orally over shaved ice or in an ice cold drink. For rectal administration, can be administered as a suppository or mixed equal parts with a vegetable oil (olive oil).

Long, continued use may lead to dependence as observed with chloral hydrate.

Although *bromides* are one of the oldest sedative drugs, their replacement by the newer sedative agents has resulted in their omission from the National Formulary.

In spite of this situation the bromides can still find useful application in the occasional patient who reacts adversely to most of the newer drugs and requires only short term therapy (five to seven days). Because of the various complications which are common following long term therapy with these drugs, the use of bromides should be restricted to single episodes requiring therapy for a number of days (five to seven). The complications include skin eruptions, usually acneiform (bromidism), conjunctivitis, fetid breath, furry tongue, gastric disturbances, anorexia and constipation.

ANTIANXIETY AGENTS*
(Minor Tranquilizers)

In the allergic patient the antianxiety drugs are useful when the sedative drugs are either contraindicated or produce unwanted side effects. This group of drugs is intended for the control of mild to moderate degrees of emotional disturbances in both normal and neurotic individuals. The antianxiety drugs

---

* This term is suggested by the AMA Council on Drugs to differentiate this group of agents from the antipsychotic drugs, e.g. (1) phenothiazines of which chlorpromazine (thorazine) is the chief example; (2) thioxanthenes which include chlorprothixene (Taractan®) and thiothixene (Novane); and (3) butyrophenone derivative (haloperidol, Haldol®).

usually induce a mild sedative action without causing drowsiness and without interference with the efficiency of the psychomotor response.

The most commonly used drugs of this group include:

Chlordiazepoxide (Librium®)
Dosage: Oral
Adults, 15 to 40 mg. daily; for elderly or debilitated patients, 10 to 20 mg daily.
Children over six years, 0.5 mg/kg of body weight divided into three or four doses daily.

Diazepam (Valium®)
Dosage: Oral
Adults, 4 to 40 mg per twenty-four hours in divided doses; smaller doses for elderly and debilitated.
Children, 0.12 to 0.8 mg/kg of body weight in three or four divided doses in twenty-four hours.

Meprobamate (Equanil® and Miltown®)
Dosage: Oral
Adults, 400 mg three or four times daily.
Children, 25 mg/kg body weight divided into three or four doses daily.

Oxazepam (Serax®)
Dosage: Oral
Adults, 30 to 120 mg daily in divided doses.
Children, no dosage established.

Hydroxyzine (Atarax-Vistaril)
Dosage: Atarax
Adults, 10 mg three or four times daily; a small number of patients may require 25 mg tid.
Children, 5 to 10 mg three times daily.

Dosage: Vistaril
Adults, 25 mg three to four times daily. Most patients will tolerate Atarax better than Vistaril with few side effects.

Note: The dosage indicated for the above drugs applies to their use in clinical allergy. For the doses required for nonallergic conditions the reader is referred to any standard text on pharmacology or the AMA Drug Evaluations.

The relative effectiveness of the various antianxiety drugs has not yet been accurately determined, but clinical experience permits a few conclusions.

The response, both favorable and unfavorable, to the various drugs of this group varies from patient to patient. Although the meprobamates (Equanil, Miltown) have enjoyed wide usage, their effectiveness seems less than that of some of the newer members of this group of agents, such as chlordiazepoxide (Librium), diazepam (Valium) oxazepam (Serax), and the hydroxyzines (Atarax and Vistaril).

Side Reactions

Any of the drugs in the antianxiety class may induce drowsiness and at times ataxia, dizziness and headaches. The occurrence of these symptoms and their intensity varies with different patients. In most cases they occur during the first few days following administration of the drug and clear after a few days of continued usage. With more serious side effects, such as gastrointestinal discomfort, dryness of the mouth, nausea, vomiting, rash, chills and fever, the drug should be discontinued. Patients on continued therapy with these agents should be checked for blood dyscrasias, which occur occasionally. Urticaria and angio-edema have been observed with meprobamate (Equanil and Miltown), chlordiazepoxide (Librium), and diazepam (Valium), while maculo-papular eruptions occur with meprobamate. On the other hand, the hydroxyzine drugs, instead of inducing urticaria and angio-edema, are frequently effective in the management of these conditions.

CROMOLYN SODIUM
(Disodium Cromoglycate) (DSCG)

Khellin, which is a chromone derived from *Ammi visnaga*, a fruit indigenous to the eastern Mediterranean area and particularly Egypt, has been used for many years as a coronary dilator. In more recent years, the observation that khellin is effective in the treatment of some cases of bronchial asthma led to numerous attempts to develop a related synthetic compound for the treatment of bronchial asthma. These studies culminated in the synthesis in England (1965) of disodium cromoglycate (DSCG), which is marketed in Great Britain as Intal,® Lomodal® and Aarane®.

DSCG is an odorless, crystalline, white powder with a slightly bitter taste. Although it is soluble in water, it is poorly absorbed from the stomach, necessitating that it be administered by inhalation. For this purpose, 20 mg of the dry powder with lactose as a vehicle are dispensed in a gelatin capsule which is fitted into a special turbo-inhaler. Following puncture of the capsule, the act of inhalation causes the turbo-inhaler to spin and vibrate which results in the delivery of the micronized powder into the bronchial tree and into the alveolar spaces. Since the particulate size of the powder is under five microns in diameter, it is reasonable to expect that the drug finds access to the aerating segment of the lung. This is supported by studies demonstrating that 1 to 2 mg of the contents of the capsule reach the alveoli. From three to six inhalations empty the capsule. Following inhalation, the major portion (91%) is deposited in the oropharynx and trachea, swallowed and then eliminated via the gastrointestinal tract. Approximately 9 per cent is absorbed systemically followed by rapid excretion through the urine and bile. The plasma half-life for man averages ninety minutes.

The exact mode of action of DSCG is not known. The many immunologic and clinical studies have demonstrated that the drug does not relax smooth muscle and has no anti-inflammatory properties. The anti-allergic actions of the drug are postulated as (1) interference with the sensitization procedure, (2) influence upon the Ag-Ab interaction, and (3) the suppression of the release of pharmacologic mediators of anaphylaxis.

The results of the many clinical studies with DSCG have been summarized by Fallier* as follows:

(1) The variations in the degree and duration of therapeutic responses were unpredictable.

(2) There was observed a more consistent improvement in symptoms such as cough, dyspnea, exercise, tolerance, *etc.*, and a much less pronounced or frequently absent amelioration in pulmonary function.

(3) A higher rate of beneficial responses among younger patients, especially those with extrinsic asthma and without evidence of bronchitis.

(4) A significant reduction in the dependence of most patients on bronchodilator and other drugs when DSCG was given.

Some recent clinical trials conducted in the United States with Aarane® (cromolyn sodium) offer promise as a profitable drug in young individuals with asthma. It is also believed to have merit in exercise-induced asthma and the asthma induced by challenge, e.g. with pollen or animal dander in human subjects.

Recent studies in England by Cox** indicate that disodium cromoglycate inhibits the immediate type of hypersensitivity in the lung before exposure to the antigen. This suggests a prophylactic use for the drug. Cox reports that cromolyn sodium does not antagonize the action of histamine or other mediators, but rather it appears to act by preventing the release of the mediators from sensitized mast cells, possibly through some specific action upon the mast cell membrane. The following conclusions are reported by this investigator:

(1) Not all patients with classic allergic asthma respond to the drug.

---

* Fallier, Constantine J., Cromylui Sodium (Disodium Cromoglygate) J. Allergy, 298, 1971.
** Cox, J. S. G. Disodium Cromoglycate—Mode of Action and Its Possible Relevance to the Clinical Use of the Drug. *Brit. J Dis Chest* 65:189, 1971.

(2) Some non-atopic asthmatics are helped.

(3) Cromolyn appears to benefit some cases of asthma induced by the Arthus type reaction.

(4) Pre-treatment with cromolyn significantly reduces the exercise-induced asthmatic reaction.

(5) Some of the observations suggest that cromolyn blocks the alpha (α) type of bronchial adrenergic receptors.

In spite of the large number of clinical studies with DSCG in asthmatic subjects, the results are still inconclusive. Further investigation of the immunologic and pharmacologic effects of the drug are necessary. Observations over a longer period are essential to determine the likelihood and the nature of complications and side effects.

The studies limited to the treatment of allergic rhinitis have been limited in number and in very small samples. The value of DSCG in allergic rhinitis cannot be estimated at the present time.

In general it may be stated that continued studies are necessary with DSCG to determine both its clinical effectiveness—its value as either a substitute or adjunct to available therapeutic measures—and the safety of the drug.

REFERENCES

1. Alexander, H. L.: *Reactions with Drug Therapy*. Philadelphia, Saunders, 1955.
2. AMA Council on Drugs: *AMA Drug Evaluations*, 1st ed., Chicago, 1971.
3. Basch, F. B., Hollinger, P. H. and Poncher, H. S.: Physical and chemical properties of sputum; influence of drugs, steam, carbon dioxide and oxygen. *Am J Dis Child, 62:* 1149, 1941.
4. Burn, J. H.: The antihistaminic compounds. *Br Med J, 2:* 845, 1958.
5. Chen, J. L., Moore, N., Norman, P. S. and Ven Meter, T. E.: Disodium cromoglycate, a new compound for the prevention of exacerbations of asthma. *J Allergy, 43:* 89, 1969.
6. Cutting, W. C.: *Handbook of Pharmacology*, 4th ed. New York, Meredith, 1969.
7. Goodman, L. S. and Gilman, A. (Eds.): *The Pharmacological Basis of Therapeutics*, 4th ed. New York, MacMillan, 1970.
8. Goth, A.: *Medical Pharmacology*, 4th ed. St. Louis, Mosby, 1968.
9. Krantz, J. C., Jr., Carr, C. J. and LaDu, B. N., Jr.: *The Pharmacologic Principles of Medical Practice*, 7th ed. Baltimore, Williams & Wilkins, 1969.
10. Lands, A. M., Arnold, A., McAuliff, J. P., Luduena, F. P. and Brown, T. G., Jr.: Differentiation of receptor systems activated by sympathomimetic amines. *Nature (Lond), 214:* 597, 1967.
11. Loew, E. R.: Pharmacologic properties of antihistamines in relation to allergic and nonallergic disease. *Boston Med Q, 3:* 1, 1952.
12. Merrill, G. A.: Aminophylline deaths. *JAMA, 123:* 1115, 1943.
13. Meyers, F. H., Jawetz, E. and Goldfien, A.: *Review of Medical Pharmacology*. Los Altos, Lange Med P, 1970.
14. Moser, R. H.: *Diseases of Medical Progress*, 3rd ed. Springfield, Thomas, 1969.
15. Nichols, C. T. and Tyler, F. H.: Diurnal variation in adrenal cortical function. *Annu Rev Med, 18:* 313, 1967.
16. Paterson, J. W. *et al.*: Isoprenaline resistance and the use of pressurized aerosols in asthma. *Lancet, II:* 426, 1968.
17. Walton, J., Watson, B. S. and Ney, R. L.: Alternate day versus shorter interval steroid administration. *Arch Intern Med, 126,* 1970.

Chapter 16

THE BOTANY OF ALLERGY

by

Morris E. Webb,* Robert W. Townsend,† Ray Nelson†

Taxonomy

Although taxonomy (science of classification) is essential for the botanist, for the physician attempting to apply this classified data to the problems of clinical allergy, the various groupings (taxa) become a very complicated, unwieldy maze of names and groupings. The confusion arises not only from the hundreds of thousands of individual plant names, but also the considerable number of systems of classification, frequently using different terminology for the taxon, plus the constant shifting from one category to another. Much of the confusion in cataloging plants is derived from the lack of precise criteria for determining the grouping or family to which the plant belongs.

It is generally accepted that all plants through their line of descent have a genetic relationship. Some of the data establishing the genetic association of plants has been derived from fossil specimens, but very few ancestors have been identified through fossil remains. This has resulted in many gaps in the phylogeny of plants which have been filled by inference based upon morphologic resemblances of plants and similarities in flower structure. Recognizing these deficiencies, it can be readily appreciated that botanical taxonomy is an inexact science. The imprecision of the guidelines of botanical taxonomy has led to a constant change in cataloging and in nomenclature not only for individual plants but also the various taxa or groupings which constitute a system.

A commonly used classification of the hierarchic groups (taxa) singular: taxon) is:

Phylum
Division
Class
Order
Family
Genus
Species
Subspecies, variety, form

Species is the basic unit in toxonomy. Species of plants have virtually identical features of plant and flower structure. Species are gathered into a larger group labelled the genus, which in turn is gathered into an even larger group termed the family, and so on up the hierarchic scale.

For the purpose of clinical allergy a taxon above the level of genus is not important. On the other hand, refinements of classification below species, e.g. subspecies, variety and form are of no practical value in clinical allergy, since they all exhibit identical allergenicity. For example, *Lolium* temulentum*, which is the darnel introduced from Europe, has awned† lemmas,‡ while a recognized subspecies *Lolium temulentum* L. var. *leptochaeton* A. Br. lacks awns. The aller-

---

* Consultant, Hollister-Stier Laboratories.
† Botanist, Hollister-Stier Laboratories.

---

* Lolium is an old Latin name for darnel. Darnel is actually synonymous with *Lolium* which is presently the more common term.

† Awn: bristle-like appendages of a plant, especially in the glume of grasses. Awns: such appendages collectively as that forming the beard of wheat, barley and some species of *Lolium*.

‡ Lemma: a bract in the grass spikelet just below the pistil and the stamens.

genicity of each form is probably identical.

For the reasons indicated, a regional manual of botany may list over a thousand species of grasses of which only two or three dozen at the most will be significant for the physician practicing allergy.

By the same token, caution must be exercised when interpreting a *local* manual of botany.

A variable population of plants may be labelled as several species when isolated specimens from a single state are examined. However, a monographer examining the entire range of a group may report only one "good" species with several recognizable varieties or forms which develop under different environmental conditions.

The point is emphasized by Benson (1962) who, commenting on a 1905 report on Eschscholtzia (California poppy) that named 112 species of poppy rather than the six or eight generally recognized, stated that "the plants named in 1905 as different species were of no more stability and distinctness in their characters than the families of a middlewestern town might be in theirs, and many of them were merely seasonal forms of the same population."

It is important for the physician to recognize the deficiencies of botanical taxonomy as applied to clinical allergy. He should not be overwhelmed and misled by the various taxa and innumerable species but should be guided by groups of closely related species labelled as a genus which will probably manifest close antigenic relationship. For example, the species name includes the genus and the specific epithet, as in *Lolium temulentum*. The specific epithet, *temulentum*, is never used alone. Any reference to *Lolium temulentum, Lolium perenne,* and *Lolium multiflorium, ipso facto* indicates a close relationship among the three and also an antigenic relationship. In this instance *Lolium,* which represents the genus, is important and not the epithet.

Ecology

The factors which govern the growth, development, adaptation and survival of plants are both regional and local. In every instance climate and soil are the chief determining factors and of these, climate is the more important since soil conditions are in great measure influenced by climate.

Vegetation types in general correspond to major climatic regions:

   Tropical and subtropical
   Warm temperate
   Cold temperate
   Arctic and subarctic

The climatic regions are based upon latitude and longitude, mean temperature and light, while important influences within any region are contributed by altitude, prevailing winds, precipitation and proximity to large bodies of water.

Plant growth and development are influenced by all the factors indicated, so that any combination of the various primary and secondary factors results in the creation of a particular plant community constituted of characteristic species indigenous to the region. Since a plant rarely exists alone, it is necessary to view any population of plants in the region in relation to its habitat, for as the habitat changes, the plant population changes. Some species are adapted to very limited and unvarying habitats. For example, the California juniper which is a moderately important hay fever tree grows in the foothills surrounding the Colorado desert in California, while the Utah juniper, which is remarkably similar to the California juniper, thrives from the Mojave Desert in southern California, through Arizona, New Mexico, Colorado, Utah, Nevada, southwestern Idaho and southwestern Wyoming.

Local ecological conditions include variations in soil resulting from habitation of an area and air pollution resulting from urban and industrial development.

With urbanization and industrialization of an area, weeds and grasses which were not important to the area may become important in clinical allergy. For example, Bermuda grass frequently becomes an important factor in hay fever and asthma as communities develop and lawns are cultivated, which provides the adequate supply of water required for profuse growth of Bermuda grass.

In like manner some weeds, such as lamb's-quarter, an annual which is sparse in the native vegetation within its range, becomes an important hay fever plant growing in disturbed soil in vacant lots and cultivated areas, while the native vegetation is prevented from reaching a climax or stability. Air pollution affects the growth and maturation of plants, resulting in a decrease in their importance as potential allergenic plants.

Pollen

In determining the importance of plants in inhalant allergy, pollen production and floral anatomy are critical factors. Some conifers may produce as much as ten thousand grams of airborne pollen per tree, while acres of cultivated alfalfa yield very little airborne pollen. This is true because the pollen of alfalfa is held within tightly overlapping petals to produce a trap-like flower whose pollen is available only to the bee (insect pollinated).

Most plants have structural and/or biochemical prevention of self-fertilization. Unisexual cones and flowers are especially effective in preventing self-fertilization. Some plants have separate staminate and pistillate flowers which are all on the same plant (monoecious), while others bear staminate flowers or cones on one plant and the pistillate flowers on another (dioecious). Such unisexual plants are called imperfect; the flowers of many allergenic plants are imperfect. Many, though not all imperfect flowers, but all cones, are wind pollinated (amenophilous).

In evaluating the allergenicity of pollens it is important to recognize that wind-pollinated plants are the primary cause of respiratory allergic disease, while insect-pollinated plants (entomophilous) are of little importance in respiratory allergy regardless of allergenicity.

Wind pollination is extremely inefficient, which accounts for nature's provision of extremely large quantities of pollen which contaminate the atmosphere, to be inhaled, with the resulting symptoms of respiratory allergy. Some windborne pollens may be carried for many miles—up to thirty or forty miles—so that absence of the plant in the immediate environment of the patient does not exclude such a plant as a potential factor in respiratory allergic disease.

On the other hand, the pollen of insect-pollinated plants is usually much less in quantity, larger in size, waxy and sticky, so that the grains adhere to the pollinating insect. The pollen of insect-pollinated plants is seldom airborne and therefore is rarely inhaled. Accordingly, regardless of antigenicity, the insect-pollinated plants rarely if ever cause respiratory allergic disease.

As a rule insect-pollinated flowers are very showy and have a marked fragrance which attracts the insects. This contrasts with the wind-pollinated plants which have obscure, usually insignificant flowers with no fragrance. Pollen of insect-pollinated plants is not carried very far from its source.

The pollens of fruit trees and most lilies do not cause respiratory allergic disease. Occasionally, when such flowers are used for ornamental displays in the house, the pollen may drop to the floor, forming part of the house dust. This occurs only rarely, since a considerable amount of pollen is required for an effective contamination of house dust.

In some cases an individual inhaling the pollens of calla, rubrum and other forms of lilies may experience a temporary nasal reaction, but these are usually transient and of minor importance.

Thommen's Postulates

The most reliable criteria for determining the importance of plants as major offenders in the management of the allergic patient are the five postulates of Thommen.

I. *Postulates related to the plant*
  1. The plant must be seed-bearing

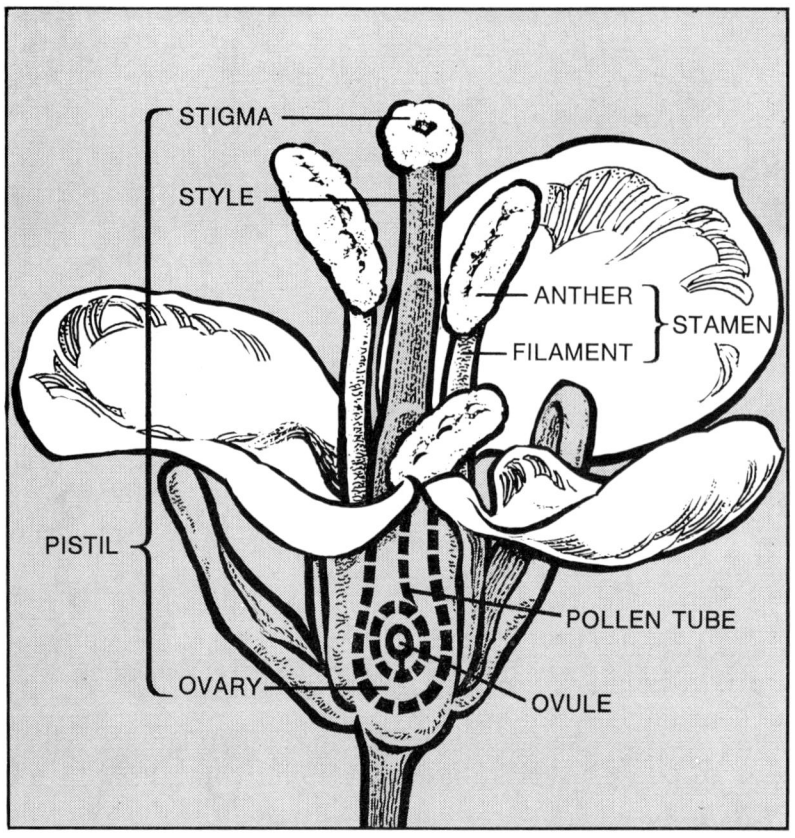

FLOWER CROSS SECTION shows a cluster of stamens, each with a pollen-filled anther at its tip, surrounding a central pistil with a sticky stigma at the tip and an ovary in the base. One pollen grain adhering to the stigma has grown a long tube reaching the ovary.

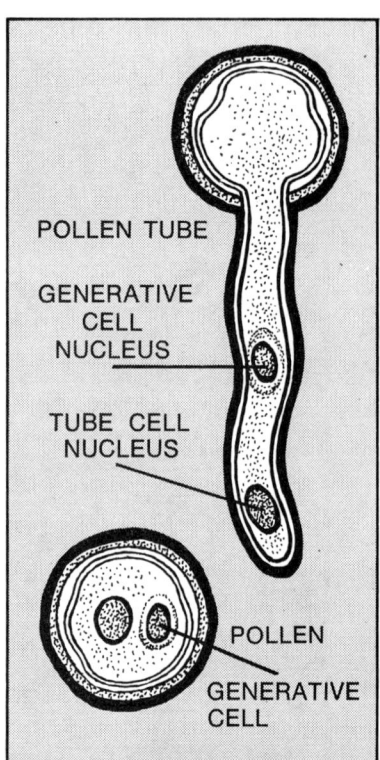

GRAIN OF POLLEN. If a free pollen grain comes in contact with a stigma, the tube cell becomes involved with the growth of the pollen tube toward the ovary and the generative cell then travels down the tube to fertilize the ovule.

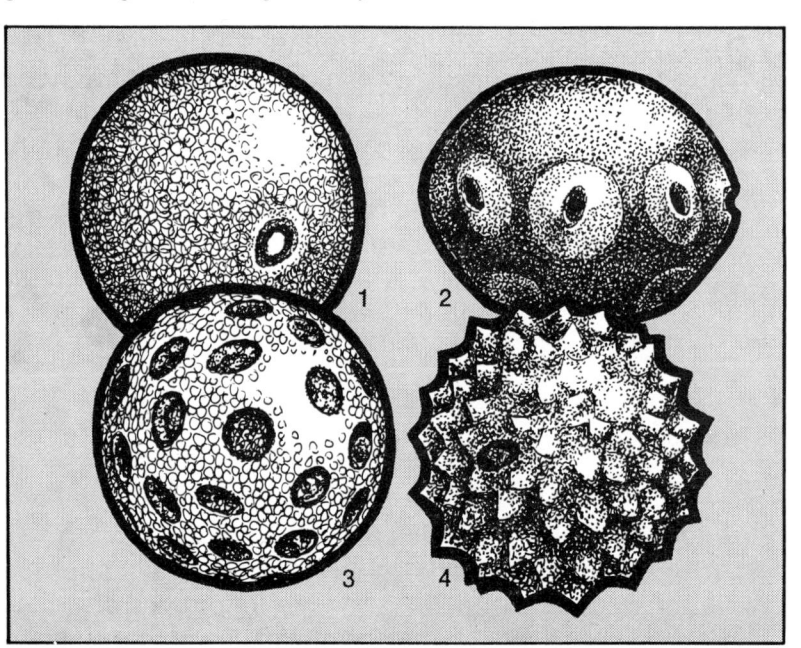

1, *PHLEUM PRATENSE*, ventral view, 35 μ in diameter.
2, *JUGLANS NIGRA*, side view dorsal side uppermost, 34 μ in diameter.
3, *SALSOLA PESTIFER*, 27.5 μ in diameter.
4, *AMBROSIA TRIFIDA*, 17.7 μ in diameter.

Figure 16-1

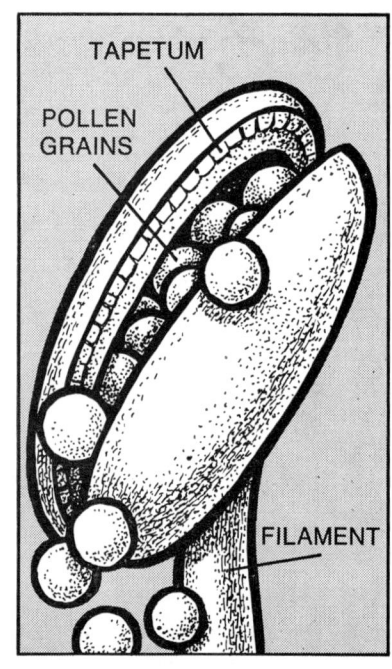

ANTHER, which splits at maturity allowing the loose pollen in its cavities to disperse.

which means it is a pollen producing plant.

2. The plant must have a wide distribution or its relation to the patient's environment must be close and dominant.

The term "wide distribution" is only relative, since judgments depend upon the species and the locality. The greater the distribution, the higher will be the pollen count and accordingly the greater the likelihood that the pollen will be a factor in the induction of symptoms, which are usually proportional to the pollen count.

II. *Postulates related to the pollen*

1. The plant must produce large quantities of pollen.

2. The pollen must be light and airborne. The size of the pollen grain is usually between fifteen and fifty microns in diameter. Many physicians wish to do "pollen counts." If counts are made once weekly throughout the year for several years, the historical data is valuable in establishing the seasons of high count. Identification of pollens must be reserved for the expert.

3. The pollen must be allergenic. Not all pollens are allergenic. What determines allergenicity is not known. For example, there is no explanation for the antigenicity of ragweed pollen which results in frequent sensitization, while pine pollen, a weak antigen, seldom causes allergic symptoms.

Recently, attempts have been made to isolate the antigen or antigens from pollens. Most research in this area has been conducted on short ragweed pollen which has led to the isolation of antigen E. Although antigen E accounts for an estimated 90 per cent of the skin reactivity, other antigens of lesser concentration but high antigenicity have also been demonstrated for ragweed.

It is important to understand there is no United States standardization of pollen extracts. Attempts are now being made to standardize short ragweed *(Ambrosia trifida)* on the basis of antigen E concentration. The whole extract contains other active antigens, each of which may be significant. The program of standardization using the "E" fraction must await the trial of experience.

Studies with timothy *(Phleum pratense)* and perennial ryegrass *(Lolium perenne)* to isolate the active antigen(s) have also been conducted, but to date the observations are inconclusive.

Allergenicity alone is not sufficient to determine the clinical importance of a pollen. The quantity of pollen produced and the ability to be disseminated throughout the atmosphere is a very important factor. Accordingly, a strongly antigenic pollen produced in very limited quantities is usually of little clinical importance.

All seed plants produce pollen in varying degrees of abundance. In general, the catkin-bearing trees (Amentiferae) like oaks, birches, alders, sycamores, cottonwoods, walnuts and many other species produce large quantities of airborne pollen. In general, conifer pollen is nonallergenic. Grasses are variable. Timothy, orchard grass, sweet vernal grass, Kentucky blue grass, meadow fescue and several rye grasses are abundant pollinators. The oats, bromes, grama grasses and most others are sparse pollinators.

The ragweeds, false ragweeds, sagebrushes, Russian thistle, cockleburs, marshelders and hemp are heavy pollinators.

The distinction between heavy and sparse pollinators is the determining factor between primary and secondary offenders (see Tables 16-I and 16-II.

It is important that the physician who treats patients with pollenosis acquaint himself with the dominant flora of the area which provides potential offenders in pollen allergy and particularly the "index plants." For assistance in identifying grasses and weeds, botany experts and farm extension agents can be helpful, while local nurserymen can be of assistance in identifying ornamental and introduced plants.

Reliable manufacturers of pollen extracts usually maintain a staff of botanists who survey and analyze the various regions and

Table 16-I: PRIMARY OFFENDERS*

Acer negundo	BOX ELDER
Acnida tamariscina	WESTERN WATERHEMP
Agrostis alba	REDTOP
Ambrosia spp. (species, plural)	RAGWEEDS
Anthoxanthum odoratum	SWEET VERNALGRASS
Artemisia spp.	SAGEBRUSHES
Carya pecan	PECAN
Cedrus spp.	CEDARS
Cynodon dactylon	BERMUDA GRASS
Dactylis glomerata	ORCHARD GRASS
Elymus spp.	RYEGRASSES (in part)
Festuca elatior	MEADOW FESCUE
Franseria spp.	FALSE RAGWEEDS
Iva spp.	MARSH ELDERS
Juglans spp.	WALNUTS
Lolium spp.	RYEGRASSES (in part)
Olea europaea	OLIVE
Phleum pratense	TIMOTHY
Poa pratensis	KENTUCKY BLUEGRASS
Quercus spp.	OAKS
Salsola kali	RUSSIAN THISTLE
Xanthium spp.	COCKLEBURS

* Primary index plants are those that fulfill the five postulates of Thommen. These include most indigenous flora and some nonindigenous. The latter are those plants introduced for economic reasons by nurserymen, growers and developers.

areas of the country. In most instances the biological laboratories that are so equipped can be very helpful in guiding the physician in the identification and selection of the important pollens for a given area or a given patient.

Collecting Pollens

Biological laboratories concerned with the preparation of pollen extracts employ various procedures for harvesting the pollen, e.g. (1) field vacuum collecting, (2) screen or rack drying of the flower and flower parts,

Table 16-II: SECONDARY OFFENDERS*

Acacia spp.	ACACIAS
Alnus spp.	ALDERS
Atriplex spp.	SALTBUSHES
Avena spp.	OATS, CULTIVATED & WILD
Betula spp.	BIRCHES
Bouteloua spp.	GRAMA-GRASSES
Bromus spp.	BROMES
Chenopodium album	LAMBS-QUARTERS
Cupressus spp.	CYPRESSES
Distichlis spp.	SALTGRASSES
Eucalyptus spp.	EUCALYPTUS, AUSTRALIAN GUM
Fraxinus spp.	ASHES
Koeleria cristata	KOEHLER'S GRASS
Ligustrum spp.	PRIVETS
Pinus spp.	PINES
Platanus spp.	SYCAMORES
Populus spp.	POPLARS
Rumex spp.	DOCKS, SORRELS

* Secondary index plants are those that do not completely fulfill the five postulates of Thommen. They may or may not be indigenous.

and (3) water set or bouquet technique. The choice of the various procedures is governed by the nature of the plant, the distribution of the plants, and the structure of the flower.

Quality control for the collection of pollen has been discussed in Chapter 17 on the preparation of pollen extracts. The deficiencies encountered in the preparation of extracts have also been discussed under the preparation of pollen extracts.

It is important to repeat that at present there are no United States standards of potency for any allergenic extracts including those prepared from pollens. There may soon be standards adopted for ragweed and grass extracts. The reliability of antigen E as a standard for ragweed extracts has been indicated above. At present, the most reliable index for standardization of pollen extracts is the quality control of the pollen supply and the reliability of the processor and evidence of biological activity.

The lack of dependability of PNU as a standard of potency has been discussed in Chapter 17 under preparation of extracts. The practical application of weight by volume (W/V) as an index of potency has also been discussed in Chapter 17 (Preparation of Extracts).

The following guidelines can be helpful in evaluating pollen-producing plants.

By giving consideration to the plant characteristics that influence distribution, pollen production and allergenicity, the plants commonly used by the physician for the diagnosis and treatment of pollen allergy can be rated on a scale from 1 to 10.

Trees rate 4
Grasses rate 7
Weeds rate 10

Trees (rating 4)

All trees have a short pollinating season. Most trees pollinate in the spring of the year which coincides with the season for heavy rains. Exceptions to this rule are olive, elm species, and some ornamental trees.

Grasses (rating 7)

The grass season extends over two to four months. The growth of the various grasses starts in early spring with an increase in mean temperature, increase in hours of sunlight and a proportional decrease in the hours of darkness.

The development of the various grasses overlaps so that pollen production is staggered. The pollen count shows a progressive rise with the maximum attained through May and often into June. During the heat of summer, most grasses are destroyed but not before completing their life cycle which includes growth, pollination, seed production and destruction. Some grasses, such as *Cynodon dactylon* (Bermuda) defy this sequence and under protected and artificial circumstances may pollinate eleven months of the year.

Weeds (rating 10)

The weeds are hardy plants, usually with a long season extending from July to October, but generally terminated by frost. False pollen showers can be created by heavy winds, especially during outdoor cleaning or with atmospheric dust contamination.

Imported plants and ornamental plants must always be considered as a possible source of antigenic pollen. A survey of the home conducted at the specific time when symptoms are being experienced will frequently identify any likely offender.

Geographical Distribution and Survey

The charts presented in this chapter have been governed by grouping contiguous states that have broad ecological factors in common. The risk of enlarging any survey area is the generalization of plant populations. However, by including the index plants (see Tables 16-I and 16-II) and including clinical surveys, coverage has been given to a plant even though it may be secondary in one section and primary in another. The index plants are never eliminated completely from the testing chart.

The floristic literature for some states is very deficient; however, the major biological laboratories with their staff of botanists have contributed their knowledge and experience with shifts in the plant population.

The features that unite a botanical area and permit broad surveys include temperature variations, latitude, soil conditions, prevailing winds, and altitude. The greater the similarity in these individual factors, the greater will be the similarity in the flora.

Plant Surveys

The precise botanical definition of a region is not possible. But because the index plants listed in the Tables constitute approximately 90 per cent of the important pollen producing plants that cause hay fever and bronchial asthma, the allergenic flora of a region can be predicted with a high degree of reliability.

Plant adaptations are usually secondary to ecologic and climatic variables, but since these factors, such as altitude, rainfall, wind, sunlight and humidity are not necessarily limited to political boundaries (states, *etc.*), the plant adaptations are not restricted to these artificial demarcations. As a rule, plant adaptations do not have sharp limitations but fade out gradually without respect for unnatural boundaries.

As has been indicated, allergenic plants produce airborne pollens (amenophilous). Accordingly, a plant with a profuse growth may not be allergenic if it is insect pollinated. For the same reason, colorful flowers which are usually insect pollinated (entomophilous) are not allergenic. Patients who do not recognize this fact may erroneously incriminate a plant or flower as the cause of their symptoms.

For example, for many years the colorful insect-pollinated goldenrod, which blooms at the same time as pollinating ragweed, was considered an important cause of hay fever.

INDIGENOUS PLANTS: Indigenous plants are those that evolved in a country, region or specific environment. The native hay fever plants usually have numerous, inconspicuous flowers that produce an abundance of windborne pollens which is undoubtedly nature's compensation for the great element of chance involved in a given pollen finding its respective stigma.

CULTIVATED PLANTS AND TREES: The cultivated plants and trees include both those grown for (1) economic purposes, and (2) those grown for ornamental or shade trees.

(1) The plants and trees grown for economic purposes include all the fruit and nut trees, the berry bushes, and the cultivated grains, sugar beets, corn, alfalfa, clover, *etc.*

Most of the fruit trees produce attractive blossoms which are usually quite fragrant. These are the characteristics of the insect pollinated plant which means they are not allergenic. The exceptions to this general rule are the olive and walnut trees, which in some areas are grown in large numbers. Since they are prolific producers of a toxic windborne pollen, these trees can be very important in clinical allergy. Olive trees are frequently used as ornamental trees.

In some areas, particularly in northern California, old walnut groves have been subdivided for acreage. In such subdivisions, the remaining walnut trees can become very important pollen producers and cause severe allergic reactions. The cultivated grains usually create no serious clinical allergy problems.

In sections of the country where large tracts of sugar beets are cultivated, the plants are usually harvested before pollination, so that they create no allergy problems. However, in some areas as in the Salinas Valley of California, or in Arizona where large tracts of sugar beets are under cultivation, an isolated pollinating plant may permit the escape of pollen. This escaped pollen leads to the growth of wild sugar beet plants that mature and pollinate and become an important cause of allergic symptoms.

(2) Ornamental trees and shade trees as well as decorative shrubs and bushes are both insect pollinated and wind pollinated.

The entomophilous trees and plants usually have colorful, fragrant flowers which attract the insects. The pollen grains are large which prevents them from being airborne, and are waxy and sticky which causes them to adhere to the foraging insect.

Some ornamental trees such as Chinese elm produce large quantities of airborne pollen.

CHANGES IN SURVEYS: Changes in surveys can occur with all types of plants, but among the indigenous flora alterations in the species are very slow. Nature permits such changes very grudgingly because of their fixed forces, such as climate, rainfall, soil and fauna. Occasionally, exceptions do occur among indigenous plants as illustrated by the introduction of Russian thistle (Salsola) into the United States via wheat seed. In a few short years this plant became a dominant contaminant in the far West and Midwest from Canada to Mexico.

Changes in the flora of cultivated plants usually follow the march of civilization with the development of urban and suburban areas. The plants in a given area usually follow the preferences of a nursery, an arboretum or the land developer. In most cases the plants are insect pollinated, such as acacia, camellia, magnolia, gardenia, honeysuckle, night blooming jasmine, privet, myrtle and many others. Occasionally, a wind pollinated tree, such as Chinese elm, willow and oak may be used for ornamental purposes.

With urban and suburban developments, changing conditions permit the increased growth of an indigenous plant. For example, Bermuda grass may become very prolific and an important allergenic offender following frequent watering and fertilizing of lawns.

In every instance, in making plant surveys a pollen should not be considered as allergenic unless it fulfills the five postulates of Thommen indicated above.

The United States will be divided into seventeen (17) regions. The regions will generally be composed of contiguous areas having similar climatic and geographical features. State boundaries may be used for easy identification whenever possible, but other boundaries may be identified by counties within states.

Region I

STATES:

Maine	New Jersey
Delaware	New York
Massachusetts	Vermont
New Hampshire	Connecticut
Pennsylvania	Rhode Island

REGIONAL TOPOGRAPHY:

A folding parallel mountain range with verdant valleys merging into rolling coastal lowlands. 40° to 47° N. latitude.

REGIONAL CLIMATE:

Low temperature in January: Vermont 17.9°, New Jersey 35.8°

High temperature in July: Maine 67.8°, New Jersey 73.6°

Rainfall: Vermont 32.22 inches, Maine 47.8 inches

Tree population is characteristic of northern tier of states. Many species are found, but distribution is spotty. Pines abound but are low in antigenicity.

Proceeding from 40° to 47° N. latitude we find an increase in rainfall and decrease in high and low temperature. Grasses are significant but limited in number of genus. Early pollinating in the south to later pollinating dates as one travels from south to north in this region.

INDEX TREES: Pollinate March to May in south and April to May in north.

(2) ASH (*Fraxinus*)
(2) HICKORY (*Carya*)

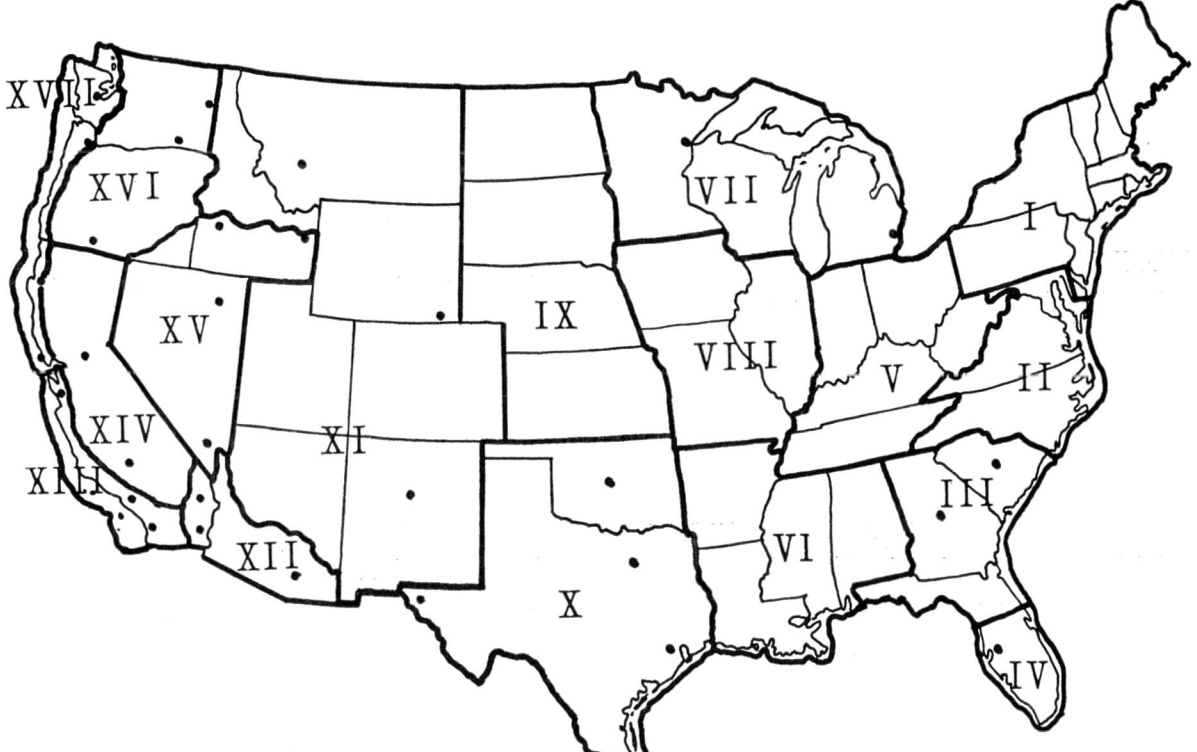

Figure 16-2. The seventeen botanical regions of the United States are indicated by bold outlines. The boundaries of the regions do not always correspond with political boundaries. See text for descriptions of the respectvie regions.

(2) POPLAR, COTTONWOOD (*Populus*)
(2) BIRCH (*Betula*)
(1) MAPLE, BOX ELDER (*Acer*)
(2) SYCAMORE (*Platanus*)
(1) ELM (*Ulmus*)
(1) OAK (*Quercus*)
(3) PINE (*Pinus*)

INDEX GRASSES: Pollinate April through June.
(1) BLUE GRASS (*Poa*)
(1) ORCHARD (*Dactylis*)
(2) MEADOW FESCUE (*Festuca*)
(1) TIMOTHY (*Phleum*)
(1) REDTOP (*Agrostis*)
(2) BERMUDA (*Cynodon*)

INDEX WEEDS: Pollinate mid-August to September and early October.
(1) RAGWEED (*Ambrosia*)
(2) LAMBS-QUARTERS (*Chenopodium*)
(1) PLANTAIN (*Plantago*)
(2) COCKLEBUR (*Xanthium*)
(2) SORREL (*Rumex*)

Note: (1) indicates primary index plants. (2) indicates secondary index plants. (3) indicates minimal importance.

Region II

STATES:

Maryland	Virginia
Washington, D.C.	North Carolina

REGIONAL TOPOGRAPHY:
Common features include coastal lowlands, central plains merging into parallel mountain ranges (Appalachian and Blue Ridge). 33° to 40° N. latitude.

REGIONAL CLIMATE:
Low temperature in January: Maryland 34.2°
High temperature in July: North Carolina 78.5°
Rainfall: all similar, 42 to 46 inches per year

The further south the heavier the rainfall and the higher the mean temperature.

The combination of moisture and temperature creates a heavy ragweed (Ambrosia) belt. Grasses are dominant. Trees are generally found to have a longer pollinating period.

INDEX TREES: Pollinate February to May.
(2) ASH (*Fraxinus*)
(2) BIRCH (*Betula*)
(2) HACKBERRY (*Celtis*)
(1) WALNUT (*Juglans*)
(1) ELM (*Ulmus*)
(2) CEDAR (*Juniperus*)
(2) MAPLE, BOX ELDER (*Acer*)
(1) MULBERRY (*Morus*)
(1) PECAN, HICKORY (*Carya*)
(1) OAK (*Quercus*)
(2) POPLAR, COTTONWOOD (*Populus*)

INDEX GRASSES: Pollinate March to July—Bermuda longer.
(1) JOHNSON (*Sorghum*)
(2) REDTOP (*Agrostis*)
(2) RYEGRASS (*Lolium*)
(1) BERMUDA (*Cynodon*)
(1) TIMOTHY (*Phleum*)
(1) VERNAL (*Anthoxanthum*)
(1) ORCHARD (*Dactylis*)
(1) BLUEGRASS (*Poa*)

INDEX WEEDS: Pollinate August to frost.
(1) RAGWEED (*Ambrosia*)
(2) KOCHIA (*Kochia*)
(2) SORREL (*Rumex*)
(1) COCKLEBUR (*Xanthium*)
(2) LAMBS-QUARTERS (*Chenopodium*)
(2) PIGWEED (*Amaranthus*)
(1) PLANTAIN (*Plantago*)

Note: (1) indicates primary index plants. (2) indicates secondary index plants.

Region III

STATES:

South Carolina	Northern Florida
Georgia	

REGIONAL TOPOGRAPHY:

Wide coastal plains compose at least 60 per cent of the states. The southern tip of the Appalachian extends into northwest Georgia with Blue Ridge Mountains in the northwest portion of South Carolina. Temperature, rainfall and latitude indicate a semitropical climate. The flora from Orlando, northern Florida compares with that found in Georgia. 28° to 33° N. latitude.

REGIONAL CLIMATE:

Low temperature in January: Columbia, S.C. 47°

High temperature in July: Macon, Ga. 82.4°

Rainfall: general throughout, 48 inches

Due to similar altitude and climatic features it is difficult to draw precise lines of floral change. There will be a blending of plants north and west of this region. Local nurseries can assist in identifying ornamentals and imports.

INDEX TREES: Pollinate February to April.

(1) ELM *(Ulmus)*
(2) MESQUITE *(Prosopis)*
(1) MAPLE, BOX ELDER *(Acer)*
(1) WALNUT *(Juglans)*
(1) PECAN, HICKORY *(Carya)*
(1) OAK *(Quercus)*
(2) BIRCH *(Betula)*
(2) COTTONWOOD, POPLAR *(Populus)*
(2) MT. CEDAR *(Juniperus)*
(2) ASH *(Fraxinus)*
(2) MULBERRY *(Morus)*
(2) HACKBERRY *(Celtis)*

INDEX GRASSES: Pollinate February to July (major season); February to December—Bermuda.

(1) BERMUDA *(Cynodon)*
(1) REDTOP *(Agrostis)*
(1) RYEGRASS *(Lolium)*
(1) JOHNSON *(Sorghum)*
(2) TIMOTHY *(Phleum)*
(1) SWEET VERNAL *(Anthoxanthum)*
(1) ORCHARD *(Dactylis)*
(1) BLUEGRASS *(Poa)*
(2) MEADOW FESCUE *(Festuca)*

INDEX WEEDS: Pollinate August to October.

(1) RAGWEED *(Ambrosia)*
(2) SAGEBRUSH *(Artemisia)*
(1) PLANTAIN *(Plantago)*
(1) COCKLEBUR *(Xanthium)*
(2) SORREL *(Rumex)*
(2) LAMBS-QUARTERS *(Chenopodium)*

Note: (1) indicates primary index plants. (2) indicates secondary index plants.

Region IV

STATES:

Southern Florida   Orlando South

REGIONAL TOPOGRAPHY:

Generally low, flat; many swamps (Everglades). Many lakes in central portion. 25° to 28° N. latitude.

REGIONAL CLIMATE:

Low temperature in January: Tampa 61.5°

High temperature in July: throughout, 81.6°

Rainfall: 47 to 50 inches

There are a number of trees and grasses peculiar to this area. Mango causes skin irritation but the pollen is heavy, waxy with no airborne quality. Austrian pine is an import that produces very little pollen but has wide distribution. Bahia grass *(Paspalum)* is an import, a perennial and produces small amounts of pollen. Melaluca is of minor importance and is insect pollinated.

INDEX TREES: Pollinate February to April.

(1) ELM *(Ulmus)*
(2) MOUNTAIN CEDAR *(Juniperus)*

- (2) MAPLE BOX ELDER *(Acer)*
- (1) OAK *(Quercus)*
- (2) PRIVET *(Ligustrum)*
- (2) PALM *(Palmaceae)*
- (2) MESQUITE *(Prosopis)*
- (2) COTTONWOOD, POPLAR *(Populus)*
- (2) SYCAMORE *(Platanus)*
- (3) AUSTRALIAN PINE *(Auracaria)*
- (1) PECAN, HICKORY *(Carya)*

INDEX GRASSES: Pollinate January to June (peak); Bermuda—January to December.

- (1) BERMUDA *(Cynodon)*
- (1) JOHNSON *(Sorghum)*
- (2) CANARY *(Phalaris)*
- (2) JUNE *(Poa)*
- (2) BAHIA *(Paspalum)*
- (2) REDTOP *(Agrostis)*
- (2) RYEGRASS *(Lolium)*
- (2) SALT GRASS *(Distichlis)*

INDEX WEEDS:

- (2) RAGWEED *(Ambrosia)*
- (2) MARSH ELDER *(Iva)*
- (2) PIGWEED *(Amaranthus)*
- (1) LAMBS-QUARTERS *(Chenopodium)*
- (1) SORREL *(Rumex)*
- (2) SAGEBRUSH *(Artemisia)*

Note: (1) indicates primary index plants. (2) indicates secondary index plants.

Region V

STATES:

Ohio	Tennessee
Kentucky	West Virginia
Indiana	

REGIONAL TOPOGRAPHY:

This region is dominated by plateaus, parallel valleys, and sloping plains to the Mississippi River Valley. Appalachian ridges found in Kentucky, West Virginia and eastern Tennessee. These give way to glacial plains in the western section. 35° to 42° N. latitude.

REGIONAL CLIMATE:

Low temperature in January: Indiana 24.6°, Tennessee 41.9°

High temperature in July: average 75°

Rainfall: Ohio, Indiana 35 inches; Kentucky, West Virginia, Tennessee 45 inches

The distinct seasons create a high pollen count and also distinct pollinating dates. Tree population is similar to other localities in this latitude. Grasses are dominant in many of the plains and valleys. Ragweed is the most dominant factor.

INDEX TREES: Pollinating March and April.

- (2) ASH *(Fraxinus)*
- (2) POPLAR, COTTONWOOD *(Populus)*
- (2) SYCAMORE *(Platanus)*
- (2) BIRCH *(Betula)*
- (1) HICKORY, PECAN *(Carya)*
- (1) ELM *(Ulmus)*
- (1) MAPLE, BOX ELDER *(Acer)*
- (1) OAK *(Quercus)*
- (1) WALNUT *(Juglans)*

INDEX GRASSES: Pollinate March to June.

- (1) BLUE *(Poa)*
- (1) TIMOTHY *(Phleum)*
- (2) JOHNSON *(Sorghum)*
- (1) ORCHARD *(Dactylis)*
- (1) RYEGRASS *(Lolium)*
- (1) FESCUE *(Festuca)*
- (1) REDTOP *(Agrostis)*
- (1) BERMUDA *(Cynodon)*

INDEX WEEDS: Pollinate late July to October.

- (1) RAGWEED *(Ambrosia)*
- (2) SORREL *(Rumex)*
- (2) LAMBS-QUARTERS *(Chenopodium)*
- (2) PIGWEED *(Amaranthus)*
- (1) WATER HEMP *(Acnida)*
- (2) PLANTAIN *(Plantago)*
- (1) COCKLEBUR *(Xanthium)*

(1) ANNUAL SAGEBRUSH
(*Artemisia*)

Note: (1) indicates primary index plants.
(2) indicates secondary index plants.

Region VI

STATES:

Arkansas   Louisiana
Alabama   Mississippi

REGIONAL TOPOGRAPHY:

Arkansas River Valley separates the Boston Mountains and Ouachita Mountains in northwest section of Arkansas. Rest of the state slopes southeast to the Mississippi River. These states are dominated by the Gulf of Mexico and Mississippi River. These influence rainfall, temperature, soil conditions. A long grass season is encouraged by mild winter and spring. 29° to 36° N. latitude.

REGIONAL CLIMATE:

Low temperature in January: Arkansas 41.8°, Mississippi 54.2°
High temperature in July: average 83°
Rainfall: Mobile and New Orleans, high 64 inches, average 52 inches

Hot humid growing seasons encourage the ragweed population. Agricultural practices can introduce pigweeds (*Amaranthus*), Lambs-quarters (*Chenopodium*).

INDEX TREES: Pollinating February through April.

(2) ELM (*Ulmus*)
(2) COTTONWOOD POPLAR (*Populus*)
(1) OAK (*Quercus*)
(1) MAPLE, BOX ELDER (*Acer*)
(1) PECAN, HICKORY (*Carya*)
(2) SYCAMORE (*Platanus*)
(1) WALNUT (*Juglans*)
(2) ASH (*Fraxinus*)
(2) HACKBERRY (*Celtis*)
(1) CEDAR (*Juniperus*)

INDEX GRASSES: Peak season February through June, Bermuda—ten months.

(1) BERMUDA (*Cynodon*)
(1) REDTOP (*Agrostis*)
(1) RYEGRASS (*Lolium*)
(2) JOHNSON (*Sorghum*)
(1) TIMOTHY (*Phleum*)
(1) ORCHARD (*Dactylis*)
(1) BLUE GRASS (*Poa*)

INDEX WEEDS: Pollinating July to November. Ragweed (*Ambrosia*) dominant.

(1) COCKLEBUR (*Xanthium*)
(2) PLANTAIN (*Plantago*)
(2) SORREL (*Rumex*)
(1) PIGWEED (*Amaranthus*)
(2) LAMBS-QUARTERS (*Chenopodium*)
(1) RAGWEED (*Ambrosia*)
(1) MARSH ELDER (*Iva*)
(1) SAGEBRUSH (*Artemisia*)

Note: (1) indicates primary index plants.
(2) indicates secondary index plants.

Region VII

STATES:

Minnesota   Michigan
Wisconsin

REGIONAL TOPOGRAPHY:

Mountain ranges in the north of Michigan and Minnesota. Much of the remaining area is rolling glaciated surfaces (plateau) dotted with lakes and moraines. This is a ridge of unstratified rock material deposited by a glacier.

REGIONAL CLIMATE:

Low temperature in January: 8° to 23°
High temperature in July: 67° to 71°
Rainfall: 26 to 30 inches

The low in January in Detroit, Michigan is 26.2°; Duluth, Minnesota 8.3°. This climate clearly defines the seasons and concentrates the pollen count in short growing periods for all plants.

INDEX TREES: Pollinate in April and May, occasionally as early as March.

- (1) ELM *(Ulmus)*
- (2) ALDER *(Alnus)*
- (2) COTTONWOOD, POPLAR *(Populus)*
- (2) ASH *(Fraxinus)*
- (1) MAPLE, BOX ELDER *(Acer)*
- (1) WALNUT *(Juglans)*
- (2) SYCAMORE *(Platanus)*
- (2) BIRCH *(Betula)*
- (1) OAK *(Quercus)*
- (1) HICKORY, PECAN *(Carya)*

Occasional spotty distribution: Juniper, Mulberry, Hackberry.

INDEX GRASSES: Pollinate April, May, June.

- (2) BROME *(Bromus)*
- (1) FESCUE *(Festuca)*
- (1) RYEGRASS *(Lolium)*
- (1) REDTOP *(Agrostis)*
- (1) TIMOTHY *(Phleum)*
- (1) KOEHLERS *(Koeleria)*
- (1) ORCHARD *(Dactylis)*
- (1) BLUE GRASS *(Poa)*
- (2) CANARY *(Phalaris)*

INDEX WEEDS: Pollinate July to frost.

- (2) SORREL *(Rumex)*
- (2) LAMBS-QUARTERS *(Chenopodium)*
- (1) PIGWEED *(Amaranthus)*
- (2) RUSSIAN THISTLE *(Salsola)*
- (1) RAGWEED *(Ambrosia)*
- (1) WATER HEMP *(Acnida)*
- (1) MARSH ELDER *(Iva)*
- (1) SAGEBRUSH *(Artemisia)*
- (1) COCKLEBUR *(Xanthium)*

Note: (1) indicates primary index plants. (2) indicates secondary index plants.

Region VIII

STATES:

Iowa   Missouri   Illinois

REGIONAL TOPOGRAPHY:

These three states are greatly influenced by the Mississippi River and to a lesser extent by the Missouri River. Upon leaving the Ozark plateau in southern Missouri and the hilly region of southern Illinois, the total area is a series of rolling plains gradually sloping to the Mississippi River. 36° to 43° N. latitude.

REGIONAL CLIMATE:

Low temperature in January: 20° to 30°
High temperature in July: 76° to 80°
Rainfall: Proximity to rivers and lakes increases rainfall. A low of 25 inches in Sioux City, Iowa to high of 41.5 inches in Springfield, Illinois. Averages 34.6 inches.

The effect of the many lakes and rivers is to stabilize the temperatures and regulate the seasons in a predictable manner. Grasses are dominant in spring and early summer, but the weed population has the greatest effect on symptomatology.

INDEX TREES: Pollinating March and April.

- (2) POPLAR, COTTONWOOD *(Populus)*
- (1) WALNUT *(Juglans)*
- (2) HICKORY, PECAN *(Carya)*
- (1) ELM *(Ulmus)*
- (2) SYCAMORE *(Platanus)*
- (2) ASH *(Fraxinus)*
- (1) OAK *(Quercus)*
- (2) MULBERRY *(Morus)*
- (2) BIRCH *(Betula)*
- (1) MAPLE, BOX ELDER *(Acer)*

INDEX GRASSES: Pollinating March through June.

- (1) ORCHARD *(Dactylis)*
- (1) REDTOP *(Agrostis)*
- (1) KENTUCKY BLUE *(Poa)*
- (1) RYEGRASS *(Lolium)*
- (1) TIMOTHY *(Phleum)*
- (2) JOHNSON *(Sorghum)*

- (2) BERMUDA *(Cynodon)*
- (3) CORN *(Zea)*

INDEX WEEDS: Pollinating July to frost.
- (2) LAMBS-QUARTERS *(Chenopodium)*
- (2) PIGWEED *(Amaranthus)*
- (2) SORREL *(Rumex)*
- (1) KOCHIA, FIREWEED *(Kochia)*
- (2) PLANTAIN *(Plantago)*
- (1) RAGWEED *(Ambrosia)*
- (1) BURWEED *(Iva)*
- (1) RUSSIAN THISTLE *(Salsola)*
- (1) SAGEBRUSH *(Artemisia)*
- (1) WEST WATER HEMP *(Acnida)*

Note: (1) indicates primary index plants. (2) indicates secondary index plants. (3) indicates minimal importance.

Region IX

STATES:

North Dakota	South Dakota
Nebraska	Kansas

REGIONAL TOPOGRAPHY:

The eastern sections of these states are glaciated plains in the north becoming undulating, sandy plains to the south. The Missouri River, Red River, Platt River and the Arkansas River create fertile plateaus and valleys. Elevation increases gradually to the westward. Black Hills in the southwest of South Dakota and the foothills of the Rockies in the west of Nebraska introduce altitude and its effect on flora. 37° to 50° N. latitude. Highest altitude 12,700 feet in west Nebraska.

REGIONAL CLIMATE:
- Low temperature in January: North Dakota 4.4°, Kansas 30°
- High temperature in July: North Dakota 71°, Kansas 80.9°
- Rainfall: North Dakota 15.4 inches, Kansas 30.7 inches

There will be a longer growing period progressing from north to south. More grass problems in the south. Distinct seasons with high pollen count.

INDEX TREES: Pollinating late March through April.
- (2) ALDER *(Alnus)*
- (2) POPLAR, ASPEN, COTTONWOOD *(Populus)*
- (1) MAPLE, BOX ELDER *(Acer)*
- (2) BIRCH *(Betula)*
- (1) ELM *(Ulmus)*
- (2) ASH *(Fraxinus)*
- (1) OAK *(Quercus)*
- (1) HAZELNUT *(Corylus)*
- (1) WALNUT *(Juglans)*
- (2) HICKORY *(Carya)*

INDEX GRASSES: Pollinating March through June.
- (1) BLUE *(Poa)*
- (1) ORCHARD *(Dactylis)*
- (1) REDTOP *(Agrostis)*
- (1) TIMOTHY *(Phleum)*
- (2) BROME *(Bromus)*
- (1) RYEGRASS *(Lolium)*
- (1) FESCUE *(Festuca)*
- (2) QUACK *(Agropyron)*
- (2) BERMUDA *(Cynodon)* (Kansas)

INDEX WEEDS: Pollinating July to frost.
- (2) COCKLEBUR *(Xanthium)*
- (2) LAMBS-QUARTERS *(Chenopodium)*
- (2) PIGWEED *(Amaranthus)*
- (2) PLANTAIN *(Plantago)*
- (1) RAGWEED *(Ambrosia) (Franseria)*
- (1) BURWEED, MARSH ELDER *(Iva)*
- (1) KOCHIA *(Kochia)*
- (1) RUSSIAN THISTLE *(Salsola)*
- (1) SAGEBRUSH *(Artemisia)*
- (1) WEST WATER HEMP *(Acnida)*
- (2) SORREL *(Rumex)*

Note: (1) indicates primary index plants. (2) indicates secondary index plants.

Region X

STATES:

Texas   Oklahoma

REGIONAL TOPOGRAPHY:

It is possible but not practical to treat Texas as two separate floral regions. The coastal plains in the east change to high rolling plateau in the west. The altitude rises from sea level to 8,000 feet (Guadalupe Peak) in the southwest.

Oklahoma follows the same contour as the rolling prairies of the east become high plains rising westward. The Ouachita Mountains are a minor influence in the southeast.

Even with this change, the flora is very similar and with minor local variations can be considered appropriate for the region. 26° to 37° N. latitude.

REGIONAL CLIMATE:

Low temperature in January: Houston 53.8°, Dallas 45.7°, El Paso 7.8°, Oklahoma City 37°

High temperature in July: Houston 83.8°, Dallas 85.8°, El Paso 81°, Oklahoma City 81°

Rainfall: Houston 46 inches, Dallas 34 inches, El Paso 7.8 inches, Oklahoma 30.2 inches

Great variations in rainfall and differences in temperature (high and low) can influence the flora and the pollinating dates, but do not induce a basic alteration of the flora. For example, Russian thistle, indigenous to an area of high temperature and copious rainfall, may produce a plant of considerable growth which is quite verdant but development of flowers that produce a lesser quantity of pollen results. On the other hand, a Russian thistle indigenous to an area of low temperature and low rainfall may produce a smaller, scrubby plant but with floral development with greater capacity to produce dry airborne pollen.

INDEX TREES: Pollinate December (Juniper), February, March and April.

(1) JUNIPER *(Juniperus)*
(2) COTTONWOOD, POPLAR *(Populus)*
(1) ELM *(Ulmus)*
(1) MAPLE, BOX ELDER *(Acer)*
(2) ASH *(Fraxinus)*
(2) MESQUITE *(Prosopsis)*
(1) MULBERRY *(Morus)*
(1) OAK *(Quercus)*

INDEX GRASSES: Pollinate April through June.

(1) BLUE GRASS *(Poa)*
(1) BERMUDA *(Cynodon)*
(2) JOHNSON *(Sorghum)*
(1) ORCHARD *(Dactylis)*
(1) REDTOP *(Agrostis)*
(1) RYEGRASS *(Lolium)*
(1) TIMOTHY *(Phleum)*
(2) WEST WHEAT *(Agropyron)*
(1) FESCUE *(Festuca)*

INDEX WEEDS: Pollinate July to October.

(2) LAMBS-QUARTERS *(Chenopodium)*
(2) PIGWEED *(Amaranthus)*
(1) RUSSIAN THISTLE *(Salsola)*
(2) SORREL *(Rumex)*
(1) KOCHIA *(Kochia)*
(2) SCALE, SALTBUSH *(Atriplex)*
(1) WEST WATER HEMP *(Acnida)*
(1) MARSH ELDER *(Iva)*
(1) SAGEBRUSH *(Artemisia)*
(1) COCKLEBUR *(Xanthium)*
(1) RAGWEED *(Ambrosia)*

Note: (1) indicates primary index plants. (2) indicates secondary index plants.

Region XI

STATES:

New Mexico	Wyoming
Utah	Colorado
Montana	Idaho (mountainous)
Arizona (mountainous)	

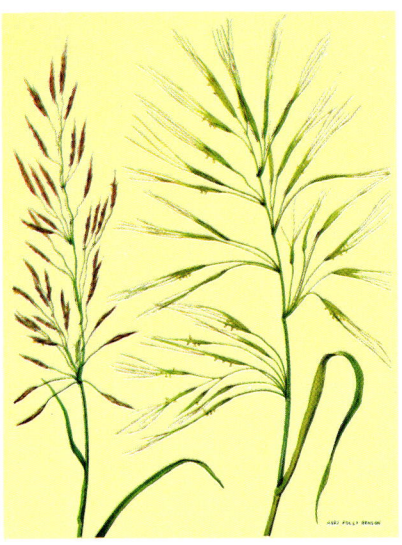

Smooth Brome
Bromus inermis
May-June

Broncho Grass
Bromus rigidus
March-June

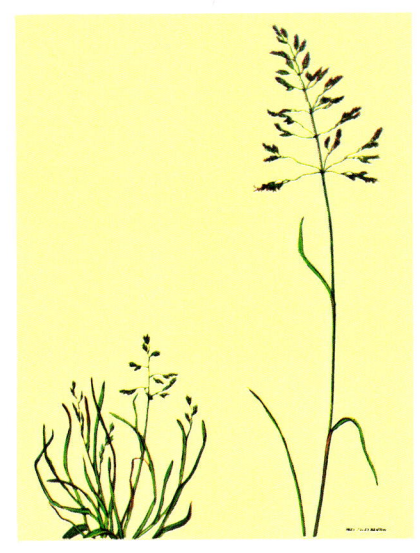

Annual June Grass
Poa annua
February-October

Kentucky Blue Grass
Poa pratensis
May-June

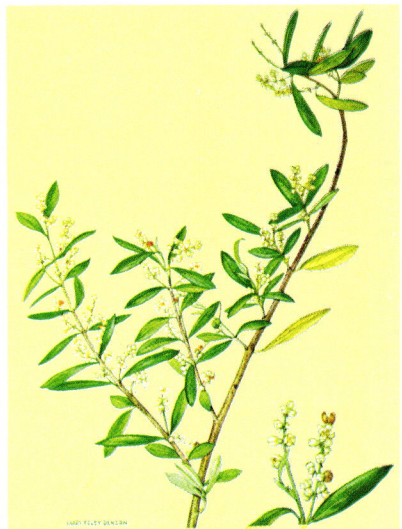

Olive
Olea europaea
April-May

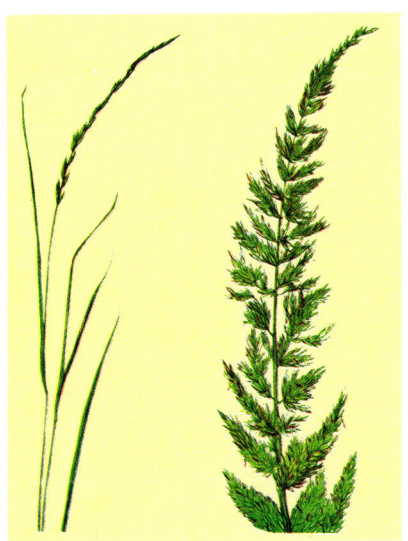

Alkali Rye
Elymus triticoides
May-June

Giant Wild-Rye
Elymus condensatus
June-August

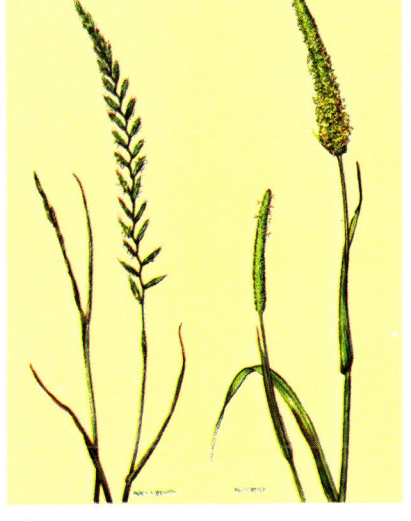

Italian Ryegrass
Lolium multiflorum
April-August

Timothy
Phleum pratense
June-July

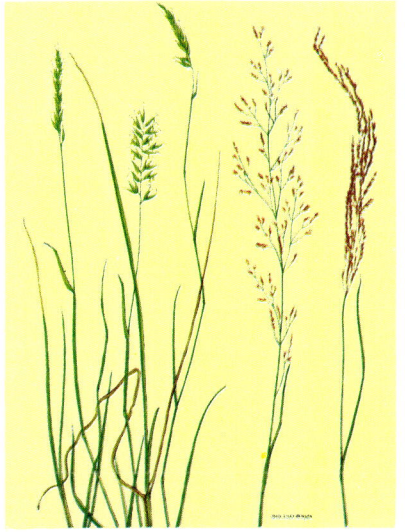

Sweet Vernalgrass
Anthoxanthum odoratum
April-July

Redtop
Agrostis alba
June-July

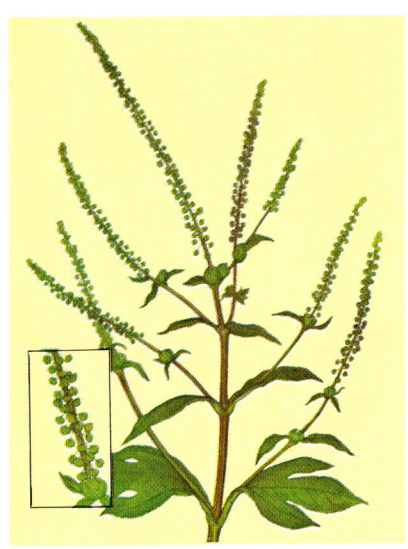

Giant Ragweed
Ambrosia trifida
August-September

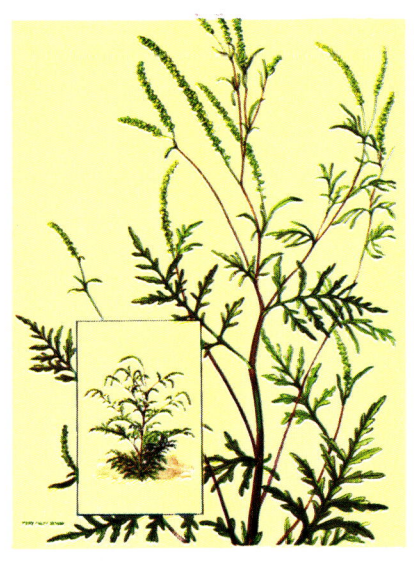

Short Ragweed
Ambrosia elatior
August-October

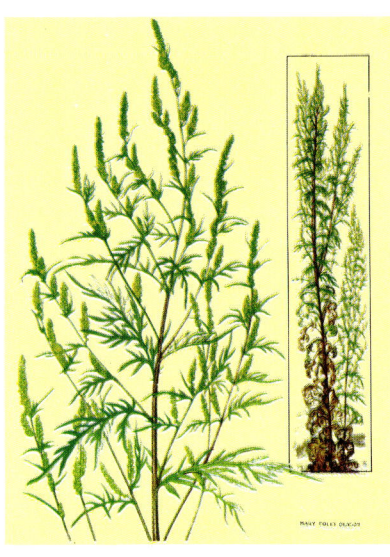

Western Ragweed
Ambrosia psilostachya
August-September

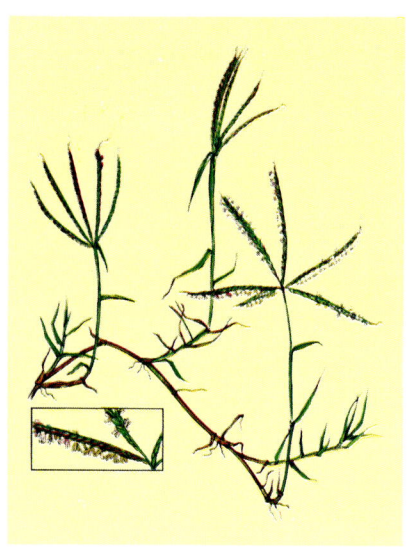

Bermuda Grass
Cynodon dactylon
April-September

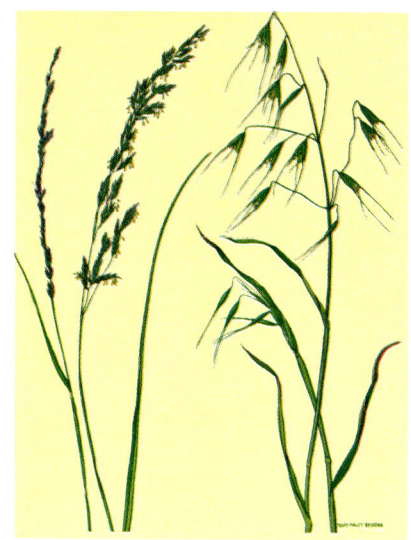

Meadow Fescue
Festuca elatior
May-July

Wild Oat
Avena fatua
June-August

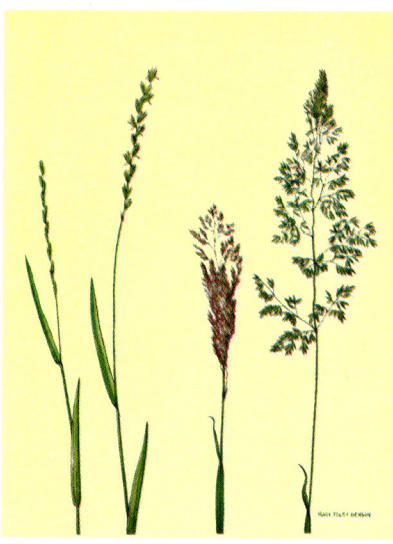

Quackgrass
Agropyron repens
July-September

Velvet Grass
Holcus lanatus
June-August

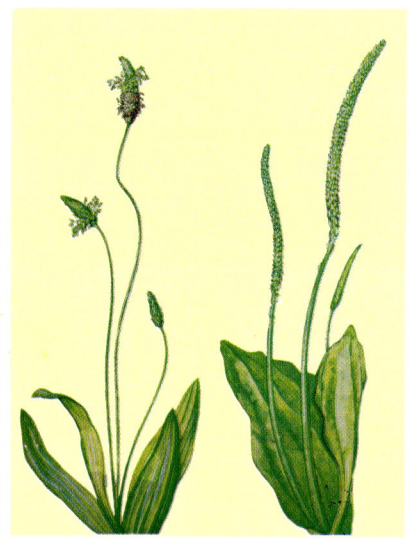

English Plantain
Plantago lanceolata
May-June

Broad-Leaf Plantain
Plantago major
April-September

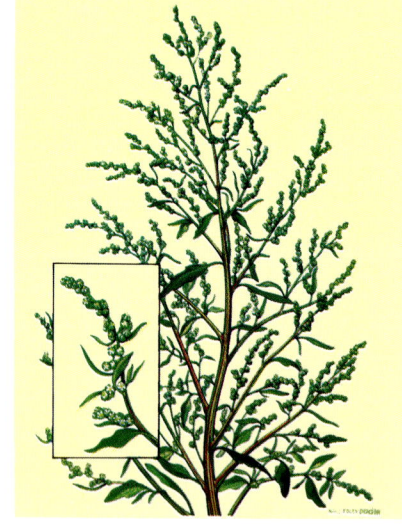

Lamb's Quarters
Chenopodium album
May-October

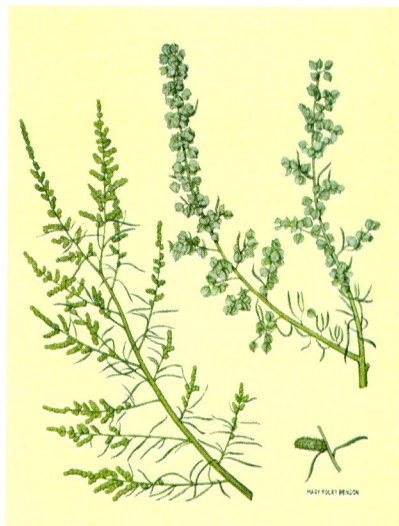

Wingscale (Shadscale)
Atriplex canescens
June-September

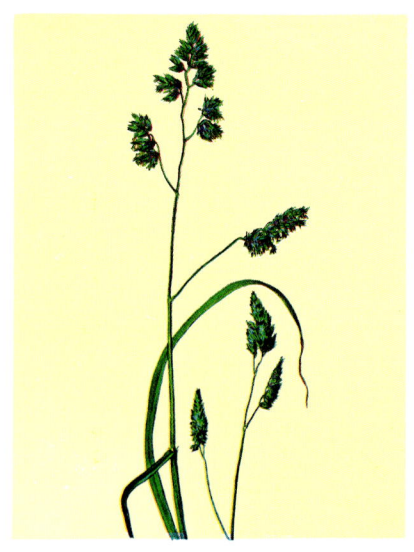

Orchard Grass
Dactylis glomerata
May-June

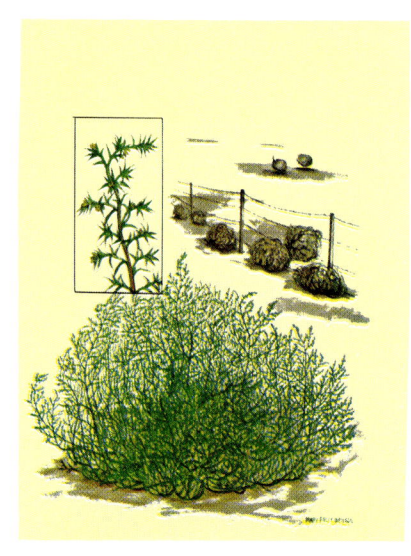

Russian Thistle (Tumbleweed)
Salsola Kali tenuifolia (Salsola pestifer)
June-September

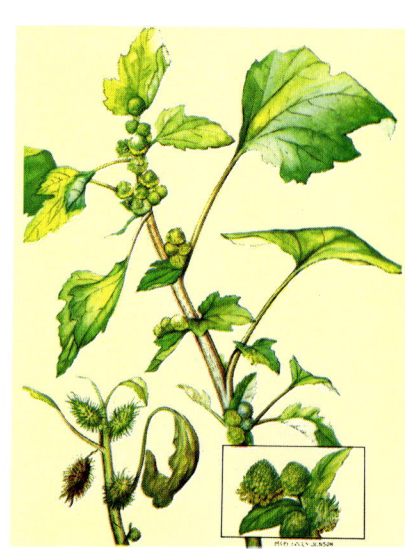

Cocklebur
Xanthium pennsylvanicum
August-September

REGIONAL TOPOGRAPHY:

Starting with scattered mountain ranges in New Mexico, the rugged Rocky Mountains dominate the total area. The Bitterroot and other ranges cover the north, east and south of Idaho.

Scattered throughout the rugged terrain will be high basins, plateaus, undulating plains. High altitudes will limit plant life, but frequently an abundant flora will be found in sheltered areas or fertile glacial rolling plains. 32° to 49° N. latitude.

REGIONAL CLIMATE:

Low temperature in January: Butte, Montana 14.2°, Cheyenne, Wyoming, 25.5°, Albuquerque, New Mexico 33.7°

High temperature in July: Butte, Montana 62.4°, Cheyenne, Wyoming 69.7°, Albuquerque, New Mexico 79.0°

Rainfall: Butte, Montana 12.6 inches, Cheyenne, Wyoming 16.25 inches, Albuquerque, New Mexico 8.6 inches

It is interesting to note the general effect of latitude on temperature. Rainfall is often influenced by local geographic conditions. Low temperature will vary more than high temperature. The predictable change from winter to spring to summer causes dramatic pollen seasons of trees, grasses and weed, in that order.

INDEX TREES: Pollinate March and April.
- (2) ALDER *(Alnus)*
- (1) MOUNTAIN CEDAR, JUNIPER *(Juniperus)*
- (2) COTTONWOOD, POPLAR *(Populus)*
- (2) BIRCH *(Betula)*
- (1) OAK *(Quercus)*
- (1) ELM *(Ulmus)*
- (1) MAPLE, BOX ELDER *(Acer)*
- (3) PINE *(Pinus)*
- (2) ASH *(Fraxinus)*

INDEX GRASSES: Pollinate April, May, June.
- (1) BLUE *(Poa)*
- (1) TIMOTHY *(Phleum)*
- (1) REDTOP *(Agrostis)*
- (1) ORCHARD *(Dactylis)*
- (1) RYEGRASS *(Lolium)*
- (1) FESCUE *(Festuca)*
- (2) BROME *(Bromus)*
- (2) WHEATGRASS *(Agropyron)*
- (2) KOELERS *(Koelaria)*
- (2) BERMUDA *(Cynodon)* (isolated spots)

INDEX WEEDS: Pollinate July to frost or late fall.
- (2) PLANTAIN *(Plantago)*
- (2) SORREL *(Rumex)*
- (1) SUMMER CYPRESS *(Kochia)*
- (1) SCALE *(Atriplex)*
- (1) PIGWEED *(Amaranthus)*
- (1) RAGWEED *(Ambrosia) (Franseria)*
- (1) MARSH ELDER *(Iva)*
- (2) LAMBS-QUARTERS *(Chenopodium)*
- (1) RUSSIAN THISTLE *(Salsola)*
- (1) COCKLEBUR *(Xanthium)*
- (1) WEST WATER HEMP *(Acnida)*
- (1) SAGEBRUSH *(Artemisia)*
- (2) SUGAR BEET *(Beta)* (where grown for seed)

Note: (1) indicates primary index plants. (2) indicates secondary index plants.

Region XII

STATES:

Desert Area of southwest California; Southern Section of Arizona

REGIONAL TOPOGRAPHY:

The majestic Sierra Nevada Range joins with the San Gabriels, Sierra Madre and San Jacinto Mountains to keep moisture from the coastal area on the western slopes. The result is the Southwest Desert. A high desert starting at the eastern base of the mountains and gradually losing altitude until the Salton Sea is below sea level. This desert region extends east and south into Arizona.

REGIONAL CLIMATE:

Mean low temperature in January: Mojave, Tucson, Palm Springs, 49.7°
Mean high temperature in July: Mojave, Tucson, Palm Springs, 86.2°
Rainfall: Mojave, Tucson, Palm Springs, 10.6 inches

This dramatic geographical change limits the indigenous flora, but irrigation and resulting agricultural development broaden. Because of the limited rainfall, plants must have efficient root structure and heat resistant stems and leaves. Most grasses will burn out unless pampered. Grasses will survive along irrigataion ditches and other types of artificial watering. This is an ideal environment for Bermuda grass (*Cynodon*), and it thrives throughout the year. Near Yuma, Arizona, Bermuda is grown for seed. Under those conditions there are two pollinating seasons that peak in May and also August or September.

The basic flora of the desert is *Atriplex*. The many colorful flowering plants are insect pollinated.

31° to 36° N. latitude in California.

INDEX TREES: Pollinate December (*Juniperus*) to May (Olive).

- (2) ARIZONA CYPRESS (*Cupressus*)
- (2) JUNIPER (*Juniperus*)
- (2) COTTONWOOD, POPLAR (*Populus*)
- (1) ELM (*Ulmus*)
- (1) OLIVE (*Olea*)
- (2) ASH (*Fraxinus*)
- (3) WILLOW (*Salix*)

INDEX GRASSES: Pollinate February to December (Bermuda).

- (2) BLUE (*Poa*)
- (1) BERMUDA (*Cynodon*)
- (2) BROME (*Bromus*)
- (1) RYEGRASS (*Lolium*)
- (2) SALT GRASS (*Distichlis*)
- (2) CANARY (*Phalaris*)

INDEX WEEDS: Pollinate May to November.

- (2) LAMBS-QUARTERS (*Chenopodium*)
- (1) RAGWEED (*Ambrosia*) (*Franseria*)
- (1) RUSSIAN THISTLE (*Salsola*)
- (1) SCALE, SALTBUSH (*Atriplex*)
- (2) IODINE BUSH (*Allenrolfea*)
- (1) SAGEBRUSH (*Artemisia*)
- (2) DICORIA (*Dicoria*)
- (1) CARELESS WEED (*Amaranthus*)
- (2) ALKALIBLITE (*Suaeda*)
- (2) HYMENOCLEA (*Hymenoclea*)

Note: (1) indicates primary index plants. (2) indicates secondary index plants. (3) indicates minimal importance.

Region XIII

STATES:

Coastal Region of California from San Diego to San Jose

REGIONAL TOPOGRAPHY:

This is a narrow coastal plain gradually rising to the limited elevation of the Coast Range. 32° to 37°N. latitude.

REGIONAL CLIMATE:

Mean low temperature in January: San Diego 54.9°, Los Angeles 55.0°, San Jose 50.1°
Mean high temperature in July: San Diego 69.3°, Los Angeles 72.5°, San Jose 70.1°
Rainfall: San Diego 10.86 inches, Los Angeles 14.54 inches, San Jose 16.5 inches

From a semitropical climate in the south to a moderate climate in the north, the area is dominated by grass and reduced weed population. Trees are complex because of the many imports and ornamentals brought to the area for shade and beauty. Most trees and bushes develop flowering parts and are insect pollinated. Indigenous trees and commercial imports are of primary significance.

INDEX TREES: Pollinate January to May (elm in September).

- (2) CYPRESS *(Cupressus)*
- (2) COTTONWOOD, POPLAR *(Populus)*
- (1) OAK *(Quercus)*
- (2) ELM *(Ulmus)*
- (2) ASH *(Fraxinus)*
- (3) ACACIA *(Acacia)*
- (1) WALNUT *(Juglans)*
- (2) SYCAMORE *(Platanus)*
- (2) MAPLE, BOX ELDER *(Acer)*
- (1) OLIVE *(Olea)*
- (3) EUCALYPTUS *(Eucalyptus)*
- (2) MULBERRY *(Morus)*

INDEX GRASSES: Pollinate January to middle June; Bermuda—January to November.

- (1) BLUE *(Poa)*
- (1) BERMUDA *(Cynodon)*
- (2) BROME *(Bromus)*
- (2) OAT *(Avena)*
- (2) SALT GRASS *(Distichlis)*
- (1) ORCHARD *(Dactylis)*
- (1) RYEGRASS *(Lolium)*
- (1) FESCUE *(Festuca)*
- (2) JOHNSON *(Sorghum)*

INDEX WEEDS: Pollinate May *(Franseria)*, July to November.

- (2) PLANTAIN *(Plantago)*
- (2) SORREL *(Rumex)*
- (2) SCALE, SALTBUSH *(Atriplex)*
- (1) RAGWEED *(Ambrosia) (Franseria)*
- (2) PIGWEED *(Amaranthus)*
- (1) RUSSIAN THISTLE *(Salsola)*
- (2) LAMBS-QUARTERS *(Chenopodium)*
- (1) SAGEBRUSH *(Artemisia)*
- (2) COCKLEBUR *(Xanthium)*

Note: (1) indicates primary index plants. (2) indicates secondary index plants. (3) indicates minimal importance.

Region XIV

STATES:

The two central valleys of California, the San Joaquin and the Sacramento. These valleys are bounded on the west by the Coast Range and on the east by the Sierra Nevada Range. A desert-like region develops on the immediate eastern slopes of the Coast Range. This quickly changes to fertile agricultural valleys of the San Joaquin and Sacramento Rivers. The valleys are closed to the north by the Siskiyou Mountains and to the south by the Tehachapi Mountains. 35° to 42° N. latitude

REGIONAL CLIMATE:

Mean low temperature in January: Sacramento 45.2°, Bakersfield 42.1°

Mean high temperature in July: Sacramento 75.3°, Bakersfield 81.2°

Rainfall: Sacramento 16.32 inches, Bakersfield 12.1 inches

Colder winters and warmer summers tend to create clearcut seasons for trees, grasses and weeds. Agricultural practices have introduced other than indigenous plants.

INDEX TREES: Pollinate February to May.

- (2) COTTONWOOD, POPLAR *(Populus)*
- (1) OAK *(Quercus)*
- (2) CYPRESS *(Cupressus)*
- (2) ALDER *(Alnus)*
- (2) BIRCH *(Betula)*
- (1) WALNUT *(Juglans)*
- (1) PECAN *(Carya)*
- (1) ELM *(Ulmus)*
- (2) SYCAMORE *(Platanus)*
- (2) MAPLE, BOX ELDER *(Acer)*
- (2) ASH *(Fraxinus)*
- (1) OLIVE *(Olea)*

INDEX GRASSES: Pollinate February to June, November (Bermuda).

- (1) BLUE *(Poa)*
- (1) BERMUDA *(Cynodon)*

- (2) BROME *(Bromus)*
- (2) OAT *(Avena)*
- (2) CANARY *(Phalaris)*
- (2) FESCUE *(Festuca)*
- (1) ORCHARD *(Dactylis)*
- (2) REDTOP *(Agrostis)*
- (1) RYEGRASS *(Lolium)*
- (2) TIMOTHY *(Phleum)*
- (2) JOHNSON *(Sorghum)*
- (2) SALT GRASS *(Distichlis)*

INDEX WEEDS: Pollinate July to November.

- (2) SORREL *(Rumex)*
- (2) SCALE *(Atriplex)*
- (2) PIGWEED *(Amaranthus)*
- (2) COCKLEBUR *(Xanthium)*
- (2) PLANTAIN *(Plantago)*
- (1) SAGEBRUSH *(Artemisia)*
- (2) LAMBS-QUARTERS *(Chenopodium)*
- (1) RAGWEED *(Ambrosia) (Franseria)*
- (1) RUSSIAN THISTLE *(Salsola)*
- (2) SUGAR BEET *(Betula)*

Note: (1) indicates primary index plants. (2) indicates secondary index plants.

Region XV

STATES:

Nevada
southeastern quarter of Oregon
southern Idaho

REGIONAL TOPOGRAPHY:

From the high Sierra Nevada on the west the land breaks into a series of roughly parallel ranges and basins. Semi-desert in nature. In the southeast quarter of Oregon are lava plateaus and basins and limited population. Southern Idaho bound on the north and east by the Bitterroot Range is a series of high Snake River plains. 36° to 44° N. latitude.

REGIONAL CLIMATE:

Mean low temperature in January: Las Vegas, Nevada 44.2°, Elko, Nevada 21.9°, Idaho Falls, Idaho 15.7°, Boise, Idaho 27.3°

Mean high temperature in July: Las Vegas, Nevada 90.5°, Elko, Nevada 70.2°, Idaho Falls, Idaho 69.2°, Boise, Idaho 74.8°

Rainfall: Las Vegas, Nevada 4.35 inches, Elko, Nevada 9.13 inches, Idaho Falls, Idaho 7.69 inches, Boise, Idaho 11.48 inches

It is obvious from the climatic record that this is primarily a dry arid area. The grass season is limited and hardy weeds predominate.

INDEX TREES: Pollinate March to April.

- (2) SYCAMORE *(Platanus)*
- (2) ALDER *(Alnus)*
- (1) ELM *(Ulmus)*
- (1) COTTONWOOD, POPLAR *(Populus)*
- (1) MAPLE, BOX ELDER *(Acer)*
- (1) JUNIPER *(Juniperus)*
- (2) BIRCH *(Betula)*
- (2) ASH *(Fraxinus)*
- (1) OLIVE *(Olea)* (Las Vegas, Nevada)

INDEX GRASSES: Pollinate April to June; Bermuda, October (Nevada).

- (1) BLUE *(Poa)*
- (1) ORCHARD *(Dactylis)*
- (2) BROME *(Bromus)*
- (1) TIMOTHY *(Phleum)*
- (1) REDTOP *(Agrostis)*
- (2) QUACK, WEST WHEAT GRASS *(Agropyron)*
- (1) RYEGRASS *(Lolium)*
- (1) FESCUE *(Festuca)*
- (1) BERMUDA *(Cynodon)*
- (2) SALT GRASS *(Distichlis)*

INDEX WEEDS: Pollinate July to October; June (Las Vegas, Nevada).

- (2) LAMBS-QUARTERS *(Chenopodium)*
- (1) RAGWEED *(Ambrosia) (Franseria)*

(1) RUSSIAN THISTLE *(Salsola)*
(2) SORREL *(Rumex)*
(1) SCALE, SALTBUSH *(Atriplex)*
(1) BURNING BUSH, KOCHIA *(Kochia)*
(2) PLANTAIN *(Plantago)*
(1) SAGE *(Artemesia)*
(1) COCKLEBUR *(Xanthium)*
(1) MARSH ELDER *(Iva)*
(2) RED PIGWEED *(Amaranthus)*
(2) RABBIT BUSH *(Chrysothamnus)*
(2) IODINE BUSH *(Allenrolfea)*

Note: (1) indicates primary index plants. (2) indicates secsondary index plants.

Region XVI

STATES:

Central and eastern Oregon and Washington

REGIONAL TOPOGRAPHY:

The broad Cascade Range and Coast Range parallel the coast and create a moisture barrier. The central sections are rolling plateau and fertile valeys. Mountain ranges hug the eastern borders. 42° to 49° N. latitude.

REGIONAL CLIMATE:

Low mean temperature in January: Klamath Falls, Oregon 29.2°, Walla Walla, Washington 32.0°, Spokane, Washington 24.9°

High mean temperature in July: Klamath Falls, Oregon 68.7°, Walla Walla, Washington 76.2°, Spokane, Washington, 69.6°

Rainfall: Klamath Falls, Oregon 13.9 inches, Walla Walla, Washington 15.07 inches, Spokane, Washington 14.9 inches

INDEX TREES: Pollinate April to May.

(2) ALDER *(Alnus)*
(2) ASPEN, COTTONWOOD, POPLAR, *(Populus)*
(1) MAPLE, BOX ELDER *(Acer)*
(2) BIRCH *(Betula)*
(2) WILLOW *(Salix)*
(2) WALNUT *(Juglans)* (Oregon)
(2) PINE *(Pinus)*
(1) OAK *(Quercus)*

INDEX GRASSES: Pollinate April to June.

(1) BLUE *(Poa)*
(1) RYEGRASS *(Lolium)*
(1) KOELERS *(Koeleria)*
(2) VERNAL *(Anthoxanthum)*
(1) ORCHARD *(Dactylis)*
(1) REDTOP *(Agrostis)*
(2) BROME *(Bromus)*
(1) TIMOTHY *(Phleum)*
(2) VELVET *(Holcus)*
(2) QUACK, WEST WHEATGRASS *(Agropyron)*

INDEX WEEDS: Pollinate July to frost.

(1) SAGEBRUSH *(Artemisia)*
(2) LAMBS-QUARTERS *(Chenopodium)*
(1) PIGWEED *(Amaranthus)*
(2) SCALE *(Atriplex)*
(1) PLANTAIN *(Plantago)*
(1) RAGWEED *(Ambrosia) (Franseria)* (Central Washington)
(2) SORREL *(Rumex)*
(1) RUSSIAN THISTLE *(Salsola)*
(1) MARSH ELDER *(Iva)*

Note: (1) indicates primary index plants. (2) indicates secondary index plants. (3) indicates minimal importance.

Region XVII

STATES:

Western edge of California (San Francisco north)
Western Oregon
Western Washington

REGIONAL TOPOGRAPHY:

Bound on the west by the Pacific Ocean and on the east by the Coast Range. Siskiyous, Cascades and the Olympics on the westerly coast of Washington. These mountains act as a moisture barrier. The result is a strip of mild climate, high rainfall. This promotes a heavy grass population and limited weed distribution. 38° to 49° N. latitude.

REGIONAL CLIMATE:

Low mean temperature in January: San Francisco 47.9°, Eureka 47.2°, Portland 39.5,° Seattle 40.7°

High mean temperature in July: San Francisco 60.4°, Eureka 56.4°, Portland 68.5°, Seattle 65.6°

Rainfall: San Francisco 17.43 inches, Eureka 36.15 inches, Portland 39.9 inches, Seattle 31.9 inches

INDEX TREES: Pollinate February to April.

- (2) ALDER *(Alnus)*
- (3) LOCUST *(Robinia)*
- (2) ASH *(Fraxinus)*
- (2) COTTONWOOD, ASPEN *(Populus)*
- (1) MAPLE, BOX ELDER *(Acer)*
- (3) WILLOW *(Salix)*
- (1) OAK *(Quercus)*
- (1) WALNUT *(Juglans)*
- (2) HAZELNUT *(Corylus)*
- (2) BIRCH *(Betula)*
- (2) ELM *(Ulmus)*
- (2) REDWOOD *(Sequoia)*
- (2) ACACIA *(Acacia)*
- (1) OLIVE *(Olea)*

INDEX GRASSES: Pollinate February to June.

- (1) BLUE *(Poa)*
- (1) BERMUDA *(Cynodon)*
- (2) BROME *(Bromus)*
- (2) OAT *(Avena)*
- (1) FESCUE *(Festuca)*
- (1) ORCHARD *(Dactylis)*
- (1) REDTOP, BENT *(Agrostis)*
- (1) RYEGRASS *(Lolium)*
- (2) SALTGRASS *(Distichlis)*
- (1) TIMOTHY *(Phleum)*
- (1) VERNAL *(Anthoxanthum)*
- (2) CANARY *(Phalaris)*
- (1) VELVET *(Holcus)*
- (2) SUDAN *(Andropogon)*

INDEX WEEDS: Pollinate June to October.

- (2) LAMBS-QUARTERS *(Chenopodium)*
- (2) PIGWEED *(Amaranthus)*
- (2) SORREL *(Rumex)*
- (1) PLANTAIN *(Plantago)*
- (1) RUSSIAN THISTLE *(Salsola)* (California mostly)
- (2) SCALE, SALTBUSH *(Atriplex)*
- (1) RAGWEED *(Ambrosia) (Franseria)*
- (1) SAGEBRUSH *(Artemisia)*
- (2) COCKLEBUR *(Xanthium)*

Note: (1) indicates primary index plants. (2) indicates secondary index plants. (3) indicates minimal importance.

A BOTANIC LIBRARY FOR PHYSICIANS

There is no need to spend a lot of money on botany books. The following are selected for their general nature and simplicity, though they are much more than little books of pretty flowers.

1. Harrington, H. D. and Durrell, L. W.: *How to Identify Plants.* Chicago, Swallow, 1957. Quality paperbound. Essentially this is an illustrated glossary of botanic terminology. For example, there are some twenty terms used to describe and distinguish plant hairs; Dr. Harrington and Dr. Durrell have given the standard definitions and descriptions, then arranged the illustrations for quick comparison. Chapter XIV shows which regional and local guides to plant identification cover *any* part of the United States.

2. *The Pictured-Key Nature Series: How to Know the—*
    Plant Families, Jaques, 1948
    Trees, Jaques, 1946
    Western Trees, Baerg, 1955
    Economic Plants, Jaques, 1958

Chapter 17

IMMUNOTHERAPY
(Desensitization—Hyposensitization)

THE TERM "DESENSITIZATION" was initially suggested by Weil (1913) for designating the refractory state due to the depletion of serum antibodies observed in anaphylactic animals following the injection of specific sera. With the recognition of the immunological nature of hay fever, the term "desensitization" was applied to the favorable responses observed following treatment with repeated injections of pollen extracts. It was soon observed that the concept of depletion of serum antibodies did not explain the favorable clinical responses following injection therapy. In 1922 Cooke proposed the term "hyposensitization" for the clinical injection procedure which implies that decreased sensitivity accounts for the favorable response. Since this is not a true interpretation of the response to the administration of specific allergenic extracts, the term "immunotherapy" is currently (1971) favored because the broader connotation recognizes that the response to injection therapy is the product of the interaction of several immunologic events, some identified and some still unexplained.

Immunotherapy consists of three phases:

I. The preparation of extracts
II. Diagnostic test procedures—skin testing
III. Injection therapy.

There are no standard procedures for the preparation of extracts, for testing and for the administration of antigens. Because of many variations in the techniques applied at each stage, there is no standard routine for the management of the allergic patient. However, in spite of differences in procedure, the objective of each program is the control of the patient's symptoms which must be accomplished without undesirable reactions that can further endanger the patient's health and even be a hazard to his life.

The discussion which follows is based upon the techniques and procedures practiced in the Allergy Department of the Kaiser Foundation Hospitals and the Permanente Medical Group (KFH-PMG) of Northern California. The techniques include the preparation of allergenic extracts, the testing experience with more than 500,000 patient visits (over 10,000,000 individual allergy tests), and the injection program applied in the management of several hundred thousand allergy patients over a period of twenty years.

When pertinent, comparisons will be made with techniques and procedures other than those practiced in the KFH-PMG program.

I. THE PREPARATION OF EXTRACTS

Satisfactory allergenic extracts for both testing and treatment are available from reliable biological laboratories. The following discussion of the preparation of allergenic extracts is intended as a guide for evaluating the quality of commercially available products rather than a recommended procedure for the preparation of extracts.

All allergenic extracts are aqueous solutions of soluble proteins derived from raw materials, such as pollens, epidermal and environmental factors, foods and molds.

Weeds, Jaques, 1959
Grasses, Pohl, 1968
Pollen and Spores, Kapp, 1969
Wm. C. Brown Dubuque, Iowa. The Pictured-Key Series is general for the United States, usually under $3.00 per volume, well illustrated, and spiral bound for quick reference.

3. Wodehouse, Roger P.: *Hay Fever Plants,* 2nd ed. New York, Hafner, 1971. This is *the* classic text on the botany of hay fever.
4. Wodehouse, Roger P.: *Pollen Grains.* New York, Hafner, 1959. This other classic by Wodehouse includes pollen morphology, palaeopalynology and hay fever.

Pollen Extracts

The first prerequisite for a good pollen extract is a reliable supply of raw pollen. The quality of the pollen supply depends upon the following factors:

(1) Control of contamination

(a) The control of contamination of pollens must begin with the harvesting of the plants. When plants are gathered, care must be exercised to assure that the specimens are not infested with smuts and other fungi. Grasses and grains are frequently smut infested which makes them unsuitable for supplying pollens for extracts. Unskilled personnel can make errors in the identification of plants which results in either adulteration of the pollens or complete substitution with an unwanted species. Such errors lead to false skin test reactions and failure in treatment.

Additional sources of contamination arise from twigs, leaves or other plant parts. These also make unsatisfactory extracts which lead to unreliable skin test reactions and decreased biological activity.

(b) Pollens can be contaminated by molds after collection, which proliferate under improper storage conditions, making the material unsuitable for extracts.

(2) The Storage of Pollens

As soon as possible following their collection, pollens should be dehydrated and stored in sealed containers under anaerobic conditions (nitrogen) at low temperature (not freezing).

Pollens have natural enzymes which at room temperature and average humidity can degrade the pollen protein which leads to either a decrease or a complete loss of biological activity.

Extracting Procedures for Pollens

The purpose of pollen extracts is to provide in concentrated form, with as little alteration in structure as possible, all the active proteins required for both testing and treatment. Each pollen usually has more than one allergenic protein. Since the specific allergens in pollens have not been identified, the extracting techniques are usually simple procedures to recover all the proteins in any given pollen. There are no standard formulae for extracting fluids and no standard procedures for extracting.

The defatting procedure which was a routine practice in the early years of the preparation of extracts has been abandoned by most laboratories. Buffered solutions for maintaining an alkaline pH are in general use. Except for Coca's solution which is indicated below, the extracting formulae provide 50 per cent glycerol which serves as a stabilizer. A pollen extract in 50 per cent glycerol will usually maintain its biological activity for several years if stored in the refrigerator. The generally accepted preservative is phenol 0.4 to 0.5 per cent. Mercurial preservatives are not recommended because of the risk of mercurial toxicity.

Buffered Glycerol Extracting Fluid*

Stock solutions are prepared as follows:
Dibasic phosphate, $K_2(HPO_4)$
52.3 gm/liter of distilled water
Monobasic phosphate, $K(H_2PO_4)$
40.85 gm/liter of distilled water

To prepare one liter of *buffered glycerol extracting fluid:*

$K_2(HPO_4)$	400 cc
$K(H_2PO_4)$	100 cc
glycerol	500 cc

Glycerol Extracting Fluid:
analytical-grade glycerol 50 per cent
distilled water 50 per cent

Glycerol-Saline Extracting Fluid:
glycerol 50 per cent by weight
sodium chloride 2 per cent by weight
water 48 per cent by weight

Extracts prepared without buffer are prone to be irritating.

---

* This formula has been used for all extractives at the KFH-PMG.

Coca's Solution:

sodium chloride	0.5 per cent
sodium bicarbonate	0.275 per cent
phenol	0.4 per cent

Extracts prepared with this solution are not very stable.

For diluents: (1) Normal saline with 0.4 per cent phenol, or (2) buffered solution as recommended for extracting media with 0.4 per cent phenol.

Extracting Technique for Pollens

(1) Add two grams of dry pollen to 100 cc of extracting fluid.

(2) Permit the mixture to stand overnight in the refrigerator (38° to 40° F).

(3) Agitate for two and one-half hours on a mechanical shaker.

(4) Stand overnight in the refrigerator.

(5) Nonextractable portion will precipitate.

(6) Handle gently to avoid unnecessary mixing of the precipitate. Decant the supernatant into a filter (either *Seitz* or *Milipore*).

(7) Collect the filtrate in sterile containers.

(8) Remove sample for culture in Sabouraud's media.

Standardization of Pollen Extracts

There are no precise techniques for the standardization of the allergenic activity of pollen extracts. If the specific allergen(s) for each pollen were known, it would offer an ideal and reliable method for the standardization of pollen extracts for both testing and injection therapy. An attempt in this direction was made by King and Norman who isolated Antigen E from eastern ragweed *(Ambrosia elatior)*. It was hoped that the antigen E content of any ragweed extract would indicate the exact biological activity. But not all patients react to antigen E. The small percentage of patients who fail to react to antigen E makes the expression of the potency of ragweed extract in terms of antigen E an unsatisfactory measure of the activity for all ragweed sensitive patients.

Noon Units: One of the earliest attempts at standardization was that proposed by Noon who attempted to develop a precise unit based upon the weight of the pollen before extraction. The Noon unit represents 0.001 mg of dry pollen per milliliter of extract. The fallacy of this unit as a standard is the failure to recognize the variability in the protein content of different supplies of pollen. Protein content of pollen may vary from one season to another depending upon conditions of plant growth, such as moisture, temperature and sunlight. In addition, the variability in activity arising from differences in storage conditions and extracting procedures must be considered. Because of these differences, an attempt at precise standardization as implied by the Noon unit is not possible.

Protein Nitrogen Units (PNU): It was recognized very early by Cook (1915) that the proteins of an extract are responsible for its biological activity. On the basis of this concept it was postulated that the PNUs of an extract should serve as the index of its biological activity.

The determination of PNU is based upon the phosphotungstic acid procedure which delivers nonallergenic nitrogenous substances in the extract as well as active proteins. The PNU is not an exact measure of allergenic activity.

Pollen proteins can become denatured and lose their biological activity, or the activity may become altered and not represent the specificity of the pollen being assayed. For this reason PNUs are not necessarily an index of biological activity.

Because of these variations, it is possible for an extract with a rating of 4,000 PNUs/cc to manifest greater biological activity than an extract derived from the same species with a rating of 40,000 PNUs/cc.

In spite of the unreliability of PNU assays as an indicator of biological activity, this index is still commonly used as the standard for extracts and a measure of dosage for treatment. It must be recognized that two extracts from the identical species of pollen with equal PNU ratings may exhibit great differences in biological activity. This condition is very important when PNU assays are applied to extracts derived from batches of pollens collected in different years.

IgE Standard: It is possible that future developments in the immunochemistry of IgE may provide more reliable techniques for standardization of allergic extracts. This is predicated upon the assumption that IgE is the only antibody involved in atopic allergy.

Weight by Volume: In the absence of reliable criteria for the standardization of allergenic extracts, the only practical index for the present is the preparation of extracts on the basis of weight by volume (w/v) with standardization for activity on known human reactors by skin testing.

General Principles

In evaluating the quality of an extract, all the production details must be considered. They include:

(1) The quality of the dry pollen.
(2) The extraction media and technique.
(3) Production controls, which include laboratory facilities, storage conditions for pollens, operational efficiency, and controls.
(4) Clinical standardization.

Routine skin test reactions are not a reliable guide for the quality of an extract. Contaminating factors can induce strong nonspecific reactions. A pollen substituted in error can give false skin test reactions and cause failures in hyposensitization. Controls must be conducted on known human reactors.

Extraction of Environmental Factors

The extraction of allergenic proteins from epidermal factors presents two conditions not encountered with pollen extractives: (1) the low concentration of active proteins in the raw material and (2) the high concentration of contaminants in the raw material.

Quills and animal hairs are keratinous in nature which makes them immunologically inactive. The allergenic material encountered with feathers and hairs is found in the dander which is of epithelial origin. The quantity of dander derived from a batch of hairs and feathers is relatively very small, so that the yield of active protein from a given supply of raw material is extremely low. For example, a kilogram of either cat hair or dog hair will yield approximately 3 to 4 gm of active protein. In order to produce an effective extract of good titer, it is advisable to resort to extracting techniques that concentrate the protein.

Both feathers and hairs have a high concentration of contaminants constituted of molds, bacteria, bacterial components and various dusts.

Feathers are subject to attack by molds and also tend to accumulate dusts. In order to prepare a good specific feather extract, it is necessary to have a supply of fresh, clean feathers, as free as possible of external contaminants. The protein yield from clean feathers is very low but the extracts are very active and specific.

Animal hairs are contaminated with bacteria and dusts. Clipping the hair from clean pets will reduce to a minimum the extraneous materials. A high concentration of bacteria in the hair supply can result in extracts with (1) a high incidence of delayed reactions in skin testing, and (2) a high incidence of reactions, both local and constitutional, due to high titers of bacterial endotoxins.

Some laboratories produce epidermal extracts by scrubbing the pelts in order to loosen epidermal cells. Extracts produced by this technique may exhibit good reactions on skin testing, but the reactivity is probably attributable to a high histamine content in the extracts released by the scrubbing process.

The preparation of good epidermal extracts requires techniques that concentrate the proteins and separate them from the contaminants. The acetone precipitation technique fulfills both requirements.

Acetone Precipitation Technique

Reagents: Buffered solution
NaCl	1 part
$NaHCO_3$	2 parts
phenol	0.5 per cent

To prepare twenty-eight liters of buffer:
NaCl	28 gm
$NaHCO_3$	56 gm
phenol	
water *q.s.* to given 28 liters	

6N HCl and 2N HCl acid

Precooled Pure Acetone Procedure

(1) Raw material is weighed out.

All extraneous material should be removed before weighing. If large quills are used, they should be broken into pieces about 5 to 6 cm in length.

(2) Place in suitable container. Mix with buffered saline, approximately 8 liters to 1 kilogram raw material.

(3) Layer with toluene.

(4) Store in cold box for eighteen to twenty-four hours.

(5) Mixture is filtered through diatomaceous earth. Squeeze out all fluid from the solid material either by hand or by means of a press.

(6) Concentrate the solution to approximately one-fourth volume.

   (a) Concentration can be achieved by placing material in a Visking casing and permitting perevaporation by exposing to air heated by infrared lanps. By this technique a reduction of 25 per cent volume can be achieved.

   (b) Concentration can be achieved more efficiently and more quickly by membrane filtration techniques. Concentration to one-tenth volume can be achieved very quickly which is extremely important to reduce the likelihood of denaturation.

(7) The concentrated solution is usually at a pH of 8.0 or above. pH is adjusted to 4.8 using 6N and 2N HCl. This represents the isoelectric point for most of the proteins to be recovered.

(8) Add three parts of precooled acetone to the mixture.

(9) Store in the deep freeze for eighteen to twenty-four hours.

(10) At this stage most of the proteins will have precipitated or will be in suspension. Filter through paper.

(11) Wash the recovered precipitate two times with cold acetone.

(12) Dry in air and store *in vacuo* over $CaCl_2$.

(13) Grind the dry precipitate in a mortar and pass through a 28 mesh screen.

(14) Place in a clean, wide-mouth reagent bottle. Store *in vacuo* over $CaCl_2$ until completely dry.

(15) When removed from *vacuo* (usually after ten to fourteen days), flood with nitrogen, cap, and seal with paraffin.

The dry precipitate which represents the protein can be stored in the cold for indefinite periods. If the bottle is opened for the removal of samples, the opened bottle should be returned *in vacuo* for about ten days before sealing. Moisture predisposes to denaturation.

The yield is usually very small. For cat and dog hair, the yield of precipitate is usually about 3 to 4 grams for 2,000 grams of *starting* raw material. The precipitate is practically pure protein which can be handled in the same manner as a pure pollen sample.

With the adjustment of the pH to the isoelectric point and the addition of precooled acetone, the proteins are precipitated, leaving behind the nonproteinaceous materials including the unwanted salts.

Membrane filtration is a more dependable technique for the removal of unwanted salts.

The dry precipitate is extracted on the basis of 2 grams/100 cc of buffered extracting fluid. The procedure from this point is identical to that outlined for pollen.

The advantages of this technique are:

(1) Recovery of a high concentration of protein.

(2) The elimination of contaminants.

(3) More specific skin responses and more effective response in hyposensitization. With the elimination of contaminants, nonspecific reactivity is reduced to a minimum.

Other environmental factors, such as cocoanut fiber, kapok, jute and wool can be processed by the same acetone precipitation technique. The same advantages are offered as experienced with the epidermal factors.

Dust Extracts

Dust extracts are extremely important in clinical allergy for both testing and treatment of patients. They empirically provide many items to which the patient may be reactive. From the standpoint of clinical allergy "dust" must be differentiated from "dirt." It is possible that a very untidy, even filthy environment may not be particularly allergenic for a patient, while a well groomed environment with down upholstered furniture, heavy jute carpet pads and one or more pets may be highly allergenic.

Many unsuccessful attempts have been made to isolate a single allergen from house dust. The likelihood of achieving that goal is very doubtful in view of the many potential components of dust and the variation in reactivity to different dust samples.

The allergenicity of dust extracts will vary with the source of the dust. For this reason it is advisable to prepare dust extracts from a pooled supply representative of many environments in any given area. The samples should be from private homes, schools, offices, hotels, motels, and at times even industrial environments. If a special industry is prominent in an area, it is advisable to include dust samples representative of the industry. Dust extracts for specific geographical districts should be available from biological laboratories. Occasionally, it may be necessary to prepare dust extracts for special environments, such as post offices, coffee dust and mill dust of various types. The necessity for preparing such dust extracts is not too frequent. A pooled sample taken from several sources in the area where the patient lives is usually satisfactory.

Special house dust extracts prepared from samples taken from the patient's home and prepared by simple direct extracting procedures are usually not reliable. These contain nonspecific irritants which give false skin reactions. It is not reasonable to expect an adequate concentration of active protein to be derived by the extraction of a cigar box or even a shoe box full of dust by means of direct extraction with *any* of the extracting media.

The extraction of dusts presents the same problem encountered with the extraction of hairs and feathers. For the same reasons the acetone precipitation technique yields the most reliable dust extract. An acetone precipitated dust can be processed on a weight by volume ratio, just as was recommended for pollens.

Commercial dust extracts are available which exhibit a high degree of reactivity in skin testing. It is usually necessary to dilute such extracts ten to one hundred times to avoid positive skin reactions with every test applied. When such extracts are used, it is important to rule out nonspecific factors which may contribute to the reactivity. PNU is not a dependable guide.

Most extracts of environmental factors, dusts and foods available on the market are not prepared by the acetone precipitation technique, but rather by the direct extraction procedure. The extracts produced by the direct method usually have a low concentration of active protein. They frequently contain a relatively high content of nonspecific factors which may induce a good skin response that is not specific and at times not even immunologic. Most of these extracts are assayed on the basis of PNU, which as has been pointed out for pollens, is not a reliable index of immunologic activity. The acetone precipitate technique which provides a concentrated protein base for extraction permits standardization on a weight by volume (w/v) basis comparable to the method recommended for pollen extracts.

Mites

There are several reports indicating that mites occur in most house dusts. The species and the number of mites in the sample of house dust varies with the geographical and regional source of the dust. Studies have demonstrated a relationship between the skin response to extracts of mites and house dust extracts. Recent observations have also demonstrated IgE antibodies specific for mites. The evidence to date is strongly in favor of mites as an important allergenic factor in house dust, but it is unlikely that mites are the only source of antigenic components in dusts. Further studies are required to determine the extent to which mites participate in the atopic reaction. Since most insects induce delayed hypersensitivity, it would be important to determine the role of mites in this type of allergic response.

Solving the problems of mite sensitivity is complicated by the difficulty in developing pure cultures of various species of mites in sufficient supply, free of contaminants, for the production of extracts.

Until more definite data become available, it is reasonable to believe that good house dust extracts prepared from samples provided by any given region will contain fractions contributed by mites indigenous in the area. If hyposensitization with mite extracts is of clinical value, the house dust extracts containing mite components should temporarily serve the clinical needs for dealing with mite sensitivity.

Vegetable Fibers

The vegetable fibers encountered in the average environment include cotton, cocoanut fiber, kapok, and jute.

All the vegetable fibers provide low yields of active proteins. For this reason the acetone precipitation technique is best suited for producing an active extract. The extracts should be prepared from fresh, clean, raw material to avoid the contaminants such as molds, bacteria and dusts. (See discussion of environmental factors for source and distribution of vegetable fibers.)

Gums

The gums listed below are those commonly used in the preparation of commercial food products.

Derived from seaweed	Country of Origin
Agar—red algae	Japan
Algin—brown algae	United States Pacific coast
Carrageenan—red algae (*Chondrus crispus*), Irish moss	Ireland
Furcellaran—red algae	Denmark

Derived from tree exudates and extracts	
Gum arabic—exudate of Acacia	West Africa
Ghatti—exudate of *Anogeissus latifolia*	India and Ceylon
Karaya—exudate of *Sterculia ureus*	India
Larch gum (Aribinogalactan)—extract of larch tree	Northwestern United States
Tragacanth—exudate of *Astragalus gummifer*	Iran, Syria, Turkey, Asia Minor

Derived from seeds	
Guar gum—seed of guar plant (*Cyarnopsis tetragonolobus*)	India, Pakistan, United States

Locust bean—seed of carob tree (St. John's bread) — Mediterranean countries

Positive skin test reactions have been reported for extracts of agar, gum arabic, karaya and tragacanth. Commercially prepared extracts for the remaining gums listed above are not available. It is very likely that reactions would be observed with Carrageenan and Furcellaran which have a very wide distribution in our food supply. There are no studies reported with these two gums.

The gums are complex, long-chain carbohydrates which, because of their structure, are very stable and probably not antigenic. It is possible that the reactions attributed to gums, both clinical and on testing may be due to contaminants rather than the gums themselves. Until these factors can be identified, the commercial extracts available can serve as a guide to determine sensitivity.

Silk

As the silk worm spins its cocoon, the fine fibers which are fibroin are held together by a glue-like substance, sericin. Fibroin is insoluble in water and accordingly is not antigenic, while sericin which is water soluble can serve as an inhalant allergen to produce allergic rhinitis, asthma and urticaria. At times dermatitis is caused by silk.

Since the use of silk has decreased appreciably with the development of various synthetic fibers, it is less important as an allergenic factor. However, it must still be considered as a possibility in situations where silk is in use.

In addition to the silk worm, it is possible that other animals, such as the arachnids (spiders) may serve as a source of silk allergens. In these situations the silk is a constituent of the house dust. Testing and treating with a dust extract derived from the patient's environment should provide the offending allergen.

Food Extracts

The most reliable procedure for preparing allergenic extracts of foods is the acetone precipitation technique which permits concentration of the protein and separation of nonproteinaceous materials which can induce nonspecific reactions on testing. Foods are never prescribed for hyposensitization.

The basic procedure as outlined for epidermal factors is suitable for most foods, but for some items, the technique must be modified in order to remove relatively high concentrations of unwanted materials, such as salts, sugars and pectins. Repeated dialysis successfully removes the salts and sugars. The viscid mass produced by the hydrophilic nature of the pectins, as in apples, apricots, grapes, can usually be handled by membrane filtration with pressure under nitrogen.

The precipitated product, properly dried, can be stored for several years in sealed bottles. The dried precipitate can be reconstituted on a weight by volume basis with 50 per cent glycerolated buffered solution. This provides a stable alkaline solution which is not irritating.

Because of the instability of the proteins in fruits and berries, the use of freshly preserved juices has been recommended for testing. The high concentration of nonproteinaceous materials induces a high number of nonspecific reactions by this procedure.

A nonirritating extract of banana has never been produced. All banana extracts are highly reactive due to nonallergenic factors which cannot be removed successfully without denaturing the banana protein. Practically everyone, whether allergic or not, will react positively with banana extract.

II. SKIN TESTING

Skin tests as a diagnostic procedure in allergy were first utilized by Blackley, a hay fever sufferer, who in 1873 tested various specimens of pollens by conjunctival instillation, application to the nasal and buccal mucosae, deep inhalation, and "by inoculating the upper arms and lower limbs with fresh moistened pollens."

The use of skin tests as a medium for making clinical tests came into vogue with the introduction of the cutaneous test for tuberculosis by von Pirquet in 1907. Von Pirquet's technique met with immediate and universal acceptance and paved the way for clinical tests in various types of allergy. Von Pirquet's scarification technique was followed very shortly by the Schick intracutaneous test for diphtheria immunity (1910).

The technique of von Pirquet as a method for demonstrating hypersensitiveness in hay fever, asthma and food allergy was permanently established by the studies of Schloss (1912) and Goodale (1914). The method referred to as the "scratch test" was popularized by Walker and his colleagues who in an extensive series of studies on hypersensitivity focused the attention of the medical profession upon the value of skin testing as a diagnostic aid.

The intracutaneous or intradermal test as currently applied in clinical allergy was developed by Cooke and his co-workers (1915).

The techniques for performing the various tests have not varied appreciably since their initial development, but the clinical significance and interpretation of the various tests has kept apace with the advancements in immunology. The allergy skin test is not a diagnostic procedure for determining whether an individual has allergic disease, but rather a technical aid to be interpreted on the basis of the patient's history and physical findings. The diagnosis of allergic disease must always be made by a carefully developed history and a thorough physical examination, while the reactions observed with skin testing serve to support the diagnosis and guide the management of the patient.

Technique

The three techniques commonly used for atopic allergy skin tests are (1) the scratch test, (2) the prick test, and (3) the intradermal (intracutaneous) test.

Scratch Test Procedure

(1) Use the flexural surface of the forearm.

(2) Prepare the area with alcohol, permitting it to dry.

(3) Tense the skin of the flexural surface by grasping the back of the arm with the left hand.

(4) With a semi-sharp scalpel or scarifier produce small abrasions (0.25 to 0.3 cm) in the superficial layer of the skin. Care must be exercised not to cut too deeply so as to draw blood which will interfere with the reaction. Special caution must be exercised with the thin skins of young children and some females.

(5) Ten to twenty tests can be performed at one session, depending upon the size of the forearm.

(6) Allow a minimum of 1.5 to 2.0 cm between tests to avoid coalescence.

(7) With either a sterile toothpick or sterile applicator stick apply a small drop of concentrated extract.* Rub in gently for one to two seconds.

(8) Use plain extracting fluid for the control.

(9) Read after twenty minutes.

See discussion below for rating of skin reactions.

Note: Excessive trauma from scarification by the scratch technique can induce a response which may be difficult to evaluate.

A second technique recommended for performing the scratch test involves placing a drop of extract upon the cleansed skin surface and introducing the instrument through the drop to scarify the skin. This technique may be satisfactory for a single test but is not practical when multiple tests are performed, since it necessitates using a separate immunologically clean instrument for each test performed to avoid the transfer of antigen from one test to another.

The Prick Test

The extract is the same concentration as for the scratch test.

---

* For 50 per cent glycerolated acetone precipitated extracts, use 1:50 concentration. For buffered extracts prepared by direct techniques. use 1:10 concentration.

There are two methods for performing the prick test.

(a) Apply a drop of extract to the prepared skin surface. With a sharp sterile darning needle introduce the point through the drop to prick the skin or produce a slight scratch.

(b) The instrument used is a solid shaft, stainless steel needle with a bifurcated tip. The points of the tip are semi-sharp (see Fig. 17-1). By dipping the tip of the needle into the vial of extract, the capillary action of the bifurcated tip will pick up sufficient extract to perform the test.

With the extract on the needle tip, place the tip at a right angle to the skin surface on the flexural surface of the forearm. Exert gentle pressure. Rotate the needle 180°. This action will fracture the skin and also introduce the test antigen.

By this technique the area of trauma to the skin is limited to the circumference of the needle tip. The degree of trauma is governed by the degree of pressure exerted and limited by the blunt nature of the needle tip. The volume of antigen delivered is limited to the quantity picked up by the capillary action of the bifurcation of the needle, which is identical with each needle. The slots in the needles are machined to be *identical* in size.

This technique produces a series of tests of uniform size, with a minimum of trauma. The size of the test and the controlled volume of antigen delivered permits accurate reproduction of the test conditions. This allows for accurate comparison of one test experience with subsequent tests.

Twenty tests with a control can be applied to the average forearm with allowance for adequate spacing between tests to prevent coalescence of neighboring reactions.

Each test site can be marked with a skin pencil.

After twenty minutes the tests are wiped clean with an alcohol sponge and the reading made.

Allow a minimum of 1.5 cm between tests.

In small children both forearms may be used.

When properly applied with a well designed needle, the prick test is not a painful procedure. It is tolerated very well by children.

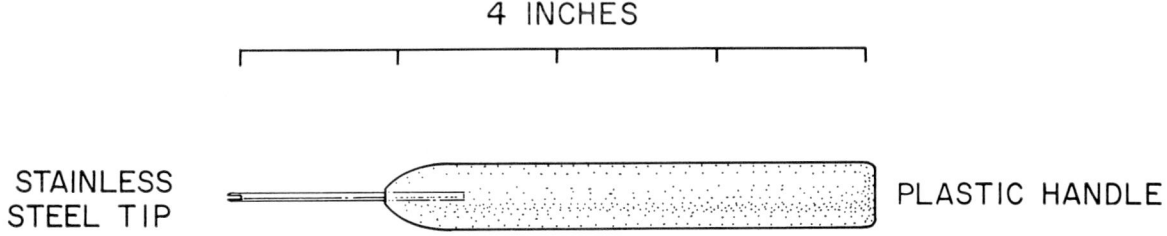

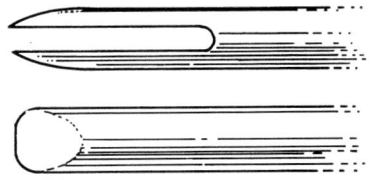

Figure 17-1

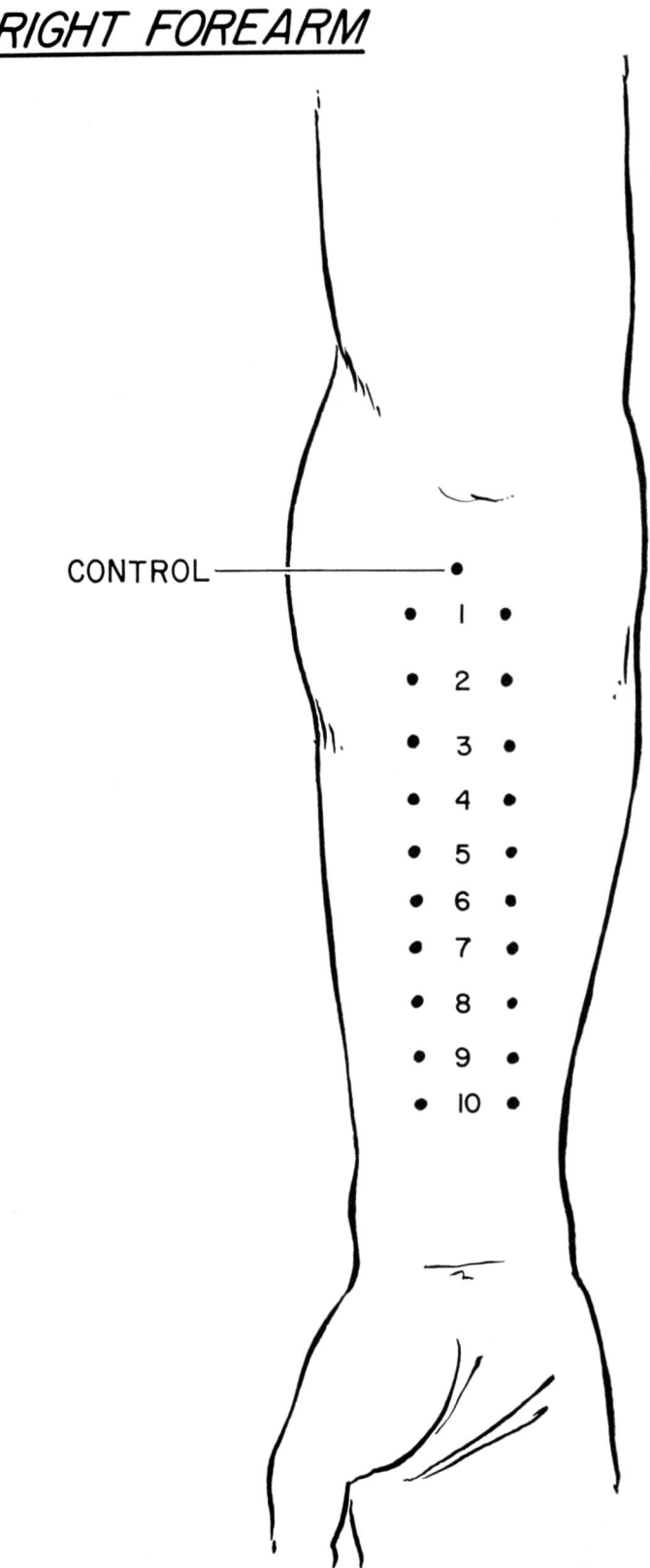

Figure 17-2. Position of prick tests on the forearm. 20 tests can be performed. Left 1–10—Rt 1–20.

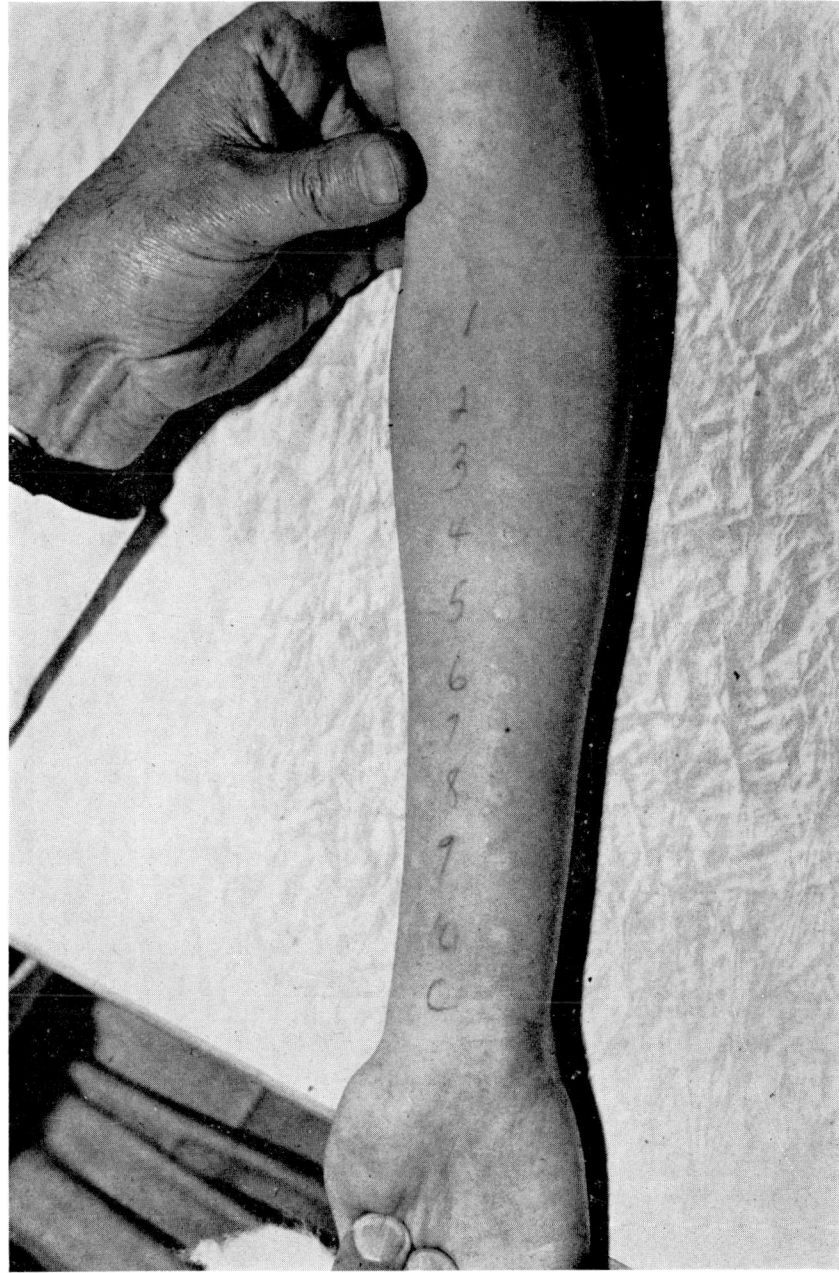

Figure 17-3. Whealing reactions following positive prick tests.

Intradermal (Intracutaneous) (I.D.) Test Procedure

(1) The lateral surface of the upper arm is the site of choice. (For indications for testing on the back, see below.)

(2) Skin surface should be cleansed with an alcohol sponge and air dried.

(3) With the left hand, grasp firmly the back of the arm. This will serve to steady the patient's arm and at the same time exert tension on the skin at the testing site.

(4) Equipment: Syringes—glass or disposable 1 ml tuberculin type needles, gauge #26, length 3/8; short intradermal type bevel. Disposable needles are frequently excessively sharp which can have a cutting action on the tissues. Disposable syringes usually do not have the smooth plunger action of a

glass syringe. The length of the syringe and the shape of the plunger cap are less suitable for a good intradermal technique.

(5) Care of the syringes: All syringes should be properly labelled to permit accurate identification of the contents. A metal bird tag is a simple and reliable method for labelling syringes.

A syringe must be used for only one antigen. Washing and autoclaving does not make a syringe immunologically clean. Residual antigen must be destroyed by acid treatment. A minute residual of antigen in the syringe may serve to produce a false reaction.

Disposable syringes can be discarded.

Glass syringes must be acid treated to destroy residual antigen.

(6) The position of the syringe in the hand: Hold the barrel of the syringe be-

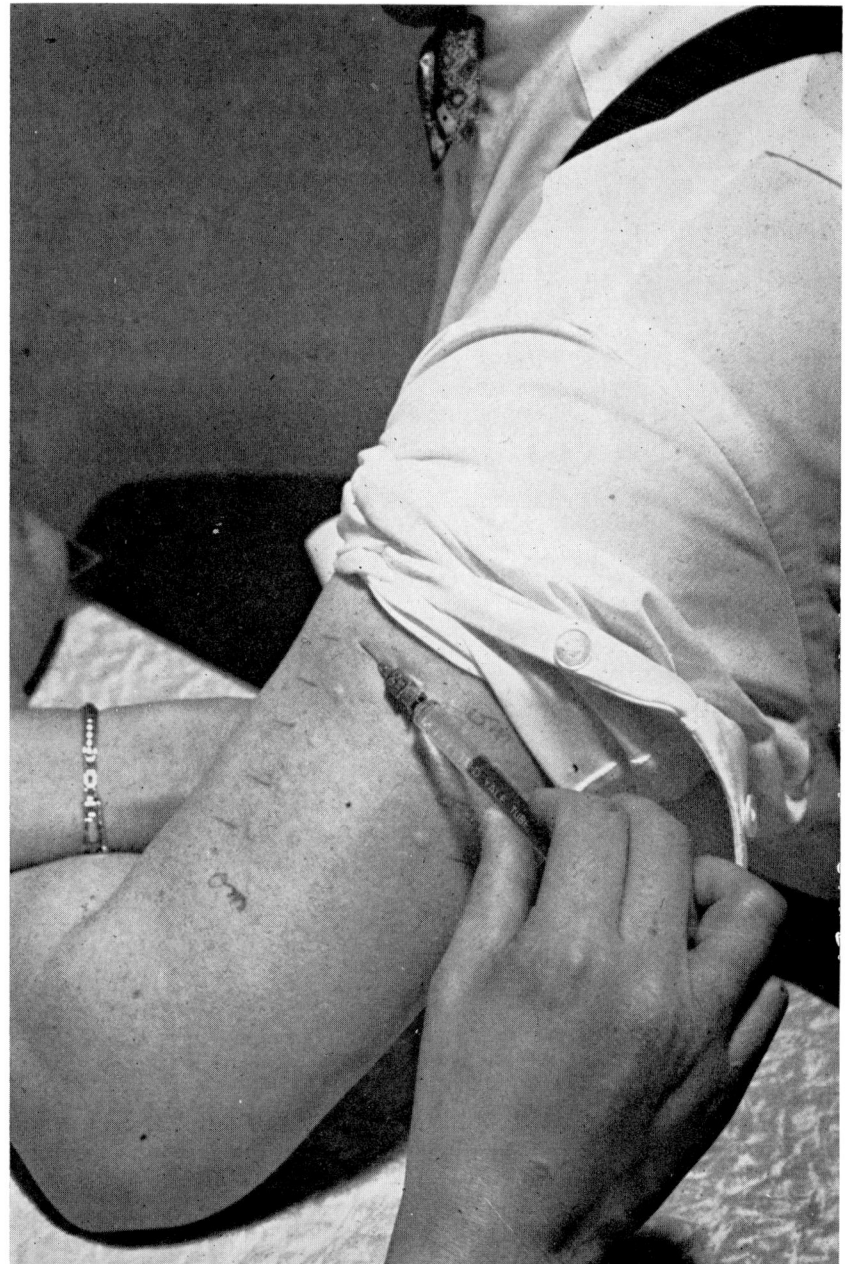

Figure 17-4. Illustrates position of needle on the arm and position of syringe in the hand.

tween the thumb and the fingers, so that the thumb and index finger grasp the barrel firmly about 2 to 3 cm above the hilt of the needle. This position will permit the syringe to be rolled freely between the thumb and the index finger. Extend the little finger so that it hooks firmly about the end of the plunger. This can only be accomplished with a partially filled syringe, not more than 0.3 cc of fluid in the syringe.

(7) From the stock vial, draw up between 0.2 to 0.3 ml of testing material into the syringe.

(8) Hold the syringe in a vertical position, with the needle upright to permit any air to rise to the top.

With the syringe in a vertical position, expel all the air from both the syringe and the needle. This step is very important. The introduction of air causes a splattering of tissue which causes a false reaction.

(9) Choose the skin site for the test. With the syringe at a 45° angle to the arm, place the point of the needle at the chosen site with the bevel of the needle facing *upward*.

(10) Very gently introduce the needle point and with a slight lifting motion as though attempting to pick up the skin, introduce the needle point.

(11) As the tip of the needle engages and enters the skin, the syringe is rotated 180° which locks the bevel against the skin, preventing leakage.

(12) After the syringe has been rotated 180°, gentle pressure is exerted upon the plunger with the little finger which introduces the test antigen. Only sufficient testing solution to produce a tiny, just perceptible wheal is injected—never in excess of 0.025 ml per test.

(13) Ten (10) individual tests and one control can be applied to each arm as indicated in Fig. 17-5. Always place 1 through 10 on the right arm and 11 through 20 on the left arm.

Controls are placed on each arm above and between the groups of tests. The same diluting fluid used for preparing dilutions of extracts serves as the control.

Tests should be spaced a minimum of 1.5 to 2.0 cm to avoid coalescing and interaction.

(14) Tests are read after twenty minutes. Wiping the tests with a moist sponge and permitting the light to cross the test tangentially from the side of the arm, in front of the observer, will frequently aid in delineating the outline of the reaction. This is especially helpful with pigmented skins.

When the above technique is mastered,

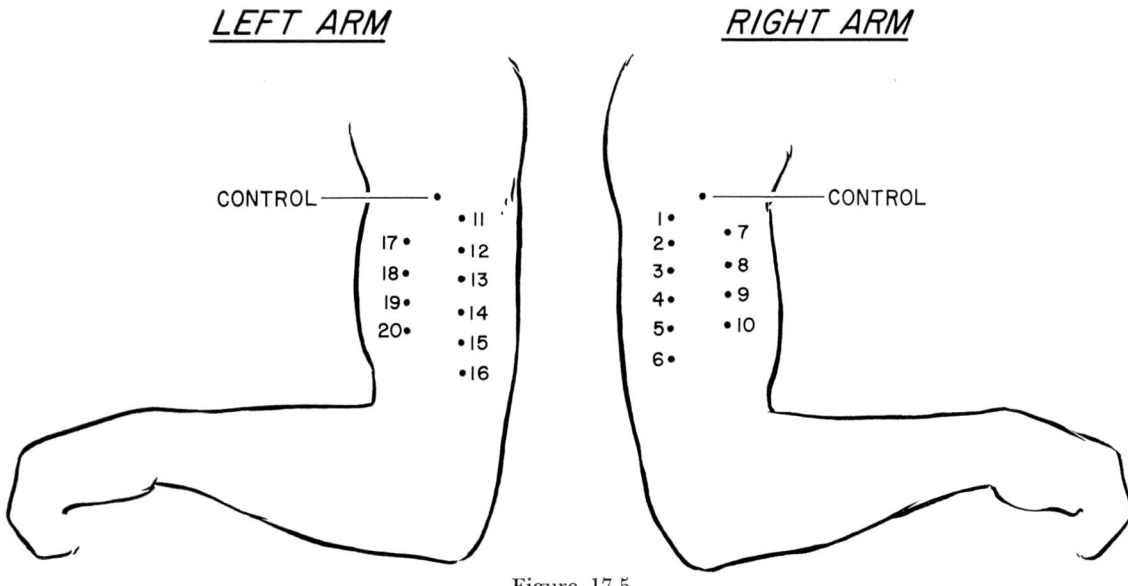

Figure 17-5.

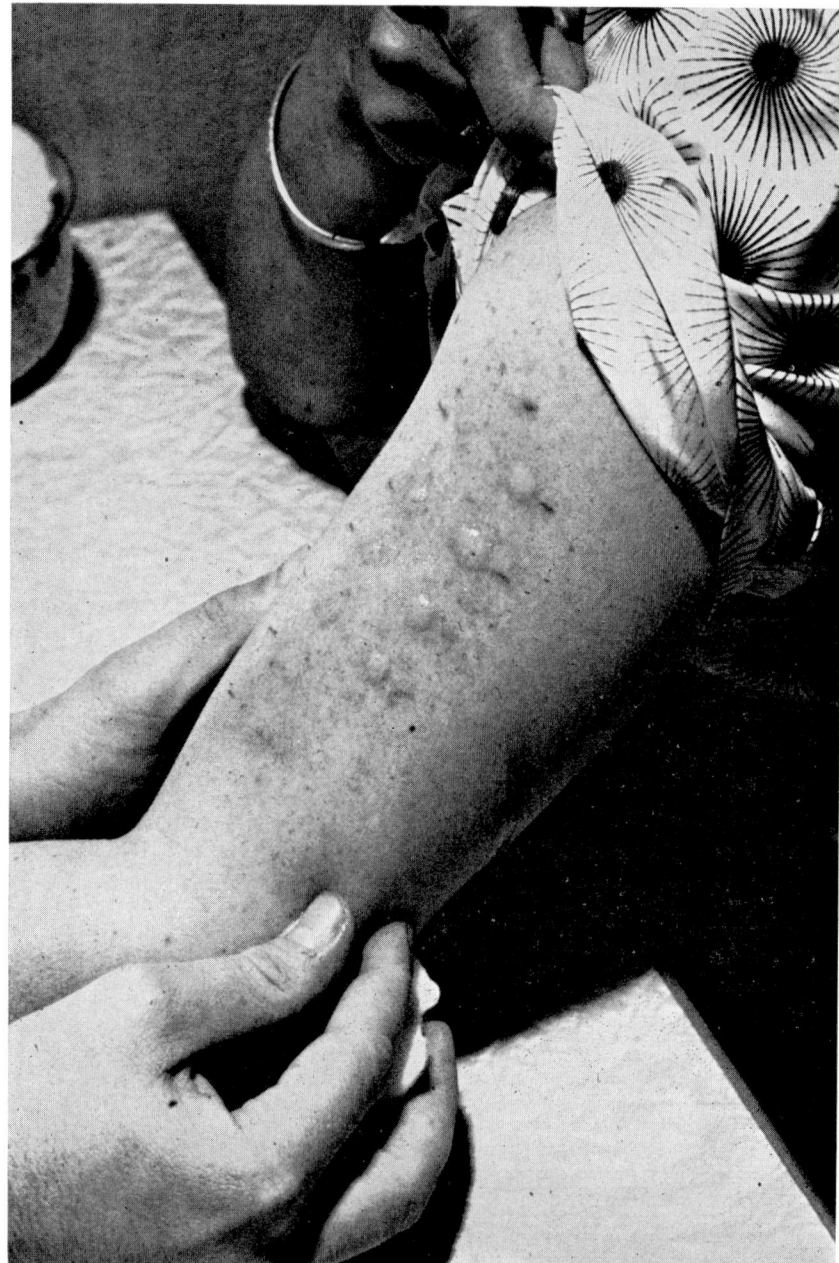

Figure 17-6. Whealing reactions following intradermal testing.

it not only permits speed of performance but also uniformity in the size of the tests as they are applied, with absence of discomfort to the patient. A properly performed intradermal test causes almost no discomfort to the patient. This is supported by the behavior of very young children when tested by this technique.

Indications for Skin Testing

Any diagnosis of allergic disease is an indication for skin testing except drug allergy and auto-allergic disease.

Choice of Allergens for Skin Testing

It has been pointed out that the allergic

constitution is inherited which means that an individual who only complains of intermittent or seasonal symptoms is actually allergic twelve months of the year. In many cases the symptoms between acute episodes may be very mild and not annoying to the patient. Careful study is usually required to detect the smoldering condition and elicit the mild symptoms. Since environmental factors are the most frequent cause of perennial allergic disease, practically every patient who manifests skin reactivity on testing will react to environmental factors. Patients with seasonal allergic symptoms who react to pollens rarely fail to show reactions to environmental factors. The converse is not observed as frequently; patients who react to environmentals very frequently fail to manifest reactivity on testing to pollens. This observation becomes very apparent in regions where pollens are present in the atmosphere for ten to eleven months of the year as occurs in California.

A similar observation is applicable to patients sensitive to foods. An individual who is allergic to foods usually manifests inhalant allergy and most frequently reactivity and sensitivity to environmental factors. Without inhalant sensitivity, a diagnosis of food allergy should be made with great caution. The patient may complain of food intolerance, but it may not necessarily be an allergic response.

Skin reactivity on testing does not always indicate that the allergen is an offender. Skin tests for pollens are very reliable in their correlation with patient's history, but food tests are very unreliable. A positive test for an environmental factor when the item is present in the patient's environment is strong support that the test indicates an offender. When the patient's history suggests either pollens or foods as causative factors, the likelihood of environmental factors as additional offending allergens is frequently overlooked. The recognition that environmental factors are important in practically every patient with *inhalant* allergic disease is very important in successful management.

On the basis of these observations, testing with environmental factors is recommended as a routine procedure for every allergic patient for whom skin testing is recommended.

The environmental factors for routine testing should include:

Feathers:
| chicken | goose |
| duck | turkey |

Animal Danders:
cat	hog
cattle	horse
dog	rabbit
goat	wool

Vegetable Fibers:
cotton	hemp
cocoanut fiber	jute
kapok	

House Dust.

Choice of pollens is discussed in Chapter 16 on pollens.

For the indications for food testing, refer to the discussion on food allergy in Chapter 8.

Choice of the Technique for Testing

Every allergy skin testing program should provide not only reliable data for the patient's management but must incorporate safeguards to prevent untoward reactions. Reliable results on skin testing depend upon the use of active allergenic extracts, which if handled improperly can be hazardous to the patient, even endangering his life. The fear of untoward reactions has undoubtedly discouraged many physicians from performing allergy skin tests. However, with a well designed testing program, the physician can obtain the data necessary for the patient's management with a high degree of safety.

The following precautions should be observed:

(1) *Do not test* by any technique if the

history is positive for highly allergenic substances, such as:

- egg white — cottonseed
- cat — shellfish
- horse — fish
- castor bean — nuts

Before testing for any of the above items, the patient must be questioned carefully to determine whether there is a history of sensitivity to them. It is *not recommended* that the history be confirmed by testing for these items.

(2) Never perform intradermal testing without preliminary screening with either the scratch or prick techniques, but preferably the prick technique. Preliminary screening will establish the patient's pattern of reactivity and determine which routine to follow for subsequent testing.

(3) Do *not* test a patient during an acute attack of hay fever, asthma, urticaria or angio-edema.

(4) Do not test during the pollinating season any patient with hay fever or asthma due to pollen sensitivity.

(5) Do not test on the *back* without preliminary screening on the arm or forearm.

(6) Do not test with bacterial extracts or vaccines which are liable to provoke constitutional reactions.

(7) Do not test patients with auto-allergic disease.

(8) Exercise great caution in testing with sera (see serum disease).

(9) Do not test for penicillin sensitivity.

The Skin Test Reaction

The response of the skin to any test antigen is governed by the type of immunologic reaction involved. Atopic allergic disease is caused by the immediate type of hypersensitivity which in skin testing is characterized by the wheal and flare reaction. The wheal is a manifestation of edema secondary to increased permeability, resulting from the interaction of IgE antibody with its specific allergen. The flare is a manifestation of capillary dilatation. In a very active test response the wheal extends its borders by pseudopodia.

The Concentration of the Test Antigen for Scratch and Prick Techniques

When acetone precipitated extracts are used, 1/50 w/v, 50 per cent glycerolated are recommended. All other types of extracts require 1/10 w/v, perferably 50 per cent glycerolated. If higher dilutions must be used to avoid nonspecific reactions, the reliability of the extract should be questioned.

For intradermal tests a 1:1000 w/v dilution in normal saline is recommended.

To prepare 1:1000 w/v from 1:50 stock, add 0.25 ml of 1:50 dilution to a vial containing 4.75 ml of normal saline with 0.5 per cent phenol for preservative.

To prepare 1:000 w/v from 1:10 stock, (a) add 0.5 ml of 1:10 to 4.5 ml of diluent (1-100); (b) add 0.5 ml of 1:100 to 4.5 ml of diluent (1-1000).

The Control Test

The same diluent used in preparing the test extract is used for performing the control. When 50 per cent glycerol is used for preparing the basic extract, the amount of glycerol introduced by either the prick or scratch test is not sufficient to influence the reaction.

When performed properly, after twenty minutes the control should be entirely negative or manifest minimal redness at the point of penetration of the skin. With the scratch test redness may be more pronounced because of the greater degree of trauma.

Dermatographia: In patients with dermatographia, whealing may be present at the control site as well as at each test site. In order to determine the degree of dermatographia, stroke the skin of the patient's back with a tongue blade or any blunt instrument. When dermatographia is present, whealing without pseudopods will appear almost immediately. The degree of the whealing serves as an index in evaluating the control and the tests. With slight or moderate dermatographia the test reactions can be discounted to allow for the degree of response at the control and each test site. In other words, if the control shows 5 to 10 mm whealing, the *test site* should be at least twice the size of the control to be considered positive. With the presence of pseudopods, the test is usually considered positive. With marked dermatographia reliable skin testing cannot be performed.

In the absence of dermatographia, a strong reaction at the control site signifies a nonspecific reaction.

Rating the Test Reaction

The immediate skin test reaction is usually rated from 1 to 4 plus (very strong reactions may be rated 4+ or 4++).

A 1+ rating is a barely perceptible whealing with a faint flare. In most cases a 1+ rating is equivocal and of little value.

The 3+ and 4+ ratings are arbitrary separations. A 3+ rating can be considered a reaction with a 10 to 15 mm diameter wheal with a flare of varying size in the presence of an absolutely negative control.

Every whealing reaction with definite pseudopods can be rated 4+ or greater depending upon the size.

The numerical rating is actually an arbitrary standard, as there are no specific criteria for evaluating the degree of reactivity. The indices for rating a test reaction are usually influenced by the personal interpretation of the observer, and although the assessment may vary slightly with each *individual* doing the reading, in most instances the positive reaction will be recognized. With experience, each observer establishes his own guideline for evaluating a test reaction. In clinics with standardized testing procedures, the ratings may differ slightly with each observer, as to the degree of reactivity, but there is usually general agreement as to what is positive and what is negative.

In rating skin test reactions there are a number of factors which every observer should consider:

(1) The region of the body is a determining factor in the degree of the response. Tests performed on the back are usually larger than tests performed on either the arm, forearm or thigh.

Tests performed on the arm and thigh are larger than tests performed on the forearm or leg.

Tests which are negative on the arm are frequently positive on the back.

The progression of testing on the forearm to the arm to the back will be discussed under clinical procedures.

(2) The age of the patient. In very young children, usually one year to two years of age, but at times even three years of age, only a flare without whealing represents a positive skin reaction. At the other extreme is the aged individual, in the sixth decade and beyond who responds to testing only with whealing, usually with no pseudopods and without a flare. This disparity corresponds to the differences in the histological structure of the skin at the two extremes of age. Between the two extremes the tests have the classical characteristics of the flare and wheal.

(3) The texture of the skin is important. The delicate skins of the young and some females show a greater tendency to flaring. Very thin skins offer difficulty in introducing the test material without traumatizing the skin and inducing bleeding. Both factors can interfere with development of a positive response.

(4) Naturally pigmented skins do not react as strongly as fair skinned individuals. Skins that are suntanned or thickened from exposure to the elements are usually poor reactors.

(5) The inherent difference in the antigenicity of different materials must be considered in the relative evaluation of skin test reactions. For example, cat is perhaps the most active of all the environmental antigens. An individual may react very strongly

to cat and exhibit only moderate reactions to the remaining epidermal factors, yet these factors may be of equal clinical importance even with their lesser reactivity. There are other highly antigenic substances which include egg white, buckwheat, flaxseed, cottonseed, fish, shellfish and nuts. Chocolate is frequently mentioned as a highly antigenic substance, but it enjoys a reputation it does not deserve (see Food Allergy in Chapter 8).

Variations in antigenicity are observed among pollens (see pollens in Chapter 16).

(6) Each patient has a characteristic reaction pattern which is governed by the titer of IgE antibody and the various nonimmunologic factors indicated above.

The patient's pattern of reactivity cannot be determined from a single test reaction or even a few tests, but must be established by his response to an entire group of allergens, such as all the environmental factors, approximately twenty in number, or to all the pollens indigenous to the environment of the patient. A patient's reaction pattern cannot be determined from a single test for house dust to the exclusion of the various environmental factors.

The reaction pattern has great value in relating the test results to the clinical picture. A patient with very severe symptoms may have a very weak skin test reaction pattern which for this patient is *very* signifcant. A patient with a mild clinical pattern or even no complaints may have a very strong reaction pattern. The reaction pattern serves to grade the importance of each individual allergen as it relates to the patient's complaints.

Clinical Procedures for Testing

The following program will provide the data desired from skin testing and also protect the patient against unwanted reactions.

1. Perform all initial testing on the forearm by the prick technique.

2. If necessary, repeat by intradermal testing on the arm, but omit all prick reactions rated 3 or above.

3. Proceed to testing on the back following screening by the intradermal technique and omitting all intracutaneous arm tests rated 3 or above.

This step by step testing from forearm to back provides (1) a reliable index of the patient's reaction pattern, and (2) offers great protection against unwanted reactions.

Rapidly developing strong reactions with large wheals and pseudopods are observed most frequently in individuals highly sensitive to pollens with a history of seasonal symptoms. These patients will very often have a very strong reaction pattern on prick testing. The environmental factors only occasionally exhibit such an exquisite reaction pattern.

If the skin response develops rapidly, within a few minutes following testing, proceed as follows:

(1) Wipe off the excess antigen at the test site with a well saturated alcohol sponge. This will help arrest the progress of the reaction and control the intense itching.

(2) Administer 0.3 to 0.4 ml of epinephrine-HCl 1-1000 by hypodermic.

(3) Read and record the reaction.

(4) Administer an antihistamine orally.

(5) Observe the patient for about thirty minutes.

Although a tourniquet to the arm is recommended for constitutional reactions following allergy skin tests, the likelihood of such an eventuality is very remote if the history is carefully developed, if the patient is initially screened by prick testing, and if the patient is under surveillance following the testing procedure to observe the rapid development of skin responses. With a negative history the likelihood of a constitutional reaction following a prick test, even with strongly antigenic substances, is quite remote. A constitutional reaction following an intradermal test which has been previously screened by prick test is also very unlikely.

Castor bean extracts should not be used for clinical tests. The extracts frequently produce constitutional reactions *following* prick tests.

Patch Tests

Indications: In the majority of cases of contact dermatitis the offending allergen can usually be identified by a careful, thoroughgoing history. The history is particularly successful in acute reactions, when the onset of the dermatitis can be related to contact with the oleoresin of a plant, a cosmetic, a chemical or local application of a drug. In acute cases symptomatic treatment and avoidance of the contactant will result in complete recovery. In more chronic and indolent reactions a high element of suspicion gathered from the pattern of distribution coupled with a careful analysis of the patient's environment on an hourly and daily basis will usually succeed in identifying the offending agent.

Avoidance of contact with the offending agent usually results in complete restitution of the skin to normal. In every instance, when the offending agent is identified, confirmation by *patch testing* is *not* justified.

Patch testing should be limited to those patients for whom a careful history and the elimination of suspected items have not been successful.

Since an element of risk accompanies all patch testing, the procedure should always be performed with caution. When the diagnosis is obscure and an extensive series is indicated, the tests should be performed by personnel experienced with the procedure.

PROCEDURE: There are two types of patch testing: (1) the "open," (2) the "closed."

(1) The *open patch testing* is performed by placing a highly diluted drop of the suspected material, e.g. plant extract, cosmetic, upon an area of skin one centimeter in diameter.

The "ring" technique utilizes a small metal ring to limit the testing area. The drop of highly diluted test material is placed within the confines of the ring. After the test material dries, the ring is removed and the test area is left uncovered.

(2) The closed patch test
 (a) The test material is placed upon the skin, covered with a small piece of cellophane or similar material and affixed with adhesive tape.

 (b) A 2-inch square plastic bandage or patches made of Dermicel® which contains "acrylic mass" adhesive are used. The suspected material is placed upon the gauze portion of the patch. The test area is kept covered until the test is read, or sooner if the patient experiences untoward symptoms, e.g. itching or burning at the test site. "Closed" patch tests are more sensitive and more likely to elicit reactions to weak allergens than the "open" tests.

The Test Site: The test site should always be normal skin, free of hair and preferably on an exposed part of the body.

When only a few tests are performed, the inner aspect of the upper arm or the upper anterior chest wall near the axillary fold are the preferred sites. It is advisable to place the test so that it can be readily removed by the patient in the event of an early acute reaction.

When a large number of tests are performed, the back is the most suitable area for testing. If great numbers of potential allergens must be considered, the number of patches applied can be reduced by using mixtures of related allergens. (For details of his technique, see Hjorth's studies.)

Evaluation of the Test Reactions

1. Factors which influence the degree of the test response
 (a) the nonspecific irritant quality of the test material
 (b) the allergenicity of the test material
 (c) the length of time the patch is permitted on the skin
 (d) a closed patch is more likely to produce a stronger reaction
 (e) persistent pressure over the test site may lead to a more intense reaction

2. Characteristics of the Test Reaction

Since contact dermatitis is the expression of delayed hypersensitivity, the positive patch test reaction will duplicate all the characteristics of this type of reactivity.

(a) The reaction appears twenty-four hours following application of the test. Any response that appears immediately or any time before twenty-four hours usually indicates a nonspecific irritant which has no diagnostic value.

(b) *Pruritus* is a constant feature of the positive response. In the absence of pruritus any skin reaction at the test site must be challenged for authenticity.

(c) The skin response at the test site is characterized by erythema, edema and vesiculation. A single bullous response is usually indicative of an irritant.

3. Reading the Test

(a) The patches are usually removed after forty-eight hours, but actual reading is delayed for twenty to sixty minutes to permit any nonspecific erythema secondary to pressure to fade. The patient should be instructed to remove immediately (before the forty-eight hour period) any patch that causes severe itching or burning.

(b) True erythema of the positive response persists for hours or even days.

(c) The test areas should be inspected five to seven days after application of the patch test. Delayed reactions are not unusual, even with highly antigenic materials and with very sensitive patients.

(d) The test response is usually graded negative for no reaction and rated 1 to 4 for varying degrees of a positive response. From a practical clinical standpoint grading on a scale of 1 to 4 is of no importance. A patch test is either positive or negative.

The following conditions should always be observed when performing a patch test:

(1) *Never perform a patch test in the presence of acute contact dermatitis.* Even a very small area of patch testing can induce a violent aggravation of an existing dermatitis. Patch testing should be performed when the skin is clear during a period of remission, or at least when the dermatitis is in a subacute stage.

(2) Never use an exposed area of the skin. Never patch test on the face. This is particularly important when testing for cosmetics.

Never patch test over the chest, upper back or thighs of women who may at times expose these areas.

A severe response to a patch test may result in longstanding pigmentation. With *very* acute responses, scarring may result.

(3) The concentration of the test material should be carefully checked. If in doubt concerning the activity of the test material, a preliminary open patch test can be performed. Lists of materials with recommended concentration are available from reliable biological literature. A list of materials with suggested concentrations has been reported by Baer and Witten.

Mucosal Tests

The mucosal tests for hypersensitivity, which include (1) the nasal mucosal test and (2) the ophthalmic test, have been applied in diagnosis for hay fever since the earliest observations on this disease. In 1835 Kirkman, a hay fever sufferer, reproduced his symptoms by sniffing the pollen of sweet vernal grass. Blackley, also a hay fever sufferer, tested himself by both nasal and ophthalmic instillation of pollen and in 1873 made his classic report "Experimental Research on the Cause and Nature of Catarrhus Aestivus."

NASAL TEST: The symptoms of allergic disease can be reproduced by introducing either dry pollen or powdered allergen onto the nasal mucosa. In hay fever subjects the test is best performed during the symptom-free interval, since during the acute stage any irritant applied to the nasal mucosa may induce a nonspecific response. A nonspecific response is also observed in chronic allergic rhinitis, when any irritant applied to the nasal mucosa may induce a reaction. An additional limitation is the restriction of the procedure to a single allergen at one sitting.

THE OPHTHALMIC TEST: This test is performed by introducing into the inner canthus of the eye a small drop of testing extract. A syringe without the attached needle may be used for this purpose.

A positive reaction will appear within one to five minutes with reddening and itching of the caruncle and conjunctiva and often associated with sneezing.

Following a reaction, it is well to instill a drop of highly diluted epinephrine-HCl (1–10,000) to arrest the response, as otherwise the reaction may cause discomfort.

Since the ophthalmic test reaction parallels the intradermal test very closely, its application in routine clinical allergy is not indicated.

III. INJECTION THERAPY

Principles of Immunotherapy

Reaginic allergic disease is the manifestation of the tissue responses induced by the interaction of IgE type antibody with its specific allergen. When an allergen contacts the mucosal surface of either the respiratory or the gastrointestinal tracts, the response is an increased production of IgE type antibody. However, when the identical allergen is administered parenterally by injection, the following immunologic events are observed:

(1) The production of blocking antibody which belongs to the IgG class of immunoglobulins. The blocking antibody has a greater affinity for the allergen than IgE antibody and in this manner prevents the reaginic reaction with allergen which is responsible for the clinical patterns of atopic allergic disease.

(2) The ultimate reduction of the serum titer of reaginic antibody which makes the patient less sensitive.

(3) A decrease *in vitro* of the allergen-induced release of histamine from the patient's leukocytes. Although this behavior of the leukocytes has not been demonstrated *in vivo,* the clinical response of the patient suggests that an identical change in the leukocytes may occur.

The precise relationship between these laboratory parameters and the clinical course of allergic disease is not known. Dumonde suggests that the activity of lymphokines may serve to regulate the immune response by acting as cellular cooperators or regulators of lymphoid cell traffic. For example, the production of IgE antibody following the stimulation of lymphocytes by specific allergen may require the participation of factors which activate lymphocytes. These factors may be generated by allergen-sensitive lymphocytes which produce no antibody. It is also suggested that a migration inhibiting factor (MIF) induced following injection therapy may act *in vivo* as an internal adjuvant for the production of blocking antibodies.

Efficacy

The injection of pollen antigens for treatment was initially proposed by Curtis in 1897, who because of irregular and uncertain results, abandoned the procedure. About the turn of the century Noon revived injection therapy and developed a practical program based upon the subcutaneous injection of timothy extract, the dosage of which was controlled by the ophthalmic test. Noon's studies were interrupted by his untimely death, but the observations were continued by Freeman. Following the reports of Freeman and Noon in 1911, injection therapy received wide acceptance and was expanded to include all types of inhalant allergens, which led to the appearance of many reports on the clinical experiences with this method of therapy.

Today, more than sixty years after the initial reports of Freeman and Noon, injection therapy is accepted as a routine procedure in clinical allergy, applied not only by allergists but by practically all the major specialities, including internal medicine, pediatrics, otolaryngology and dermatology. Yet in spite of the extensive application of injection therapy for more than two generations, questions regarding the efficacy are constantly raised.

Until 1954, when the first controlled clinical studies were reported by Frankland and Augustine and then by Frankland in 1955, the evaluation of injection therapy was based almost entirely upon empiricism. The general attitude of the profession during this period was expressed by Van de Veer, who in 1947 reported in Cooke's text, *Allergy in Theory and Practice*: "With proper care and experience 80 per cent of treated patients should have at least 80 per cent relief from hay fever and nearly half of them will be entirely free. Fifteen per cent will have slight or moderate relief and 5 per cent will have no relief at all. These figures are gathered from reports of many physicians over the entire country and cover many years of experience, so they may be considered reliable." The general experience today of physicians properly trained and experienced with injection therapy supports the position expressed by Van de Veer in 1947.

It is interesting to note that the results of the double blind controlled clinical studies of Frankland and Augustine and of Frankland paralleled very closely the incidence of favorable response reported by Van de Veer for the physicians he surveyed.

In a double blind study in 1965 by Laurel and Franklin, the conclusion was drawn that ragweed pollen extract was not only effective but specific.

Contrary to the experiences of the above investigators was a report in 1966 by Fontana, Holt and Mainland in a double blind study conducted over a five year period on children with ragweed hay fever. Since the methods of evaluation of this study were quite different from those of previous clinical double blind studies comparative conclusions cannot be drawn.

The first attempt to utilize serologic studies to demonstrate efficacy with pollen injection therapy was that of Cooke and Howard in 1931 who, utilizing passive transfer techniques with various serum dilutions were able to titrate the skin sensitizing factor in the patient's serum. By mixing a fixed amount of sensitizing sera with known graduated amounts of antigen, these observers were able to demonstrate the neutralization of the skin sensitizing property of the patient's serum.

Cooke* reported that, using these simple tests to compare the serum of a patient before any treatment with the serum of the same patient after treatment, it was possible to observe if any alteration had occurred as a result of the injection of antigen used in the treatment. From such comparative studies it was apparent that the amount of ragweed pollen antigen needed to neutralize the antibody of the post-treatment serum was out of proportion to the amount of skin sensitizing antibody shown by the dilution test, suggesting the presence of a second immune body in serum, the blocking antibody.

The properties of blocking antibody which were demonstrated by Cooke include (1) stability to heat, (2) specificity for its antigen, (3) ability to combine with the specific antigen *in vitro*, (4) ability to be induced in nonallergic individuals, and (5) the ability to pass the placental barrier. The observations of Cooke have been confirmed by many investigators who in addition have identified blocking antibody as belonging to the IgG class.

In spite of numerous studies the relationship of blocking antibody to clinical improvement has not been established. Some reports indicate a definite relationship while other studies fail to correlate blocking antibody titer with a favorable clinical response. However, the efficiency of blocking antibody has been demonstrated by the administration of globulin preparations containing high titers of blocking antibody which have been produced in nonallergic individuals.

Several groups of investigators (Van Ars-

---

* Cooke, Robert A.: *Allergy in Theory and Practice*. Philadelphia, Saunders, 1947, p. 57.

dale and Middleton; Pruzansky and Patterson; Norman and Lichtenstein) have observed a decrease in the basic activity of target cells (leukocytes and basophils) in response to injection therapy. The decreased activity is manifested by either a diminished release or failure to release histamine, which has no obvious relationship to IgE antibody level. In other words, cell responsiveness may be diminished in the presence of elevated IgE.

Sherman and Connell have observed that continued, perennial injection therapy, over a period of several years can produce a diminution in the skin test response. The author has observed a similar effect following several years of therapy, usually eight to ten years, but occasionally after two to three years. Initially, the strong reactions on prick testing gradually diminish in degree of response until no reaction can be elicited by this technique. The patient continues to react on intradermal testing on the arm. Following several additional years of therapy, this response gradually diminishes until the only skin response elicited is by intradermal testing on the back. With continued therapy all skin tests may become negative. Clinical improvement is observed for a long period before a change in skin reactivity, but once the skin response shows a decrease, the complete abolition of the skin test response occurs rapidly, within a period of a year or two of continued injection therapy. In no case was a decreased response or a complete failure to react observed in a patient who failed to have a satisfactory clinical response.

The significance of each immunologic event in immunotherapy is not yet clearly defined nor is the interrelationship of the various parameters understood. Even in the absence of clear definition of immunologic function, clinicians throughout the world feel that injection therapy is an effective procedure in the greater majority of patients whose allergic condition is accurately diagnosed and carefully managed. Successful management is contingent upon the availability of reliable raw materials, biologically active extracts and experienced supervision of the patient. It is true that some individuals fail to respond to immunotherapy. It is possible that a number of these failures may be due to mechanisms other than reaginic allergy, or if they are the victims of atopic hypersensitivity, the solution of their problem may require a further clarification of the mechanisms involved and an understanding of the interrelationship of various immunologic phenomena.

With the advances in immunology it is foreseeable that new procedures will be developed, perhaps involving the principle of low molecular therapy or even less specific tools, such as utilization of the Fc fraction of the IgE antibody to block the attachment of a complete antigen.

The Clinical Program

Environmental Control

Strict environmental control is an important prerequisite in the management of every allergic patient. The hereditary atopic constitution predisposes the individual to reactions to every potential allergen in his environment. The patient who experiences intermittent symptoms is allergic during the interval between acute episodes, and in like manner the patient with seasonal pollenosis is actually allergic perennially. In view of this basic characteristic of the atopic individual, it is important in management of the patient to evaluate all factors in the environment as well as all inhalants and ingestants.

Recognizing the perennial nature of reaginic allergy, it is interesting to note the following observations:

(1) Most pollen sensitive individuals will also react to environmental factors.

(2) Individuals who react to environmental factors do not always react to pollens. This observation is quite apparent in areas such as California where pollens may be in the atmosphere for ten to eleven months of the year.

(3) Food sensitivity (allergic) is rarely observed without inhalant allergy, either environmentals or pollens, or both.

(4) Most patients with seasonal symptoms will fail to experience a good response to treatment unless the environmental factors are controlled; the same observation applies when patients exhibit an *allergic* sensitivity to foods.

Environmental control should consider every exposure of the patient which includes not only the home, but also the occupational environment of the patient as well as that of other members of the family; the school environment of children and all places visited by the patient, such as the homes of friends and relatives, parks, playgrounds, *etc*.

The commonly encountered environmental factors are listed in Table 17-I.

All articles in the patient's environment that correlate with positive skin reactions should be removed.

Control of the home should not be restricted to the patient's room but must be comprehensive and include all areas of the home including the basement and garage. Limiting environmental control to the bedroom or one room occupied by the patient offers a sense of false security. Dust generated in one room can be carried to all parts of the home by convection of air currents, via hot air heating ducts or inefficient air conditioning systems.

Following the removal of offending environmental items, such as feathers, carpet pads, pets, *etc*., it is advisable to thoroughly clean the ducts of hot air heating systems. Filters used in heating systems are usually ineffective in eliminating allergenic dusts which are too fine to be withheld by the filter. Electronic precipitators are frequently helpful in controlling dusts in the home.

Patients do not confine themselves strictly to one room of the house. This is particularly true of children who will often visit the parents' bed with either down or feather items of bedding, or play on the carpeted floor of an uncontrolled area of the house. Carpeted floors with felt paddings provide a rich source of highly allergenic materials derived from jute and animals hairs, usually cattle hair. The dust generated from carpet pads seeps through the carpeting and contrary to common belief, this dust is not contained by wall-to-wall carpeting.

Children attending kindergarten are frequently exposed to the dander of pet animals and the feather pillows on the cots used for napping.

Since occupational environments vary widely, each situation must be analyzed individually.

The emotional attachment to animals presents one of the most difficult problems in programming environmental control. It is difficult for patients to accept that an animal that has been in the environment for years can be the determining factor in the successful control of the patient's symptoms. Parents are frequently fearful that separation from a pet dog or cat will cause an emotional upheaval in the child, but do not recognize that failure to control the child's allergic symptoms can serve as an even greater potential for causing emotional disturbances.

The failure to exercise environmental control is one of the most frequently encountered reasons for the failure of immunotherapy in the treatment of allergic disease. The immunologic interaction between persistent environmental factors and the administration of allergens is supported by the observations of Connell who demonstrated the triggering mechanism of allergens. By applying a measured quantity of a known pollen to the nasal mucosa of a specifically sensitive individual, Connell was able, through repeated challenges to decrease the quantity of pollen required to induce a response. If the challenge was limited to one side of the nose, only the side that was challenged manifested this variation in response. This decreased tolerance or increased sensitivity, whichever the preference in labelling it, is not specific. In other words, a ragweed pollen will decrease the tolerance for other pollens, or a pollen allergen will decrease the tolerance for dusts or environmental allergens. This important observation strengthens the concept that failure to control the environment in a pollen-sensitive individual decreases the patient's tolerance for pollens and accordingly influences the success of the response to therapy. When the environment is not controlled, local and constitutional reactions following injections are more frequent, increased doses of antigen are not tolerated, and not infrequently symptoms are aggravated rather than improved with the administration of antigens.

The Injection Procedure

In the absence of controlled studies to serve as guidelines, the programs for injection therapy as practiced in clinical allergy have developed empirically which explains the lack of a single standard procedure. Programs vary with the experience of the clinician which accounts for the variety of routines reported in the literature.

The following program has been developed over the past twenty years in the Allergy Department of the KFH-PMG.

The primary objective of every allergy treatment program is the control of the patient's symptoms, but in addition, this program was designed to permit, to the fullest extent possible, the utilization of paramedical personnel. To achieve this objective, the injection routine incorporates numerous safeguards to (1) avoid administering the wrong mixture to the patient, and (2) to prevent adverse responses and particularly constitutional reactions. The paramedical personnel who administer the injections are never permitted to deviate from the established routine without authorization from a physician who is always present within a few feet from the patient.

The program gives consideration to the following basic elements of injection therapy:

(1) The formulation of the treatment extract.

(2) The technique for administering antigens.

(3) The dosage schedule for treatment extracts.

(4) The interval between injections.

(5) The indications for perennial, pre-seasonal and co-seasonal treatment.

(6) The duration of the treatment program.

(7) Reactions—local and constitutional, immediate and delayed.

1. The Formulation of Treatment Antigens

Only environmental (see list of environmental factors in Table 17-I) and pollen extracts are used for injection therapy.

No mold extracts are used for treatment under this program (see discussion on molds in this chapter). The response to therapy with mold extracts is generally considered less satisfactory than with other aeroallergens.

The response to bacterial vaccines* has been very unfavorable and perhaps not without hazard.

Environmental extracts and pollen extracts are never combined in the same mixture.

Each mixture is usually limited to eight extracts but never more than ten extracts. An excessive number of extracts in one mixture results in dilution, which reduces the effectiveness of the antigen. An increased number of allergens in the mixture, because of dilution, necessitates the administration of larger volumes of antigen to be effective. Large volumes of antigen, greater than 0.5 ml, predispose to local reactions. Larger volumes of extract contain an increased quantity of preservative, either glycerol or phenol 0.4 per cent, which also predisposes to local reactions and local discomfort following the injection.

---

* A recent regulation of the Division of Biologics Standards of N.I.H. has stopped the distribution of bacterial vaccines for injection therapy because of the failure to demonstrate efficacy.

Table 17-I: CHECKLIST OF SIGNIFICANT FACTORS CAUSING YOUR ALLERGIC SYMPTOMS

Avoid Items Checked:	Where Found
Grass Pollens	
Weed Pollens	
Tree Pollens	
Cotton Linters	Not the same fibers used in cotton cloth. Linters are used in cotton wadding or batting to make pads, cushions, comforters, mattresses, upholstery and some varnishes.
Feathers & Down	Pillows, down cushions, couches, and other upholstered articles, birds, sleeping bags.
Cocoanut Fiber	Tropical furniture, doormats, gymnasium mats, mattresses, box springs.
Cat Hair	Cats, toy animals, "imitation" furs, some fur caps, ear muffs, slippers, gloves.
Cattle Hair	Rugs, rug pads, blankets, carpet padding.
Dog Hair	Dogs—all dogs produce dander.
Goat Hair	Mohair, angora, cashmere, alpaca.
Hog Hair	Rug and carpet pads, hair brushes, furniture stuffing, mattresses, auto cushions.
Horse Hair	Horses, carpet padding, some blankets, some antique furniture.
Rabbit Hair	Fur coats, trimmings sold under trade name Coney® or Lapin,® toy animals, fabrics, some felts.
Hemp	Rope, carpet pads, used as sisal in mattresses and box springs, rugs.
Kapok	Kapok is a plant fiber used in cushions, mattresses, sleeping bags, pillows, upholstery.
Wool	Raw wool and coarse woolens of all kinds should be avoided. Avoid wool blankets and knitting with wool yarn.
Flaxseed	Some cereals, laxatives, wave sets, paints, varnishes, linseed oil, furniture stuffings.
Jute	Carpet pads, carpet backing, burlap, gunny sacks, crocus cloth, "Polynesian" articles such as grass skirts, handbags, place mats, cushions.
House Dust	A mixture of all the above agents. In addition, it in itself has factors that cause allergy. Control of the above factors in part controls the potency of house dust.
Orris Root	All ladies' and men's cosmetics, talcum, dusting powder, perfume, deodorants, gin factories, bakeries, toothpaste and powders.
Pyrethrum	Insect sprays (almost all—check label).
Vegetable Gums Acacia Gum	Mucilage, bakery products.
Karaya Gum	In denture adhesive—check labels; also in cream cheeses.
Tragacanth Gum	Confections, gum drops, pastries and pies.
Molds (Fungi & Mildew)	Dark, damp, cool places as shower stalls, bathrooms, cabinet under sinks, refrigerators, basement, windows, eaves of houses; also in the air and in cheeses. Check around for musty (mildew) odors. Clean thoroughly and spray repeatedly with Lysol.®

The environmental mixture should contain the items to which the patient shows positive skin reactions which correlate with the history of symptoms caused by the allergen or a history of the allergen present in the environment at the time of the initial interview. For example: a history that reveals the presence of hairy pets (dogs,† cats), feather or down pillows, upholstered furniture with down, felt carpet pads, *etc.* is an indication for including the respective allergens in the mixture. The patient should not receive injections with an allergen unless the offending factor(s) has been removed from the environment.

Treating with environmental antigens in the presence of these items in the environment is comparable to pollen injection therapy during the pollinating season. It is usually unsatisfactory and leads to reactions or aggravation of symptoms. Without strict environmental control, it is to the patient's advantage to receive no injection therapy.

Dust extract should always be included in the environmental mixture. At times, if justified by the history, more than one sample of dust extract may be included, as, for example, an extract to cover the average home environment, and a special dust extract for occupational situations.

Dusts that require high dilutions in order to avoid a skin test response in all individuals are not recommended. Such skin responses are usually nonspecific and can be demonstrated in all individuals tested unless the extract is reduced to very high dilutions.

Dust extracts are not a substitute for each environmental factor, but rather an adjunct. Extract mixtures which include the individual environmental factors are more effective.

This concept is supported by the observation of Berg and Johansson who report that different types of allergens might be more or less potent in their ability to stimulate IgE production. Thus dust and mold allergens

---

† Dogs—The belief that hairless dogs are not allergenic is a myth. It is the dander and not the hair that is allergenic. There is no difference among species of dogs.

have been regarded as weak allergens by these allergists, whereas common animal danders and pollen allergens have been regarded as strong allergens. In a study by Berg and Johansson* of children with asthma, it was found that eleven children with positive skin and provocation tests for dust and/or mold had a mean IgE level of only 104 per cent of the mean for their age compared to 338 per cent for forty-two children allergic to other common allergens.

PREPARATION OF EXTRACT MIXTURES:

Basic extract 1–50 w/v of 50 per cent glycerolated extract.
Add 0.5 ml of each ingredient.
With 8 items, the final volume will be 4.0 cc.
With 10 items, the final volume will be 5.0 cc.

Remove 0.5 ml for preparing higher dilulutions, 1–500 w/v and above. This will leave either 3.5 ml or 4.5 ml of basic extract, 50 per cent glycerolated 1–50 w/v, which when kept under refrigeration will retain its potency for at least two to three years. This assures the patient of a uniform supply of antigen for several years Higher dilutions are less stable. Very high dilutions, 1–5,000,000,000 or 1–500,000,000 w/v, if not refrigerated will lose their activity within a matter of days. Under refrigeration, activity is preserved for several weeks.

Higher dilutions are prepared by adding 0.5 ml of the preceding dilution to a 4.5 ml vial of diluting fluid. For example, 0.5 ml of 1–500 w/v to 4.5 ml of dilution fluid produces a 1–5,000 w/v dilution.

Color coding the cap of the vial and the label of each dilution serves as an added protection against using an improper concentration.

A program that provides an individual antigen mixture for each patient offers several advantages. It assures the patient of a uniform supply of extract. With the procedures presently applied in the manufacture of commercial extracts, it is almost impossible to duplicate precisely the composition of an allergenic extract from one lot to another. Johansson, et al.,* have reported that the characterization of a number of commerically available pollen and epidermal allergens using the radio-allergo-sorbant test (RAST) † reveals both qualitative and quantitative differences between different products as well as batches of one and the same allergen. PNU determinations and Noon units are not reliable indications of biological activity. At the present time the standardization of extracts on a weight by volume w/v basis is the most satisfactory procedure.

The basic supply of extract for each patient which can be stored under refrigeration for several years (a) permits a more precise regulation of the dose administered, (b) permits a more exact evaluation of the patient's response to the specific therapy, (c) reduces the incidence of untoward reactions to injections, and (d) permits labelling the vials with the patient's name. When the patient's treatment dose is derived from different lots of extract, all the advantages indicated are lost.

---

* Johansson, S.G.O., Bennich, H., Berg, T. and Forecord, T.: *Adv Immunol. 13:* 48, 1971.

† Radio-allergo-sorbant Test (RAST)

(1) Antigen (allergen) is conjugated to a suitable sorbent, e.g. Sephadex® particles.

(2) The conjugated material is incubated with the patient's serum. Allergen will combine with its specific reaginic antibody if present in the serum.

(3) Anti-IgE sera are produced in sheep or rabbits labelled with radioactive iodine.

(4) Patient's allergen-serum complex (item #2) + radioactive IgE serum (item #3) ⟶ radioactive complex.

(5) Components of serum not combined with allergen are washed out.

(6) Specific reaction is determined quantitatively by means of scintillator counter.

The test is not fully developed for clinical application. The lack of immunologically pure antigens detracts from clinical efficacy. Reference: Bennich, H. and Johansson, S.G.O.: Structure and biological function of human IgE. *Adv Immunol, 13,* 1971.

---

* Berg, T. and Johansson. S.G.O., *Acta Paediatr Scand,* 58: 513, 1969. Bennich, Hans and Johansson, S.G.O. Structure and function of human immunoglobulin E. *Adv Immunol, 13,* 1971.

The preparation of separate mixtures for each type of antigen permits a more exact regulation of the dosage. Patients who are exquisitely sensitive to pollens, as is frequently observed with marked seasonal symptoms, require a considerably higher dilution for the initial injection of the pollen extract than the environmental extract. For example, it is not uncommon to observe a patient who at the initial injection will tolerate a starting dose of the environmental antigen of 0.05 ml of 1–5,000,000 w/v, while the same patient will require a starting dose of 0.05 ml of 1–5,000,000,000 w/v of a pollen antigen.

A program providing individual environmental and pollen antigens is well suited for treating patient groups of moderate size—three hundred daily visits or less. When confronted with very large numbers of patients, five hundred to one thousand patient visits per day, the program presents the problem of adequate refrigeration space for the various formulae. To meet this situation a compromise can be adopted by preparing individual environmental mixtures for each patient and stock mixtures for pollens. This is not the ideal situation, but for the treatment of large groups of patients, such an arrangement is feasible. If pollens are collected properly, stored under controlled conditions and processed by a standard technique, an extract can be prepared which will be reasonably similar in activity but not identical. Because of the great variation in the raw material used in the preparation of environmental extracts, the duplication of extracts is quite unreliable. They may all have biological activity but of varying degree and varying specificity.

2. The Injection Technique

For the injection of allergenic extracts tuberculin type syringes, 1 ml capacity with 26 gauge, one-half inch hypodermic needle, are recommended.

Although the hypodermic injection of antigens is a simple procedure, if improperly administered it can be a determining factor in producing either local or constitutional reactions.

The top of the vial should be wiped with an alcohol sponge.

The required amount of extract is drawn into the syringe.

Before proceeding with the injection, the air is expelled from the syringe by holding the needle upright and forcing a small amount of extract into the needle. If the syringe has a faulty plunger, it should be discarded for an efficiently operating syringe.

With the finger of the right hand (reverse the procedure for left handed individuals) grasp the syringe at the end so that the thumb rests upon the plunger. The syringe is held as though grasping a dart. With the left hand, the patient's arm is held firmly with the fingers positioned posteriorly and the thumb anteriorly. The arm should be elevated so that it is almost at a right angle to the shoulder. This position relaxes the arm and diminishes resistance to the needle from muscle contraction. The needle is positioned at an angle of 45 degrees or slightly less over the upper one third of the outer aspect of the arm, just below the apex of the deltoid. Grasping the arm firmly prevents movement of the arm which diminishes excessive tissue trauma and also avoids the risk of breaking the needle.

With a very rapid action of the plunger, the extract is injected subcutaneously. As the needle is removed, the thumb which occupies a position on the anterior surface of the arm, immediately exerts pressure upon the puncture point. This prevents escape of extract through the puncture and immediately controls any punctate hemorrhage.

The injection should be performed rapidly to avoid unnecessary wriggling of the tip of the needle. Excessive motion of the needle tip may cause undue tissue trauma which can produce hemorrhage at the site which in turn may predispose to local reactions and at times even constitutional reactions because of too rapid absorption of the antigen. Intramuscular injections of the antigen may also lead to too rapid absorption which may lead to reactions. By elevating the arm and with proper angulation of the needle, intramuscular injections can be avoided. Special precautions must be observed with children and individuals with a thin subcutaneous layer, to avoid intramuscular injections.

3. The Dosage Schedule for Injections

THE INITIAL INJECTION: Since exact methods for designating the biological activity of allergenic extracts are lacking, it is not possible to standardize the degree of a patient's reactivity or tolerance for an antigenic mixture on the basis of a mathematical formula. However, tolerance for a mixture can be gauged by the response of intracutaneous testing with the allergenic mixture. This procedure is labelled the "dilution test."

The technique involves the injection of 0.025 ml of the extract to be tested in the same manner as any intracutaneous test. The diluting vehicle of the extract serves as a control solution.

On dilution testing the manifestation of even a slight flare and wheal response indicates a critical level of tolerance which should be heeded as a warning *not* to exceed the level of concentration and the dose of the test material. It is even advisable to retreat to a higher level of dilution to assure the safety of the patient. A marked flare and wheal with pseudopods indicate unequivocally a level above the tolerance of the patient which demands retreating to at least two lower levels of dilution.

The initial concentration for the *first dilution* test must be determined arbitrarily.

It is known from experience that patients who react strongly, but not exquisitely to intradermal testing on the arm will tolerate a starting dilution of 1–5,000,000 w/v.

With strong reactions observed on prick testing as occurs commonly with seasonal pollen sensitivity, the starting level is frequently 1–5,000,000,000 w/v.

It is usually safer to start at the higher dilution level. With a negative dilution test the next concentration can be tested. It is not advisable to administer more than two dilution test doses for any mixture at one visit. As many as four or five different mixtures can be tested at one time.

Treatment injections always begin with the first dilution that manifests no response on testing.

The program as outlined permits the clinician to arrive at the *starting concentration* with a high degree of safety and with no fear of hazardous constitutional reactions.

A dilution test is performed with each extract mixture to determine the starting level. The starting level may not be the same for all the extracts required for the patient's treatment.

Patients with perennial symptoms and no pollen sensitivity require only one antigen—an environmental mixture.

Patients with pollen sensitivity will require pollen mixtures that will be determined by the history of symptoms and their reactivity.

In some sections of the country, as the Midwest and eastern states, the pollen seasons are more limited than in the western regions such as California where pollens are present in the atmosphere eleven months of the year. In the East and Midwest the spring grasses and trees and the fall weeds will usually cover the patient's needs. In areas such as California it is usually necessary to provide mixtures covering the spring (grasses and trees, late spring (grasses), and fall (weeds). In every patient the type and number of the mixtures required are governed by the history and skin reactions. (See Chapter 16 on pollens.)

A program providing multiple extract mixtures permits greater flexibility in treatment. An intolerance to one group of antigens at a given level can be identified and does not require restricting the progression in dosage of the remaining mixtures. The dosage of each mixture is entirely independent of that of the other mixtures in the treatment program.

Following the determination of the nonreactivity or tolerance level for each antigen mixture ordered for the patient, treatment progresses according to the schedule listed in Table 17-II.

If during the course of treatment, the patient experiences a local reaction to any antigen mixture, the dose is reduced one dilution. If a reaction still occurs, the patient is dilution tested to determine his level of tolerance. The dilution test is always ordered by the physician who on the basis of the patient's history, reactivity pattern on testing and treatment prescribes the level for the dilution test.

In evaluating the patient's tolerance to an antigenic mixture, consideration must be given to factors which influence the clinical response such as failure to control the environment, infection, puberty, menses, preg-

Table 17-II

NAME_____

DATE_____

INSTRUCTIONS: Give pollen antigens at 3–5 day interval until dosage of 1–500 is reached, and then give at 5–7 day intervals. Give epidermal antigen at 5–7 day interval only.

FOLLOW THIS SCHEDULE OF INCREASING DOSAGES

W/V
1—5,000,000,000
  0.05cc
  0.1
  0.2
  0.3
  0.4
1—500,000,000
  0.05cc
  0.1
  0.2
  0.3
  0.4
1—50,000,000
  0.05cc
  0.1
  0.2
  0.3
  0.4
1—5,000,000
  0.05cc
  0.1
  0.2
  0.3
  0.4
1—500,000
  0.05cc
  0.1
  0.2
  0.3
  0.4
1—50,000
  0.05cc
  0.1
  0.2
  0.3
  0.4
1—5,000
  0.05cc
  0.1
  0.2
  0.3
  0.4
ONCE A WEEK
1—500
  0.025cc
  0.05
  0.1
  0.15
  0.2
  0.25
  0.3
  0.35
  0.4
1:50
  0.025
MAINTAIN

Antigen:_____Arm			Antigen:_____Arm			Antigen:_____Arm		
Date	Dose	Dilution	Date	Dose	Dilution	Date	Dose	Dilution
BEGIN WITH:			BEGIN WITH:			BEGIN WITH:		

nancy and changes in the life style of the patient.

An uncontrolled environment in a patient sensitive to environmental factors will interfere with the patient's tolerance to antigen and be manifested as reactions following injections.

Infection influences the clinical pattern of allergy (see infection and allergy in Chapter 4).

Puberty, menses and pregnancy may influence the clinical pattern in either direction, i.e. either an improvement or an aggravation of symptoms. When symptoms are aggravated, tolerance is decreased which will be manifested as a reaction when antigen is administered. Injections are not contraindicated during pregnancy. They are usually tolerated very well, but the patient must be managed very carefully to avoid reactions.

A change in the patient's living habits, his residence, his occupation and changes in diet contribute new allergenic factors that exacerbate the degree of reactivity which is manifested by reactions. These must be evaluated in determining the patient's tolerance when reactions are experienced following injection.

With constitutional reactions the level for resuming treatment is never determined arbitrarily but always by a dilution test. The patient is reviewed by a physician to determine if possible the reason for the constitutional reaction (see constitutional reactions below).

Following the dilution test, when a new level of tolerance has been determined, injections are resumed and the dose increased according to the normal schedule. If the patient again manifests reactions, and it may occur at the same level as previously experienced, the injection dose is decreased and maintained at the nonreactive level. Following several weeks of injection at a maintenance level, the tolerance of the patient may increase and permit progression in dosage in accordance with the regular schedule.

Not infrequently patients are observed who do not tolerate a concentration beyond a given level. Any attempt to exceed the level causes reactions. It is important to maintain the treatment injections at the level of tolerance or nonreactivity. It is important that the patient be questioned carefully before each injection to determine his response to the previous injections before proceeding. It is not necessary for the patient to receive the higher or highest concentration in order to experience a good response. A patient who has reactions will do well when maintained at the sub-reaction level, i.e. the dose just below a level that causes a reaction, while any attempt to force higher concentrations of antigen may aggravate his symptoms or even risk inducing a constitutional reaction.

In the treatment schedule indicated in Table 17-II the volume of extract administered in a single injection never exceeds 0.4 ml, but the combined volume of several extracts may be as much as 2.0 ml. Treatment with multiple mixtures permits the administration of smaller volumes which has definite advantages. Smaller volumes because of less pressure upon the tissues are less painful to the patient. They are also not as likely to produce local reactions. Larger volumes have a greater tendency to disrupt the tissues which can lead to hemorrhage, local reactions, and even a higher incidence of constitutional reactions.

Another factor to consider with larger volumes of extract in a single injection is the increased quantity of preservative, either glycerol or phenol. Increased quantities of preservative at one site are more likely to cause discomfort to the patient.

4. The Interval Between Injections

There are no specific guidelines for determining the most desirable interval between injections. The spacing must be arbitrary but based upon experience.

For higher dilutions as indicated in the

schedule, an interval of three to five days is recommended, while at higher concentrations, i.e. less dilute antigens, the interval of five to seven days is advisable.

It is important to observe the intervals as strictly as possible for both effective response and protection of the patient against either local or constitutional reactions. If the injection program has been interrupted for several weeks or more, it is advisable to determine the patient's nonreactivity level by dilution testing.

When the interval between injections is extended beyond the recommended seven days, the risk of reaction is increased greatly and the efficacy of therapy is decreased. This observation is supported by Levine and Chan,* who studied the "Effect of time interval between antigen injections on reagin and IgG titers in low phase immunization in mice." These investigators observed that frequently repeated antigen doses (every week) favored higher IgG titers, whereas less frequent doses (three to four weeks) favored lower reagin titers. Thus, a given dose of antigen resulted in two to four fold or higher IgG antibody titer, if the dose was divided among weekly injections, than if it was given every four weeks. Generally, comparing the one week interval groups with the four week interval groups, IgG antibody titers were four to eight times as high and reagin titers were one-fourth and one-half as high.

Since both a high IgG blocking antibody titer and a low titer of reaginic antibody are advantageous immunologic features, it would seem from clinical studies, immunologic investigation and animal research, that the short interval between injections is not only preferable but a safer procedure.

Notwithstanding the advantages of short interval schedules for injection over long interval injection programs, it is common practice to extend the period beyond seven days and at times even up to three weeks or more. It is also common practice to require the patient to remain under observation for twenty to thirty minutes following the injection, which permits immediate treatment for any evidence of an unfavorable reaction. A period of surveillance may be practical when treating small groups of patients; however, when dealing with large numbers of patients, 150 or more per day, it becomes impractical to require a period of observation which is necessary when the interval is expanded.

With the program outlined, when all the details are observed, i.e. individual mixtures of antigens which can be controlled, a careful injection technique, meticulous attention to local reactions, titration of reactivity by dilution testing, and observance of the recommended intervals between injections, it permits the administration of allergenic extracts with a high degree of safety which does not necessitate having the patients wait for twenty to thirty minutes for observation following injections. Under this program patients are released immediately and the safety of the program is supported by the experience of over twenty years with several million injections with no severe adverse reactions.

5. The Indications for Perennial, Pre-seasonal and Co-seasonal Treatment

Perennial therapy is the procedure of choice. Since most patients are reactive to environmental factors and experience perennial symptoms, it is advisable that treatment should be continued throughout the year. It has been indicated that patients with distinct seasonal complaints experience mild perennial symptoms, so that the seasonal pattern is usually an exacerbation of the perennial pattern. On the basis of this observation, it is advisable that patients with seasonal symptoms due to pollens be treated perennially. In most instances this requires treatment with both environmental and pollen extracts.

---

* Levine, B.B. and Chan, H., Jr.: Effect of time interval between antigen injections on reagin and IgG antibody titers in low dose immunizations in mice. *Int Arch Allergy Appl Immunol*, 40: 113–116, 1971.

Although pre-seasonal treatment is practiced commonly, especially in areas with a sharply limited seasonal pollen pattern as with *Ambrosia elatior* (dwarf ragweed or Eastern ragweed), there are many disadvatages to such a routine. The difficulty in anticipating the season to permit maximum effective dosage just prior to onset of the pollen season can lead to inadequate treatment or to the risk of reactions. If the higher concentrations coincide with the onset of the pollinating season, the incidence of reactions may be much higher.

Co-seasonal therapy in most instances is not only less satisfactory but also carries with it great risk of reactions, especially constitutional reactions.

With the availability of antihistamines and steroids for the control of very severe symptoms over a brief period, co-seasonal therapy is not recommended at any time.

It is generally recognized that perennial injection therapy is not only more satisfactory but also is a much safer routine.

6. The Duration of Treatment

Injection therapy does not cure the allergic patient but merely modifies his immunologic responses so that he fails to react adversely upon exposure to allergens. The time required to convert clinical reactivity to nonreactivity varies considerably.

The degree of clinical reactivity is one of the most important factors that influence the duration of treatment. Although the degree of the patient's clinical response usually correlates well with the intensity of the skin test reactions, this is not a constant observation. Patients with only moderate and at times a very slight reaction on skin testing may experience severe clinical patterns. In most cases regardless of the degree of skin reactivity, patients with a severe clinical pattern require longer periods of injection therapy.

It is not always necessary to achieve the highest level of concentration of the antigen to experience control of symptoms. Patients may have an intolerance to high concentrations of antigen which aggravates their symptoms, while the administration of weak dilutions of antigen are effective in controlling symptoms. Most patients with a low tolerance for antigen require long periods of injection therapy (over 10 years), while many of these patients are never able to discontinue therapy without a recurrence of symptoms.

Although the intensity of skin test reactions does not always correlate with the degree of clinical response, skin tests can serve as an index for terminating injection therapy. Sherman and Connell have reported that following long periods of injection therapy (several years), skin reactions are diminished. In our experience it has been noted that following long periods of injection therapy, usually from ten to fifteen years, but rarely after two or three years, the skin test reactions are either diminished or completely reversed (no reactivity). The gradual diminution in skin reactivity is a common observation after several years of injection therapy. The sequence is first the loss of prick test reactivity followed by a loss of intracutaneous reactions on the arm, and then weak reactivity or complete failure to react on the back, which is the most sensitive site for skin testing. Clinical improvement usually parallels the decreased or absent skin reactivity. In some patients following many years (ten to twenty years) of uninterrupted injection therapy the skin response remains strongly positive, although the patient is entirely free of symptoms.

Adequate studies to explain the immunologic events involved in these clinical observations are lacking, yet on the basis of clinical experience, it is possible to set up guidelines for the safe termination of injection therapy.

(a) The control of symptoms associated with negative skin test reactions in patients with a history of positive skin reactions can safely terminate therapy. This usually requires over ten years of uninterrupted therapy. These patients may remain symptom-free for ten years or more and many for indefinite periods.

(b) The control of symptoms associated with persistent skin reactivity requires continued injection therapy. These patients usually experience an early recurrence of symptoms (a few months to almost one year) following the cessation of injection therapy.

(c) If symptoms recur following an interruption of therapy of more than one year, the patient should be retested and a new antigen ordered before resuming therapy. If the interruption is less than one year, a dilution test with the patient's extract will suffice to determine the level of tolerance.

Constitutional Reactions

(1) IMMEDIATE: The immediate form of constitutional reactions is the most serious and requires measures of treatment without delay. With the sudden onset of symptoms the person administering the antigen should immediately inject 0.5 ml of epinephrine-HCl 1–1000 by hypodermic and then notify the physician. When the program as outlined is strictly observed, the likelihood of such reactions is exceedingly rare. However, it is because of the extraordinary situation, when a violent constitutional reaction may occur, that it is important that a physician should always be in close proximity to the treatment area.

The symptoms are those of anaphylactic shock (see discussion on anaphylaxis in Chapter 1 for symptoms and treatment).

(2) DELAYED: The delayed constitutional reaction although frightening and disturbing to the patient is rarely fatal. The experience among allergists indicates that constitutional reactions that occur fifteen to thirty minutes following the injection of the antigenic extract are rarely fatal.

The symptoms include:

(a) An exacerbation of the patient's symptoms which include nasal congestion; itching, rhinorrhea and sneezing; itching of the eyes with lacrimation and conjunctival injection; cough, dyspnea, wheezing

(b) Itching of the palms and soles

(c) Flushing, urticaria and angio-edema.

Treatment

Epinephrine-HCl 1-1000 0.4 ml which can be repeated in twenty to thirty minutes if necessary.

For mild reactions antihistamines orally may be sufficient to control the symptoms. For more severe reactions steroid therapy is recommended.

Both antihistamines and steroids are too slow for emergency treatment and do not replace epinephrine-HCl.

Epinephrine may be repeated in small doses if necessary. *Depot* epinephrine (Sus-Phrine® 0.25 ml) may be administered to provide prolonged action until the antihistamines or steroids become effective.

Adjuvant Therapy

Since its inception, physicians have attempted to correct some of the undesirable features of injection therapy, either by a modification of the procedure or the product. Many patients resist the necessity for long periods of repeated injections at frequent intervals, while some patients because of occupational situations or residence in remote areas cannot avail themselves of the conventional programs of therapy.

Although a number of modifications of the conventional procedures have been suggested, three programs currently in use illustrate the modifications indicated above.

(1) The emulsion repository technique which is a modification of administration of the allergenic extract

(2) Alum precipitated extracts

(3) Pyridine-alum precipitated extracts[*] which are modifications of the basic allergens.

---

[*] Allpyral,® Dome Chemicals, Inc., New York, New York.

1. Emulsion Repository Therapy

Following Freund's discovery of the adjuvant property of mineral oil in the sensitization of animals, Lovelace applied the principle to the treatment of hay fever by incorporating pollen extracts into mineral oil emulsions. The favorable reports of Lovelace's experience encouraged other physicians to apply the priniciple to a variety of allergens for the treatment of both perennial and seasonal allergic disease, as well as sensitivity to hymenopterous insects.

By this technique a water-in-oil emulsion is produced by incorporating the aqueous extract of the allergen into a highly refined mineral oil (Drakeol) with isomannide mono-oleate (Arlacel A) as an emulsifying agent. The dose of the antigen is calculated in terms of PNUs and administered intramuscularly in either single or multiple injections at monthly intervals.

The principle of the procedure is based upon the slow release of antigen which induces an IgG blocking antibody response.

The proponents of emulsion therapy point out the following advantages:

(1) The number of injections for seasonal therapy is reduced to one, two or three monthly injections. This abbreviated program is less hardship for many patients.

(2) The slow release of antigens provides a persistent level of IgG blocking antibody.

(3) The slow release of antigen decreases the incidence of constitutional reactions.

(4) The slow release of antigen permits treatment of patients who cannot tolerate aqueous extracts at any dilution.

The opponents of emulsion therapy point out the following disadvantages:

(1) Antigens incorporated into mineral oil induce the delayed type of hypersensitivity. This is comparable to the delayed hypersensitivity induced experimentally with Freund's adjuvant.

(2) Cracking of the emulsion (breakdown) results in the rapid release of an overwhelming dose of antigen which can cause severe constitutional reactions.

(3) Cysts, nodules and abscesses at the site of injection are a common complication.

(4) Arthralgia is not an uncommon complaint.

(5) The carcinogenic potential of the mineral oil has not been evaluated to the satisfaction of the Food and Drug Administration (FDA).

(6) The failure to license the products required for preparing emulsions makes emulsions unavailable commercially. Emulsions must be prepared by the physician, which involves controls to assure sterility of the emulsion, completeness of emulsification and elimination of contaminating irritants.

In order to evaluate emulsion repository therapy, under an Investigational New Drug (IND) license from the Food and Drug Administration, an experimental study was instituted in the KFH-PMG Allergy Department in the fall of 1963 in preparation for the spring season of 1964. This program was continued annually through the spring season of 1969.

PATIENT SAMPLE: The patient sample included 592 adults with seasonal hay fever and/or asthma. Only patients who had pre-

Table 17-III: COMPARATIVE RESULTS WITH EMULSION THERAPY PROGRAM AT KFH-PMG

Year	No. Patients	Excellent	Good	Poor
1964	592	16.5%	74.2%	22%
1965	489	14.4%	63.6%	11.1%
1966	350	30.0%	58.0%	12.0%
1967	347	20.5%	67.0%	12.5%
1968	328	11.1%	75.7%	5.0%
1969	301	24.2%	67.8%	7.8%

Table 17-IV: 1964 SPRING SEASON EMULSION THERAPY

Patients	Reviewed	Local Reactions†	Systemic†	Excellent	Good	Poor
592*	478	92 19.2%	32 6.6%	79	355	42

* Five-hundred ninety-two patients were treated, but only 478 reported for review in July 1964 following the spring season. Percentages are based upon the patients interviewed following the season.
† Local Reactions were: (1) small areas of erythema at the site of the injection which persisted for periods varying from several hours to several days, (2) nodules which appeared within days and persisted for periods varying from days to months; these varied in size from a shot to a bean.

viously received conventional aqueous therapy were selected. This policy was adopted as a safeguard against severe reactions, since emulsion therapy offers no procedure for determining the patient's tolerance for antigen. Excluded from the program were individuals with perennial symptoms, chronic bronchitis, emphysema; pregnant women; or any one with evidence of foci of infection.

PROCEDURE: Patients offering a history of early spring symptoms received their initial injection in November and followed with monthly injections through February. In California the peak of the spring grass season is usually April and May to mid-June. This group of patients started injections in January and continued at monthly intervals through February and March.

Various grass and tree pollen mixtures were prepared to meet the requirements of the patient, determined by history and skin reactions.

The total dose of antigen for the patient determined on the basis of PNUs was calculated to deliver a small initial priming dose followed by divided doses so that the last injection was roughly 50 per cent of the total PNUs ordered for the patient.

The results for the 1964 spring season are indicated in Table 17-III.

In the first series of treatments one abscess was observed. This occurred in a male following the second injection of emulsified antigen. The first injection was administered in the left sub-deltoid region on January 9, and the second injection was administered in the right sub-deltoid on February 17. On March 4 the patient had a hot, tender, fluctuant mass which was drained. Following drainage, the course was uneventful.

Systemic reactions usually occurred within thirty to sixty minutes following the administration of the antigen. Symptoms included generalized blushing, pruritus, tingling, urticaria, angio-edema, and in a few cases, mild asthma. Since all patients were premedicated with 4 mg of Chlor-Trimeton® and 5 mg of prednisone, they responded quickly to a repetition of their medication. A few cases required the administration of adrenalin. No instance of severe anaphylaxis was observed.

In one patient following the initial injection, which was a small priming dose (818 PNUs) of spring grasses, painful joints of the hands and feet developed but no redness or swelling.

The patient was placed on steroid therapy and further emulsion injections were discontinued. The patient's joint symptoms cleared completely, and his hay fever for the season 1964 was exceptionally well controlled.

One patient complained of coldness and tingling of the extremities intermittently for three weeks following the first and second injections, but no such complaints following the third and fourth injections.

One patient complained of rather ill-defined symptoms of malaise and "not feeling well" following each injection, but no other symptoms of a systemic response were observed.

(a) An *excellent* response was a complete absence of symptoms requiring no medication.

(b) A *good* response was one comparable to the control of symptoms experienced with conventional therapy. The symptoms in this group varied from those requiring very little medication during the season to more moderate symptoms requiring more frequent medication. In every instance the grading was based upon an anecdotal evaluation of the patient. In some cases of this group, results were actually less satisfactory than with conventional therapy, but because of the convenience of the program the patients were frequently prejudiced in their appraisal.

(c) *Poor* meant complete failure. These patients were returned to conventional therapy.

The results obtained with emulsion therapy are quite comparable to those obtained with conventional aqueous therapy, but the risk of reactions is far greater.

of allergic individuals as reported by Hyde and associates in Wales, to 21 to 29 per cent reported by Prince in Texas. Intermediate are the reports by Nilsby in Sweden who considers the incidence to be 10 per cent, while Feinberg in the United States reports that 20 per cent of patients with inhalant allergy are sensitive to molds. Statistics for the incidence of mold sensitivity are derived from skin test surveys which in turn are influenced by: (1) variations in both mold populations and mold concentration which are governed by climatic differences and weather changes, (2) the variation in antigenicity that exists among species and genera of molds, and (3) the inherent ability of the individual to react to mold antigens.

Immunology of Molds

Except for studies conducted on extrinsic allergic bronchopneumonia (see Chapter 4), investigations on the immunology of the molds involved in allergic diseases have been very limited.

Mold Antigens and Antibodies

An excellent study from Arbesman's laboratory by Bonilla-Soto and Rose on the antigenic and allergenic properties of *Alternaria tenuis* indicates the complexity of the mold antigen and accordingly the multiplicity of the antibody response. The observations of these investigators are helpful in forming an approximate judgment regarding some of the characteristics of mold antigens other than Alternaria and the antibodies they evoke.

The presence of multiple bands, as many as six, by agar gel diffusion, indicates that Alternaria has a number of antigenic determinants of which some are in common with determinants of other members of the Dematiaceous group of molds (see Table 17-VII). The common determinants explain the cross reactivity observed clinically with various species of Alternaria as well as the cross reactivity observed among members of a family or among members of a genera. In addition to the common determinants, Alternaria has specific determinant(s) not shared with other members.

The failure of trypsin, diastase and pepsin to exert a detectable digestive action upon Alternaria antigens suggests that the chemical structure of Alternaria, and perhaps other mold antigens, differs *fundamentally* from that of pollen antigens which are subjected to enzymatic digestion (Augustine 1959). This is consistent with the dual response observed on skin testing with mold antigens. The dual immunologic mechanism is well illustrated in extrinsic allergic bronchopneumonia in which syndrome the response may be either a combination of IgE and precipitating IgG or a dual response with delayed hypersensitivity and precipitating IgG. Occasionally, delayed skin test reactions are observed with pollen extracts which could be attributed to contaminants, such as bacterial components or molds. This fundamental difference in chemical structure may also explain the higher incidence of both local and constitutional reactions encountered with mold extracts.

Bonilla-Soto, Rose and Arbesman observed that following injection therapy, patients showed an increased titer by the indirect hemagglutination test, using cells sensitized with heated Alternaria antigen. It is undetermined whether the antibodies detected belong to the precipitating IgG class encountered in the Arthus mechanism or whether they are the blocking antibodies observed with pollen allergens. It is also important to note that these investigators detected a low level of Alternaria antibodies in some normal individuals. This indicates that the presence of antibodies does not always indicate active disease. A similar situation is observed with Aspergillus and the thermophilic Actinomyces. A positive skin test reaction (Arthus type) may be accompanied by low titers of precipitating antibody, but the patient experiences no active disease. The antibody response to molds may be similar to that observed with IgE, i.e. an increased titer does not indicate active disease. In auto-allergic disease apparently normal individuals may have auto antibodies and at times with rather high titers.

Skin Test Reactions to Mold Extracts

There is an extensive literature on the skin reactions to mold extracts which is in general agreement that mold antigens may induce:

(1) An immediate whealing type response which is observed in atopic individuals within twenty minutes.

(2) An early (Arthus type) delayed skin reaction observed about six hours following the challenge, and

(3) The classical delayed response observed twenty-four hours following the challenge.

The immediate reaction is observed most commonly, followed by the Arthus type and then by the classical delayed reaction. In a study of one hundred subjects by Warren, Paul, and Rose in the Montreal area, only six patients showed a delayed (Arthus type) reaction. No reactions for DH were reported.

Patients usually show skin reactivity to more than one mold. In the Canadian study the average for all patients was twelve positive skin reactions. No statistical difference was observed in the number of reactions for patients with rhinitis as compared with asthma. In some measure, the multiplicity of reactions may be attributed to the cross reactivity observed, particularly among species of a given family (see Table 17-VII) and also among genera. The demonstration of antigenic determinants in common explains the high degree of cross reactivity.

It is important to recognize that positive reactivity on skin testing does not indicate active disease. A patient may manifest reactivity to numerous allergens with no clinical evidence of disease. Reactivity merely signifies that the individual has been sensitized to the respective antigen and under

Table 17-VII: BOTANICAL RELATIONSHIPS OF AIRBORNE MOLDS AVAILABLE IN MMP* ALLERGENS†

PHYCOMYCETES
Mucor racemosus
Rhizopus nigricans

FUNGI IMPERFECTI
Dematiaceae
  Alternaria
  Curvularia spicifera
  Spondylocladium sp.
  Helminthosporium interseminatum
  Hormodendrum cladosporioides
  Stemphylium botryosum
  Nigrospora sphaerica
  Pullularia pullulans

Moniliaceae
  Aspergillus fumigatus
  Aspergillus glacus
  Aspergillus nidulans
  Aspergillus niger
  Aspergillus sydowi
  Aspergillus terreus
  Botrytis cinerea
  Monilia sitophila
  Mycogone sp.
  Paecilomyces varioti
  Penicillium atramentosum
  Penicillium biforma
  Penicillium carmino-violaceum
  Penicillium intricatum
  Penicillium luteum
  Penicillium notatum
  Trichoderma viride
  Gliocladium fimbriatum

Sphaerioidaceae
  Phoma herbarum

Tuberculariaceae
  Fusarium vasinfectum

Cryptococcaceae
  Rhodotorula glutinis

ASCOMYCETES
Saccharomycetaceae
  Saccharomyces cerevisiae
Chaetomiaceae
  Chaetomium indicum

Note: It is very fortunate that only a limited number of the several thousands of individual molds have been identified as factors in allergic disease. It is further fortunate that the cross reactivity observed among various genera and species permits limiting skin testing for diagnostic purposes to a comparatively small number as recommended in the list compiled by Prince and Morrow. These investigators state, Multiple sensitization to several related species or genera is most striking insofar as the most frequently reacting group of molds, the Dematiaceae, is concerned. It is a matter of common knowledge that when one species of a genus, such as the genus Alternaria of this family reacts on a sensitive patient, species of one or more of the other genera may react similarly... We feel that reaction patterns are highly diagnostic. In our search for such patterns we continue to test with representative genera of the dematiaceous molds and several genera or even species in the larger moniliaceous group. We prefer the mutually confirmatory aspect of multiple reactions to related genera or species rather than any convenience afforded by testing with mold mixtures.

The list of references suggests several references which present in detail the structural bases for the classification of fungi.

* *MMP:* Morrow, Meyer and Prince have developed an extracting procedure recommended and licensed by the Association of Allergists for Mycological Investigations. MMP mold extracts are available from Hollister-Stier Laboratories.

† From Prince, H. E. and Morrow, M. B.: A logical approach to mold allergy. *Ann Allergy, 27:*79, 1969.

proper circumstances, exposure to the antigen can produce disease.

Most atopic individuals who react to mold extracts usually react to other allergens, such as pollens, epidermal and environmental factors. In the Montreal study of Warren, William and Rose seven of the one hundred patients studied failed to react to other inhalant allergens including ragweed pollen, but each of the seven patients reacted to seven mold extracts.

The concomitant reaction to other allergens makes the incrimination of molds in active disease more difficult. Feinberg contends that in most cases a positive reaction to mold extracts can be evaluated on the basis of criteria derived from the patient's history, such as:

(1) Hay fever and asthma that fail to correlate with the pollen season. Symptoms that persist beyond the pollinating season (see Chapter 16, The Botany of Allergy for regional distribution and seasons for pollens).

In colder climates the patient's symptoms may fail to clear with the first frost and may persist until the first snowfall.

Symptoms may occur only during pollen-free periods.

The patients are usually worse in hot windy weather preceded by rain.

Note: In tropical and semitropical regions, such as California, where pollens are present in the atmosphere for eleven months of the year, a diagnosis of mold allergy on the basis of history is not practical.

(2) A history of acute allergic attacks occurring in special environments, such as barns, haylofts, strawstacks, musty damp rooms and basements, during sleigh rides (straw is present for the protection of the feet), or at the time of threshing. *Note*: These exposures constitute the exciting circumstances associated with extrinsic allergic bronchopneumonia (see Chapter 4).

(3) The failure of environmental control plus immunotherapy with pollen, epidermal and environmental extracts. *Note*: Before mold sensitivity is considered, those substances which cannot be demonstrated by positive skin testing, such as food chemicals and food parts, must be excluded (see Chapter 8, Adverse Reactions to Foods and Food Chemicals).

Treatment with Mold Antigens

The administration of mold extracts is a common practice among physicians who employ injection therapy for the management of allergic disease. In most instances the indication for therapy with mold extracts is based upon the history, the immediate skin reactivity observed on testing and occasionally on a provocative challenge.* In some cases the response to testing is correlated with the demonstration of the organism on culture plates exposed to the patient's environmental atmosphere. The composition of the treatment extract is determined on the basis of history, skin sensitivity and the incidence of the organism in the region where the patient resides.

In general, the tolerance for mold extracts is much lower than that observed with other inhalant allergens. As a result lower concentrations and smaller doses of mold extracts must be administered in order to avoid reaction. Both local and constitutional reactions are more frequent with the injection of mold extracts.

The procedure for the management of allergy patients at the Kaiser-Permanente (KP) Medical Care Program of Northern California provides for routine skin testing with a selected group of molds indigenous to the region. Included are Alternaria, Hormodendrum, Aspergillus and Penicillium. Although skin tests are performed for diagnostic information, no mold extracts are administered for treatment.

---

* The provocative challenge consists of the direct challenge of the patient with the allergen by (1) applying the allergen in the nasal mucosa, (2) permitting the patient to sniff the dry allergen, and (3) confining the patient to a room into which is blown a measured quantity of the allergen.

Over the past twenty-one years, hundreds of thousands of allergy patients, at times as many as two thousand to three thousand daily patient visits, have been treated in the combined Allergy Departments of KFH-PMG, but injection therapy has always been limited to inhalant factors with the exclusion of mold extracts. The success of the patient response under this program justifies the exclusion of mold extracts for the treatment of patients in the San Francisco Bay area.

Management of Mold Allergy

Programs for the control of mold allergy are usually not as easily carried out as those applied to other inhalant allergens because: (1) environmental control for molds is usually more difficult to exercise, and (2) fundamental differences exist in the chemistry of mold antigens which result in more complex immunological responses.

(1) *Environmental Control*: It is important to recognize that isolated mold sensitiviy, without reactiviy to other inhalant factors, is not a common observation. In the studies of Warren, William and Rose in one hundred patients who reacted to mold antigens, only seven patients failed to reacted on skin testing to other commonly encountered inhalant allergens, including ragweed pollen. In view of the high incidence of reactivity to antigens other than molds, it is important to exclude all potential environmental factors before incriminating mold as the etiologic agent.

Basically, the principles for environmental control in mold allergy are identical with those outlined for other inhalant allergens.

When premises (residences or other structures) frequented by the patient are infested with molds, improvement in the patient's illness can frequently be effected by control of the conditions which predispose to inordinate growth of the organisms. This includes dampness, inadequate light and ventilation in dark rooms and basements. Chemical and mechanical drying procedures are at times helpful. When carefully programmed environmental control fails, consideration must be given to removing the patient from the environment, at times necessitating a change in residence.

Exposure to inordinate doses of mold, as encountered in some occupational environments, particularly agricultural, must be strictly avoided by the patient. The risks from undue exposure to such environments, which may be either persistent or intermittent, are too serious to justify even occasional contact. For some patients such absolute control may necessitate a change in occupation (see Extrinsic Allergic Bronchopneumonia in Chapter 4).

When all measures for environmental control fail in situations where the atmospheric distribution and concentration are persistently high for molds to which the patient shows reactivity, consideration must be given to moving the patient to an area which is entirely free of the offending species of mold or to one with a mold concentration sufficiently low to be tolerated by the patient.*

There is general acceptance that in some patients molds may be the etiologic agent of allergic disease. However, it is important to recognize that compared with other allergens, fundamental differences exist in the chemistry of mold antigens which result in a different immunologic response. Because of these differences the management of mold sensitivity cannot be identical with that for other inhalant allergens.

(2) *Fundamental Differences*: The clarification of the immunological aspects of the problem would be helpful for the clinician in the management of mold-sensitive patients and in making a decision as to the advisability of employing mold extracts for treatment.

(a) Does the particular mold in question evoke reaginic antibody? Apparently all molds do *not* have this capacity even in the atopic individual. In allergic aspergillosis the Aspergillus antigen can evoke IgE anti-

---

* For regional distribution of molds, see Morrow, Meyer and Prince: A summary of air-borne mold surveys. *Ann Allergy*, 22: 575–587, 1964.

bodies in atopic individuals, while the thermophilic Actinomyces which causes farmer's lung cannot induce IgE antibodies in any individual, either atopic or nonatopic. The response to thermophilic Actinomyces is with delayed hypersensitivity combined with precipitating IgG class antibodies.

(b) Can a mold that evokes IgE antibody do so without concomitant production of IgG antibody? This question is unanswered.

An isolated IgE response to mold antigen would support the incrimination of molds as the cause of uncomplicated bronchial asthma (without extrinsic allergic bronchopneumonia) in patients manifesting immediate skin reactivity to extracts of the mold.

(c) It would seem advisable to screen all patients with positive skin reactions, and particularly those with the early (Arthus type) delayed for precipitating antibodies. In the survey of Warren, William and Rose, patients with the Arthus type reaction had precipitating antibodies in their sera and also a history supporting a diagnosis of farmer's lung.

Experience with extrinsic allergic bronchopneumonia indicates that the administration of mold extracts aggravates the condition. Is it possible that in some patients with mold sensitivity and particularly those with the Arthus type delayed skin response, with or without demonstrable precipitin in the sera, the administration of mold extracts may aggravate the patient's condition?

(d) The studies of Bonilla-Soto et al. indicate that injection therapy with mold extracts induces increased IgG titers. It would be important to determine the nature of the IgG antibodies. Are they blocking antibodies as encountered in routine injection therapy, or are they precipitating antibodies as encountered in the Arthus mechanism? They could be both.

As has been indicated, mold sensitivity involves a more complex immunologic response than that encountered with other inhalant allergens. Accordingly, the management is more complex. The decision to administer mold extracts for treatment should be governed by not only the patient's history and skin reactivity, but also a serological survey to determine the patient's immunologic response.

REFERENCES

General Texts and References

1. Aas, K.: Hyposensitization in house dust allergy asthma. A double-blind study with evaluation of the effect on the bronchial sensitivity to house dust allergens. *Acta Paediatr Scand, 60:* 264, 1971.
2. Arbesman, C. E., Reisman, R. E. Bonstein, H. S. and Rose, N. R.: Allergic and immunologic studies of a "purified" fraction of ragweed pollen. *J Immunol, 90:* 612, 1963.
3. Augustin, R. and Hayward, B. J.: Human reagins to grass pollens and molds: Their purification and physio-chemical characterization. *Immunology, 3:* 45, 1960.
4. Augustin, R. and Hayward, B. J.: Grass pollen allergens: IV. The isolation of some of the principle allergens of *Phleum pratense* and their sensitivity spectra in patients. *Immunology, 5:* 424, 1962.
5. Baer, H., Godfrey, H., Maloney, C. J., Norman, P. S. and Lichtenstein, L. M.: The potency and antigen E content of commercially prepared ragweed extracts. *J Allergy, 45:* 347, 1970.
6. Beers, Ray F., Jr.: Skin tests. In Samter, M. and Alexander, H. L. (Eds.): *Immunologic Disorders.* Boston, Little, 1965, pp. 539–548.
7. Blanton, W. B. and Sutphin, A. K.: Death during skin testing. *Am J Med Sci, 217:* 169, 1949.
8. Brown, E. A.: The conjunctival test. *Ann Allergy, 20:* 608, 1962.
9. Citron, K. M.: Injection treatment for desensitization in asthma, hay fever and allergic rhinitis. *Br J Dis Chest, 60:* 1, 1966.
10. Claman, H. N.: Does injection therapy produce tolerance or immunity? *J Allergy, 35:* 371, 1964.
11. Colldahl, H.: A study of provocative tests in patients with bronchial asthma. III. The interpretation of the provocation tests and the value of the test for allergy diagnosis and treatment. *Acta Allergol, 5:* 154, 1952.
12. Connell, J. T., Sherman, W. B. and Meyers, P. A.: Antibody studies in constitutional reactions resulting from injection of ragweed pollen extract. *J Allergy, 33:* 365, 1962.
13. Connell, J. T. and Sherman, W. B.: Skin sensitizing titer. III. Relationship of skin sensitizing antibody titer to the intracutaneous skin test, to the

tolerance of injections of antigens, and to the effects of prolonged treatment with antigen. *J Allergy, 35:* 109, 1964.
14. Connell, J. T.: Sensitization of human subjects after multiple intracutaneous injections of aqueous ragweed extract. *J Allergy, 40:* 268, 1967.
15. Connell, J. T. and Sherman, W. B.: Hay fever symptoms related to immunological findings. *Ann Allergy, 25:* 239, 1967.
16. Connell, J. T. and Sherman, W. B.: Changes in skin sensitizing antibody titers after injection of aqueous pollen extract. *J Allergy, 43:* 22, 1969.
17. Connell, J. T.: Quantitative intranasal pollen challenge. III. The priming effect in allergic rhinitis. *J Allergy, 43:* 33, 1969.
18. Fontana, V. J., Holt, L. E., Jr. and Mainland, D.: Effectiveness of hyposensitization therapy in ragweed hay fever children. *JAMA, 192:* 985, 1966.
19. Frankland, A. W. and Augustine, R.: Prophylaxis of summer hay fever and asthma. Controlled trial comparing crude grass pollen extracts with isolated main protein component. *Lancet, 1:* 1055, 1954.
20. Hjorth, N.: Routine patch tests. St. John's Hospital. *Derm Soc, 49:* 99, 1963.
21. Inhalation Tests. Proceedings of two symposia held during the Sixth Congress of Allergology. *Acta Allergol, 22,* Suppl. 8, 1967.
22. Johnson, P. and Marsh, D. G.: Allergens from common rye grass pollen (*Lolium perenne*). I. Chemical composition and structure. *Immunochemistry, 3:* 91, 1966.
23. Johnson, P. and Marsh, D. G.: II. The allergenic determinants and carbohydrate moiety. *Immunochemistry, 3:* 10, 1966.
24. Johnstone, D. E. and Dutton, A.: The value of hyposensitization therapy for bronchial asthma in children. A 14 year study. *Pediatrics, 42:* 793, 1968.
25. Kilburn, K. H. (Ed.): Pulmonary responses to inhaled materials. An evaluation of model systems. *Arch Intern Med, 126:* 1970.
26. King, T. P. and Norman, P. S.: Isolation studies of allergens from ragweed pollen. *Biochemistry, 1:* 709, 1962.
27. King, T. P. and Norman, P. S.: Chemical studies of the predominant allergen from ragweed pollen. *Abstracts VI International Congress of Biochemistry, II.* 160, 1964.
28. King, T. P., Norman, P. S. and Lichtenstein, L. M.: Studies on ragweed pollen allergens, IV. *Biochemistry, 6:* 1992, 1967.
29. Levy, D. A. and Osler, A. G.: Studies on the mechanisms of hypersensitivity phenomena. XIV. Passive sensitization *in vitro* of human leukocytes to ragweed pollen antigen. *J Immunol, 97:* 203, 1966.
30. Levy, D. A. and Osler, A. G.: XVI. *In vitro* assays of reaginic activity in human sera. Effect of therapeutic immunization on seasonal titer changes. *J Immunol, 99:* 1068, 1967.
31. Lichtenstein, L. M. and Osler, A. G.: Studies on the mechanisms of hypersensitivity phenomena. IX. Histamine release from human leukocytes by ragweed pollen antigen. *J Exp Med, 120:* 507, 1964.
32. Lichtenstein, L. M., Norman, P. S., Osler, A. G. and and Winkenwerder, W. L.: *In vitro* studies of human ragweed allergy: Changes in cellular and humoral activity associated with specific desensitization. *J Clin Invest, 45:* 1126, 1966.
33. Lichtenstein, L. M. and Osler, A. G.: Studies on the mechanisms of hypersensitivity phenomena. XII. An *in vitro* study of the reaction between ragweed pollen antigen, allergic human serum and ragweed sensitive human leukocytes. *J Immunol, 96:* 169, 1966.
34. Lichtenstein, L. M., Norman, P. S. and Connell, J. T.: Comparison between skin sensitizing antibody titers and leukocyte sensitivity measurement as an index of the severity of ragweed hay fever. *J Allergy, 40:* 160, 1967.
35. Lichtenstein, L. M., Norman, P. S. and Winkenwerder, W. L.: Clinical and *in vitro* studies on the role of immunotherapy in ragweed hay fever. *Am J Med, 44:* 514, 1968.
36. Lichtenstein, L. M.: *In vitro* approach to problems in clinical allergy. *N Y State J Med, 68:* 2168, 1968.
37. Lowell, F. C. and Franklin, W.: A "double blind" study of the effectiveness and specificity of injection therapy in ragweed hay fever. *N Engl J Med, 273:* 675, 1965.
38. Lowell, F. C. and Franklin, W.: A "double blind" study of treatment with aqueous allergenic extracts in cases of allergic rhinitis. *J Allergy, 34:* 165, 1963.
39. Lowell, F. C. and Franklin, W.: Letter to the editor: Criticism of the Fontana, Holt and Mainland report. *JAMA, 195:* 1071, 1966.
40. Lowell, F. C. and Franklin, W.: Criticisms and rebuttal. *JAMA, 195:* 1071, 1966, *196:* 1025, 1966.
41. Lowell, F. C., Gaillard, G. E. and Lichtenstein, L. M.: Current status and effectiveness of hyposensitization therapy. Symposium. *Westchester Allergy Soc,* New York, May 1968.
42. Malley, A., Reed, C. E. and Lietze, A.: Isolation of allergens from timothy pollen. *J Allergy, 23:* 534, 1965.
43. Marsh, D. G., Milner, F. H. and Johnson, P.: The allergenic activity and stability of purified allergens from the pollen of common rye grass (*Lolium perenne*). *Int Arch Allergy Appl Immunol, 29:* 521, 1966.

44. Noon, L.: Prophylactic inoculations against hay fever. *Lancet, 1:* 1572, 1971.
45. Norman, P. S.: A rational approach to desensitization. *J Allergy, 44:* 129, 1969.
46. Osserman, E. F.: Plasma cell dyscrasias. Current clinical and biochemical concepts. *Am J Med, 44:* 256, 1968.
47. Palmstiema, H.: On the purification of allergens. I. *Phleum pratense* allergen. *Sci Tools, 7:* 29, 1960.
48. Peeler, R. N., Kadull, P. J. and Cluff, L. E.: Intensive immunization of man. Evaluation of possible adverse consequences. *Ann Intern Med, 63:* 44, 1965.
49. Popoc, V. et al.: The value of inhalation tests in perennial bronchial asthma. *J Allergy, 42:* 130, 1968.
50. Pruzansky, J. J. and Patterson, R.: Histamine release from leukocytes of hypersensitive individuals. II. Reduced sensitivity of leukocytes after injection therapy. *J Allergy, 39:* 44, 1967.
51. Pruzansky, J. J. and Patterson, R.: Immunologic changes during hyposensitization therapy. *JAMA, 203:* 805, 1968.
52. Reisman, R. E., Bonstein, H. S., Rose, N. R. and Arbesman, C. E.: Studies of purified fractions of ragweed pollen. *J Allergy, 35:* 227, 1964.
53. Reisman, R. E., Wicker, K. and Arbesman, C. E.: Immunotherapy with antigen E. *J Allergy, 44:* 82, 1969.
54. Richter, M. and Sehon, A. H.: Studies on the allergens of ragweed pollen. *J Allergy, 31:* 111, 1960.
55. Rimington, C., Stilwell, D. E. and Maunsell, K.: The allergen(s) of house dusts: Purification and chemical nature of active constituents. *Br J Exp Pathol, 28:* 309, 1947.
56. Sadan, N., Rhyne, M. B., Mellits, D., Goldstein, E. Q., Levy, D. A. and Lichtenstein, L. M.: Immunotherapy of pollenosis in children: An investigation of the immunological basis of clinical improvement. *N Engl J Med, 280:* 623, 1969.
57. Salvaggio, J. E., Cavanaugh, J. J. A., Lowell, F. C. and Leskowitz, S.: A comparison of the immunologic responses of normal and atopic individuals to intranasally administered antigen. *J Allergy, 35:* 62, 1964.
58. Sherman, W. B.: Changes in serological reactions and tissue sensitivity in hay fever patients during the early months of treatment. *J Immunol, 40:* 289, 1941.
59. Spiegelman, J., Friedman, H. and Tuft, L.: Immunologic responses of pollenosis patients treated with alum-precipitated pyridine ragweed extract. *Ann Allergy, 25:* 262, 1967.
60. Spiegelman, J. and Friedman, H.: The effects of central air filtration and air conditioning on pollen and microbial contamination. *J Allergy, 42:* 193, 1968.
61. Sprecace, G. A., Pomper, S. G., Sherman, W. B., Lemlich, A. and Ziffer, H.: The effect of antigen injections on skin reactivity to antigens. *J Allergy, 38:* 9, 1966.
62. Stanworth, D. R.: The mechanisms of reaginic reaction. In *Proceedings VIIth European Congress of Allergology.* Berlin, 1968.
63. Swineford, O., Jr.: Anaphylactic shock from skin testing. *J Allergy, 17:* 24, 1946.
64. Woodruff, A. J.: Multiple myeloma associated with long history of hyposensitization with allergen vaccines. *Lancet, 1:* 99, 1972.

Mites

1. Brown, H. M. and Filer, J. L.: Role of mites in allergy to house dust. *Br Med J, 3:* 646, 1968.
2. Spieksma, F. Th. M.: The house dust mite, *Dermatophagoides pteromyssinus*. Doctoral thesis, 1967.
3. Spieksma, F. Th. M.: Cultivation of house dust mites. *J Allergy, 43:* 151, 1968.
4. Spieksma, F. Th. M.: Biological aspects of the house dust mite (*Dermatophagoides pteromyssimus*) in relation to house dust atopy. *Clin Exp Immunol, 6:* 61, 1970.
5. Voorhorst, R., Spieksma-Boezman, M. I. A. and Spieksma, F. Th. M.: Is a mite (*Dermatophagoides*, sp) the producer of house dust allergen? *Allerg Asthma (Leipz), 10:* 329, 1969.
6. Voorhorst, R. et al.: The house dust mite (*Dermatophagoides pteromyssimus*) and the allergies it produces. Identity with the house dust allergen. *J Allergy, 39:* 325, 1967.

Adjuvant Therapy

1. Arbesman, C. E. and Reisman, R. E.: Repository pollen therapy: Clinical and immunologic studies. In Brown, E. A. (Ed.): *Allergology.* London, Pergamon Pr, 1962.
2. Arbesman, C. E. and Reisman, R. E.: Hyposensitization therapy including repository therapy. *J Allergy, 35:* 12, 1964.
3. Caplan, I. and Hayns, J. T.: Allpyral and aqueous extracts in ragweed hay fever and asthma: A comparison. *J Asthma Res, 4:* 105, 1966.
4. Connell, J. T. and Sherman, W. B.: The effects of treatment with the emulsions of ragweed extract on antibody titers. *J Immunol, 91:* 197, 1963.
5. Department of Health, Education and Welfare, F. D. A.: A letter regarding mineral oil preparations. *Ann Allergy, 23:* 555, 1965.

6. Feinberg, S. M. and Feinberg, A. R.: Desensitization therapy with emulsified extracts: Its present status. In Holub, M. and Jarosková, L. (Eds.): *Mechanisms of Antibody Formation.* Czecho-Slovak Acad Sci, Prague. New York, Grune & Stratton, 1960, p. 161.
7. Feinberg, S. M., Becker, R. S., Slavin, R. G., Feinberg, A. R. and Sparks, D. B.: The sensitizing effects of emulsified pollen antigens in atopic subjects naturally sensitive to an unrelated antigen. *J Allergy, 33:* 285, 1962.
8. Holzman, R. S. and Norman, P. S.: The effect of alum concentration on the repository and adjuvant properties of alum-precipitated antigens. *J Allergy, 38:* 65, 1966.
9. International symposium on pyridine extract and alum-precipitated extract. *N Y Acad Med,* 1967.
10. Lichtenstein, L. M., Norman, P. S. and Winkenwerder, W. L.: Antibody response in ragweed hay fever: Allpyral vs whole ragweed extract. *J Allergy, 41:* 49, 1968.
11. Marsh, D. G., Lichtenstein, L. M. and Campbell, D. H.: Studies on "allergoids" prepared from naturally occurring allergens. I. Assay of allergenicity and antigenicity of formalized rye group I allergen. *Immunology, 18:* 703, 1970.
12. Norman, P. S., Winkenwerder, W. L. and Lichtenstein, L. M.: Trials of alum-precipitated pollen extracts in the treatment of hay fever. *J Allergy, 50:* 31, 1972.

Molds

1. Austwick, P. K. C.: The role of spores in allergies and mycoses in man and animals. *Colston Research Society, Bristol Symposium, 18:* 8321, 1966.
2. Bonilla-Soto, O., Rose, N. R. and Arbesman, C. E.: Allergenic molds. Antigenic and allergenic properties of *Alternaria tenuis. J Allergy, 32:* 241, 1961.
3. Cohen, J., Van Arsdel, P. P., Jr., Pasnick, I. J. and Horan, J. D.: Observations on the experimental reproduction of asthma with mold antigen. *J Allergy, 35:* 331, 1964.
4. Feinberg, S. T.: *Allergy in Practice.* Chicago, Year Bk, 1944.
5. Hyde, H. A., Richards, M. and Williams, D. A.: Allergy to mold spores. *Br Med J, 1:* 886, 1956.
6. Hyde, H. A.: Atmospheric pollen and spores in relation to allergy. *Clin Allergy, 2:* 153, 1972.
7. Ingold, C. T.: *Biology of Fungi.* Oxford, Clarenden Pr, 1961.
8. Ingold, C. T.: *Spore Liberation.* Oxford, Clarendon Pr, 1965.
9. Jones, E. A., Jr. *et al.:* Comparison of environmentally cultured molds with positive skin tests to mold antigens. *Ann Allergy, 29:* 525, 1971.
10. Magnusson, B. *et al.:* Routine patch testing, IV. *Acta Derm Venerol (Stockh), 48:* 110, 1968.
11. McGovern, J. P., McElheney, T. R. and Brown, R. M.: Airborne algae and their allergenicity. Part I. Air sampling and delineation of the problem. *Ann Allergy, 23:* 47, 1965.
12. McGovern, J. P., Hayward, T. J. and McElheney, T. R.: Airborne algae and their allergenicity. Part II. Clinical and laboratory: Multiple correlative studies with food genera. *Ann Allergy, 24:* 145, 1966.
13. Morrow, M. E., Meyer, G. H. and Prince, H. E.: A summary of airborne mold surveys. *Ann Allergy, 22:* 575, 1969.
14. Nilsby, I.: Allergy to molds in Sweden. A botanical and clinical study. *Acta Allergol, 2:* 57, 1949.
15. Penny, R. and Hughes, S.: Repeated stimulation of the reticuloendothelial system and the development of plasma cell dyscrasias. *Lancet, 1:* 77, 1970.
16. Pepys, J.: *Hypersensitivity Diseases of the Lungs Due to Fungi and Organic Dusts.* Basel, Karger, 1969.
17. Prince, H. F., Arbesman, C. E., Sellers, E. D., Petit, P. T., Brown, E. A. and Morrow, M. B.: Mold fungi in the etiology of respiratory allergic diseases. XII. Further studies with mold extracts. *Ann Allergy, 7:* 597, 1949.
18. Prince, H. E., Morrow, M. B. and Meyer, G. H.: Molds in occupational environments as causative factors in inhalant allergic diseases. *Ann Allergy, 22:* 688, 1964.
19. Prince, H. E., Talbott, G., Browning, W. H., Holman, J., Weiner, A. and Morrow, M. B.: Comparative skin tests with two stem phylum species. *Ann Allergy, 29:* 1971.
20. Prince, H. E. and Morrow, M. B.: A logical approach to mold allergy. *Ann Allergy, 27:* 79, 1969.
21. Prince, H. E. and Morrow, M. B.: Skin reaction patterns to Dematiaceous mold allergens. *Ann Allergy, 29:* 535, 1971.
22. Ripe, E.: Mold allergy, IV. A study of mold allergy in the respiratory tract. *Acta Allergol (Kbh), 21:* 370, 1966.
23. Tomsikova, A., Dura, J. and Nováčková, D.: Antikörperbildung und allergische nekrotisierende Arteriolitis im Hauttest nach Inhalation von Pilzsporen. *Med Monatsschr, 23:* 276, 1969.
24. Van der Werff, P. J.: *Mold, Fungi and Bronchial Asthma.* Springfield, Thomas, 1958.
25. Warren, William-Paul and Rose: Airborne fungi and respiratory allergy. A Montreal study. *Can Med Assoc J, 99:* 827, 1968.

Chapter 18

AUTO-ALLERGIC DISEASE

IF IMMUNITY IS the protective mechanism of the body, and "allergy" is altered reactivity of the immune mechanism, then "auto-allergy," rather than autoimmune (AA) should be the appropriate term to apply to the diseases induced by the direct interaction of the body's tissues (self) with either a sensitized lymphocyte (T-cell) or a specific antibody (auto-antibody). This definition is applicable whether the mechanism of auto-involvement proves to be increased involvement, decrease involvement or both.

The hypotheses proposed to explain the mechanism of auto-allergic disease (AAD) are:

(1) The sequestered protein
(2) Cross-reacting AD for bacteria and tissues
(3) Environmental factors
   (a) Infection
   (b) Drugs and chemicals
   (c) Trauma
(4) Genetic and Somatic factors
   (a) Burnett's theory of the "forbidden clone"
   (b) Fudenberg's concept of immunologic deficiency
(5) Breakdown of the mechanism of tolerance

1. The Sequestered Protein Concept

The mechanism by which body proteins are recognized as *self* is not explained. During the period of development when *self-recognition* is being established, some body proteins, such as lens, thyroid (thyroglobulin) and sperm are sequestered within their respective organs which prevents them from making contact with the recognition cells of the immune system to establish their identity as *self*. In later life when sequestered proteins, secondary to either infection or trauma, are released into the circulation, the lymphocytes recognize them as foreign and respond by producing specific antibodies, such as anti-thyroid, anti-lens, *etc.*, which are injurious to the specific organs.

This hypothesis has been disproved by increasing evidence of the presence in clinically healthy subjects, of antibodies to various cell constituents, such as nuclei of lymphocytes and granulocytes, gammaglobulin, smooth muscle, gastric parietal cells and adrenal cortical cells. Whittingham and his associates (1969) have reported that in a random population the percentage of apparently healthy subjects with antibody to one or more specific tissue antigens increased proportionately with age up to an incidence of more than 50 per cent in persons over sixty years.

2. Cross Reacting Antigenic Determinant (AD) For Bacteria and Tissues

This hypothesis was developed by Stevens who in 1964 associated chronic microbial infections with a number of diseases of doubtful etiology, such as rheumatic fever, glomerulonephritis and multiple sclerosis. He extended his concept of microbial etiology to auto-allergic disease on the premise that certain common bacteria possess chemical groupings which serve as antigenic determinants (AD) that are identical with chemical groupings or AD on body tissues, e.g.

basement membranes of kidney, synovial membranes and myelin sheaths of nerves.

Following an infection, the antibodies produced against the organism interact with AD on tissue to produce disease.

This concept received support from the observation of Kaplan who demonstrated a cross reactivity between AD in streptococcal antigen and cardiac muscle. The cross reactivity was supported by the fact that when rabbits are immunized with cell wall material from an A (type S) strain of streptococci, approximately 25 per cent of the rabbit sera reacts with human cardiac muscle as demonstrated by complement fixation and immunofluorescence. Following streptococcal infection, similar antibodies are found in the sera of 24 per cent of individuals with no manifestation of rheumatic fever and more than 50 per cent of patients with rheumatic fever. This is strong evidence in support of a streptococcal etiology in rheumatic fever, but the concept fails to explain the selectivity of auto-immune disease among individuals with active streptococcal infection and the presence of similar antibodies in many individuals who are apparently healthy. The theory also presumes that auto-allergic disease is caused by humoral antibodies which are damaging to tissues. Neither of these two contentions has been proved.

3. Environmental Factors

(a) Environmental factors include bacteria, various drugs, chemicals, sunlight and other forms of radiation, any one of which may alter the steric structure of the protein molecule so that it fails to be recognized as *self* and then can serve as an antigen to activate either T-cells or B-cells which leads to tissue changes manifested as AAD. The change in the molecule may result in complete denaturation of the protein or the modification may be slight but sufficient to expose a sequestered AD. It is generally recognized that infection may play an important role in the induction of AAD but only when predisposing conditions exist that permit infection to be effective.

Bacteria and viruses may become attached to body cells and serve as haptens. Many immunologists do not consider this mechanism as truly auto-allergic.

(b) Drugs and physical agents such as sunlight and other forms of radiation may activate long-standing intracellular viral infections, resulting in tissue alterations which serve as antigens to induce AAD.

Drugs and chemicals may conjugate with body proteins, resulting in steric changes in structure which expose sequestered antigenic determinants. (See Fig. 1-2 and 1-3.) Sunlight seems to facilitate such a union which explains the sudden development of systemic lupus erythematosis (SLE) in patients following sun tanning while ingesting a drug. In most of these cases, if the drug is discontinued, the process is arrested as the antigen is eliminated from the body. However, if administration of the drug is continued in the face of developing signs and symptoms, the condition may become irreversible AAD.

(c) The role of trauma in AAD is supported by the demonstration of auto-antibodies to cardiac tissue following heart surgery and infarction.

4. Genetic and Somatic Factors

Lymphocytes are constantly undergoing somatic mutations which are governed by hereditary factors and a number of environmental influences, such as infections, drugs, chemicals, sunlight and other forms of radiation.

The alterations in tissue proteins induced by genetic and somatic mutations result in the failure of the body to recognize these tissues as *self*. The tissue proteins may be completely degraded so that the entire molecule becomes antigenic, or through partial alteration in steric structure, a sequestered AD may be uncovered to become available for action upon a receptive lymphocyte.

The chemical groupings capable of cross

reacting with antibodies evoked by bacteria are part of the individual's hereditary pattern. This can explain the auto-allergic response of some individuals to infection, while others weather the assault of infection without the complication of auto-allergic disease.

The variations in both the quantity and the quality of antibodies observed between animal species and among individuals may also in great measure be attributed to alterations induced by genetic and somatic mutations. This can account for the ability of some individuals to produce a particular type of antibody as well as the ability of some individuals to manifest a good antibody response, while in others the antibody response is weak.

(a) The Forbidden Clone (Burnett)

A clone is a population of cells derived from a single cell. Under normal circumstances any newly differentiated immunocyte capable of reacting with an accessible AD on a normal body component will be destroyed soon after it is differentiated. If following differentiation an immunocyte with a receptor capable of reacting with an AD on normal tissue, i.e. forbidden cell, escapes destruction and instead proliferates, the *forbidden cell* can give rise to a *forbidden clone*. The involvement of either T or B lymphocytes by the *forbidden clone* can give rise to tissue changes manifested clinically as auto-allergic disease.

This does not mean that only a single progenitor cell develops or that the forbidden cell is the product of a single mutation. It is conceivable that several forbidden cells develop but only one escapes the surveillance mechanism. Further, it is likely, as Burnett points out, that the progenitor with the necessary qualities to produce AAD may be the product of several mutations. However, the ability to change is always governed by inherited features which explains susceptibility.

It is conceivable that secondary to infections or some other environmental agent as a drug, a number of forbidden cells are produced through the process of mutation. The number of forbidden cells produced by mutation at any given time may be beyond the capacity of the body's surveillance mechanism. If only a single cell escapes as the progenitor of a *forbidden clone,* AAD may develop. This concept could explain the occurrence of AAD in a selective group of individuals exposed to the identical environmental factor. For example:

(1) An infection or a single dose of a drug, either large or small, in an individual with the proper genetic predisposition could induce the mutation of large numbers of *forbidden cells* far beyond the surveillance capacity of the body. Only one pathogenic cell need escape to proliferate and produce AAD.

(2) Chronic infection or protracted administration of a drug could provide the environment for the constant production of *forbidden cells*. Only a single pathogenic immunocyte need escape to serve as the progenitor of a *forbidden clone*. Such events could explain the sudden appearance of AAD in individuals who have tolerated a given drug for long periods with no obvious ill effects.

(3) Burnett believes that more than a single mutation may be required before a cell acquires all the necessary qualities which permit it to emerge as the progenitor of a pathogenic or *forbidden clone*. Chronic infections or the prolonged administration of a drug could serve as the trigger for such conditions. All the events in the concept of the *forbidden clone* imply a productive or active response on the part of the newly formed cells.

(b) Immunologic Deficiency Concept of Fudenberg

Fudenberg predicates his concept on the identical genetic and somatic mutations which operate in the theory of the *forbidden clone* but with one added feature. The incidence of AAD is extremely high in individuals with immunologic deficiency disease. Agammaglobulinemic individuals manifest a high incidence of AAD. In view of these observations Fudenberg postulates that the immunologic *incompetence* associated with a deficiency disease permits the development of AAD.

Immunologic deficiency means failure of an immunologic response. For example, a bacterial antigen normally can stimulate either TD cells or B cells which eventually lead to destruction of the bacterial antigen. With immunologic deficiency no such protective response develops. In a similar manner, when a *forbidden cell* develops in an immunologically deficient individual the protective lymphocytes cannot be stimulated to destroy the *forbidden cell*. As a result, the mutant or *forbidden cell* proliferates to form a *forbidden clone* which leads to AAD. In Fudenberg's hypothesis, the *forbidden cell* is immunologically inactive (failure to induce a response), while in the clonal theory of Burnett, the *forbidden cell* is active (proliferates) and not destroyed.

Complete absence of auto-antibodies in AAD occurs when immunologic deficiency is general, while the development of AAD in the presence of an apparently normal globulin profile occurs with selective immunologic deficiency.

In the absence of immunologic competence, many microorganisms in the circulation are not destroyed and serve as a constant supply of environmental agents to induce mutations. The microorganisms, unaltered by antibody, are free to attack body tissues to which they may be specifically attracted. Tissue damage follows with the exposure of sequestered AD which interacts with competent lymphocytes to produce AAD. Organisms at times may adhere to body tissues to serve as haptens which can initiate the sequence of events that lead to AAD.

The concept of immunologic deficiencies can explain the high incidence of AAD in older individuals, particularly the aged, who have a decreased capacity to produce new types of antibodies. The aged also have a decrease in the number of lymphocytes. When a new AD appears, antibodies against it cannot be produced, resulting in survival of the mutant and proliferation which leads to AAD.

This concept fails to explain the function of auto-antibodies as observed in normal individuals or in patients with AAD. The concept implies a loss of competence which permits survival of the mutant cell, yet permits activity that destroys it.

5. Breakdown of the Mechanism of Tolerance

In neonatal life complete tolerance can be induced to any foreign substance. Beyond neonatal life tolerance to either cellular or humoral immunity can be induced but not to both. This would suggest that the protection of the individual against destruction of his own body tissues is achieved through either an alteration of the neonatal mechanism or the development of a new protective mechanism. The explanation of the behavioral pattern responsible for the protective response must await clarification of a number of fundamentals in immunology, such as:

(a) Does maternal IgG or some other factor present in the blood of the newborn influence the development of the immune mechanism postnatally?

(b) Does the lack of cortical center development in the spleen and lymph nodes of the newborn influence in any manner the mechanism of tolerance?

(c) What chemical prperties of a substance dictate whether it will be a good immunogen or a good tolerogen?

(d) What is the nature of the induction of antibody production?

(e) What is the nature of the induction process of tolerance?

(f) What is the role of auto-antibody? Are they protective or destructive?

In the interpretation of the auto-allergic mechanism, consideration must be given to both genetic and somatic mutations which are affected by both external and internal affronts. The mutations, governed by genetic and somatic factors are influenced by environmental agents, such as infection, drugs, chemicals, trauma and radiation of various types. The complete degradation of a body protein or the partial denaturation with exposure of a sequestered AD provides new antigenic stimuli which specifically activate thymus dependent (TD) lymphocytes to initiate DH or B lymphocytes for antibody production.

Whether tissue specific antibodies (auto-antibodies) are protective or injurious is still unsettled, but recent studies in tolerance and particularly the *in vitro* investigations of Diener and his associates suggest a possible answer. Diener *et al.* have demonstrated in tissue culture that low zone tolerance is antibody mediated and is dependent upon a critical ratio between antigen and antibody.

The required ratio between antigen concentration and antibody titer is still undetermined, but the following have been observed:

(a) High concentrations of antigen require higher antibody titer.

(b) Low antibody titers, such as observed with low concentration of antigens or with very weak immunogens are sufficient to induce low zone tolerance.

If these observations can be confirmed *in vivo*, they will explain several clinical observations, such as:

(c) The high incidence of AAD in immunologic deficiency diseases may result from the failure to provide the antibodies necessary for low phase tolerance.

(d) The auto-antibodies observed in healthy individuals may be required to maintain low zone tolerance which could be the mechanism for homeostasis when low grade tissue damage occurs.

(e) The increasing titers of auto-antibodies observed with aging may be necessary to provide the critical Ag-Ab ratio for low zone tolerance, the mechanism for homeostasis.

(f) Variations in titer of auto-antibodies may be related to the degree of temporary tissue damage induced by one of the environmental factors, such as infections, drugs, chemicals, *etc.* This variation is essential for maintaining the critical Ag-Ab ratio required for low zone tolerance.

(g) The sudden release of large quantities of antigen could result in the production of an antibody titer far in excess of the low concentration required for low zone tolerance. Under such conditions the antibodies could become injurious, causing tissue damage which is manifested clinically as auto-allergic disease.

For example, recent studies on the immunochemistry of collagen have demonstrated that although this protein is antigenic, it is very weakly immunogenic. Michaeli has observed that the DH induced by collagen as an antigen is accompanied by very low titers of humoral antibodies. The induction of a humoral antibody response by DH is generally recognized. This observation suggests that when collagen acts as an antigen, it induces both DH and a humoral antibody response which provides the optimal conditions for the induction of low phase tolerance. Since collagen is a weak immunogen, it is particularly adapted to the mechanism of low phase tolerance. Since collagen represents about 50 per cent of all body tissues and 70 per cent of lung tissue, it is eminently suited as a candidate for mutation by various environmental factors. The mutations could serve as weak immunogens which induce DH and auto-antibodies to establish a system of low zone tolerance which would serve to maintain the homeostasis required for the healthy individual.

Sudden severe damage to collagen could release a large amount of denatured collagen which could evoke a high titer of anti-collagen antibodies. The titer of these antibodies, above the critical level required for low zone tolerance, could result in tissue damage manifested clinically as auto-allergic disease, or in this example as collagen disease.

Types of Auto-Antibodies

Any body protein that experiences structural alterations is no longer recognized as *self*. The altered protein may serve as an antigen to evoke auto-antibodies. A variety of changes can occur in the structure of the protein molecule which can make available one or many antigenic determinants. Each antigenic determinant evokes its own specific antibody. The protein of a given organ can have an antigenic determinant specific for the organ, as, for example, kidney, skin or basement membrane. In addition, the protein molecule can have determinants which are nonspecific but are common or cross reactive with other tissues. For example, antibodies for synovial joint membranes may be found in the sera of lupus erythematosis, while thyroid auto-antibodies may be found in rheumatoid arthritis.

Because of this complex response, there are no specific profiles of the patients' sera for any auto-allergic disease. There is considerable overlapping of the pattern from one auto-allergic disease to another, but for any given patient the pattern is very distinct. This great variation and cross reaction among the sera from patients with different auto-allergic diseases makes diagnosis on an immunological basis extremely difficult and at times impossible.

The following classification represents the auto-antibodies which have been identified. It is conceivable that many other auto-antibodies occur which, although not prominent in the serological pattern, could play an important role in the production of disease.

A. Anti-nuclear Antibodies Induced by the Following Antigens

(1) Deoxyribonucleic Acid (DNA)
(2) Histone
(3) Nucleoprotein
(4) Phosphate extract—multiple components

DNA antibodies are highly specific in sera of patients with systemic lupus erthematosis (SLE). They are not always present in SLE sera but are observed more frequently following treatment of the disease with steroids. Occasionally, DNA antibodies occur in rheumatoid arthritis (RA) if the pateints have manifestations of SLE.

Antibodies to histone are found in isolated cases of SLE. When observed, they are specific.

Nucleoproteins and phosphates are found in a variety of auto-allergic conditions.

B. Anticytoplasmic Antibodies

Anticytoplasmic antibodies are difficult to demonstrate. Samples of cytoplasm are usually contaminated with nuclear components which makes the dissociation of anticytoplasmic antibodies from anti-nuclear antibodies very difficult.

Complement fixation reactions with various cytoplasmic cell fractions have indicated the presence of gammaglobulins reacting with microsomes, mitochondria and other elements.

Extracts of cytoplasm with lipid solvents are found in SLE sera, liver disease, Sjögren's syndrome, scleroderma and a variety of hyperglobulinemic states.

C. Anti-Gammaglobulin Antibodies

The presence in sera of antibodies against gammaglobulins is supported by the following physical, chemical and antigenic characteristics of IgM (19S) antibodies:

(1) characteristic sedimentation rate
(2) dissociation with mercaptoethanol

(3) cross reaction with IgG (7S) in the light (L) chain

(4) antigenic individuality in the heavy (H) chain

(5) specificity for various determinants on the IgG molecule, particularly the Gm genetic factors

The following types of anti-gammaglobulin antibodies are found in man:

(1) Antibodies to gammaglobulin genetic characters: iso-specific and auto-specific

(2) Rheumatoid factor (RF) with primary specificity for Ag-Ab complexes and aggregates of gammaglobulin.

(3) "Anti-antibodies" or Milgram's factors

(4) Antibodies to buried determinants revealed by enzymatic splitting.

1. ANTIBODIES WITH GM AND INV SPECIFICITY: It has been demonstrated that within a species, individual variants of immunoglobulins occur which have been named *allotypes* by Oudin, who was the first to demonstrate their presence in rabbits. Since Oudin's studies, it has been observed that in humans sensitized following transfusions, the sera contain antibodies specific for genetically controlled antigenic determinants on the IgG molecule. These determinants constitute the *allotypes* of the human IgG molecule.

In humans two allelic expressions have been determined: (1) the so-called "Gm locus" which governs the amino acid sequence on the F_c segment of the heavy (H) chain portion of the IgG molecule (see Figs. 1-6 through 1-10), and (2) another genetic locus has been found to determine light (L) chain structures and is termed "Inv locus."

Antibodies to the two genetic loci, the Gm and the Inv, were initially demonstrated in the sera from patients with rheumatoid arthritis, but subsequently similar antibodies have been found in a small percentage of normal individuals. The antibodies found in rheumatic sera appear quite different from others found in normal sera, and it seems probable that the mechanism by which they are produced is also different.

They have been termed "serum normal agglutinator" (SNAgg) and "rheumatoid agglutinator" (RAgg). The various Gm factors have been found in both groups, but anti-Inv antibodies have not been found in rheumatoid sera.*

2. RHEUMATOID FACTOR (RF): The exact nature of rheumatoid factor is not known. It appears that only the heavy chain fragment of the antibody molecule separated by papain digestion is involved (see Figs. 1-6 through 1-10). The form that the γ globulin molecule takes when it serves as an antigen to produce RF is not known, but two possibilities exist:

(a) Either aggregation of the IgG molecule or complexes of IgG with an antigen may serve as an antigen to react with IgG or IgM to form an aggregate with the characteristics of RF. Such aggregates may represent the IgM (19S RF) demonstrated in rheumatic sera.

(b) Small components of the antibody molecule with the exposure of sequestered AD may react with IgG to form smaller aggregates with characteristics of RF. These may represent the IgG (7S) factors observed in rheumatic sera.

For example, collagen could react with IgG or a component of IgG to form a complex which in turn reacts with either IgG or IgM to form aggregates with the characteristics of RF.

There are two types of RF recognized immunologically:

(1) Those that react with human sera.
(2) Those that react with rabbit sera.

This group is believed to be associated with reactions induced by sequestered AD.

---

* For a complete discussion of the genetic factors involved in the two groups, the reader is referred to Kunkel and Tan: Review of auto-antibodies and disease, *Adv Immunol*, 4, 1964.

The complex antibody molecules with many AD, both those on the surface and the sequestered, offer a variety of possibilities for forming the RF either through the development of complexes or aggregation of the globulin molecule. Elucidation of this problem must await increased knowledge of the behavior of proteins and greater refinements in immunological techniques.

(c) *Factors found in normal sera and those of other diseases:* Rheumatoid factors are found in normal sera as well as in the sera from patients with other diseases, such as liver disease, subacute bacterial endocarditis, parasitic disorders and some other diseases.

All normal individuals possess definite RF that can be isolated. These increase in titer with age and may represent the responses to the constant insults to body tissues and as such, perhaps serve as protective antibodies for maintaining homeostasis through tolerance.

The RF in non-rheumatoid sera is always the type that reacts with human γ globulins which differentiate them from true RF which reacts with rabbit γ globulin.

3. ANTI-γ GLOBULINS OF THE NON-RHEUMATOID TYPE (MILGRAM FACTORS): The major characteristic of RA sera and RF is the great variation in agglutination obtained with different incomplete Rh coats attached to red cells. Rh antibodies from one serum may serve as an excellent coat for one RA serum but very weak with another RA serum with identical titers for other components. Milgram described other factors, like a rabbit Coombs* serum which reacts nonselectively with all coats. These are only inhibited by γ globulin in either aggregated form or complexed with antigen. Recent studies indicate that these anti-γ glubulins represent the larger fractions of the Ab molecule separated by papain digestion.

4. ANTIBODIES TO BURIED DETERMINANTS OF γ GLOBULIN: Another anit-γ globulin has been observed in normal sera, RA and other diseases which reacts only with γ globulin that has been digested by enzymes, such as papain. Their activity is explained by the exposure of sequestered AD by the enzymatic digestion.

The incidence of this factor is reported as:
normal sera—20 per cent
subacute bacterial—43 per cent
rheumatoid arthritis—57 per cent

These anti-γ globulins are usually of the IgG (7S) variety as would be expected from their involvement with only a small portion of the antibody molecule.

D. Anti-Collagen and Anti-Elastin Antibodies

Both collagen and elastin have wide distribution in the body and together represent at least 50 per cent of cell body tissue and approximately 70 per cent of lung tissue. Current studies have demonstrated that both collagen and elastin are antigenic and weakly immunogenic. Again, organ specificity for collagen has been demonstrated by several investigators, which may explain the localization of involvement in certain diseases, such as RA, subacute bacterial endocarditis or perhaps the involvement of basement membranes in glomerulo-nephritis and SLE.

Antibodies for both collagen and elastin have been demonstrated in normal sera, while particularly high titers for anti-collagen antibodies in RA have been demonstrated by Michaeli. With the increased

---

* The Coombs test is an antiglobulin test. Univalent antibodies which are attached to RBC cannot be demonstrated by agglutination, because they do not form a lattice to precipitate. By producing an antiglobulin in rabbits by the injection of serum and then adding the rabbit antiglobulin serum to the RBC, the antibodies can be demonstrated by precipitation. The procedure is known as the Coombs test.

observations reported in the field of immunochemistry on collagen and elastin, the role of collagen as an important factor in auto-allergic diseases will be revived, and collagen disease as an entity will again receive recognition in clinical medicine.

SPECIFIC DISEASES ASSOCIATED WITH AUTO-ANTIBODIES INCLUDE:

    Rheumatoid arthritis
    Sjögren's syndrome
    Systemic lupus erythematosis
    Thyroiditis (Hashimoto's disease)
    Pernicious anemia
    Myasthenia gravis
    Scleroderma and dermatomyositis
    Pancreatic disease
    Addison's disease
    Ulcerative colitis

REFERENCES

1. Autoimmunity: Experimental and clinical aspects. *Ann N Y Acad Sci, 124:* 1.
2. Burnett, F. M.: Autoimmune disease. *Br Med J, 2:* 645, 1959.
3. Fudenberg, H. H. and Franklin, E. C.: Rheumatoid factor and the eiology or rheumatoid arthritis. *Ann N Y Acad Sci, 124:* 884, 1965.
4. Fudenberg, H. H., Good, R. A., Hitzig, W. et al.: Classification of the primary immune deficiencies: WHO recommendation. *N Engl J Med, 283:* 656, 1970.
5. McCombs, R. P.: Systemic "allergic" vasculitis: Clinical and pathological relationships. *JAMA, 194:* 1059, 1965.
6. McDevitt, H. O. and Benacerraf, B.: Genetic control of specific immune responses. *Adv Immunol, 11:* 31, 1969.
7. Natvig, J. B. and Kunkel, H. G.: Genetic markers of human immunoglobulins. The Gm and Inv system. *Ser Hematol, 165:* 66, 1968.
8. Whittingham, S. J., Irwin, I. R., Mackay, S. and Cowling, D. C.: Autoantibodies in healthy subjects. *Aust Ann Med, 18:* 130, 1969.

Chapter 19

IMMUNE DEFICIENCY STATES

by

ALAN S. LEVIN,[*] LYNN E. SPITLER,[†] H. HUGH FUDENBERG[‡]

Introduction

IMMUNE DEFICIENCY STATES have taken on greater importance in clinical allergy with the recognition that these conditions may either complicate allergic disease or occur as isolated entities which induce clinical patterns simulating allergic diseases. When an immune deficiency state complicates the allergic pattern, the resulting recurrent and persistent infections prevent successful allergy management. On the other hand, the occurrence of an immune deficiency state in a nonatopic individual may induce respiratory and dermatological disturbances which resemble true atopic involvement that can lead to error in both diagnosis and management.

Immune Deficiency States

Immune deficiency states are either congenital or acquired. The congenital immune deficiency states have been recognized since the antibiotics have come into general use. Prior to the era of antibiotics the majority of the patients with congenital immune deficiency states died of infectious diseases. The acquired immune deficiency diseases have gained prominence since the development of transplantation surgery, the use of immunosuppressant therapy and treatment of various malignant disorders with lympholytic agents.

I. Congenital Immune Deficiency States

A. DEFECTIVE CELLULAR (T-CELL) SYSTEM WITH AN INTACT HUMORAL (B-CELL) SYSTEM

1. *Thymic and parathyroid agenesis: DiGeorge Syndrome:* During embryogenesis, epithelial components derived from the third and fourth pharyngeal pouches form the upper portion of the pinna of the ear, part of the mandible, a portion of the aortic arch as well as all of the parathyroid glands and the epithelial lattice of the thymus.

Defects in the developmental stages of these embryonic components result in deficiencies of the developing organ system. One such defect is the *DiGeorge Syndrome* which is characterized by agenesis of the thymus and parathyroid glands which is commonly associated with defects in the aortic arch and characteristic mandibular, ear lobe and facial stigmata. The children with the DiGeorge syndrome commonly manifest neonatal tetany which is uncontrollable with calcium infusions, and therefore require therapy with parathyroid hormones. Following control of the hypoparathyroidism, the patients usually develop recurrent infections from which they eventually die if untreated. Patients with the Di George syn-

---

[*] Director, Laboratory of Immunology, Kaiser Foundation Research Institute, San Francisco. Adjunct Instructor, Department of Pediatrics, University of California Medical Center, San Francisco. Supported by American Cancer Society Faculty Research Award PRA-88.

[†] Assistant Professor of Medicine, University of California Medical Center, San Francisco. Supported by NIH Career Development Award I-K4-AI 43012.

[‡] Professor of Medicine, University of California Medical Center, San Francisco. Supported by NIH Grant AI 09145.

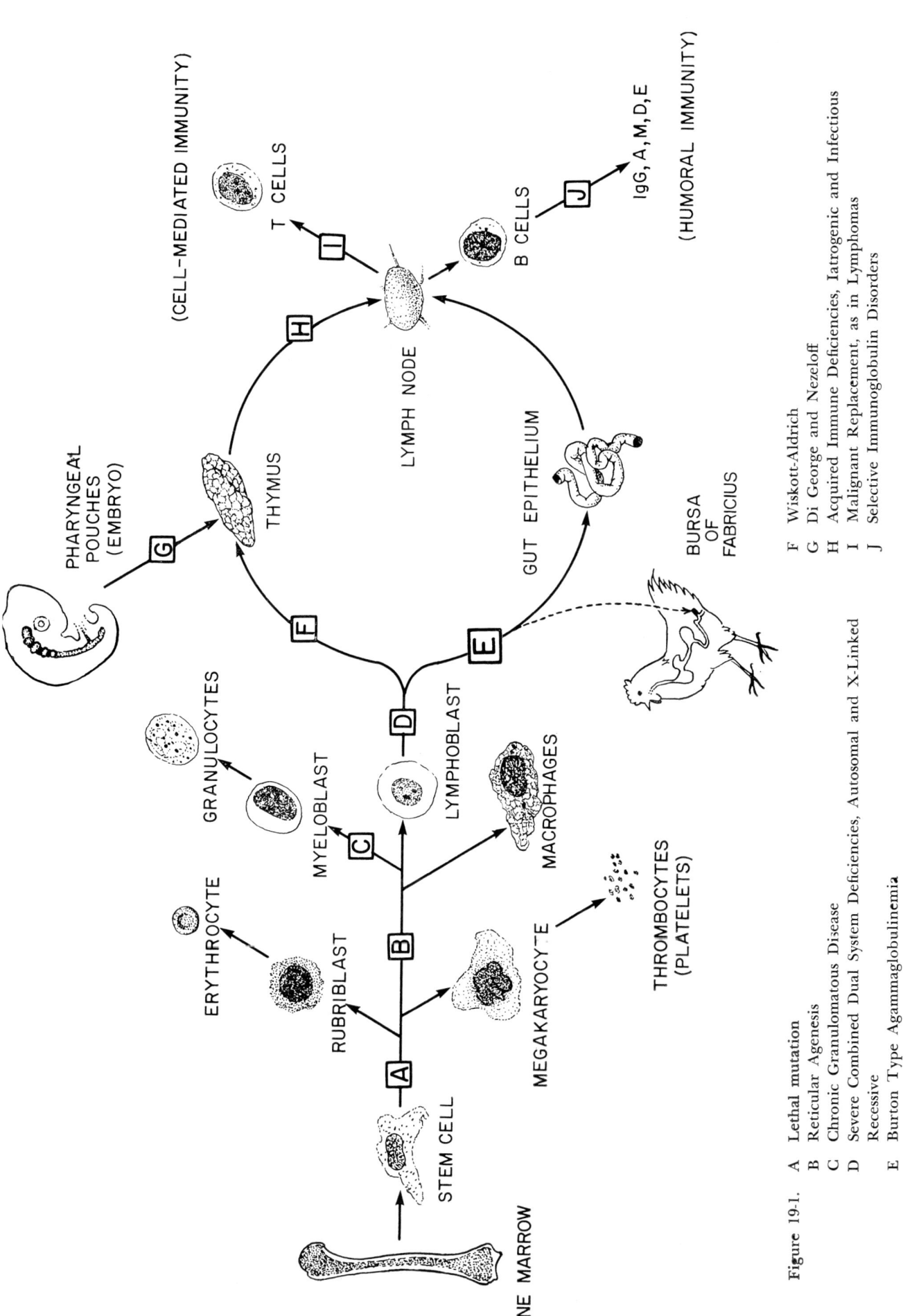

Figure 19-1.
A Lethal mutation
B Reticular Agenesis
C Chronic Granulomatous Disease
D Severe Combined Dual System Deficiencies, Autosomal and X-Linked Recessive
E Burton Type Agammaglobulinemia
F Wiskott-Aldrich
G Di George and Nezeloff
H Acquired Immune Deficiencies, Iatrogenic and Infectious
I Malignant Replacement, as in Lymphomas
J Selective Immunoglobulin Disorders

Table 19-I: CLASSIFICATION OF IMMUNE DEFICIENCY STATES

I. Congenital Immune Deficiency States.
  A. Defective Cellular (T) and Intact Humoral (B) Cell Systems.
    1. Thymic and Parathyroid Agenesis: *Di George Syndrome*.
    2. Autosomal Recessive Thymic Aplasia with Lymphopenia: *Nezeloff*.
  B. Defective Antibody Mediated (B-cell) System with Intact Cellular (T-cell) System.
    1. Infantile X-Linked Agammaglobulinemia: *Bruton*.
    2. Selective Immunoglobulin Disorders.
      (a) Selective IgA Deficiency.
      (b) Selective IgG Deficiency.
      (c) Selective IgM Deficiency.
      (d) Specific Immune Paralysis with Normal Immunoglobulin Levels.
    3. Transient Hypogammaglobulinemia of Infancy.
    4. Non-Sex Linked Primary Immunoglobulin Aberration: Adult "Acquired" Hypogammaglobulinemia.
  C. Mixed Deficiencies.
    1. Ataxia Telangiectasia.
    2. X-Linked Dual System Deficiency: *Thymic Alymphoplasia*.
    3. Autosomal Recessive Dual System Deficiency: *Swiss Type*.
    4. Variable Deficiencies.
      (a) Mucocutaneous Candidiasis.
      (b) Wiskott-Aldrich Syndrome.
  D. Granulocyte Defects.
    1. Chronic Granulomatous Disease.
    2. Job's Syndrome.
    3. Chediak-Higashi Syndrome.
II. "Acquired" Immune Deficiency States.
  A. Infectious "Acquired" Immune Deficiency States.
    1. Sarcoidosis.
    2. Tuberculosis.
    3. Coccidiomycosis.
    4. Leprosy.
  B. Malignant "Acquired" Immune Deficiency States.
    1. Carcinoma.
    2. Sarcoma.
  C. Iatrogenic Immunosuppressive Therapy.

drome have either normal or elevated serum immunoglobulin associated with a lymphopenia; however, in some cases the lymphocyte count may be normal during the first few months. In addition they have absence of skin reactivity to all antigens for delayed hypersensitivity and diminished *in vitro* parameters of cellular immunity, such as blastogenesis evoked by phytohemagglutinin and/or specific antigens. Robinson and Rosen of Boston feel that this disease may be related to some intra-uterine viral infections at some time during gestation. A large number of these patients were recognized in the northeastern section of this country during the middle 1960's; however, there have been very few new case reports from that region. These observers feel that the decrease in new cases is suggestive of an epidemic of a mutagenic virus which passed through the population of that geographical area and has dissipated itself. Several patients with this syndrome have been treated successfully with thymus transplants.

2. Autosomal Recessive Thymic Aplasia with Lymphopenia: Nezeloff: The Nezeloff syndrome appears to be a mild variation of the Di George syndrome. The patients in this group appear to have normal parathyroids and normal aortic arches; however, they do have thymic aplasia with markedly diminished T-cell systems.

B. DEFECTIVE ANTIBODY MEDIATED (B-CELL) SYSTEM VITH INTACT CELLULAR (T-CELL) SYSTEM.

1. Infantile X-linked Agammaglobulinemia: Bruton: Infantile X-linked agammaglobulinemia was first reported as a clinical entity by O. C. Bruton in 1952 when he noted a child who had recurrent infection and an abnormal immunoelectrophoresis, showing a marked absence of the gammaglobulin fractions. This is a rare X-linked disease characterized clinically by marked susceptibility to recurrent pyogenic infections, such as conjunctivitis, otitis, pneumonia, cellulitis, and gastrointestinal infections (especially *Giardia lamblia*). Laboratory findings include markedly diminished levels of all measurable immunoglobulins.

Most of these patients have small amounts of one or more classes of immunoglobulins. However, they cannot be immunized by routine antigens used to induce humoral immune responses. This implies that although they have the primordial machinery to make immune globulins, those that are made may be "nonsense immunoglobulins."* The cellular immune system in these patients appears to be generally intact. Bone marrow

---

* "Nonsense immunoglobulins" is a term which implies synthesis of immunoglobulins which manifest no known antibody activity.

aspirations show a marked paucity of mature immunoglobulin-containing plasma cells. Lymph node biopsies revealed abundant small mature lymphocytes in the pericortical and deep cortical regions with a significant absence of plasma cell and large lymphocyte-containing germinal centers.

These children also have a marked paucity of lymphoid and adenoid tissues which should raise the suspicion of the clinician that the child may not be allergic in the classical sense of the term.

Patients with this syndrome, although they have a markedly diminished humoral immune system, often manifest the clinical patterns of rheumatoid arthritis and atopic allergy.† This suggests that the rheumatoid arthritis observed in these patients may be primarily a cellular immune response. The symptoms resembling atopic allergy may be in response to a non-antibody mediated reaction such as triggered by either the properidin or plasma-kinin systems.

2. Selective Immunoglobulin Disorders

(a) SELECTIVE IgA DEFICIENCY: The most common selective immunoglobulin disorder is one in which IgA is markedly diminished or absent while the other immunoglobulins are normal. This disorder is found in one in five hundred of the population. These patients, although previously considered to be asymptomatic, have a high incidence of respiratory infections, asthma, gastrointestinal disorders of various types, and autoimmune diseases. A high frequency of anti-ruminant‡ antibodies is also seen in these patients, presumably due to the lack of the protective "blocking" activity of secretory IgA which is also diminished in these patients. Cellular immunity in these patients also appears to be reasonably intact.

(b) SELECTIVE IgG DEFICIENCY: Another selective immunoglobulin disorder involves a diminished IgG level with elevated IgM and at times elevated IgA levels. These patients suffer from recurrent pyogenic infections.

(c) SELECTIVE IgM DEFICIENCY: Selective IgM deficiencies have also been reported. These patients generally have difficulty with Gram negative organisms, since many of the protective antibodies directed against these organisms are from the IgM class.

(d) SPECIFIC IMMUNE PARALYSIS WITH NORMAL IMMNOGLOBULIN LEVELS: A new and possibly common selective immunoglobulin disorder is now being recognized at several medical centers. This involves patients with recurrent infections having "normal" levels of immunoglobulins. These patients, when investigated further, appear to have specific immune paralysis, or the inability to respond to certain selective antigenic stimuli, rendering the patient immune deficient to that pathogenic moiety. These patients will often be recognized by their failure to respond to immunization following a full dose of DPT as demonstrated by a non-immune Schick response. (See J in Figure 19-1.)

3. *The Transient Hypogammaglobulinemia of Infancy*: The normal newborn infant is endowed with adult levels of IgG derived from placental transport of maternal immunoglobulins. Maternal immunoglobulins disappear from the infant's circulation by four months of age. Endogenous synthesis of IgG begins slowly in the third semester of pregnancy and gradually builds up until the third month of age when the infant's own IgG becomes the dominant IgG protein in the circulation. The levels then rise gradually until the early teens when it plateaus at the adult level. IgM synthesis begins very late in the third trimester of pregnancy and detectable levels are often noted in cord blood.

---

† The term "atopic allergy" is used in the sense described in Chapter 1, which implies the immediate type of tissue response induced by reaginic antibody which to date is synonymous with IgE.

‡ Anti-ruminant antibodies refers to those antibodies which develop in response to the ingestion of proteins derived from ruminant animals, such as cattle.

Circulating IgA is often undetectable in the normal newborn cord blood but appears shortly after birth and rises gradually until the teenage period.

In transient hypogammaglobulinemia of infancy, the onset of endogenous synthesis of these immune globulins is retarded. These children rarely have problems before age three months and are often asymptomatic. Probably a majority of infants with this disorder escape detection since they never arouse the suspicion of the clinician. Infants with hypogammaglobulinemia in infancy and infections generally present themselves to the pediatrician between four and six months with recurrent pyogenic infections, mostly minor in nature. A routine immunoelectrophoresis usually reveals the diagnosis.

Therapy of these patients is controversial. One school of thought states that treatment with injections of IgG will reduce the recurrent infections and thereby tide the child over until endogenous synthesis begins. Another school of thought contends that no exogenous IgG should be used, since it may retard endogenous synthesis. The decision as to whether or not these patients should be treated with injections of gammaglobulin depends upon (1) the severity of the recurrent infections, and (2) the clinical discretion of the practicing physician. These children generally recover at approximately one year of age, and appear normal after that. Any child with an IgG level of less than 200 mg per cent after one year of age should be suspected of having a permanent form of hypogammaglobulinemia.

The basic defect in the disease of these children may be a result of the iso-immunization during pregnancy, e.g. maternal antibodies directed against genetic markers of the infant's own immunoglobulin (those inherited from the father) may destroy or retard the maturation of plasma cells which would eventually secrete these immunoglobulins.

4. *Non-sex Linked Primary Immunoglobulin Aberrations: Adult "Acquired" Hypogammaglobulinemia*: This disease is generally recognized in patients at the end of their second decade or through the third decade of life. It is characterized by an insidious onset of recurrent pyogenic infections. Upon routine examination, diminished or absent immunoglobulins of all classes are found. The patients apparently had normal immunoglobulin levels during infancy and childhood, since they did not develop these recurrent infections at that time. A carrier state in this disease can be recognized in relatives of these patients. As the disease progresses, this group of patients often develops lymphoreticular malignancies.

C. Mixed Deficiencies

1. *Ataxia Telangiectasia*: Ataxia telangiectasia is an autosomal recessive disease characterized clinically by a progressive familial choreoathetosis, cutaneous telangectasia and recurrent sinopulmonary infection. These patients have a high incidence of reticuloendothelial neoplasms. Laboratory findings indicate a markedly diminished serum IgA, apparently caused by a decreased synthesis of the immunoglobulin. Some patients have detectable antibodies directed against allogeneic IgA. Some patients with this disorder also have markedly diminished IgG levels. These patients have diminished cellular immunity (T-Cell systems) measured by absent skin reactivity to skin test antigens and diminished *in vitro* parameters of cellular immunity.

2. *X-Linked Dual System Deficiency: Thymic Alymphoplasia*: Patients with severe dual combined deficiency disorders generally have diminished immunoglobulin levels in all classes. Some patients with these disorders, however, may have low normal-to-normal levels of one class of immunoglobulin. These patients also have several severely deficient cellular immune systems with absent skin test reactivity and diminished *in vitro* responsiveness of lymphocytes to nonspecific mitogens, such as phytohemagglutinins and to specific antigens. These patients are gen-

erally very ill and have problems with pyogenic bacteria, viruses, fungi and microbacteria. Untreated, these patients rarely survive their early infancy.

3. *Autosomal Recessive Dual System Deficiency: Swiss Type*: Autosomal recessive alymphocytic agammaglobulinemia is clinically and pathologically very similar to the thymic alymphoplasia. The major differentiating factor is the inheritance pattern.

4. *Variable Deficiencies*

(a) MUCOCUTANEOUS CANDIDIASIS: The term "mucocutaneous candidiasis" is used to describe a broad variety of disease states, all characterized clinically by candidiasis involving the skin and mucus membranes. Defects in cellular and humoral immunity have been reported among different populations of patients. Differences in response to specific therapeutic regimes and nonspecific immunologic induction regimes have been reported. This disease has also been associated with other forms of epithelial agenesis such as cartilage, hair aplasia and fingernail aplasia.

(b) WISKOTT-ALDRICH SYNDROME: The Wiskott-Aldrich syndrome is an X-linked recessive disorder characterized by thrombocytopenia, eczema and recurrent infections. The thrombocytopenia appears to be the result of an intrinsic platelet defect, resulting in early senescence. Normal platelets injected into Wiskott-Aldrich patients have a near normal half-life, while Wiskott platelets have a shortened half-life when injected into normal subjects. Bone marrow aspirations reveal normal numbers of megakaryocytes.

The recurrent infections appear to be caused by defects in both cellular and humoral immunity. The cellular immune defects can be measured by absence of skin reactivity of the delayed type and also diminished *in vitro* parameters of cellular immunity. The humoral defect appears to be an inability to recognize certain carbohydrate antigens, which is characterized by a low level of serum IgM that is often accompanied by a compensatory elevation of serum IgA.

It has recently been reported that despite the recurrent pyogenic infections experienced by these children, the immunoglobulin levels are either normal or low normal. When compared with "normal immunity" (cystic fibrosis) and recurrent pyogenic infections, these children appear to have markedly lower levels of IgG which would indicate a possible humoral defect in the IgG fraction. It is presumed that these children are born with a normal complement of cellular immune constituents; however, because of the inability to recognize antigenic stimulation, the normal constituents atrophy which leaves the child with a nonfunctional cellular immune system (T-cell system). Our group has successfully treated a number of these patients with transfer factor.

D. GRANULOCYTE DEFECTS

1. *Chronic Granulomatous Disease*: Chronic granulomatous disease was first defined as a clinical entity in 1957. Patients with this syndrome were found to have defective bactericidal capacity of polymorphonuclear leukocytes associated with failure of respiratory bursts and subsequent H_2O_2 production following microbial ingestion. Although the precise biochemical lesion is controversial, various groups have described nucleotide adenosine diphosphate (NADH) and glucose-6-phosphate dehydrogenase defects.

Neutrophils from these patients fail to reduce nitroblue tetrazolioum dye (NBT) when stimulated by polysterene ingestion. They also have a significantly diminished intracellular bactericidal activity on *in vitro* testing. These patients suffer with recurrent pyogenic infections caused by a variety of pathogens, primarily *Staphylococcus aureus* and Gram negative bacilli and various fungi. Granulomata formed in the liver, lungs and lymph nodes are filled with lipid-laden histiocytes. The pleomorphic genetic and clinical forms of this disease have suggested the more general term, *neutrophil dysfunction syndrome,* in order to describe this heterogeneous group.

2. *Job's Syndrome*: Job's syndrome appears to be very similar in both laboratory and clinical pictures to chronic granulomatous disease but affects primarily red-headed females from Mediterranean descent. These patients suffer primarily from furunculosis, "boils," hence the name.

3. *Chediak-Higashi Syndrome*: Chediak-Higashi syndrome is a disease characterized by partial albinism and recurrent pyogenic infections. Large abnormal cytoplasmic organelles are seen in all granule-containing cells. These organelles are in the nervous system, skin, ocular pigment, epithelium, peripheral nerve, hair, adrenal and pituitary glands. These patients appear to have some lysomal defect; however, they have normal NBT and leukocyte bactericidal assays. A recent report indicates that the immunologic defects may be a quantitative defect in leukocyte intracellular bactericidal activity.

II. "Acquired" Immune Deficiency States

A. INFECTIOUS "ACQUIRED" IMMUNE DEFICIENCY STATES. Infectious "acquired" immune deficiency states manifest themselves as variable deficiencies in both humoral and cellular immunity. For the sake of brevity, we will discuss only four disease states in which "acquired" immune deficiency plays a role: (1) sarcoidosis, (2) tuberculosis, (3) coccidiomycosis, and (4) leprosy.

1. *Sarcoidosis*: Sarcoidosis is an inflammatory disease of unknown etiology characterized by the formation of non-caseating granulomas in many organs and tissues of the body. The lymphoid and hematopoietic organs and the lungs tend to be affected most serverely. The pathology of this disease is well documented in many texts. In sarcoidosis one may see the loss of normal skin test reactivity (DH) to antigens other than the sarcoid. In other words, a patient who has a positive tuberculin test before developing sarcoidosis may lose his tuberculin reactivity, as measured by skin test, blastogenesis, and MIF production.

Of significant interest is the fact that these patients, although they lose reactivity to other antigens, develop what appears to be cellular immune reactivity to the Kveim antigen (an extract of sarcoid spleen). The exact nature of this anergy (lack of reactivity) is unclear and at present still controversial; however, it is currently held that this phenomenon is a result of the patient's lymphoreticular system being overwhelmed by the sarcoidosis antigen, rendering it incapable of responding to other antigenic moieties. Patients with sarcoidosis when treated (paradoxically with immunosuppressant drugs, such as steroids) will redevelop their normal skin test reactivity, such as tuberculin and candida.

2. *Tuberculosis*: The reciprocal of the above is true with tuberculosis. During the course of the disease, patients will first develop skin test reactivity against the tuberculin antigen. If the disease becomes overwhelming, they will lose reactivity to the tuberculin antigen and may maintain reactivity to other antigens, such as candida and other fungi. As the disease progresses, however, they may lose reactivity to these other antigens also. Again, the exact biochemical basis for this phenomenon is unclear. However, it appears that the tubercle bacillus is capable of rendering those lymphoid cells responsive to them tolerant, possibly on the basis of antigen overload anergy. As the disease progresses, the broad spectrum anergy may be on the basis of total debilitation of the patient.

3. *Coccidiomycosis*: Coccidiomycosis is an infectious disease caused by *Coccidioides immitis*. The clinical disease is quite variable in severity and has cutaneous and pulmonary localization. The reader is referred to standard pathology textbooks for descriptions of

the disease state. Immunologically, one can follow the course of the disease in a patient by the loss of cellular immune responsiveness against the antigen with reciprocal increase in humoral immune activity. As the disease begins, the patient will develop skin test reactivity against the coccidioides antigen. If the disease is to progress and disseminate, one sees a gradual diminution of cellular immune responsiveness against that particular antigen with a reciprocal rise in complement fixing IgM and IgG type antibodies (directed against that antigen).

The exact relationship between these two phenomena is unclear. However, it appears to be that one of the systems of host resistance is overwhelmed; the remaining system may respond in a hyperactive way in order to overcome the overall immunologic deficit. If the patient is to recover from the disease state, a gradual return of cellular immune responsiveness with a diminution of humoral immune reactivity will be seen.

4. *Leprosy*: Leprosy is a low grade indolent infection which is caused by *Mycobacterium leprae*. Two forms of this disorder are recognized: (1) tuberculoid and (2) lepromatous. These variants reflect differences in host susceptibility to the infection.

Tuberculoid leprosy occurs in the more resistant host and is principally characterized by symmetrical, raised lesions of the skin and peripheral nodes which on biopsy appear to be granulomatous lesions. These patients classically respond on skin testing to the lepromin (Mitsuda) antigen.

In lepromatous leprosy the disease begins with a raised red rash which is symmetrical and resembles that present in the tuberculoid type. However, the rash rapidly changes to nodular lesions in the dermis (lepromata) that vary in size. This form represents a more virulent infection, and the prognosis of patients with this disease is significantly poorer than those with the tuberculoid form. These patients classically do not respond with skin test reactivity against lepromin antigen.

In lepromatous leprosy, one often observes hyperglobulinemia with large quantities of antibodies directed against *M. leprae*. In the tuberculoid form, however, the patients have normal levels of immunoglobulins with significantly lower levels of specific anti-lepra antibodies.

Immunologic reactions in infectious diseases are dependent upon (1) the virulence and pathogenicity of the invading organism, and (2) the status of host resistence at the time of invasion. It appears that in the "normal" host most slow growing low grade pathogens are generally not markedly affected by humoral immune responses against them. These organisms are generally attacked by elements of the cellular immune system. If the cellular immune system is overwhelmed, such as in antigen overload anergy, and the disease progresses, a reciprocal hyperactivity (albeit nonprotective) in the humoral immune system is often seen.

The host is protected from high grade pathogens, such as staphylococci, streptococci, and toxin-producing pathogens such as diphtheria and clostridial organisms, by the humoral immune system. Cellular immunity against these pathogens can be demonstrated, but it appears not to play a major role in host protection. In selected situations such as neutrophil dysfunction syndrome and cystic fibrosis where host cellular and humoral immunologic systems appear to be reasonably intact but some other facet of resistance is defective, virulence of these high grade pathogens may be significantly changed. The high grade pathogen which would normally be pyogenic may now change to low grade pathogenicity and be attacked by the cellular immune system, causing granuloma formation.

B. MALIGNANT "ACQUIRED" IMMUNE DEFICIENCY STATES: In certain situations such as in congenital immune deficiency states, the immune deficiency disorder may be antecedent to and possibly related to the subsequent lymphoreticular malignancy. In lymphomas and reticulum cell sarcomas a defect in cellular immunity may be apparent. This may be a result of replacement of the normal cellular immune system by tumor cells or some specific depression of normal cellular immunity.

These patients have an increased susceptibility to organisms which normally infect patients with cellular immune defects, such as *Pneumocystis* and fungal diseases. In patients with malignancies of the myeloid system, such as granulocytic leukemia, the immune deficiency appears to be a lack of normally functioning myeloid cells. These patients are susceptible to a variety of organisms but particularly the high grade pathogens, such as staphylococci and pseudomonas.

Malignant plasma cell dyscrasias appear to induce several forms of immune deficiency in the patient. The replacement of normal immunoglobulin producing plasma cells by malignant cells may reduce the normal immune responses. Tumor cells may secrete an inhibitor of the normal immune response, possibly an RNA-type molecule which can passively transfer immunosuppression into non-tumor bearing animals. This mechanism may also render the myeloma-bearing human immune deficient.

1. *Carcinoma*: In carinoma, which is a malignancy involving tissues of epithelial origin, cellular immunity appears to play a very great role. Patients with carcinomas, which on biopsy show significant inflammatory reactions with lymphocytic infiltrates around the tumor, have much better prognoses than those without reaction.

2. *Sarcoma*: Sarcomas, which are malignancies of mesothelial origin, are very interesting tumors. The experiments of the Helstroms and Morton indicated that cellular immunity plays a large role in the protection of hosts from tumor progression, and some immune globulin "blocking or enhancing" antibodies appear to enhance tumor growth.

Very detailed descriptions of these factors can be found in the latest cancer research literature.

C. IATROGENIC IMMUNOSUPPRESSIVE THERAPY

Immunosuppressive therapy has become a prominent mode of treatment for patients with allogeneic transplants, "autoimmune" disorders, and malignant disorders. Many varieties of immunodeficiencies affecting both the humoral and cellular immune systems may be seen depending upon:

(1) the drug utilized
(2) the state of host resistance of the recipient
(3) the disease state for which the drug has been used.

All variants of immune deficiency disorders can be seen in patients on immunosuppressive therapy.

EVALUATION OF IMMUNOLOGIC COMPETENCE

An example of a detailed immunologic study of competence is illustrated by the procedure practiced at the Kaiser Foundation Hospital in San Francisco, California.

Kaiser Foundation Hospital Procedure

A. Initial Evaluation

1. History and physical examination
2. Nonimmunologic status:

  Liver function: SGOT, SGPT, bilirubin, alkaline phosphatase, BSP
  Renal function: Urinalysis, BUN, creatinine clearance, Addis count,

Table 19-II: GLOSSARY

BSP	Bromsulphalein
DNCB	Dinitrochlorbenzene
GVH	Graft versus host
KLH	Keyhole limpet hemocyanin
NBT	Nitroblue tetrazolium
PHA	Phytohemagglutinin
PPD	Partial protein derivative of tuberculin
SGOT	Serum glutamic oxaloacetic transaminase
SGPT	Serum glutamic pyruvic transaminase
SK-SD	Streptokinase-streptodornase

urine culture, 24 hour urinary protein

Endocrine function: Sodium, potassium, CO_2, chloride, calcium, phosphorus, 2-hour postprandial blood sugar, protein bound iodine

3. Hematologic evaluation: complete blood count, reticulocyte count, platelet count, serum iron, total iron binding capacity, Coombs' test, prothrombin time, and bone marrow (morphologic evaluation, culture, immunofluorescence).

4. Radiologic evaluation: x-rays of chest and abdomen, tomograms of mediastinum, spleen scan.

5. Cellular immunity: *In vivo*, skin tests with candida 1:100 and 1:10 (Dermatophytin "O"® Hollister-Stier); Coccidioidin® 1:100 and 1:10 (Cutter Laboratories); Mumps® (Eli-Lilly Company); PPD® intermediate and second test strength (Merck, Sharp and Dohme); SK-SD: Varidase® 4/1 units and 40/10 units (Lederle Laboratories); Trichophytin, Dermatophytin® 1:30 (Hollister-Stier). Sensitization with DNCB when indicated. Skin graft when indicated. (See Table 19-III.)

In vitro, mitogenic response of lymphocyte cultures to PHA and specific antigens; ability to produce migration inhibitory factor (MIF).

6. Humoral immunity: Immunoglobulin levels: IgG, IgA, IgM, IgD, IgE; complement level, Schick test, serum immunoelectrophoresis; anti-thyroid, adrenal, gastric, nuclear and cytoplasm antibodies, cytotoxic antibodies, anti-platelet antibodies. Blood type and isohemagglutinin titers, anti-*Salmonella* H and O titers, immunization with oral polio (IgA response), tetanus (IgG response). Blood group A and/or B substance (carbohydrate antigen, IgM response), KLH.

7. Granulocyte function: NBT test, bacterial killing test, poly adherence to nylon fiber column.

8. Monocyte receptors for IgG and complement.

9. Platelet function (when appropriate: O_2 consumption, pyruvate kinase level, aggregation, platelet adhesiveness).

The preceding protocol is intended as a procedure for a medical center. The clinician who is confronted with a problem, such as a history of recurrent infections, which may indicate the need for an immunologic evaluation, can successfully perform preliminary studies to indicate either humoral or cellular incompetence or both.

Preliminary Evaluation of Immune Competence

1. Humoral Immunity

In routine clinical practice the level of circulating immunoglobulins of various classes is generally relied upon for the assessment of humoral immune competence. The Schick test is a valuable procedure to assess humoral immunity, since it will demonstrate whether the patient can mount an immune response against diphtheria toxoid, generally in the 7S IgG fraction.

2. Cellular Immunity*

Instructions for Skin Testing for the Evaluation of Cellular Immunity

Skin testing is an important aspect in the evaluation of patients for possible defects in cellular immunity. The observation of a positive skin test indicates the integrity of the afferent, central, and efferent limits of the cellular immune system. The keys to success in the use of these tests are:

(1) The use of the complete battery of six skin test antigens.

(2) Repetition of the tests in higher antigen concentration when the tests are negative with the intermediate strength.

(3) Careful observation and recording of the results in millimeters of erythema and induration at twenty-four and forty-eight

---

* These instructions comply with the World Health Organization recommendations pubished in *Pediatrics, 47:* 927, 1971.

hours. This will aid future observers much more than a simple recording of positive or negative.

Notes on the Antigens

There are two preparations of candida antigen available from Hollister-Stier Laboratories. One, called monilia antigen, is prepared by grinding the organism. This antigen is generally used for testing for immediate sensitivity. The other is the preparation called Dermatophytin "O" which is prepared from a culture filtrate of the organism. This is recommended for testing for delayed sensitivity. It is suggested that for uniformity of observations in these patients that the Dermatophytin "O" preparation be used. For the second strength test (1:10) it is necessary to obtain the Dermatophytin "O" from Hollister-Stier undiluted and prepare a 1:10 dilution from it.

The streptokinase-streptodornase (SK-SD) antigen is a preparation used in patients for its fibrinolytic activity. However, the preparation contains the streptococcal antigens, and, when appropriately diluted, the fibrinolytic activity is insignificant, and the antigens are ideal for skin testing. For the intermediate strength test, the preparation is diluted so that it contains 40 units of SK and 10 units of SD per milliliter. Thus the injected dose in 0.1 ml will be 4 units SK and 1 unit SD. For the second strength test the solution contains 400 units SK and 100 units SD per milliliter. If the diluted SK-SD antigen is kept in the refrigerator overnight, nonspecific reactivity will be reduced.

The antigens described all appear to be relatively stable in solution and can be kept in solution in the refrigerator for periods up to one year. This is true even of the preparation of PPD, although the package insert states it must be prepared fresh each time it is used. To prevent contamination, a solution containing phenol as a preservative is usually used in preparing the dilutions.

Technique of Testing

1. Place 0.1 ml of each intermediate strength antigen in separate labelled tuberculin syringes, with 27 gauge, one-half inch needles. Be sure all air is expressed from the needle (it holds almost 0.05 ml of air and could reduce the antigen dose by one half if not filled). If the patient has a history of strong sensitivity to any antigen, start with a lower dose of this antigen.

2. Inject the test antigen intradermally in the forearms, positioned alphabetically as illustrated in Figure 19-2. (Use different sites, such as the back or legs if the arms are affected by any skin involvement.)

3. Immediately circle the injection site with an indelible marking pencil and label with the initial of the antigen.

4. At twenty-four and forty-eight hours carefully record the results in millimeters erythema and induration on the attached sheet.

5. Repeat any negative tests, using the second strength antigens. If a test site does not show 5 mm of erythema and induration at either the twenty-four or forty-eight hour reading, the test should be repeated with the second strength antigen. Make the injections, labelling and recording in the same fashion as described above.

Table 19-III: ANTIGENS

Antigen	Trade Name	Intermed.	Strength Second.	Source
Candida	Dermatophytin "O"	1:100	1:10	Hollister-Stier Labs., Spokane, Washington
Cocci	Coccidioidin	1:100	1:10	Cutter Laboratories, Berkeley, California
Mumps	Mumps	—	—	Eli Lilly and Co., Indianapolis, Indiana
PPD	PPD	$2\mu gm/cc$	$50\mu gm/cc$	Merck, Sharp and Dohme, West Point, Pennsylvania
SK-SD	Varidase	$40\mu/10\mu$	$400\mu/100\mu$	Lederle Laboratories, American Cyanamid Co.
Trichophytin	Dermatophytin	1:30	—	Hollister-Stier Labs., Spokane, Washington

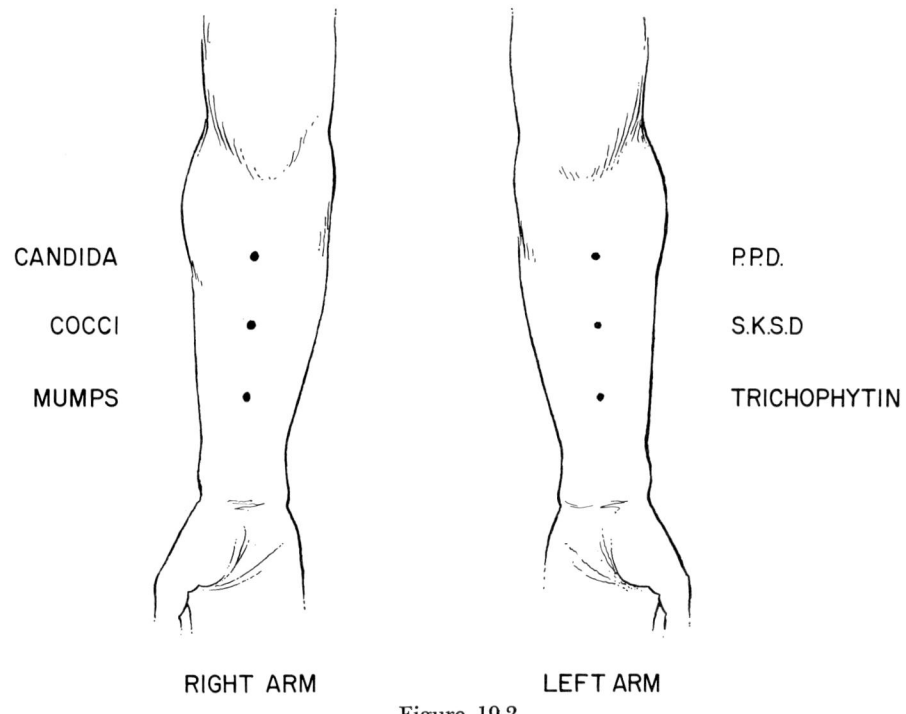

Figure 19-2

Complications of Testing

Occasionally patients who are very sensitive will have severe local reactions at the test site. These include pain, erythema, induration, and there may be blister formation and necrosis. There may be associated epitrochlear or axillary adenopathy which is usually tender. Systemic effects, such as fever, in association with skin testing have not been observed. The occurrence of severe local reactions is reduced by using the intermediate test strength antigens first (or lower strengths if the patient has a history suggesive that he may react strongly). This is followed by the second strength test only if the intermediate is negative.

Severe local reactions usually reach a peak at forty-eight to seventy-two hours, then regress rapidly. They can usually be managed by having the patient apply saline soaks three times a day. If the reaction is especially severe, it can be controlled by administering prednisone, 60 mg orally each day for two days. The prednisone is stopped immediately without tapering.

Interpretation of Results

In a large series of control subjects which have been tested with this battery of antigens, failure to react to at least one of them is exceedingly rare. Thus, if a paient does not show skin reactivity when tested as described, it is strong evidence that he probably has a defect in the cellular immune system. These patients can then be further evaluated by means of attempting sensitization with dinitrochlorbenzene (DNCB) and with *in vitro* tests such as lymphocyte stimulation and production of macrophage migration inhibitory factor (MIF).

Table 19-IV: EVALUATION OF THE PROCEDURES USED IN THE TREATMENT OF CELLULAR IMMUNE DEFECTS

Types of Materials
1. WHOLE PLASMA
2. SUB-CELLULAR COMPONENTS OF LYMPHOID CELLS
3. VIABLE WHOLE CELLS

1. WHOLE PLASMA

Advantages	Disadvantages
1. Availability	1. *Must* be leukocyte free
2. Easily collected	2. *Must* be IgA and ?IgG compatible
3. Source for IgA and IgM	3. Hepatitis
4. Easily administered	4. Does not restore cellular immune competence

2. SUB-CELLULAR COMPONENTS OF LYMPHOID CELLS

Transfer Factor

Advantages	Disadvantages
1. Induces cellular immunity without humoral response	1. Works in 50–60 per cent of patients
2. Non-antigenic	2. Laborious preparation
3. *Never* have GVH	3. Requires host cells to work
4. Need be given 2 to 3 times per year	
5. No reported untoward side effects	
6. Onset of immunity early	
7. Can be given on out-patient basis	
8. Requires minimal monitoring	

Lymphokines

Advantages	Disadvantages
1. Easily prepared	1. Immunogenic
2. May work where dialyzable Transfer Factor does not	2. Requires host cells

3. VIABLE WHOLE CELLS

Bone Marrow Transplant

Advantages	Disadvantages
1. May restore or constitute complete immune competence (humoral and cellular	1. More often fatal than curative
2. May restore or constitute normal erythropoiesis	

Peripheral Blood Leukocytes

Advantages	Disadvantages
1. May repopulate depleted lymphoid organs	1. Immunogenic
2. May partially restore cellular and humoral competence	2. Often requires host immunosuppression
3. Can be used to fight off fulminant infection or malignancy	3. Will induce GVH

Fetal Thymocytes

Advantages	Disadvantages
1. Less hazardous than above	1. Immunogenic
2. May restore partial cellular immune competence	2. GVH still possible
3. Could restore epithelial component (whole thymus)	3. Less likely to induce restoration

Salmon Technique*

Advantages	Disadvantages
1. May restore immunocompetence and hematopoietic competence without GVH	1. Still experimental and may not work

* Salmon, S. E., Mogerman, S. N., Perkins, H. A., Smith. B. A., Lehrer, R. I., and Shinefield, H. R.: Transplantation of treated lymphocytes in lymphopenic immunologic deficiency. *Am J Dis Child* 123: 111–115, 1972.

REFERENCES

1. Aldrich, R. A., Steinberg, A. G. and Campbell, D. C.: Pedigree demonstrating a sex-linked recessive condition characterized by draining ears, eczematoid dermatitis and bloody diarrhea. *Pediatrics,* 13: 133, 1954.
2. Bach, F. H., Albertini, R. J., Anderson, J. L., Joo, P. and Bortin, M. M.: Bone marrow transplantation in a patient with the Wiskott-Aldrich syndrome. *Lancet,* 11: 1364, 1968.
3. Blaese, R. M., Brown, R. S., Strober, W. and Waldmann, T. A.: The Wiskott-Aldrich syndrome. *Lancet,* 1: 1056, 1968.
4. Britton, O. C.: Agammaglobulinemia. *Pediatrics,* 9: 722, 1952.
5. Cleveland, W. W., Fogel, B. J., Brown, W. T. and Kay, H. E. M.: Foetal thymic transplant in a case of Di George's syndrome. *Lancet,* 11: 1211, 1968.
6. Cooper, M. D., Chase, H. P., Lowman, J. T., Krivit, W. and Good, R. A.: Wiskott-Aldrich syndrome. *Am J Med,* 44: 499, 1968.
7. de Konig, J., van Bekkum, D. W., Dickie, K. A., Dooren, L. J., van Rood, J. J. and Radle, J.: Transplantation of bone marrow cells and foetal thymus in an infant with lymphopoenic immunological deficiency. *Lancet,* 1: 1223, 1969.
8. Di George, A. M.: Congenital absence of thymus and its immunologic consequences: Occurrence in congenital hypoparathyroidism. In Bergsma, D. (Ed.): *Immunologic Deficiency Diseases in Man* (Birth Defects Original Article Series). New York, National Foundation, 4: 116, 1968.
9. Gatti, R. A., Meuwissen, H. J., Allen, H. D., Hong, R. and Good, R. A.: *Lancet,* 11: 1366, 1968.
10. Hill, R. L., DeLaney, R., Fellows, R. E. and Lewitz, H. E.: The evolutionary origins of immunoglobulins. *Proc Nat Acad Sci,* 56: 1762, 1966.
11. Hitzig, W. H., Kay, H. E. M. and Cottier, H.: Familial lymphopenia with agammaglobulinemia ("Swiss type of agammaglobulinemia"). Attempt of treatment by implantation of foetal thymus. *Lancet,* 11: 151, 1965.
12. Hong, R., Cooper, M. D., Allan, M. J. G., Kay, H. E. M., Meuwissen, H. and Good, R. A.: Immunological restitution in lymphopenic immunological deficiency sydrome. *Lancet,* 1: 503, 1968.
13. Kempe, C. H.: Studies in smallpox and complications of smallpox vaccination. *Pediatrics,* 26: 176, 1960.
14. Kretschmer, R., Jeannet, M., Mereu, T. R., Kretschmer, K., Winn, H., and Rosen, F. S.: Hereditary thymic dysplasia: A graft versus host reaction induced by bone marrow cells. *Pediatr Res,* 3: 34, 1969.
15. Kretschmer, R., Say, B., Brown, D. and Rosen, F.S.:

Congenital aplasia of the thymus gland (Di George's sydrome). *N Engl J Med, 279:* 1295, 1968.
16. Lawrence, H. S.: Transfer factor. *Adv Immunol, 11:* 195, 1969.
17. Lawrence, H. S.: Transfer factor and cellular immune deficiency diseases. *N Engl J Med, 283:* 411, 1970.
18. Lawrence, H. S. and Valentine, F. T.: Transfer factor and other mediators of cellular immunity. *Am J Pathol, 60:* 000, 1970.
19. Levin, A. S., Spitler, L. E., Stites, D. P. and Fudenberg, H. H.: Wiskott-Aldrich syndrome, a genetically determined cellular immunologic deficiency: Clinical and laboratory responses to therapy to transfer factor. *Proc Nat Acad Sci, 67:* 821, 1970.
20. Levin, A. S., Spitler, L. E., Stites, D. P. and Fudenberg, H. H.: Molecular intervention in genetically determined cellular immune deficiency disorders. *J Clin Invest, 50:* 59a, 1971.
21. Miller, M. E.: Thymic dysplasis (Swiss agammaglobulinemia). I. Graft versus host reaction following bone marrow transfusion. *J Pediatr, 70:* 730, 1967.
22. Nezeloff, C., Jammet, M. L., Lortholary, P., Labrune, B. and Lamy, M.: L'hypoplasie hereditaire du thymus: Sa place et sa responsabilité dans une observation d'aplaisie lymphocytaire, normalplasmocytaire et normoglobulinemie du nourrisson. *Arch Fr Pediatr, 21:* 897, 1964.
23. Rosen, F. S.: The lymphocyte and the thymus gland—congenital and hereditary abnormalities. *N Engl J Med, 279:* 643, 1968.
24. Rosen, F. S., Gotoff, S. P., Craig, J. M., Ritchie, J. and Janeway, C. A.: Further observations on Swiss type of agammaglobulinemia (alymphocytosis). *N Engl J Med, 274:* 18, 1966.
25. Rosen, F. S., Kevy, S., Merler, E., Janeway, C. A. and Gitlin, D.: Recurrent bacterial infections and dysgammaglobulinemia, deficiency of 7S gammaglobulins in presence of elevated 19S gammaglobulin. Report of two cases. *Pediatrics, 28:* 182, 1961.
26. Spitler, L. E., Levin, A. S. and Fudenberg, H. H.: In Bush, H. (Ed.): *Human Lymphocyte Transfer Factor in Methods in Cancer Research.* New York, Acad Pr, 1972.
27. Stiehm, E. R. and Fudenberg, H. H.: Serum levels of immune globulins in health and disease. *Pediatrics, 37:* 715, 1966.

INDEX

A

Aarane, see Cromolyn sodium, and DSCG
Abdominal symptoms, in migraine, 142
Acanthosis, due to scratching, 123
Acetone precipitation technique, description, 295
Acetyl cysteine, caution in bronchitis use, 251–252
Acetylcholine,
  in hornet venom, 204
  in migrainous reactions, 143
  vasodilation effect, 204
Acid-base balance, in blood, 98
Acidosis, with epinephrine fastness, 246
Acinus, description, 96
Acne, due to ACTH, 254
Acrodermatitis chronica enteropathica, characteristics, 128
ACTH, see Corticotropin
Acute allergic conditions, epinephrine's value, 245
AD, cross reacting 338–339
Adenoid, description, 56
Adenopathy, atopic dermatitis complication, 126
Adjuvant therapy, procedures, 325–329 with tables
Adolescent, contact dermatitis, 132
Adrenalin fastness, symptoms, 85
Adults,
  allergy patterns, 223
  contact dermatitis, 132
  epinephrine dosage, 245
Aerosol inhalation preparations, uses and dangers, 251–252
Aerosol sprays,
  asthmatic deaths attributed to, 246
  epinephrine, self-medication, 246–247
AFC, antibody formation role, 24
Ag-Ab,
  agglutination tests, 18–20
  definition and action, 17–20 with figs.
  demonstration techniques, 19–20
  immunoelectrophoresis, 17–18 with figs., 20 fig.
  in drug reaction, 41
  precipitation reactions, 17, 18 figs.
  role in immune action, 116
Agammaglobulinemia, infantile X-linked, 249–250

Agglutinating antibody titer, definition, 19
Agglutination tests, Ag-Ab complex, 18–20
Air: oxygen, nitrogen content, 96
Airborne allergens, in allergic reaginic conjunctivitis, 62
Airway resistance, in pulmonary function, 90
Airways, swelling, death due to, 136
Albinism, Chediak-Higashi syndrome, 353
Alcoholic beverages, accentuation, antihistamine's effects, 243
Alevaire®, evaluation for mucus liquefaction, 252
Allergen preparations, standardization, 318
Allergenic substances, skin test contraindicated, 307
Allergenic factors, check list, 337
  choice for skin tests, 305–306
  in allergic alveolitis 101 with table
Allergic alveolitis, description, 101
Allergic bronchitis, characteristics, 77
Allergic bronchopneumonia, in infants, 235
Allergic bronchial disease, "cold" remedies contraindicated, 253
Allergic bronchitis, recurrent, 79
Allergic bronchopneumonia, extrinsic, description, 101
Allergic bronchopulmonary disease, description, 101 with table
Allergic conditions, acute, epinephrine's value, 245
Allergic dermatitis,
  oral glucocorticoid treatment, 260
  types, 121–123
Allergic disease,
  ACTH not drug of choice, 253
  diagnosis, eosinophils' role, 24
  in infancy,
    clinical manifestations, 230–238
    prognosis, 232
    treatment, 231–232
  psychological factors, 189–197
  simulations, ix
  upper respiratory tract, 53–61
Allergic ear, infants, 232–233
Allergic factors, in symptoms, 193
Allergic headaches, cause and management, 139
Allergic laryngitis, diagnosis, 59–60
Allergic persons,

psychological heterogeneity, 193–194
  treatment, 195
Allergic pulmonary aspergillosis, causes, 76
Allergic reactions,
  classifications, 4
  to ACTH, 254
  to antihistamines, 243
  to triatoma bites, 202
Allergic reaginic conjunctivitis, description and treatment, 62–64
Allergic response,
  complement's role, 24, 25 fig.
  in contact dermatitis, 130–131
Allergic rhinitis,
  children, 222
  contributing factors, 54
  description, 53–55
  infants, 232
  therapy, 258
Allergic skin disease, factors in, 121–123
Allergic patterns, 220
Allergy,
  arthropods as inhalants, 211–213
  definition, 3
  differences in ingestion and inhalation, 149
  foods, symptoms, 147 table
  infants, 235–236
    acute condition management, 235–236
  immunology, 3–52 with figs.
  insect bites, 198–211 with figs.
  migraine, 192–193
  prophylaxis, in infancy, 237–238
  scope, vii
  stress response, 190–191
Allergy studies, of children, 238
Allergy symptoms, emotional precipitation, 192–193
Allotypes, immunoglobulin variants, 344
Allpyral®, see Alum-pyridine
Allyl-isopropyl, thrombocytopenia, 176
Alum precipitated extracts, evaluation, 328–329 with tables
Alum-pyridine extracts, uses, 329
Alveolar ventilation, see V_A
American Academy of Allergy, densensitization recommendations, for insect stings, 210
AMA Drug Evaluations, expectorant mixtures, 253

American Negroes,
 primaquine's effect, 172
Amino acids in molecular
 configuration, fig 8
Aminophylline,
 composition and clinical use,
  248-249
 contraindicated for children, 249
 intravenous use, serious
  reactions, 249
 side effects, 249
 status asthmaticus use, 86
Ammonium chloride, expectorant
 drug, 252-253
Amphetamine,
 addiction risk, 243
 contraindications, 144, 246
 side effects, 172
Ampicillin, reactions, 184
Amytal®, see Amobarbital, 263
Anamnestic reaction, description, 33
Anaphylactic allergy, classification, 4
Anaphylactic shock, due to
 oral ampicillin, 184
 penicillin, 182
 prick test with egg white, 151
 therapy by injection, 325
Anaphylaxis,
 antigens involved, 30
 characteristics, 29-30
 drug relationship, 177
 emergency treatment, 30
 local, characteristics, 29
 treatment, 30
 see also Systemic anaphylaxis
Anatomical dead space, see V_D
Anatomical features, lower
  respiratory tract, 71-76
  with fig.
Anemia, see Hemolytic anemia
Anergy, definition, 3
Anesthetic topical agents,
 contact dermatitis, 175
Angio-edema,
 characteristics and management, 136
 drug reaction, 173
 epinephrine and steroid therapy,
  259-260
 hereditary, characteristics, 136-137
Animal studies,
 allotypes, in rabbits, 344
 asthma conditioning, 194-195
 bronchial asthma, 81-82
 fetal sheep, homograft rejection, 229
 flea bite dermatitis, 134
 humoral antibody production, 21
 hypersensitivity to histamine, 81
 IgA in mammals' milk, 228
 reaginic type reaction, 29
 SRS-A action, 28
 thymus gland action, 23
 see also Birds

Antazoline, sedative action, 243
Antianxiety agents,
 side reactions, 265
 varieties, action and dosage,
  264-265
Antibiotics,
 allergic reaction to, 179-185
  with figs.
 moniliasis with, 172
 topical application not
  recommended, 262
 use in
  acute bronchial allergy of
   infants, 236
  infection due to dermatitis,
   133
  infection in bronchial allergy,
   83
  status asthmaticus, 86
 use limited in dermatitis, 129
Antibodies,
 anti-collagen, 345-346
 anticytoplasmic, 343
 anti-elastin, 345-346
 anti-gammaglobulin, 343-345
 antinuclear, antigens inducing, 343
 definition and classification,
  10-11 with tables
 Gm specificity, 344
 identification, technique, 17, 18 figs.
 Inv specificity, 344
 RF, 344-345
 techniques for demonstrating, 19-21
Antibody, defective, 349-351
Antibody, function, 24
Antibody forming lymphocytes,
 see AFC
Antibody molecule, papain
 treatment, 13 fig.
Antibody production, in serum
 sickness, 42-43
Antibody secretion, B-cells' action, 23
Antibody stimulating function, 40
Antibody suppression, effects of
 inducing, 41
Antigen, distribution in insect,
 205-206
Antigen-antibody complex, see
 Ag-Ab complex
Antigens,
 anaphylaxis involvement, 30
 complete, description, 5
 identification technique, 17, 18 figs.
 incomplete, description, 5-10
  with figs.
 injection treatment, 316
 preparation of mixtures, 318
 types described, 5-10 with figs.
 use in corneal allergy, 67-68
 use in sensitivity tests, 357
  with table
Antigen reactive cells, see ARC

Antihistamines,
 absorption, fate and excretion, 240
 adverse reactions, 242-243 with
  figs.
 allergic reactions, 243
 anaphylaxis therapy, 30
 blood dyscrasias, 243
 common cold medication,
  243-245 with tables
 contraindicated in
  allergic infant, 286
  bronchial involvement, 83, 245
  dermatitis, 129
  pulmonary involvement, 245
  status asthmaticus, 86
 drug sensitivity therapy, 187
 gastrointestinal side effects, 243
 hypnotic effect, 172
 ineffective in
  bronchial asthma, 245
  migraine therapy, 145
 overdose, serious effects, 243
 use in
  cold remedies, cautions, 253
  cough syrups not recommended,
   245
  upper respiratory allergic
   disease, 262
  conjunctivitis, 64
  drug and chemical allergy,
   118, 260
  fire-ants stings, 215
  hay fever, 55
  insect stings, 209, 215
  respiratory tract treatment, 60
  serum sickness, 44
  systemic anaphylaxis, 31
  treatment of mild reactions,
   325
  urticaria, 135
 value doubtful in contact
  dermatitis, 133-134
Antihistaminic preparations, names
 and dosages, 244 tables
Antipruritics,
 medications, 130
 value doubtful in contact
  dermatitis, 134
Antistine®, see Antazoline
Antitussives, contraindicated in
 bronchial allergy, 83
Anti-γ globulins, non-rheumatoid, 345
Apamin, in bee venom, 205
ARC, antibody reactive cells, 24
Art of Medicine, definition, viii-ix
Arthropods, as inhalants, 211-213
Arthus mechanism,
 in infants, 235
 in lung allergic disease, 74, 76
 role in immune reaction, 116
Arthus reaction,
 description, 4, 31-34 with fig.

diagnosis, 76
drugs' relationship, 177
food allergy, 118
in cases of
    bronchitis, 87
    corneal allergic disease, 68
    drug allergy, 173
    eyelid allergy, 66
    farmer's lung, 105
    interstitial pneumonitis, 105
    penicillin hypersensitivity, 182
    pulmonary aspergillosis,
      106–108 passim
    inflammatory nature, 42
    pathological features, 33–34
    prevented by corticosteroids, 257
    steroids in management, 260
    to food additives, 157–158
Aspergillosis, see Pulmonary aspergillosis
Aspergilloma, characteristics, 109
Aspergillus fumigatus, in human reactions, 108
Aspirin,
    buffered, toleration, 159
    nasal discharge cause, 60
    nasal polyps' association, 159
    sensitivity,
      asthma control with triamcinolone, 178
      diet restrictions, 165
      features, 178–179 with table
      identifying, 159
      nasal polyp connection, 55
      not salicylate intolerance, 179
      patient history importance, 159
      sensitivity signs, 157, 186
      tartrazine and Indomethacin involvement, 158–159 with fig.
    steroid relationship, 258
    urticaria due to, 174
    use in migraine, 144
Asthma,
    aminophylline in therapy, 249
    animal conditioning, 194–195
    attacks and emotional factors, 192
    children, 318
    constitutional reactions, 177
    cromolyn sodium therapy, 266
    deaths, aerosol sprays blamed, 247
    dependency conflict association, 192
    due to penicillin, 182
    extrinsic and intrinsic, 79–81
    in aspirin sensitivity, control with triamcinolone, 178
    May fly as cause, 211
    patients,
      dyspnea due to drugs, 172
      lung aeration variations, 100
      therapy, 99
    psychogenic association theories, 190
    psychosis association, 191
    respiratory increase, wheezing relationship, 192
    uncomplicated, pulmonary aspergillosis testing, 106
    with pulmonary eosinophilia characteristics, 106
Asthmatic bronchitis, characteristics, 77
Asthmatic patients, management, 100
Asthmatic therapy, opiates, morphine and barbiturates contraindicated, 86
Atarax®, use in
    bronchospasm, 83
    contact dermatitis, 134
    urticaria, 135
    see also hydroxyzine
Ataxia telangiectasia, characteristics, 351
Atelectasis, cause, symptoms and therapy, 87–88
Atmosphere: content and pressure, 96
Atopic allergy,
    classification, 4
    Ig E antibody involvement, 221
Atopic dermatitis,
    beyond infancy, description and management, 124
    breast-fed infants, 237–238
    characteristics, 128–129
Atopic dermatitis
    complications, adenopathy, 126
    etiology, 124–126
    in infancy, onset and course, 123–129
    management with steroids, 260
Atopic individuals, pulmonary aspergillosis, 106–107
Atopic infantile eczema, characteristics, 127
Atropine, side effects, 172
Atropine-like actions, antihistamines, 243
Atopy, characteristics, 29
Aureomycin®, see Chlortetracycline
Australia, asthma deaths, 82–83
    aerosol sprays blamed, 247
Auto-antibodies,
    diseases associated with, 346
    types, 343–346
Autosomal deficiency, Swiss type, 352

B

Bacteria
    food contamination as cause, 147
Bacterial infection, in infantile eczema, 126
Bakers, grain dust allergy, 149
Barbiturates,
    contraindicated in asthmatic, 86
    dependency danger, 83
    description and action, 263
    drawbacks in pruritus, 130
    exfoliative dermatitis relationship, 178
    inadvisable in bronchial asthma, 236
    necrosis increased by antihistamines, 243
    pruritus due to, 173
    reactions to, 174
    serum sickness relationship, 177
    side effects, 172
    use in migraine, 144
B-cells,
    animal studies, 21
    antibody formation role, 21
    T-cells as "helpers," 23
Bed bugs,
    allergic reactions, 200
    as inhalant allergen, 212
    bites' treatment, 200–201
Bee stings,
    identification, 208
    stinger removal, 208
Bee venom,
    components, 204 table
    immunoelectrophoretic pattern, 206 fig.
Behavioral disturbances, attributed to food additives, 193
Belladonna, use in migraine therapy, 144–145
Bellergal®,
    composition, 146
    use in migraine therapy, 145
Benadryl® use in
    edema therapy, 31
    serum sickness management, 44
    see also Diphenhydramine
Berger's disease, ergotamine therapy contraindicated, 144
Bermuda grass, hay fever relationship, 270
Beta-adrenergic blockade hypothesis, in bronchial allergy, 81–82
Beta-Chlor®, see Chloral betaine
Bird fanciers disease, characteristics and treatment, 109
Birds, humoral antibody production, 116
Blacks, see American Negroes
Blepharitis, characteristics and therapy, 66
Blocking antibody, properties, 313
Blood,
    acid-base balance, 98
    carbon dioxide, content, 98
    changes due to steroids, 257
    dyscrasias
      drugs' side effect, 172
      due to antihistamines, 243
    eosinophilia, in pulmonary

aspergillosis, 107
Blood oxygen, tension relationship, 97–98 with fig.
Blood vessels, Arthus reaction, 32 fig., 33
Board of Allergy, creation, vii
Body lice, allergic reactions, 200
Bone marrow, involvement in hematology, 176
Bone marrow cells, see B-cells
Boric acid, contraindicated for tub soaks, 129
Botanic library, selected for physicians, 289–290
Bradykinin, description and immunotherapy, 28
Bradypnea, side effect of drug reaction, 172
Breast feeding,
  atopic dermatitis, 237–238
  infection in, 228
Breast milk, variation due to mother's diet, 151
Breathing difficulty, muscle spasm relationship, 72
British studies, aspirin sensitivity, 179
Bromides, usefulness, 264
Bronchial allergy,
  effect on lung action, 74
  etiology, 78
  in children, 223, 235
  in infants, 233–237
    definitive treatment, 236
    diagnosis, 234
    dietary management, 236–237
    differential diagnosis, 234
    laboratory findings, 233–234
  management, 259
  mild and moderate, treatment of, 83–84
  mucus, 75
  pathology in infants, 233
  symptoms and signs in infants, 233
  thiopental contraindicated, 263
Bronchial asthma,
  aerosol medication dangers, 251
  airway resistance, 90
  characteristics, 77–78
  characteristics and deaths due to, 82–83
  description and patient classification, 99
  effect on lung action, 74
  epinephrine therapy, 245
  etiology, 78
  food reaction, 147
  in children, 223
  khellin in therapy, 265
  local anaphylaxis, 29
  management, 259
  muscle spasm, 75
  severe involvement, treatment, 84

SRS-A relationship, 28
  symptoms and therapy, 77–78
  term's inaccuracy, 72
  thiopental contraindicated, 263
  water as expectorant, 251
  VC exceeds FVC, 93
Bronchial disease,
  allergic, pulmonary function, 99–101
  asymptomatic patient, 99–101
Bronchial involvement, antihistamines contraindicated, 245
Bronchial secretions, eosinophils' presence, 24
Bronchial tree, allergic disease,
  beta-adrenergic blockade hypothesis, 81–82
  characteristics, 76–82
  complications, 82–88
  extreme involvement, 77–78
  infectious agents, 78–81 with figs.
  status asthmaticus, 82–83
Bronchial tree disease, "cold" remedy mixtures contraindicated, 253
Bronchiectasis, bacterial infection's role, 81
Bronchiolar lesions, in interstitial pneumonitis, 104
Bronchiolitis,
  asthma following, 235
  in infants, diagnosis, 235
Bronchitis,
  chronic,
    emulsion repository therapy contraindicated, 327
    VC exceeds FVC, 93
  clinical patterns, therapy, 86–87
  in infants, diagnosis, 235
Bronchodilator,
  aid to asthma patients, 99
  use in status asthmaticus, 86
Bronchopneumonia, in infants, 78
Bronchospasm, drugs to counteract, 83
Buckwheat, skin test hazardous, 149
"Buffalo hump," due to glucocorticoids, 254
Buffered glycerol extracting fluid, preparation, 292–293
Bursa cells, see B-cells
Butabarbital sodium (Butisol sodium®, dosage, 263
Butterflies, stinging hairs, 211

C

Caddis fly, as allergy cause, 211
Cafergot®, composition, 146
Cafergot P-B®, composition, 146
Caffeine, use in migraine therapy, 144
California juniper, hay fever relationship, 269

California poppy, see Eschscholtzia
Cankers, therapy, 118
Cantharides, effects on schizophrenics, 191
Carbon dioxide,
  acid base balance relationship, 98
  blood content and action, 98
  see also CO_2
Carcinoma, immune deficiency relationship, 355
Cardiac arrest,
  corticosteroids' relationship, 257
  in status asthmaticus, 82
Cardiac arrhythmias, due to corticosteroids, 257
Cardiac disease, serum sickness relationship, 43
Case history, urticaria attributed to food additives, 193
Cataracts,
  due to corticosteroids, 257
  in eczema patients, 127
Cat flea, bites' characteristics, 199
Caterpillars, stinging hairs, 211
CO_2 retention, variance in patient, 100
C' activating sites, fig. 15
Cell mediated reaction, description, 3–4
Cellular elements, immunological competence role, 20–24 with fig.
Cellular immune reaction, classification, 4
Cellular immunity evaluation, immunologic competence, 356
Cellular immunity in fetus, 228–229
Cellular immunity, skin tests in evaluation, 356–357
Central nervous system, corticosteroids' effect on, 257
Cephalosporins, toxicity, 181
Cereal-free diet, for adults and infants, 168
Cerebral symptoms, in allergic headaches, 140
Cerebrospinal fluid, IgE antibodies not present, 17
CF, description and procedure, 26
Chediak-Higashi syndrome, albinism, infections characteristics, 353
Cheese,
  dangers in penicillin sensitivity, 163
  penicillin content, 183
Chemicals,
  food reactions, 147
  gastrointestinal allergy, diagnosis and management, 117, 118
Chest x-rays, infants, in Heiner's syndrome diagnosis, 235
Chickenpox and other viral infections, 126

Children,
  adenoid facies, 56
  allergic bronchitis, recurrent, 79
  allergic involvement of nasopharynx, 58
  allergy patterns, 222–223, 238
  aminophylline therapy contraindicated, 249
  amobarbital dosage, 263
  antihistamine therapy, overdosage dangers, 243
  asthma, 318
  atelectasis, 88
  behavior and allergy, 221
  boys, hypogonadism, 65
  bronchial allergy, 88
    infection complication, 83
    management, 259
  butabarbital sodium dosage, 263
  chlordiazepoxide dosage, 264
  chronic bronchitis infrequent, 87
  conjunctivitis, diagnosis, 64
  contact dermatitis, 132
  cyanosis in asthma, 101
  dermatitis, steroid therapy contraindicated, 130
  diazepam dosage, 265
  environmental role, 224, 315
  epinephrine dosage, 245, 246
  expectorant medication, 252
  food allergy, 148, 150
  growth retardation, due to glucocorticoids, 254
  hay fever, 313
  hydroxyzine dosage, 265
  hyperactivity due to food additives, 193
  immunoglobulin deficiency, 350
  infections, Wiskott-Aldrich syndrome, 352
  insect bite reactions, 198
  laryngitis, recurrent, 222–223
  lower respiratory tract involvement, 223
  malocclusion, allergy connection, 222
  meprobamate dosage, 265
  nasal obstruction, 55
  pentobarbital dosage, caution with allergy, 263
  phenobarbital dosage, 263
  prick test, toleration good, 300
  recurrent otitis, 222
  scratch test procedure, 299
  secobarbital dosage, caution with allergy, 263
  serous otitis, recurrent, 163
  sinus development, 57
  skin manifestations, 223
  skin tests, 308
  steroids, not recommended with respiratory allergy, 259
  syrup of ipecac not recommended, 253
  tension fatigue, 222
  tension fatigue syndrome, 221
  upper respiratory symptoms, 222
  vernal conjunctivitis, 65
Chloral betaine, action and dosage, 264
Chloral hydrate, relatively safe, action and dosage, 263–264
Chlordiazepoxide, dosage, 264
Chlorothiazides, thrombocytopenia association, 176
Chlorpheniramine, see Chlor-Trimeton®
Chlorpheniramine, sedative action, 243
Chlortetracycline, reactions to, 184
Chlor-Trimeton®, use in systemic anaphylaxis, 31
Chocolate, sensitivity to, 152–153
Choledyl, see Oxtriphylline
Choline theophylline, see Oxtriphylline
Cholinergic urticaria, cause and treatment, 135
Choroiditis, diagnosis, 69
Chronic bronchitis, diagnosis, 69
Chronic reaginic-atopic conjunctivitis, characteristics, 63
Chronic symptoms, causes, 224
Chronic tissue changes, in immediate reactivity, 28–30
Ciba, see Esidrix®
Cinchonism, with quinine, 171
Circulation disturbances, ergotamine therapy contraindicated, 144
Clara cells, mucus source, 75
Classifications, allergic reactions, 4
Climacterium, effect on symptoms, 224
Climatic regions, plant growth relationship, 269
Clinical allergy, patterns and examination, 220–225
Clinical application, TF of Lawrence, 37
Clinical considerations, gastrointestinal allergy, 116–117
Clinical immunology, scope, vii
Clinical pattern, infection's influence, 322
Clinical program, environmental control, 314–316
Clone, see Forbidden clone
Coca's solution, description and drawback, 293
Coccidioidomycosis, characteristics, 354
Codeine,
  contraindicated in migraine, 144
  side effects, 172
Coeliac disease, in infants, 231
Coffee, use in migraine therapy, 144
Cold remedies, evaluation as expectorants, 253

Colic,
  gastrointestinal allergy symptom, 230
  in infants, due to soy milk, 237
Colors, artificial, elimination in salicylate-free diet, 165
Common cold, antihistamine use, 243–245 with table
Complement, description and functions, 24–25 with fig.
Complement fixation reaction, see CF
Complete antigens, see Antigens, complete
Compresses,
  therapy in contact dermatitis, 130, 133
Congenital ichthyosis, not allergic, 122
Conjunctivitis,
  allergic, diagnosis, 63
  atopic reaginic, 62–64
  chronic reaginic-atopic, 63, 64
  contact dermatitis, causes and diagnosis, 66–67
  follicular, characteristics, 64
  vernal, characteristics and symptoms, 64–65
Consciousness, alterations in, 140
Constipation in infants, gastrointestinal allergy symptoms, 230
Contact dermatitis,
  animal studies, 134
  characteristics and treatment, 127, 130–132
  due to drugs, 172, 175
  factors inducing, 126
  in children, adolescents, and adults, 132
  in infants, 131–132
  patch testing, 132
  prophylactic treatment, 134
Contact dermatitis and conjunctivitis, causes and diagnosis, 66–67
Control test, technique, 307–308
Convulsions, due to antihistamines, 243
Cor pulmonale, in farmer's lung, 104
Corn, sources, 152 table, 153
Corn-free diet, foods eliminated, 167
Cornea,
  allergic disease, characteristics, 67–68
  allergy, types and symptoms, 68
Coronary dilator, khellin, 265
Coronary disease, ergotamine therapy contraindicated, 144
Corticosteroids,
  adverse effects, 257
  choice in therapy, 260–262 with table
  ophthalmic preparations, cautions, 262
  production and types, 254
  relative potencies, 261 table

use in
  bird fanciers' disease, 109
  bronchial asthma, 84
  conjunctivitis, 64
  drug sensitivity, 187
  eye allergies, 69
  eyelid allergy, 66
  farmer's lung, 104, 105
  fire-ants stings, 215
  food allergy control, 118
  hay fever, 60
  phlyctenules, 66
  pulmonary aspergillosis, 108
  status asthmaticus, 86
Corticotropin, action and disadvantages, 253–254
Co-seasonal therapy, risk, 324
Cosmetics, involvement in conjunctivitis, 67
Cough,
  in bronchial tree allergy, 76, 77
  in infants, bronchial allergy symptom, 233
  persistent in farmer's lung, 104
  severe in atelectasis, 88
Cough mixtures,
  inadvisable in bronchial allergy, 83
  not recommended in infant's allergy, 236
  with antihistamines, not recommended, 245
Council for International Organization of Medical Sciences, drug reaction symposium, 171
Cramping, food reaction, 147
Cromolyn sodium, clinical studies, 265–267
Cross reaction,
  bacteria and tissues, 338–339
  insect stings, 206
Croup, in allergic children, 222–223
Ctenocephalides canis, see Dog flea
Ctenocephalides felis felis, see Cat flea
Cutaneous anaphylaxis, skin test reaction, 29
Cyanosis,
  causes and indications, 100–101
  due to fire-ant sting, 215
  in farmer's lung, 104
  in infants, bronchial allergy symptom, 233
  in moldy hay allergy, 103, 104
  in status asthmaticus, 82, 101
  oxygen administration helpful, 31, 84
Cystic fibrosis in infants, 231
  diagnosis, 234
Cytolytic immune reaction, classification, 4
Cytolytic response, description and management, 40–44

Cytotoxic immune reaction, classification, 4
Cytotoxic response, description and management, 40–44

D

"Dandruff," seborrheic dermatitis, 128
Death,
  due to
    angio-edema, 136
    antihistamine overdose, 243
    serum sickness relationship, 43
Declomycin®, see Dimethylchlortetracycline
Definitive treatment, bronchial allergies of infants, 236
Dehydration,
  in adrenalin fastness, 85
  treatment for, 85
Delayed hypersensitivity, see DH
Delayed immune reaction, alternate names, 4
Delayed reaction,
  food allergy, 148
  skin tissue response, 122
Dental malocclusion, due to adenoid obstruction, 56–57
Dependency, danger with barbiturates, 83
Depot corticosteroids, contraindicated in status asthmaticus, 86
Depot penicillin, description and hazards, 183–184 with tables
Depot penicillin, vaculitis relationship, 177
Dermatitis,
  definition, types and treatment, 121–137
  in infants, 221
  plants' involvement, 133
Dermatological conditions, eosinophilia observed, 24
Dermatological preparations, steroids, dangers, 262
Dermographia,
  in aspirin sensitivity history, 136
  skin test evaluation, 307–308
Dermographism,
  characteristics, 135–136
  presence in penicillin disease history, 136
Desensitization,
  definition, 291
  procedure for penicillin, 183
Dexamethasone, in anaphylaxis, 31
DH,
  characteristics in insect bite allergy, 198, 199
  description and therapy, 34–40 with figs.

experimental induction, 34
  farmer's lung relationship, 105
  impaired, TF therapy, 37
  in bronchopulmonary disease, 101
  mediators participating in, 36
Diabetes, aggravation by glucocorticoids, 254
Diagnosis,
  allergic patient, 221
  aspirin sensitivity awareness essential, 179
  bronchial allergy in infants, 234
  bronchitis in infants, 235
  conjunctivitis, 63
  contact dermatitis, 131
  cystic fibrosis in infants, 235
  dermatitis due to poison plants, 133
  drug sensitivity, 185–186
  farmer's lung, 105
  gastrointestinal allergy in infants, 231
  history's importance, 220
  physical examination's importance, 225
  triatoma bite, 203
Diagnostic features, eosinophils, 24
Diarrhea,
  immune deficiency relationship, 116
  in infants
    coeliac disease, 231
    gastrointestinal allergy symptoms, 230
    Heiner's syndrome, 235
    immune deficiency disorders, 231
    soy milk reaction, 237
Diazepam, dosage, 265
Diet, see Elimination diet
Diet diary,
  procedure, value in food management, 164–165
Diet management,
  inhalant factors, 163–164
  of infants with bronchial allergies, 236–237
DiGeorge syndrome, characteristics, 347–348
Digitalis, sensitization, 171
Dilantin®, see Hydantoins
Dimethylchlortetracycline, adverse reactions, 184
Dipalmitoyl Lecithin (DPL), 90
Diphenhydramine, sedative action, 243
  see also Benadryl®
Diphtheria antitoxin, use for treatment, 42
Disaccharidase deficiency, in infants, 231
Disaccharide intolerance, food reaction, 147
Disodium cromoglycate, action, 266
  see also DSCG

Diuretics, use in migraine, 145
Dizziness, in migraine, 142
Doctor-patient relationship, viii
Dog flea, bites' characteristics, 199
Dopamine, in bee venom, 204
Dornavac®, see Pancreatic dornase
Dosage, role in drug allergy, 172
Drakeol, emulsion respository therapy, 326
Drivers, warning of antihistaminic effects needed, 243
Drowsiness, due to antihistamines, 240, 243
Drug allergy, antihistamines in therapy, 260
Drug reactions,
  allergic, immunology and mechanism, 172-173
  ampicillian, 184
  anaphylaxis, 184
  antibiotics, allergy, 178-185 with figs.
  aspirin sensitivity, 178-179 with table
  clinical manifestations,
    generalized involvement, 174-175 with tables
    photosensitivity, 175 with table
    skin, 173-174
  corticosteroid therapy, 187
  depot penicillin, 183-184 with tables
  description, 41
  disease simulation, 171
  exfoliative dermatitis, 177
  hematological manifestations, 175-176
  hemolytic anemia, 176-177
  histamine release, 172
  idiosyncracy, 172
  interactions, 171
  interference with enzyme system, 172
  intolerance, 171
  macrolides, 185
  overdosage, 171
  penicillin hypersensitivity, 182-183
    diagnosis of, 183
  excretion prevention in renal disease, 171
  secondary effects, 172
  sensitivity diagnosis, 185-186
  serum sickness syndrome, 177
  side effects, 172
  streptomycin, 185
  sulfonamides, 185
  tetracyclines, 184-185
  thrombocytopenia, 176
  vasculitis, 177
Drug sensitivity,
  tests for and treatment, 187
  urticaria due to, antihistamine therapy, 187
Drugs,
  auto-allergy, 339
  gastrointestinal allergy,
    diagnosis and management, 118
    disease relationship, 117
  interactions in allergy, 173
  use in allergic disease therapy, 240-267, with tables
  see also specific drugs
DSCG,
  description and action, 266
  synthesis, 265
Dust,
  commercial extracts, 296
  differentiation from dirt, 296
Dust extracts, preparation and problems, 296-297
Dyspnea,
  bronchial asthma cardinal feature, 78
  drugs' side effect, 172
  in atelectasis, 87-88
  in bronchial tree allergy, 76-77
  in emphysema, 88
  in farmer's lung, 104
  in infants, bronchial allergy symptom, 233

E

Ear drum, see Tympanic membrane
Ecology, factors governing plant growth, 269-270
Eczema,
  cataract development association, 127
  description, 121
  infantile, onset and course, 123-129
  respiratory allergy symptoms, 124
Edema,
  bronchial tree, due to histamine, 76
  control, antihistamine use, 30
  counteraction measures, 31
  due to glucocorticoids, 254-257
  effect on tonsils, 56
  forces affecting, 89-90
  in lung, effect, 74
  in nasal allergies, 54
EEG studies, migraine, 143-144
Egg albumin, animal studies, 82, 194
Egg allergies, skin tests contraindicated, 117, 149, 151, 163, 307
Egg-free diet, eliminated foods listed, 166-167, 169
Egg sensitivity, chicken non-tolerance relationship, 152
Egg white,
  animal studies, 82, 194
  experimental studies, 194
  in glazing chocolate, 153
  reaction, 163
  skin test hazardous, 117, 149, 151, 163, 307
  see also Albumin, and Egg albumin
Egg yolk, intolerance in infants, 238
Ig E antibody, in atopic allergy, 221
Elastic recoil, in expiration, 89
Electrical theories, of migraine, 143-144
Elimination diet,
  additions possible in two months, 164
  aid in diagnosis and allergy management, 118
  bakery goods selection, 165
  cereals permitted, 165
  guidelines for prescribing, 162
  improvement within 10-14 days usual, 164
  in management of urticaria, 135
  infants, 237
  meat selection, 165
  procedure for, 162-165
  salad dressing preparation, 165
Elixophyllin,
  composition and dosage, 249
  use in bronchial asthma therapy, 84
Embryo, immunity development deficiency, 347
Emergency situation, status asthmaticus, 85
Emergency treatment, hymenoptera stings, 208
Emotional disturbances, involvement in urticaria questioned, 135
Emotional precipitation, allergic symptoms, 192-193
Emphysema,
  airway resistance and FEV, 99
  bacterial infection's role, 81
  description, 88
  emulsion repository therapy contraindicated, 327
  VC exceeds FVC, 93
Emulsion repository therapy, advantages and disadvantages, 326-328 with tables
Encephalitis, infantile eczema complication, 126
England,
  asthmatic deaths, aerosol sprays blamed, 247
  disodium cromoglycate studies, 266
  DSCG synthesis, 265
Environment,
  effect on infants' allergies, 238
  factor in status asthmaticus, 85
Environmental changes, role in patients' complaints, 224
Environmental control,
  importance and procedures, 314-316
  mold allergy, 333
Environmental factors,
  auto-allergy, 339

extraction technique, 294–295
gastrointestinal allergy, 117
Enzyme deficiency,
  drug overdose relationship, 171
  food reactions, 147
  gastrointestinal disease relationship, 116
Enzyme system, drugs' interference with, 172
Eosinophil chemotactic factor, 24
Eosinophils,
  diagnostic importance, 24
  in conjunctival secretions, 65
Ephedrine,
  counteraction of antihistamine's effects, 243
  effectiveness limited, 246
  in infants' acute allergic conditions, 236
  use in bronchospasm, 83
Epinephrine,
  action and dosage, 245–246
  use in
    anaphylaxis treatment, 30
    bronchial asthma therapy, 84
    serum sickness management, 43–44
    status asthmaticus, 85
    systemic anaphylaxis, 30–31
Epinephrine fastness, danger and correction, 246
Epinephrine-HCl,
  asthma therapy, 90
  dosage, 77
  use in
    acute allergic conditions of infants, 236
    emergency treatment of hymenoptera stings, 208
    therapy in fire-ant stings, 215
    treatment of reactions, 325
Equanil®, see Meprobamate
Ergotamine,
  contraindications to use, 144
  preparations available, 146
  side effects, 145
  use and caution in migraine, 144, 145
ERV, definition, 91 with fig.
Erythroblastosis fetalis, Rh antibody as cause, 40
Eschscholtzia, recognition, 269
Esidrix®, reaction to tartrazine, 157
Esophagram, diagnostic value in infants' wheezing, 234
Ether-in-oil, rectal administration in status asthmaticus, 86
Etiology, pulmonary aspergillosis, 106
Eustachian tube, description and allergic involvement, 57–58
Evaluation, immunologic competence, 355–359 with tables
Exercise, response in diagnosis, asymptomatic bronchial disease, 99
Exfoliative dermatitis, description and drug relationship, 178
Exocrine IgA, see IgA
Expectorant drugs,
  aerosol inhalation preparations, 251–252
  ammonium chloride, 252-253
  description and varieties, 250–253
  glycerol guaiacolate, 253
  mixtures, drawbacks, 253
  potassium iodide, 83, 252
  sodium iodide, 252
  steam inhalation, 251
  syrup of hydriodic acid, 252
  syrup of ipecac, 253
  use in status asthmaticus, 86
  varieties and actions, 251–253
  water by mouth or IV
"Experimental asthma," animal studies, 194
Expiration, muscle relaxation, 89
Expiratory reserve volume, see ERV
Extract mixtures, preparation, 318
Extracts, allergenic, preparation, 291–298
Extrinsic asthma, identification, 80
Extrinsic materials, examples, 3
Eye allergies, 62–70
  management, 69
Eye conditions, corticosteroid therapy cautions, 262
Eyelids,
  margins' involvement, 66
  reaginic-atopic involvement, 66
Eyes, swelling due to fire-ant sting, 215

F

Facial appearance, in migraine headache, 141
Familial tendency,
  angio-edema, 136
  atopic allergic disease, 125, 128
  disaccharidase deficiency, 163
  infantile eczema, 127
  migraine, 139
  vernal conjunctivitis, 65
  see also Heredity
Familial history,
  cystic fibrosis, 231
  IgE, 29
  immune deficiency disorder, 231
  milk intolerance, 162–163
Farmer's lung,
  Arthus type reaction, 105
  chronic phase, 104, 105
  clinical description, 101–105 with figs.
  delayed hypersensitivity relationship, 76
  diagnosis, 105
  histopathology, 104
  immunology, 105
  treatment, 105
Fat accumulation, due to glucocorticoids, 254
Fauces, description, 57
FCA (Freund's Complete Adjuvant) in DH, 34
FDA, Food report, 154
FEF, in respiration, 92 figs.
FES, measurements, 93 with fig.
Fetus,
  cellular immunity, 228–229
  homograft rejection possible, 229
  immune response, 227
  see also Neonatal life
FEV,
  in asthmatic subjects, 99
  in emphysema, 99
  normal adult values, 93
  normalization by corticosteroids, 108
Fever, due to fire-ant sting, 215
Fibrosis, in pulmonary aspergillosis, 107
Fingers, clubbing in farmer's lung, 104
Fire-ants' painful sting, 213–215
  anaphylaxis danger, 213
  signs and symptoms, 214–215 with table
  treatment, 215 with table
Fish, skin test hazardous, 117, 149
Fixed drug reaction, characteristics, 174
Flatulence, food reaction, 147
Flavors, artificial, elimination in salicylate-free diet, 165
Flea bites,
  allergic response, 198–199
  hyposensitization, 200
  infection due to, 199–200
  preventive measures, 134
  treatment, 199–200
Fluid retention, in migraine, 142
Follicular conjunctivitis, characteristics, 64
Food additives,
  behavioral disturbances attributed to, 193
  children's hyperactivity relationship, 193
  gastrointestinal disease relationship, 117
  see also Food chemicals

Food allergy,
  management by elimination, 162
  reactions, changes with age, 237
  skin tests' dangers, 149
Food chemicals,
  stabilizers, 154–156 with table
  varieties, 153–160 with tables
Food colors, 156–157 with tables
  red, Russians' adverse reports, 156
  yellow tartrazine, adverse responses, 156–157 with table
Food flavors, 156–157 with table
Food fragments, sensitivity induced by, 163
Food intolerance, in infants, treatment and prognosis, 231–232
Food sensitivity,
  as cause of urticaria, 135
  environmental factors, 315
Foods,
  adverse reactions to, 147–153
  allergies, diseases and symptoms, 147 table
  allergenic extract preparation, 298
  antibodies to, 150–153 with table
  colors and flavors, 157–158
  identification of those causing reaction, 148
  involvement in allergic reaginic conjunctivitis, 62
  gum content, 297–298
  penicillin contaminants, 174
  role in gastrointestinal allergy, 117–118
  skin tests, cautions, 148–150
Forbidden clone, auto-allergy, 340
Foreign body, in infant, wheezing cause, 234
Foreign substance, definition, 3
Fractures in osteoporosis, due to glucocorticoid therapy, 257
FRC,
  definition, 91 with fig.
  increase in asthma patients, 99
Freund's Complete Adjuvant, see FCA
Fruit-free diet, Rowe diet, 168
Functional residual capacity, see FRC
Fungal diseases, immune deficiency relationship, 355
Fungal infections, corticosteroids' relationship, 257
FVC, 92 fig.
  description, 93, with fig.

G

GALT,
  antibody production, 116
  function, 21
GALT system, allergic disease, 56
Gastric symptoms, due to corticosteroids, 257
Gastrointestinal allergy,
  drugs and chemicals, diagnosis and management, 118
  environmentals and molds, 117
  etiological agents, 117–118
  foods involved, 117–118
  immunological considerations, 116
  in infants, diagnosis, and differential diagnosis, 230–231
  pollens' involvement, 117
  role in drug reactions, 172
Gastrointestinal disturbances, in infancy, 221
Gastrointestinal side effects, with antihistamines, 243
Genetic component, in DH, 34
Genetic factors,
  auto-allergy, 339–340
  drug hypersensitivity, 172
  see also Familial, and Hereditary
Geographical distribution, plants, 274
Glaucoma, due to corticosteroids, 257
Glucocorticoids,
  actions, 254–257 with figs.
  antiinflammatory, dosage difficulties, 261
  choice in therapy, 260–262 with table
  dosage schedule, 258 with table
  duration of treatment, 261
  intravenous, not preferred method, 261
Glycerol guaiacolate, dosage and side effects, 253
Glucose-6-phosphate deficiency, oxidant drug susceptibility, 176
Glucose-6-phosphate dehydrogenase deficiency,
  drug sensitivity, 176–177
Grain dust allergy, bakers' experience, 149
Granulocyte defects, characteristics, 352–353
Granulocyte function evaluation, immunologic competence, 356
Granulocytic leukemia, in immune deficiency, 355
Granulomatous disease, chronic, characteristics, 352–353
GRAS,
  food approval, 154
  saccharin removed from list, 160
Grasses, pollens, 274
  see also United States grasses
Great Britain, asthma deaths, 82–83

Gums,
  derivations and geographic origins, 297–298
  in foods, allergic symptoms due to, 155–156 with table
Gut Associated Lymphoid Tissue, see GALT

H

Hairs, contaminants, in epidermal extracts, 294-295
Hallucinations, varieties, 140
Haptens,
  action, 10 fig.
  auto allergy, 339
  role in
    drug reactions, 172, 173, 176, 181, 182, 185
    food additive reaction, 157–158
    food allergies, 160, 163
    insect bite allergy, 198, 200
  term's derivation and meaning, 5
  see also Antigens, incomplete
Hay fever,
  California juniper relationship, 269
  description, 53–55
  emotional factors, 192
  eye involvement, 62–63
  in children, 222
  local anaphylaxis, 29
  plants causing, 270
  seasonal, treatment, 60
  steroid therapy, indications for, 259
Hay mold, allergic symptoms due to, 103
Headaches,
  allergic, cause and management, 139, 221
  aura characteristics, 140
  prodromal symptoms, 140
Hearing, eustachian tube's role, 57
Heart failure in infants, bronchial allergy symptom, 233
Heiner's syndrome in infants, diagnosis, 235
Helium dilution method, breath measurement, 96
"Helper" T cells, action, 21–23
Hematologic evaluation, immunologic competence, 356
Hematological manifestations, bone marrow involvement, 175–176
Hemogram,
  eosinophils in bronchial allergy, 234
  in diagnosis of infants' immunological disorders, 235
Hemolytic anemia,
  drug relationship, 176–177

penicillin therapy as cause, 40–41
Rh antibody as cause, 40
Henderson-Hasselbach equation, blood CO_2 relationship to pH, 98
Hereditary angio-edema, characteristics and familial aspects, 136–137
Hereditary component, in DH, 34
Heretary predisposition, IgE, 29
Heredity in,
  allergic disease, 220
  infant allergies, 229
  see also Familial, and Genetic
Heterogeneity of antigens description, 9 fig.
Histamine,
  actions induced by, 26–28 with fig.
  as cause of
    urticaria, 135
    lung edema, 76
  effect on
    bronchial tree, 76
    lung action, 74
    schizophrenics and controls, 191
  in bee venom, 204
  in migraine, 143
  release due to drugs, 172
  skin response to, 16
"Histamine headaches," description, 143
Histiocytosis X, see Letterer-Siwe syndrome
Histopathology, of farmer's lung, 104
History,
  accuracy important, 186
  importance in diagnosis and management, 220
    allergic laryngitis, 59
    infants with wheezing, 234
  in penicillin sensitivity diagnosis, 183
House dust,
  extracts often unreliable, 296
  mites present, 297
Homogeneity of antigens description, 9 fig.
Homograft rejection, in infants, 229
Hornet venom, acetylcholine content, 204
House fly, as contaminants carrier, 212
Hypogonadism, boys, in vernal conjunctivitis, 65
Human flea, bites' characteristics, 199
Humoral immunity evaluation, Schick test use, 356
Humoral response, definition and classes, 4

Hyaluronidase in bee venom, action, 205
Hydantoins, side effect, 172
Hydration, in acute allergies of infants, 235–236
Hydroxyzine,
  dosage, 265
  use in urticaria, 135
Hymenoptera,
  antigens potent, 209–210
  emergency treatment, 203
  injection schedule, 210
  venoms, 203–207 with tables
Hymenoptera stings,
  avoidance procedures, 211
  clinical patterns, 207
  diagnosis and identification, 208
  emergency kit use, 211
  emergency treatment, 208
Hyperglycemia, due to glucocorticoids, 254
Hyperkeratosis,
  description, 122
  due to scratching skin, 123
Hyperplasia, due to scratching, 123
Hypersensitivity,
  chronic, tissue changes, 28–30
  delayed,
    diagnosis difficulty, 125
    lymphocytes' role, 21
    monocytes action, 23
  immediate, description, 26–31
  immediate or delayed, 101
  intermediate, 31–34 with fig.
Hypertension, hostility conflict association, 192
Hypoergy, definition, 3
Hypogammaglobulinemia,
  diagnosis, immunoelectrophoresis, 351
  infants, 350–351
Hyposensitization,
  explanation of term, 291
  protection delay, 210–211
  stings of insects, 209
Hypotension, management, 31
Hypoxemia,
  sedatives contraindicated, 86
  studies, 100

I

Iatrogenic immunosuppressive therapy, considerations, 355
Ice packs, use in migraine therapy, 145
I. D. tests, technique, 302–305 with figs.
IgA antibodies, in pulmonary aspergillosis, 107
  presence in cornea, 68

IgA, defense against infection, 116
  deficiency, immunoglobulin disorder, 350
  in ataxia telangiectasia, 351
  description and action, 11–12 with table
  function undetermined, 12 with fig., 17
  in mother's milk, 228
  infant's production, 228
  role, 21
  tears' content, 63
IgD, description, 11 with tabl., 12
  in rectal muscosa, 116
  role in immunity action, 116
IgE, allergens' stimulation, 317
  antibodies, combination with specific antigens, 26
  in pulmonary aspergillosis, 106, 107, 108
  increase in atopic skins, 125
  skin test reaction, 307
  cell responsiveness influence, 314
  characteristics, 11 with fig., 16–17
IgE, familial predisposition, 29
  formation and action, 17
  in serum disease
  in atopic dermatitis, 128
  pollen extract measurement, 294
  role, 21
  in allergy, 116
  in bronchial allergy, 78
  in immunity action, 116
  in nasal allergies, 53
  skin tests, 318
IgE antibodies, in penicillin hypersensitivity, 182
  in reaginic allergic disease, 312
  role in allergies, 213
  mite specificity, 297
IgG, Arthus reaction association, 31
  description and functions, 11 with tabl., 12, with fig., 17
  in drug reactions, 41
  fetus, 227
  in gastrointestinal mucosa, 116
  in infants, 228
  in lung allergy disease, 76
  in neonate, 228
  in penicillin hypersensitivity, 183
  in serum disease, 42
  model of molecule, 13 with fig.
  production by plasma cells, 21
  role in immune action, 116
  antibodies, in coccidiomycosis, 354
    in farmer's lung, 105
    in mold allergy, 334
    presence in cornea, 68
    in pulmonary aspergillosis, 107, 108

deficiency, immunoglobulin
    disorder, 350
  in ataxia telangiectasia, 351
immunoglobins, production of, 312
  titers, antigen injection
    relationship, 323
IgM, Arthus reaction association, 31
  description and function, 11 with
    tabl., 12
  functions, 12 with fig., 17
  in drug reactions, 41
  in fetus, 227
  in gastrointestinal mucosa, 116
  neonate's lack, 228
  production, 21
  role in immune action, 116
  antibodies, in coccidioidomycosis,
    354
    in fetus, 227
    in pulmonary aspergillosis, 107
  deficiency, immunoglobulin
    disorder, 350
  Wiskott-Aldrich syndrome, 352
Immediate reaction, chronic tissue
    changes, 28-30
  food allergy, 148
  foods allergy, skin tests hazardous,
    149
  skin response, 122
  types, 4
Immune defects, relationship to
    gastrointestinal disturbances,
    116
  treatment, evaluation, 359 with
    tabl.
Immune deficiency, "acquired,"
    353-354
  classifications, 349 with tabl.
  congenital, defective cellular
    system, 347-349 with tabl.
    intact humoral system, 347-349
      with tabl.
  defective antibody, 349-351
  in infants, 231
Immune paralysis, description, 350
Immune reaction, immediate and
    delayed types, 4
  in fetus, 227
  in infants, 227
  lymphocytes involved, 21
  types, ix
  variations, vii
Immune system, types of response, 3
Immunity, definition, 3
  see also viral immunity
Immuno-autoradiography, Ag-Ab
    demonstrating, 20
Immunoelectrophoresis, Ag-Ab
    complex, 17-18 with fig., 20
    with fig.
  diagnosis of
    hypogammaglobulinemia, 351

Immunofluorescent staining, Ag-Ab
    demonstrating, 19
Immunogenicity, characteristics, 5
Immunogens, definition and
    description, 4-5
Immunoglobulin, deficiencies,
    disorders, 349
  disorders, mixed deficiencies, 351-
    352
    granulocyte defects, 352-353
    IgA deficiency, 350
    IgG deficiency, 350
    IgM deficiency, 350
Immunohematology, description, 40-
    41
Immunological competence, cellular
    elements, role, 20-24 with fig.
  evaluation, 355-359 with tabl.
  evaluation, preliminary steps,
    356-359 with tabl.
  testing, complications, 358
    results' interpretation, 358
    techniques, 357
  thymosin's role, 23
Immunological deficiency, auto-
    allergy, 340-341
Immunological disorders, in infants,
    diagnosis, 235
Immunological responses,
    classifications, 3-4
Immunological tolerance, mechanisms
    involved, 41
Immunology, in farmer's lung, 105
  of allergy, 3-52 with figs.
Immunotherapy, ix-x
  connotation of term, 291
  efficacy, 312-314
  fire-ants, 215
  in respiratory system allergies, 60
  principles, 312-314
Incomplete antigens, see Antigens,
    incomplete
Increased permeability factor, see IPF
Indian meal moth, as allergy cause,
    212
Indomethacin, as nasal discharge
    cause, 60
Infants, agammaglobulinemia, 349-350
  allergy, 227-239
    clinical manifestations, 230-238
    disease, ear, 232-233
    environment's relationship, 238
    management, 235-236
    patterns, 221-222
    treatment, 231-232
    rhinitis, 232
    acute condition, 235-236
  asthma, allergic, 78
  atopic dermatitis, onset and
    course, 123-129

  breast-fed, atopic dermatitis less,
    237-238
  bronchial allergy, 233-237
    definitive treatment, 236
    diagnosis, 234
    dietary management, 236-237
    laboratory findings, 233-234
    pathology, 233
    skin tests unreliable, 236
    symptoms and signs, 233
  bronchial asthma, acute, antibiotics
    in therapy, 236
    differential diagnosis, 234
  bronchiolitis, diagnosis, 235
  bronchitis, diagnosis, 235
  cereal-free Rowe diet, 168
  coeliac disease, 231
  contact dermatitis, 131-132
  cows' milk as source of allergy, 229
  cystic fibrosis, 231
    diagnosis, 234
  disaccharidase deficiency, 231
  eczema, complications, adenopathy,
    126
    complications, infection, 126-127
    misdiagnosis possibility, 125
    onset and course, 123-129
    varieties, 127-128
  elimination diet, 237
  environmental factors, as
    allergens, 229
  feeding disturbance, 221
  intolerance, treatment and
    prognosis, 231-232
  gastrointestinal allergy, diagnosis, 231
    differential diagnosis, 231
    symptoms, 230-231
  Heiner's syndrome, diagnosis, 235
  homograft rejection, 229
  hypogammaglobulinemia, 350-351
  immune disorders, deficiency, 231
    diagnosis, 235
  immune response, 228
  infection, factor in allergy, 230
  meat base formula, 237
  milk intolerance, 162
  milk substitute, 237
  nasal obstruction, 55
  prophylaxis of allergy, 237-238
  respiratory allergic disease, 232
  skin, response to irritation, 122, 123
  thymic alymphoplasia, 352
  tracheoesophageal fistula,
    diagnosis, 234
  undigested food as allergens, 229
  vomiting, 231
    forceful, 231
  see also Newborn
Infection, allergy factor, in
    infancy, 230
  Chediak-Higashi syndrome, 353
  clinical pattern influenced, 322

chronic infection in auto-allergy, 340
complication in brochial allergy, 83
defense against IgA's role, 12
due to Di George syndrome, 347
early studies, 3
foci, emulsion repository therapy excluded, 327
in status asthmaticus intravenous therapy, 85
infantile eczema complication, 126–127
influence on allergic reactions, 81
patterns induced by, 78–81 with figs.
recurrent, granulomatous disease, 352
in agammaglobulinemia, 349
in Wiskott-Aldrich syndrome, 352
treatment of, 129–130
Infectious agents, affecting bronchial tree, 78–81
Infectious diseases, effect on bronchial tree, 78, 79 with fig.
Inflammatory process, glucocorticoids' effect, 257
Inflammatory tissue response, in Arthus reaction, 31
Inhalant factors in diet management, 163–164
Inheritance, autosomal deficiency, 352
Injectable products, corticosteroids, clinical use not recommended, 261
Injection therapy, constitutional reactions, 325
dosage schedule, 320–324
duration, 324–325
evaluation, 313
initial injection, 320
intervals between treatments, 322–323
procedure, 316
technique and evaluation, 312-329 with table
Insect Allergy Committee, desensitization recommendations, 210
surveys on insect stings, 209
Insect bites, allergic response, 198–211 with figs.
sensitivity to, tests for, 209–211
treatment, 199–200, 200–203
Insect repellant, thiamine chloride, 199
Insect stings, antihistamine and steroids in therapy, 209
clinical patterns, delayed reaction, 207

cross reactivity, 206
hyposensitization, 209
sensitivity, densensitization procedure, 209–211
skin tests, 206–27
tourniquet use, 208–209
Inspiration, muscle action, 89
Inspiratory capacity, 91
Intal®, see DSCG
Intermediate hypersensitivity, see Hypersensitivity, intermediate
Intermediate immune response, classification, 4
Intermediate reactions, skin lesions, 122
Intermediate type allergic reaction, IgG's action, 12
Interstitial inflammatory changes, characteristics and treatment, 104–105
Interstitial pneumonitis, characteristics and treatment, 104–105
vascular lesions, 104–105
Intracutaneous tests, see I. D. tests
Intradermal tests, see I. D. tests
Intravascular reaction, description, 40–41
Intravascular transfusion reaction, description, 40
Intravenous fluids, use in bronchial asthma therapy, 84
Intravenous therapy, in status asthmaticus, 85
Intrinsic asthma, characteristics, 80–81
IgE increase not demonstrated, 81
Intrinsic materials, examples, 3
Iodides, not recommended, 83
Ipecac, see Syrup of ipecac
Increased Permeability Factor, description, 40
Iridocyclitis, signs and symptoms, 69
Irritant contact dermatitis, description and treatment, 130
Ischemia, danger in systemic anaphylaxis, 31
Isoproterenol, asthma therapy, 90
dosage in status asthmaticus, 86
limited use in bronchial asthma, 246
Isuprel®, see Isoproterenol
Itching, control, antihistamine use, 30
due to flea bites, control measures, 199
in eye allergy, 63
in seborrheic dermatitis, 128
in skin allergy, 122
scratching due to, 123
treatment of, 130
see also Pruritus

J

Jaundice, phenothiazine side effect, 172
Job's syndrome, characteristics, 353
Joints, swelling, due to penicillin, 174
Journal of Allergy, name change, vii
Journal of Allergy and Clinical Immunology, name change, vii
Junipers, differentiation, 269

K

Kaiser Foundation Hospital, Allergy Department, patients' primary complaints, 117
immunologic competence, evaluation, 355–356 with tabl.
allergy techniques, 297
Kaposi's varicelliform infection, in infantile eczema, 126
Keflin®, see Cephalosporins
Keratinocytes, response to irritants, 122–123
Keratitis, characteristics and cause, 67
KFH-PMG, injection procedure program, 316
KFH-PMG, mold allergy treatment, 332–333
techniques, 291
Khellin, description and action, 265
KI, see Potassium iodide
Kinin, wasp venom, action, 205
Kinins, clinical picture resembling anaphylaxis, 30
"Kissing Bug" bites, reaction, 202

L

Laboratory procedures, in status asthmaticus, 85–86
Laboratory tests, respiratory tract allergy diagnosis, 60
Laryngeal edema, management of, 31
Laryngitis, in children, 22–23
Leiner's disease, not allergic, 122
seborrheic dermatitis, in severe form, 127
Leprosy, characteristics, 354
Letterer-Siwe syndrome, characteristics, 127–128
Levarterenol, action in alpha receptors, 246
Librium®, see Chlordiazepoxide
Lice, treatment of bites, 200
Lichenification, description, 122
due to scratching skin, 123
Lichen simplex chronicus, see Neurodermatitis
Ligand, definition, 10
Lingual tonsils, location, 56
Lips, allergic symptoms, 118
Liver extract, anaphylactic reaction, 177

Lower respiratory tract, allergy
disease, sedative therapy, 263
allergic diseases, 71–115 with figs.
anatomical features, 71–76 with figs.
involvement in children, 223
pathophysiology, 71–76 with figs.
LTF, description and actions, 37–40
with figs.
Lung, allergic tissue reactions, 74
cartilaginous portion, characteristics,
71–72
collapse of, blood diversion
resulting, 97
damage of, in pulmonary
aspergillosis, 108
edema in, 74
fibromuscular segment, 72–75 with
tabl.
gas exchange segment, 75–76 with
fig.
mucus production, 74–75
parenchyma disease in, "cold"
remedy mixtures
contraindicated, 253
segments, 71
smooth muscle spasm, 74, 75
smooth muscle tonus, factors
governing, 74
ventilatory portion, 96–99 with figs.
volume, subdivisions of, 90–91
with fig.
Lymph nodes, enlargement, infection
indication, 60
Lymphocyte transforming factor,
See LTF
Lymphocytes, description and
function, 20–23 with fig.
Lymphocytopoietic factors, thymosin,
23
Lymphoid tissues, antibody
production, 116
Lymphopenia, thymic aplasia, 349
Lymphoreticular malignancy, cellular
immunity deficiency, 355
Lymphotoxin, action, 40
Lysergic acid, butanolamide, use and
caution in migraine therapy,
143, 145–146

M

Macrolides, toxicity variance, 185
Maculo-papular eruptions, in drug
reactions, 174
Malabsorption, immune deficiency
relationship, 116
Malignant immune deficiency
characteristics, 354–355
Management, of serum sickness, 43–44
Mannitol, sweetener, 160
Manure, as allergy sources, 212
Marax®, content, dependence
danger, 250
use in bronchospasm, 83
Mast cell degranulating, see MCD
Mast cells, types and function
Maturation rate, thymosin's role, 23
Maximal breathing capacity, see MBC
May fly, asthma cause
MBC, definition, 93
MBD, relation to food additives, 194
MCD peptide, in bee venom, 205
Meat, milk sensitivity relationship,
152
sensitivities, 152
Mecholyl®, psychotic patient's
reaction, 191
Mediators, antibody function, 24–26
with fig.
Medication, in acute allergic
conditions of infants, 236
Medicine, definition, vii
Medihaler-Ergotamine®, migraine
therapy preparation, 146
Megaloblastic anemia, drugs side
effect, 172
Melittin, effects, 204
in bee venom, 204
Menarche, effect on symptoms, 224
Menses, influence of, 322
Mephyton, side effect, 172
Meprobamate, dosage, 265
Meprobamate suppositories, therapy
in nausea, 145
Mesantoin®, see Mephytoin
Metabolic breakdown, role in drug
allergy, 172
Methicillin toxicity, 181
Methoxyphenamine hydrochloride,
tolerated better than ephedrin,
246–247
Methylphenidate, counteraction of
antihistamine's effect, 243
Methyl prednisolone, dosage, 261
with tabl.
Methyl xanthines, use in
bronchospasm, 83
Methysergide, use and cautions in
migraine therapy, 143, 145–146
Mexican bean weevil, role in allergy,
212
Microorganisms, IgM's role against, 12
Middle ear, allergic involvement, 58
Migraine, abdominal symptoms, 142
allergy theory, 142–145
characteristics, 139–140
chemical theory, 143
diagnosis important, ix
distribution, 140–141
duration, 141
drugs in therapy, 143
electrical theories, 143–144
etiology, 142–146
fluid retention, 142
nausea, 141
facial appearance, 141
intensity, 141
mechanism, theories, 142–144
nasal symptoms, 142
relief measures, 141
therapy, 143
treatment, 144–146
ocular symptoms, 142
vasomotor theory, 143
composition, 146
Migration inhibiting factor, see MIF
Milk, see also breast milk
allergy, 150–151
antibodies for, 150
beef sensitivity relationship, 152
casein, whey differences, 151
dangers in penicillin sensitivity, 163
food allergy in infancy, 229
intolerance, family history, 162–163
in infants, 162
penicillin contamination, 151
penicillin content, 183
substitutes for, 151
substitutes for in elimination
diets, 237
Milk fractions, skin tests unreliable,
151
Milk-free diet, eliminated foods
listed, 166
foods to be avoided, 169–170
Mill dust, role in allergy, 212
Miltown®, see Meprobamate
Mineralocorticoids, action, 254
MIF, in injection therapy, 312
Minimine, in bee venom, 205
Mites, in house dust, 297
role in allergy, 213
Mold allergy, antigens and antibodies,
330–331
immunology, 330
incidence, 329–330
management, 333–334
skin test reactions, 331–332 with
tabl.
treatment with antigens, 332–333
Mold-free diet, foods to be avoided,
167
Molds, airborne, botanical
relationships, 331 tabl.
gastrointestinal allergy, 117
Moniliasis, with oral antibiotic
therapy, 172
Monocyte receptors evaluation,
immunologic competence, 356
Monocytes, description and action,
23–24
Mood, changes in, 140
Morphine, contraindicated, in asthma,
86
in migraine, 144
side effects, 172
Mosquitoes, allergic reaction, 200

Mosquito bites, treatment, 200
Moths, stinging hairs, 211
Mouth breathing in children, 222
Mucocutaneous candidiasis, characteristics, 352
Mucomyst®, see Acetyl cysteine
Mucosal tests, use and varieties, 311–312
Muscle spasm, in bronchial asthma, 78
  in bronchial tree allergic disease, 77
  in lung, 74
Muscle weakness, due to corticosteroids, 257
  in farmer's lung, 104
  induced by SRS-A, 76, 85
Mucus, in lung, effects of, 74
Mull-Soy®, milk substitute, 237
Mushroom fly, as inhalant allergy source, 212
Myalgia of legs, allergy symptom, 221
Mycobacterium leprai, leprosy caused by, 354

N

Nausea, due to fire-ant sting, 215
  in migraine headache, 141
  therapy in migraine, 145
Nasal decongestants, allergy treatment, 60
Nasal discharge, allergy indications, 60
Nasal obstruction, in allergic rhinitis, 54–55
Nasal polyposis, aspirin sensitivity relationship, 163
  salicylate free diet indicated, 163
Nasal polyps, aspirin association, 159
  description and diagnosis, 55–56
  due to aspirin, 178
  therapy, 258
Nasal secretions, eosinophils' presence, 24
Nasal snuffles, in infancy, 221
Nasal sprays, contraindicated in allergy treatment, 60
Nasal symptoms, in migraine, 142
Nasal tests, technique, 311
Nembutal®, see Pentobarbital
Negroes, see American Negroes
Neonatal life, tolerance to foreign substance, 341
Neonatal thymectomy, cell mediated reactions prevented, 21
Neo-Mull-Soy®, milk substitute, 237
Neonate, see Infants, Newborn
Neo-Synephrine®, use in conjunctivitis, 64
Neurodermatitis, description, 128–129
Neuroses, association with allergic asthma, 190
Newborn, BCG response, 229
  inducing immunological tolerance, 41
  IgM appearance, 12
  immune response, 228
  sensitization, 229
New York Academy of Sciences Conference, decision on terms "acidosis" and "alkalosis," 100
Nezeloff syndrome, description, 349
Nitrogen clearance method, breath measurement, 96
Nonallergic dermatitis, description and treatment, 130
Nonatopic subjects, in pulmonary aspergillosis, 108
Non-barbiturates, comparison and dosage, 263–264
Noncatecholamines, amphetamine, not indicated in clinical allergy, 246
  ephedrine, effectiveness limited, 246
  methoxyphenamine hydrochloride, usefulness, 246–247
Nonimmunologic mechanisms, feed reactions, 147
Noninfectious agents, bronchial allergy relationship, 81–82
Nonmedical chemicals, reactions confused with drugs, 171
Noon units, pollen measurement, 293
Noradrenalin, in bee venom, 204
Norepinephrine®, see Levarterenol
Norinyl, reaction due to tartrazine, 157
Nose, allergic diseases, 53–56
  histology, 53
  involvement in allergic headaches, 139
  itching, in children, 222
Nummular dermatitis, characteristics, 129
Nuts, skin test hazardous, 149

O

Older persons, chronic pulmonary disease common, 81
Ophthalmic preparations with corticosteroids, cautions, 262
Ophthalmic test, technique, 312
Ophthalmologist, consultation with in eye allergy, 69
Opiates, avoidance in pruritus, 130
  contraindicated in asthmatic conditions, 86
Oranges, penicillin contaminating, 163
Orthopnea, in farmer's lung, 104
Orthoxine®, see Methoxyphenamine hydrochloride
Osteoporosis, due to glucocorticoid therapy, 257
Otic preparations, steroids not recommended, 262
Otitis, recurrent, in children, 222
Oxazepam, dosage, 265
Oxtriphylline, description, 249–250
  theophylline mixtures, varieties and disadvantages, 250
Oxygen, cautions in status asthmaticus, 86
  need in exertion, 88–89
  requirement at rest, 96–97
Oxygen therapy, helpful in cyanosis, 84
Oxytetracycline, reaction to, 184

P

Palate, description, 57
Pancreatic dornase, evaluation for asthma, 252
Papain, treatment's effect on antibody, 13 fig.
Papaya, sensitivity to, 152
Paraldehyde, action and dosage, 264
Parasitic infestations, eosinophilia observed, 24
Parathyroid agenesis, characteristics, 347
Patch tests, contraindications for, 311
  in contact dermatitis, 132
  technique and risks, 310
Pathological features, Arthus reaction, 33–34
Pathophysiology, of lower respiratory tract, 71–76 with fig.
Patients, see also Allergic patients
  age, corticosteroid therapy duration, 261
  allergy, hereditary, 220
  bronchial disease, 99–101
  changes affecting allergy, 224–225
  clinical allergy, chief complaint, 223–225
    adult patterns, 223
    childhood patterns, 22–23
    infancy patterns, 221–222
    patterns, 220–225
    physical examination, 224
    tension fatigue syndrome, 221
  cooperation essential, vii–ix
  diagnosis of allergy, 221
  history, value in aspirin sensitivity, 159
  immunoglobulin deficiency, 350
  management, 221
  no reaction to skin tests, 159–160
  reaction to skin tests, 160
  self-medication problems, 186
Pavlovian conditioning, in asthmatic studies, 194
pCO_2, elevation in asthma, 100
  increase's effects, 100
Pulmonary hypertension, in farmer's lung, 104

Penicillin, see also Depot penicillin
  allergic reactions to, 180–181
  antibodies to, 181–182
  anaphylaxis due to, 177
  angio-edema response, 136
  contaminants, 182
  desensitization procedure, 183
  dosage increase, 183 and tabl.
  food contamination, 174
  hemolytic anemia, resulting, 40–41
    due to, 176
  hypersensitivity, clinical patterns, 182–183
  immunological considerations, 181
  in milk, 151
  pruritus due to, 173
  pulmonary aspergillosis aggravated by, 108
  sensitivity, milk, cheese, dangers, 163
    diagnosis, 183
    oranges sometimes contaminated, 163
  urticaria due to, 174
  reaction to, 136, 174
  skin test contraindicated, 307
  varieties compared, 180–181
  vasculitis relationship, 177
Penicillin disease, 31
Pentobarbital, dosage, caution with allergic patient, 263
Pentothal®, see Thiopental
Pepsin, digestion, 14 with figs.
Perennial treatment, indications for, 323–324
Permanente Medical Group, 291
Peyer's patches, action, 116
Personality problems, solved by allergy treatment, 193
Personality traits, psychosomatic relationship, 192
Pets, restrictions, emotional difficulties, ix
Pharyngeal granulations, description, 56
Pharyngeal lymphoid structures, see Waldeyer's ring
Pharyngeal tonsil, see Adenoid
Phenergan®, see Promethazine
Phenindamine Thephorin®, least sedation with, 243
Pheniramine, intermediate sedative action, 243
Phenobarbital, dosage, 263
  use in bronchospasm, 83
  use in migraine therapy, 145
Phenothiazines, photosensitivity due to, 175
  side effects, 172
  vascular relationship, 177
Phospholipase A, in bee venom, action, 205

Photophobia, in conjunctivitis, 63
  in migraine, 144
Photosensitivity, allergic, characteristics, 175 with tabl.
  nonallergic, characteristics, 175 with tabl.
Physical examination, in clinical allergy, 225
Physiology, respiratory, terms, 90–96 with figs.
Phlyctenules, characteristics and treatment, 65–66
PK reaction, IgE relationship, 16
Placenta, IgE antibodies do not pass, 17
  IgM antibodies do not pass, 12
Plant surveys, changes in, 285–276
  cultivated plants and trees, 275
  indigenous plants, 274–275
  United States, 276 fig., 276–289
Plants, dermatitis involvement, 133
  pollens, offending, 273 with tabl.
Platelet function evaluation, immunologic competence, 356
Plethysmograph method, breath measurement, 96
Plethysmography, asthma patient study, 99
Pneumocytis, immune deficiency relationship, 355
PNU, allergen preparations, 318
  pollen extract measurement, 293
  undependability, 296–297
pO_2, level lowered in asthma, 100
Poison ivy, contact dermatitis, 133
Poison oak, contact dermatitis, 133
Poison plant sensitivity, preventive measures, 134
Pollen allergy, skin tests, 149
Pollen extracts, botanists' aid to manufacturers, 272–273
  contamination control, 292
  evaluation, 294
  IgE standard, 294
  mold avoidance, 292
  Noon units, 293
  PNU, 293–294
  standardization, 293–294
  storage, 292
  weight by volume measurement, 294
Pollen sensitivity, procedures to diminish exposure, 84
Pollens, clinical importance, criteria, 272
  collecting, 273–274
  defatting procedure abandoned, 292
  experimental studies, 194
  extracting procedures, 292, 293
  floral anatomy knowledge importance, 270
  gastrointestinal disease relationship, 117

not all allergenic, 272
  plants, offenders, 373 with tabl.
  postulates related to, 272–273
  skin reactions, 65
  varieties, **270**
  wind blown, 270
Potassium iodide, dosage and adverse reactions, 252
  for expectorant action, 83
Polyhydric alcohol, sweetener, 160
Polypeptides, diagrammatic description, 7 with figs.
"Postnasal drip," in nasal allergies, 54
Post-transfusion thrombocytopenia, description, 40
Prausnitz-Küstner reaction, see PK reaction
Precipitation reactions, Ag-Ab complex, 17, 18 with figs.
Precipitins, in pulmonary aspergillosis, 107
Prednisolone, sodium retention cause, 261 with tabl.
Prednisone®, hypotension therapy use, 31
  sodium retention cause, 261 with tabl.
Pre-seasonal treatment, evaluation, 324
Preservatives, few adverse reactions, 154
Pregnancy, effect on symptoms, 224
  emulsion repository therapy excluded, 327
  ergotamine therapy contraindicated, 144
  influence, 322
  iso-immunization, effect on infant, 351
  potassium iodide contraindicated, 252
Prick test, antigen concentration, 307
  technique, 299–302 with figs.
Primaquine, effect on American Negroes, 172
Promethazine, sedative action, 243
Prophylactic drugs, use in migraine, 145–146
Prophylaxis, in contact dermatitis, 134
Prostaglandins, role in capillary flow control, 100
Proteins, fibrous, description, 6 with figs.
Protein nitrogen units, see PNU
Proteins, synthesis inhibited by glucocorticoids, 254
Provera®, reactions due to tartrazine, 157
Provest®, reactions due to tartrazine, 157
Pruritus, see also itching
  drug reaction, **173**

mechanisms involved, 123
"Pseudoasthma," bronchiolitis, 235
Pseudomonas susceptibility, in immune deficiency, 355
"Psychiatric" allergic patients, compared to non-neurotics, 189
Psychosomatic illness, response to specific stresses, 192
Psychosomatic specificity, hypotheses, 191–192
   personality traits, 192
Psychological behavior, allergic disease relationship, psychoanalytic view, 190
Psychological factors, in allergic disease, 189–197
Psychological treatment, allergic individuals, 195
Psychosis, asthma association, 191
Psychotherapy, value in migraine treatment, 145
Psoriasis, neurodermatitis association, 129
Puberty, effect on allergy symptoms, 224
   influence of, 322
Pulex irritans, see Human flea
Pulmonary involvement, antihistamines contraindicated, 245
Purpuric lesions, in drug reactions, 174–175 with tabl.
Pulmonary aspergillosis, course of disease, 108
   etiology and course, 106–108
   invasive form, 108
   treatment, 108
Pulmonary dipalmitoyl lecithin, see DPL
Pulmonary function, 88–96
   in allergic bronchial disease, 99–101
   with exercise, abnormal in farmer's lung, 104
   respiration mechanics of, 88–89
Pulmonary surfactants, description and action, 89–90
Pyloric stenosis, vomiting due to, 231
Pyogenic infections, immunoglobulin disorder, 350
Pyribenzamine®, see Tripelennamine
Pyrosis, food reaction, 147

Q

Quincke's disease, see Hereditary angio-edema
Quinine, cinchonism with, 171
   effects on bone marrow, 176
   hemolytic, anemia relationship, 176
   Thrombocytopenia association, 176

R

Radiation, AAD role, 339
Radioactive Xenon, use in asthma studies, 100
Radio-allergo-sorbant test, see RAST
Radiological method, breath measurement, 96
Radiologic evaluation, immunologic competence, 356
Ragweed, studies, 272
RAST, allergen preparations, 318
Rat flea, bites' characteristics, 199
Raynaud's disease, ergotamine therapy contraindicated, 144
RBC, destruction in drug reaction, 176
Reactions, in injection therapy, 325
Reactions, treatment, 325
Reaginic allergy, characteristics, 28–29
   classification, 4
Reaginic antibody, see IgE
Reaginic-atopic conjunctivitis, treatment, 64
Reaginic complexes, anaphylaxis induced by, 29
Reaction, cell mediated response, description, 3–3
Rectal suppositories, with steroid side effects consideration, 262
Red ants, see Fire-ants
Renal deficiency, role in drug allergy, 172
Renal disease, drug excretion prevention, 171
   in serum sickness, 43
Residual volume, see RV
Resistance, in pulmonary action, 90
Respiration, normal values, 91 with tabl.
   mechanics of, 88–89
   normal value prediction, 94–95 with figs.
Respiratory acidosis, description, 100
Respiratory alkalosis, description, 100
Respiratory allergic disease, infancy, allergic rhinitis, 232
Respiratory allergy, eczema association, 124
Respiratory disease, chronic, in infants, 235
Respiratory functions, decrease in moldy hay allergy, 103
Respiratory infections, in cystic fibrosis, infants, 234
   in infants, description, 235
Respiratory physiology, terms, 90–96 with figs.
Respiratory rate, ventilation relationship, 96
Respiratory tract, see also lower respiratory tract
   allergic diseases, 53–61
Respiratory tract, lower, allergic diseases, 71–115 with figs.
Respiratory tract allergy, treatment, 60
Resting minute ventilation, see V_E
RF, description and action, 344–345
Rh antibody, effects, 40
Rheumatoid factor, see RF
   IgM's relationship
Rh mechanism, IgG's action, 12
Rhus diversilobia, see Poison oak
Rhus toxicodendron, see Poison ivy
Ritalin®, see Methylphenidate
Robitussin®, Glycerol guaiacolate
Roentgenogram, appearance in farmer's lung, 104
   hyperaeration in bronchial allergy, 234
   in atelectasis, 88
   in diagnosis on infant's wheezing, 234
Rowe elimination diets, cereal-free and fruit-free, 167–168
RV, definition, 91 with fig.
   explanation, 93–96 with figs.
Ryegrass, studies, 272

S

Saccharin, adverse reaction to, 60
Saccular bronchiectasis, in pulmonary aspergillosis, 106–107
Salbutanol, description and use, 246
Salicylate-free diet, artificial diet, flavors omitted, 166
   beverage list, 166
   drugs and miscellaneous list, 166
   indicated in nasal polyposis, 163
   list of eliminated foods, 165
   permitted fruits listed, 165
   restrictions, 165
Salivation, increase in migraine headache, 141, 142
Sand fleas, allergic reactions, 200
Sand flies, treatment of bites, 201
San Francisco, Kaiser Foundation Hospital, pyloric stenosis cases, 230
Sarcoidosis, pathology and treatment, 353
Sarcoma, immune deficiency relationship, 355
Scalp, seborrheic dermatitis, 128
Scarification technique, origin and uses, 299
Schizophrenic patients, allergens, histamines tested, 191
Scratch test, antigen concentrattion, 307
   history, 299
   technique, 299
Seasonal changes, effect on symptoms, 224
Seasonal characteristics, vernal conjunctivitis, 65

Seasonal symptoms, food sensitivity, 148
   foods suspected, 163
   pollen allergy, skin tests, 149
Seborrheic dermatitis, characteristics, 128
   infants, characteristics, 127
Secobarbital, dosage, caution with allergic patient, 263
Seconal®, Secobarbital
Sedation, due to antihistamines, 240, 243
   migraine therapy, 144
Sedatives, barbiturates, 263
   contraindicated in hypoxemia, 86
   cautions in status asthmaticus, 86
   non-barbiturates, 263–264
   undesirable in bronchial allergy, 83
   uses and drug choice, 262–263
   use in lower respiratory allergic disease, 263
Sedormid®, Allyl-isopropyl
Senescence, of thrombocytes early in Wiskott-Aldrich syndrome, 352
Sensitization, in infants, 229
Sensitivity to drugs, diagnosis, 185–186
Sensory threshold, alterations, 140
Sequestered protein concept, auto-allergy, 338
Sera, technique for testing with, 43
Serax®, see Oxazepam
Serotonin, in bee venom, 204
   role in migraine, 143
   as inhibitor, use in migraine, 143
Serous otitis, in allergic infant, 232–233
   recurrent, in children, 163
Serum disease, description and management, 42–44
   early studies, 3
   mechanism, 42–43
Serum potassium level, digitalis effects relationship, 171
Serum sickness, drug relationship, 177
Seborrheic dermatitis, not allergic, 122
Shellfish, skin test contraindicated, 117, 307
   skin test hazardous, 149
   allergic diseases, 120–138
Skin, anatomy, 120
Skin, dryness, cause and therapy, 121
   histological variations, 122
   response to irritants, 122
   stratum corneum, hygroscopic nature, 121
   structure corium, 120–121
   structure epidermis, 120
Skin manifestations, in children, 223
Skin reaction, in local anaphylaxis, 29
Skin response, histamine induced, 16
Skin testing, contraindicated for hymenoptera sensitivity, 208
   diagnostic value limited, 60
Skin tests, allergen choice, 305–306
   in arthropod inhalant allergy, 212
   cautions in foods allergy, 117
   contraindicated for egg allergy, 151
   contraindications, 307
   clinical procedure, 309–312
   diagnostic value, 162
   eggs, cautions, 163
   factors in diminution, 314
   food allergy, false positive reaction, 149–150
   foods, in allergic headaches, 139
   history and technique, 298–312 with figs.
   indications for, 221, 305
   in food sensitivity, hazards, 148–150
   in pulmonary aspergillosis, 107
   insect sting sensitivity, 206-207
   limitations, 80
   milk fractions, unreliable, 151, 221
   negative reaction, explanations, 150
   patients, failure to react, 159–160
   reaction, 160
   pollen extract variations, 294
   reactions, 307–309
      control, 309
      evaluations, 310–311
      rating, 308–309
   reading of, 311
   strong reactions, psychological disturbances fewer, 193
   technique choice, 306–307
   unreliable in infants, 234, 236
   variation with ingestion or inhalation sensitivity, 149
Silk, as allergy source, 213
   testing and treating for allergy, 298
Single breath measurements, terms explained, 93–96
Sinuses, function, 57
   involvement in allergic headaches, 139
SLE, development, 339
Slow reacting substance-A, see SRS-A
Smallpox, characteristics, 126
Smallpox vaccination, contraindicated in infantile eczema, 126–127
Smoke, in burning poison plants, allergic reactions, 133
Synalar®, uses in allergic dermatitis, 260
Soaks, see Tub soaks
   treatment of contact dermatitis, 133
Sodium bicarbonate, use in status asthmaticus, 86
Sodium iodide, asthma therapy dosage, 252
Solu-Cortef®, hypertension therapy use, 31
Somatic factors, auto-allergy, 339–340
Somnolence, due to antihistamines, 243
Soil dust, inhalation, allergy due to, 211
Sorbitol, sweetener, 160
Soy milk, adverse effects on infants, 237
Specialization, drawbacks, viii
Spores, in allergies and mycoses, 102 with fig.
Sputum, in pulmonary aspergillosis, 107
SRS-A, antihistaminic drugs ineffective, 28
   bronchospasm, relationship, 77
   muscle spasm induced by, 76, 85
   onset and action, 28
Staphylococci, susceptibility, in immune deficiency, 355
Status, compliance in, description, 89
Status asthmaticus, aminophylline in therapy, 249
   dangers, 246
   cyanosis, life threatening indication, 101
   emergency situation, 85
   intravenous therapy, 85
   laboratory procedures, 85–86
   medication, 85
   treatment, 85–86
Steam inhalation, in expectorant therapy, 251
Steroid therapy, in contact dermatitis, 133
   in dermatitis infection, cautions, 129–130
   indications for, 258
   in hay fever, 259
   not recommended in child's respiratory allergy, 259
   treatment of reactions, 325
Steroids, child patients, rarely indicated for, 259
   dermatological preparations, danger, 262
   effect on blood, 257
   in angio-edema therapy, 259–260
   in urticaria therapy, 259–260
   otic preparations, not recommended, 262
   rectal suppositories, side effects consideration, 262
   use in atopic dermatitis, 260
   use in drug allergy, 260
   use in migraine therapy, 145
   symptomatic relief sole role, 259
   therapy in allergies to drugs and chemicals, 118
   therapy in angio-edema, 136
   topical uses, 261–262
Stinging hairs and spines, reactions to, 211

Streptomycin, anaphylactic reaction, 177
  allergic reactions, 185
Sulfonamides, allergic reactions, 185
  contact dermatitis, 175
  exfoliative dermatitis relationship, 178
  photosensitivity, due to, 175
  serum sickness relationship, 177
  reactions to, 174
  sensitivity signs, 186
  vasculitis relationship, 177
Sunlight, AAD role, 339
Surface tension, lung in respiration, 89
Symptomatology, food reactions, 147–148 with tabl.
Sus-Phrine®, action, 245
  use in bronchial asthma therapy, 84
  use in serum sickness management, 44
Sweating, itching aggravation, 130
  suppression, use of drugs and dangers, 124
Sweeteners, non-nutritive, 160
Swelling, of airways, death due to, 136
Sympathomimetic drugs, catecholamines, epinephrine, action and dosage, 245–246
  alpha receptors action, 245
  beta receptors' action, 245
  classes and actions, 245
  noncatecholamines, amphetamine, 246
    ephedrine, 246
    methoxyphenamine hydrochloride, 246–247
    use in bronchospasm, 83
Symposium on Sensitivity Reactions to Drugs, comment on problem, 171
Symptoms, allergic factors, 193
  bronchial allergy, in infants, 233
  corneal allergy, 68
  fire-ant stings, 215 tabl.
  pulmonary aspergillosis, 106
  vernal conjunctivitis, 65
Syr. H. I., see Syrup of hydriodic acid
Syrup of Hydriodic acid, expectorant drug, 252
Syrup of ipecac, dosage as expectorant drug, 253
Systemic anaphylaxis, clinical picture and treatment, 29–30
  management procedure, 30–31
Systemic lupus erythematosis, see SLE

T

Tachycardia, due to antihistamines, 243

Tang®, reaction due to, 157
Tartrazine, as nasal discharge cause, 60
  elimination in salicylate-free diet, 165
  involvement in allergies, 193
Taxonomy of plants, importance to physician, 268–269
T-cells, derivation and action, 21–23
  types, 23
Tea, use in migraine therapy, 144
Tedral®, content, dependence dangers, 250
  use in bronchospasm, 83
Teldrin®, see Chlorpheniramine
Tenderizer, meat sensitivity relationship, 152
Tension fatigue, in children, 222
  syndrome, characteristics, 221
Terramycin®, see Oxytetracycline
Testing, immunologic competence, 357
  complications, 358
Tetracyclines, reactions to, 184–185
TF of Lawrence, characteristics, 36–37
  clinical application, 37
  DH mediator, 34–37 with figs.
  therapy uses, 37
Theophylline, use in bronchospasm, 83
Theophylline mixtures, with expectorants, disadvantages, 250
Thephorin®, see Phenindamine
Thiopental, contraindicated with bronchial allergy or asthma, 263
Thiouracil, vasculitis relationship, 177
Thommen's postulates, plants' allergy relationship, 270–274 with figs.
Throat, allergic diseases, 56–57
Thrombocytopenia, drugs associated with, 176
Thymic agenesis, characteristics, 347
Thymic alymphoplasia, immunoglobulin disorder, 351–352
Thymic aplasia, autosomal recessive, 349
Thyroidism, in vernal conjunctivitis, 65
Thymosin, description and function, 23
Thymus dependence, see T-cells
Thymus, role in DH response, 34
Tidal Air, V_T description,
Tidal volume, see V_T
Timothy extract, injection therapy, 312
Timothy, studies, 272
TLC, definition, 90
  increase in asthma patients, 99
Tolerance, see Immunological tolerance

allergic phenomenon?, 41
  breakdown of mechanism, 341–343
Tolerogen, definition, 41
Tongue, swelling, due to fire-ant sting, 215
Tonsils, description, 56
Topical medication, contraindicated in contact dermatitis, 133
Topical therapy, contraindicated in nasal allergies, 60
Topical treatment, contraindicated in eyelid allergy, 66
Total lung capacity, see TLC
Total plasma serotonin, see TPS
Toxic reactions, to foods, 147
TPS, study in migraine, 143
Tracheoesophageal fistula, in infants, diagnosis, 234
Tranquilizers, minor, varieties, action, and dosage, 264–265
Tranquilizers, use in migraine, 144
  useful in contact dermatitis, 134
Transfer factor of Lawrence, see TF of Lawrence
Transfusion, see also Intravascular transfusion and Post-transfusion
Transfusions, sensitization following, 344
Treatment, acute allergic conditions, in infants, 235–236
  bed bug bites, 200–201
  contact dermatitis, 133–134
  dermatitis, 129–130
  drug reactions, 187
  farmer's lung, 105
  fire-ant stings, 2–5 with tabl.
  itching, 130
  flea bites, 199–200
  immune defects, 359 with tabl.
  lice bites, 201
  migraine, 144–146
  mosquito bites, 200
  pulmonary aspergillosis, 108
  respiratory tract allergy, 60
  sand fly bites, 201
  triatoma bite, 203
Trees, pollens, 273
  see United States, trees
Triamcinolone, dosage, 261
Triatoma, varieties, bite reaction and treatment, 201–203 with fig.
Trichoptera, as allergy cause, 211
Trimeton®, see Pheniramine
Tripelennamine (PBZ), intermediate sedative action, 243
Tuberculin reaction, corticosteroids, relationship, 257
  DH lesion, 34
Tuberculin type immune reaction, 4
Tuberculosis, characteristics, 353
  delayed hypersensitivity relationship, 76

early studies, 3
morbidity, Viennese, 19th C., 3
Tub-soaks, boric acid contraindicated, 129
　in contact dermatitis, 130
　with MgSO$_4$ for dermatitis, 129
Tympanic cavity, see Middle ear
Tympanic membrane, anatomy, 58–59

U

United States,
　asthmatic deaths, aerosol sprays blamed, 247
　climate, by regions, 276–289
　cromolyn sodium studies, 266
　grasses, by regions, 277–289
　regions in plant surveys, 276 with fig., 276–289
　topography, by regions, 276–289
　trees, by region, 277–278
University of Buffalo, Elliot's bee venom studies, 205
Upper respiratory tract, see also Respiratory tract
　allergic disease, antihistamine use in, 263
　allergic disease, 53–61
　symptoms, in children, 222
Urinary retention, due to antihistamines, 243
Urticaria, antihistamine and steroid therapy, 259–260
　attributed to food additives, case history, 193
　counteraction of, 31
　description, pathology, etiology, and treatment, 134–135
　drug reaction, 173–174
　due to caterpillar hairs, 211
　due to antihistamines, 243
　due to penicillin, 182
　epinephine in therapy, 245
　food reaction, 147
　in anaphylaxis, 177
　low in children, 223
　papular, in insect bites, 198
　symptomatic treatment, 135
Urticating hairs and spines, reaction to, 211
Uvea, allergic disease, 68–69

V

V_A, definition, 91
Valium®, see Diazepam
Vascular lesions, in interstitial pneumonitis, 104–15
Vascular rings, in infants, diagnosis, 234
Vasculitis, drug relationship, 177
Vasocon-A®, use in conjunctivitis, 64
Vasomotor aspects, in migraine, 143
VC, asthma patients, 99
　definition, 90
V_D, definition,
V domain sites, 15 with fig.
V_E definition, 91
Vegetable fibers, extract preparation, 297
Venom sacs, desensitization use, 210
Venoms, antigen presence, 206
Ventilation measurements, terms used, 91–93 with figs.
Vernal conjunctivitis characteristics, 64–65
Vertigo, in anaphylaxis, 177
Viral immunity, see also Immunity
Viral infections, effect on bronchial tree, 78, 79 with fig.
　In infantile eczema, 126–127
　masked by corticosteroids, 257
Viral immunity, IgA's role, 12
Viremia, infantile eczema, complication, 126
Vision, blurring, in migraine headache, 142
　hazards to, 62
Vision blurring, due to antihistamine, 243
Vistaril,® see Hydroxyzine
　use in contact dermatitis, 134
　use in urticaria, 135
Vital capacity, see VC
Vitamin B$_{12}$, anaphylactic reaction, 177
Vomiting, by infants, diagnosis, 231
　by infants, gastrointestinal allergy symptoms, 230
　forceful, in infants, diagnosis, 231
　Heiner's syndrome, in infants, 235
　in migraine, 141, 1745
V_T, definition, 91 with fig.

W

Waldeyer's ring, antibody production, 116
　description and allergic diseases, 56–57
　function, 21
Wasp, venom kinin, action, 205
Wasp stings, identification, 208
Water, in expectorant therapy, 251
WBC, destruction in drug reaction, 176
　in drug reactions, 41
Weeds, see United States, weeds pollens, 274
Wessely phenomenon, characteristics, 68
Wheat-egg-milk free diet, forbidden foods listed, 169–170
Wheat-free diet, forbidden foods, 168–169
Wheezing, factors inducing, 81
　in infants, allergy bronchial symptom, 233, 235
　　Epinephrine-HCl use, 236
　　with tracheoesophageal fistula, 234
Wiskott-Aldrich syndrome, characteristics, 352
　TF use in therapy, 37
Wound healing, impaired by glucocorticoids, 254

X

Xanthines, aminophylline, content and clinical use, 248–249
　elixophyllin, content and dosage, 249
　uses and actions, 247–248 with fig.
Xenopsylla cheopsis, see Rat flea

Y

Youths, puberty's effect on symptoms, 224

NAME INDEX

A
Aas, K., 233, 239, 334
Ackyrod, 176
Alexander, F., 190, 191, 195
Allansmith, M., 68, 69, 227, 230, 238
Alquist, 245
Arbesman, C. E., 205, 206, 218, 329, 330, 334, 336, 337
Augustin, R., 313, 334, 335
Austwick, P. K. C., 103, 337

B
Baer, H., 334
Baer, R. L., 175, 187, 311
Balyeat, R. M., 142, 146
Barber, G. W., 68, 70
Barnard, J. H., 207, 218
Bathmank, D., 207, 218
Bazaral, M., 228, 238
Benton, 209
Berg, 317, 318
Berglund, E., 91, 112
Blackley, 298, 311
Bonilla-Soto, O., 330, 334, 337
Brambell, F. W. R., 228, 238
Bray, G. W., 233, 239
Bronson, 250
Brown, A., 209, 216
Brown, E. A., 334
Bunce, 103
Bruton, O. C., 349
Burnett, F. M., 340, 346
Bursten, B., 192, 195
Buynak, E., 227, 238

C
Campbell, J. M., 101, 109, 114
Caplan, I., 329, 336
Caro, M. R., 214, 219
Carr, C. Jeleff, 244, 267
Chafee, F. H., 157, 160, 187
Chan, H., Jr., 323
Chase, Merrill W., 41, 137
Childers, Mrs. Ivanelle, xi
Clein, N. W., 229, 239
Clements, A. N., 90, 218
Coca, A. F., 29, 147
Cocoa, Arthur H., 61
Cohen, I. H., 102, 114
Colacicco, 90
Collins-Williams, C., 168
Connell, J. T., 190, 314, 315, 334, 335, 336
Cooke, C. S., 103, 112, 150, 291, 293, 313
Cooke, Robert A., 299, 313
Coombs, R. R. A., 4, 44
Corda, 103
Cox, 266
Criep, 157

Curtis, 312
Cutting, Cecil C., xi

D
Darling, 102
Davis, S. D., 231, 239
Deamer, Wm. C., 221, 225
De Bary, 103
De Candolle, 103
Dekker, E., 192, 194, 195
Derbes, V. J., 174, 214, 219
Diener, 342
Diner, W. C., 235, 239
Doward, B., 227, 238
Dumonde, Dudley C., 36, 45, 49
Dunbar, F., 191, 195
Durrell, L. W., 289
Dutton, A. M., 238, 239, 335

E
Edelman, Gerald M., 15, 47
Eisen, A., 235, 239
Elliot, 205, 207
Ellis, 103
Emmons, 103
Eschenhagen, 194
Evans, D. G., 227, 238
Everhart, 103
Eyerman, Charles H., 139, 146

F
Falier, Constantine J., 266
Farr, Richard S., 159, 179, 186, 187
Feinberg, Samuel, 331
Fennell, 102
Fink, C. W., 227, 238
Fisher, David, W., 13, 14, 44, 132
Fontana V. J., 313, 335
Ford, D. K., 18
Frankland, A. W., 313, 335
Franklin, E. C., 313, 346
Freedman, D. H., 191, 195
Freeman, G. L., 233, 239, 312
Fregert, S., 132, 137
French, T. M., 190, 191, 195
Frenkel, E. P., 22, 45
Fresenius, 102
Freund, 326
Friedman, Alice D., xi
Fries, J. H., 103, 226
Fudenberg, H. High, xi, 46, 340-341, 346
Fuller, 243
Funkenstein, D. H., 191, 195, 196

G
Gaisford, W., 229, 239
Gell, P. G. H., 4, 44
Geraci, J. E., 184, 187

German, Donald F., xi, 227
Giacona, Mary Ann Warr, xi
Gilchrist, 102, 103
Gilman, Alfred, 180, 185, 240, 263, 264
Glaser, Jerome, 237, 238, 239
Goldstein, 23
Good, Robert A., 13, 14, 44, 51, 346
Goodale, 299
Goodman, Louis S., 180, 185, 240, 263, 264, 267, 329
Gordon, B. L., II, 18
Gordon, H., 160
Graham, D. T., 192, 196
Green, David E., 82
Green, G. R., 184, 187
Gregory, P. H., 103, 114
Griffon, 103
Groen, J., 192, 194, 195, 196

H
Haberman, E., 203, 204, 218
Hapke, E. J., 104, 114, 115
Harber, L. C., 175, 187
Harrington, H. D., 289
Harrison, 328
Hayes, 329
Helstrom, 355
Henrici, 102
Herbert, W. J., 25
Herman, 68
Higginbotham, R. D., 204, 218
Hjorth, N., 132, 137, 188, 310, 335
Hogg, J. C., 233, 239
Holt, L. E., Jr., 313, 335
Horton, B. T., 143, 146
Howard, 313
Hyde, H. A., 330, 337

I
Igersheimer, W. W., 191, 195
Ishizaka, K., 16, 28, 46, 48, 49, 116
Ishizaka, T., 16, 28, 46, 48, 49, 116

J
Jack, Robert, xi
Jackson, Chevalier, 234
Jacques, 205
Jamieson, 212
Jellison, 103
Johansson, S. G. O., 228, 238, 317, 318
Johnstone, Douglas E., 237, 238, 239, 335
Jung, R. C., 214, 219

K
Kaplan, 339
Karger, S., 103
Karnella, S., 204, 218
Karsten, 103
Katz, J., 231, 239

Keen, 212
Keene, Clifford H., xi
Kemper, H., 200, 217
King, T. P., 293, 335
Kirkman, 311
Knapp, P. H., 192, 194, 196
Kory, Ross C., 94, 95
Krantz, John C., Jr., 244, 267
Kunkle, E. C., 143, 146
Küster, 102

L

Lance, J. W., 143, 146
Langlois, C., 205, 206, 218
Laurel, 313
Lawrence, H. S., 36, 37, 38, 39, 44, 50, 52, 360
Leigh, D., 189, 196
Lender, 103
Levin, Alan S., 347
Levine, Bernard B., 181, 188, 323
Lichtenstein, L. M., 314, 329, 335, 337
Lindt, 102, 103
Link, 103
Locci, 102
Lockey, S. D., 157, 161
Lovelace, 326
Luce, R. A., 191, 197

M

Mac Connell, J. G., 213, 219
McGovern, J. P., 232, 239, 337
Mainland, D., 313, 335
Marley, E., 189, 196
Marshall, W. H., 36
Martensson, L., 227, 238
Maublanc, 103
Mellanby, 200
Michaeli, 342, 345
Miller, W. E., 227, 238, 360
Moeschlin, 176
Morton, 355

N

Nagy, M. R., 68, 70
Nast, A., 139, 146
Nelson, Ray, 268
Nemetz, S. J., 192, 196
Neuhaus, E. C., 181, 196
Nilsby, I., 330, 337
Noelpp, B., 194, 196
Noelpp-Eschenhagen, 194, 196
Noon, L., 293, 312, 336
Norman, P. S., 293, 314, 328, 335, 336, 337
Nossal, G. J., 227, 238

O

Ottenberg, P., 194, 196
Oudin, 344

P

Paquiez, P., 139, 146

Parlato, 211
Patterson, 314
Pattle, 89, 90
Paul, 331
Pelser, H. E., 194, 195, 196
Pepys, J., 103, 104, 106, 115, 337
Persoon, 103
Peters, G. A., 184, 187
Pirquet, 3, 42
Prince, 330
Pruzansky, 212, 314

R

Raper, 102
Redlich, F. C., 191, 195
Reilly, C. M., 227, 229, 238
Reisman, R. E., 329, 334, 336
Ring, F. O., 192, 196
Rixford, 103
Robinson, 349
Rose, Brahm, 331
Rose, N. R., 330, 331, 332, 334, 336, 337
Rosen, F. S., 349, 360
Rosenheim, M. L., 171, 188
Rowe, Albert H., 147, 170, 226
Rowe, Albert, Sr., 167–168

S

Sabbath, J. C., 191, 197
Saccardo, 102
Sacks, Oliver W., 140, 142, 146
Samter, Max, 157, 159, 161, 170, 179, 188
Sansert, 145
Scarpelli, E. M., 90, 110
Schachter, 205
Schiavi, R. C., 194, 197
Schick, 3, 42
Schinneer, Robert, xi
Schloss, O. M., 150, 161, 299
Schuurmans, 102
Seal, R. M. E., 104, 115
Self, T. W., 231, 239
Selye, 190
Sery, T. W., 68, 70
Sethi, B. B., 194, 197
Settipane, G. A., 157, 160, 187
Shear, 103
Sherman, W. B., 147, 314, 328, 334, 335, 336
Shields, T. L., 202, 218
Shulman, S., 41, 205, 206, 218, 219
Sicuteri, F., 143, 146
Silverstein, A. M., 229, 239
Simon, G., 235, 239
Smillie, John G., xi
Smith, J. W., 227, 238
Sommers, Sheldon C., 75
Speer, F., 147, 226
Spitler, Lynn E., xi, 347, 360
Stein, M., 194, 196, 197
Steinberg, 212
Stevens, 338

Stiehm, E. R., 227, 228, 238, 360
Stoelting, Eric, xi
Stokes, J., 102, 227, 238
Stone, M. J., 22, 45, 114
Szentivanyi, A., 81, 112

T

Tada, 116
Thom, 102
Thomas, Payne, xi, 104
Thurlbeck, W. M., 75
Townsend, Robert W., xi, 268
Triplett, R. Faser, 215, 219
Trot, 102
Tsiklinsky, 102
Tulasne, 103

U

Uhr, J. W., 229, 239
Usinger, R. L., 200, 218

V

Valentine, F. T., 36, 37, 360
Vallery-Radot, P., 139, 146
Van Arsdale, 313–314
Van de Veer, 313
Vane, John R., 97
Van Furth, R., 227, 238
Van Tieghem, 103
Vaughn, W. T., 139, 146, 147
Von Höhnel, 103
Von Neergaard, 89
Von Pirquet, 299

W

Waksman, 102
Walker, 299
Waller, 103
Walsh, E. N., 202, 218
Walzer, M., 150, 161
Wang, 250
Warren, William Paul, 331, 332, 334, 337
Webb, Morris E., xi, 268
Weil, 291
Weiss, E., 191, 197
White, 23
Whittingham, S. J., 338, 346
Wilkinson, P. C., 25 fig.
Williams, G. M., 227, 238, 332, 334
Wilson, A. B., 211, 218
Winberg, J., 228, 238
Witten, 311
Wittich, 212
Wittig, H. J., 235, 239
Wodehouse, Roger P., 290
Wolf, S., 192, 197
Wolff, H. G., 142, 143, 145, 146, 190
Wright, Robert, 73
Wulfen, 103
Wylie, 97

Z

Zak, S. J., 228, 238